Periparturient Diseases of Cattle

Periparturient Diseases of Cattle

Edited by

Tanmoy Rana, M.V.Sc & PhD
Assistant Professor, Department of Veterinary Clinical Complex
West Bengal University of Animal & Fishery Sciences
Kolkata, West Bengal, India

WILEY Blackwell

Published by John Wiley & Sons, Inc., Hoboken, New Jersey.
Published simultaneously in Canada.

Library of Congress Cataloging-in-Publication Data
Names: Rana, Tanmoy, editor.
Title: Periparturient diseases of cattle / edited by Tanmoy Rana.
Description: Hoboken, New Jersey : John Wiley & Sons, [2025] | Includes bibliographical references and index.
Identifiers: LCCN 2024026582 (print) | LCCN 2024026583 (ebook) | ISBN 9781394203970 (hardback) | ISBN 9781394203987 (Adobe PDF) | ISBN 9781394203994 (epub)
Subjects: MESH: Cattle Diseases | Pregnancy Complications–veterinary | Pregnancy, Animal–physiology | Parturition–physiology | Cattle
Classification: LCC SF961 (print) | LCC SF961 (ebook) | NLM SF 961 | DDC 636.2/0896–dc23/eng/20240719
LC record available at https://lccn.loc.gov/2024026582
LC ebook record available at https://lccn.loc.gov/2024026583

Cover Design: Wiley
Cover Images: Courtesy of Tanmoy Rana

Set in 9.5/12.5pt STIXTwoText by Straive, Pondicherry, India

Printed in Singapore
M 125643_070824

Contents

List of Contributors

Aakanksha Bhoker
Department of Veterinary Surgery and Radiology
Bihar Veterinary College
Patna, Bihar, India

Abdul Reshma
Department of Veterinary Gynaecology and Obstetrics
Veterinary College and Research Institute
Tamil Nadu Veterinary and Animal Sciences University
Salem, Tamil Nadu, India

Abhijeet Fernandes
Department of Veterinary Gynaecology and Obstetrics
College of Veterinary Science, Rampura Phul
Guru Angad Dev Veterinary and Animal Sciences University
Bathinda, Punjab, India

Abhinav Suthar
Department of Veterinary Medicine
College of Veterinary Science and Animal Husbandry
Kamdhenu University
Sardarkrushinagar, Gujarat, India

Abhishek Bhardwaj
College of Veterinary Science
Guru Angad Dev Veterinary and Animal Sciences University
Ludhiana, Punjab, India

Abhishek Pathak
Apollo College of Veterinary Medicine
Rajasthan University of Veterinary and Animal Sciences
Bikaner, Jaipur, Rajasthan, India

Adeniyi Njideka
Department of Biological Sciences
Alabama A&M University
Normal, Alabama, USA

Akhter Rasool
Department of Veterinary Gynaecology and Obstetrics
Madras Veterinary College
Chennai, Tamil Nadu, India

Allam Lukshiake
Veterinary Medicine
Ahmadu Bello University
Zaria, Kaduna, Nigeria

Ambica Gadige
Department of Veterinary Medicine
College of Veterinary Science, Rajendranagar
Hyderabad, Telangana, India

Aminu M. Galadima
Usmanu Danfodiyo University Sokoto
Sokoto, Nigeria

Amita Tiwari
Department of Veterinary Medicine
College of Veterinary Science and Animal Husbandry
Nanaji Deshmukh Veterinary Science University
Jabalpur, Madhya Pradesh, India

Amitava Roy
Livestock Farm Complex
West Bengal University of Animal & Fishery Sciences
Kolkata, West Bengal, India

Ankesh Kumar
Veterinary Clinical Complex
Bihar Veterinary College
Bihar Animal Sciences University
Patna, Bihar, India

Anil Kumar
Department of Veterinary Medicine
Bihar Veterinary College
Patna, Bihar, India

Ankit S. Prajapati
Department of Veterinary Medicine
College of Veterinary Science and Animal Husbandry
Kamdhenu University
Sardarkrushinagar, Gujarat, India

Annadurai Thangamani
Department of Veterinary Gynaecology and Obstetrics
Veterinary College and Research Institute
Tamil Nadu Veterinary and Animal Sciences University
Salem, Tamil Nadu, India

Apoorva Mishra
Department of Veterinary Surgery and Radiology
College of Veterinary Science and Animal Husbandry
Nanaji Deshmukh Veterinary Science University
Jabalpur, Madhya Pradesh, India

Apra Shahi
Department of Veterinary Surgery and Radiology
College of Veterinary Science and Animal Husbandry
Nanaji Deshmukh Veterinary Science University
Jabalpur, Madhya Pradesh, India

Arash Kheradmand
Department of Clinical Sciences
School of Veterinary Medicine, Lorestan University
Khorram Abad, Lorestan, Iran

Arkaprabha Shee
Dhaanyaganga Krishi Vigyan Kendra, Sargachi
Murshidabad, West Bengal, India

Aruna Maramulla
Department of Veterinary Clinical Complex
College of Veterinary Science, Mamnoor
Warangal, Telangana, India

Arunmozhi Narayanaswamy
Veterinary Clinical Complex, Veterinary College and Research Institute, Orathanadu
Tamil Nadu Veterinary and Animal Sciences University
Thanjavur, Tamil Nadu, India

Ashok Ashwini
Department of Veterinary Medicine
Veterinary College
Bangalore, Karnataka, India

Ayyasamy Elango
Department of Veterinary Gynaecology and Obstetrics
Veterinary College and Research Institute
Tamil Nadu Veterinary and Animal Sciences University
Salem, Tamil Nadu, India

Babita Das
Department of Veterinary Surgery and Radiology
College of Veterinary Science and Animal Husbandry
Nanaji Deshmukh Veterinary Science University
Jabalpur, Madhya Pradesh, India

Bagur K. Bhagya
Department of Veterinary Medicine, Veterinary College
Bangalore, Karnataka, India

Bashir Maryam Darma
Veterinary Teaching Hospital
Faculty of Veterinary Medicine
Bayero University
Kano, Kano State, Nigeria

Bhavna Priya
Department of Veterinary Gynaecology
Bihar Veterinary College
Patna, Bihar, India

Bhoopendra Singh
Department of Veterinary Gynaecology and Obstetrics
College of Veterinary Science and Animal Husbandry
Acharya Narendra Deva University of Agriculture and Technology
Ayodhya, Uttar Pradesh, India

Chhavi Gupta
Department of Veterinary Gynaecology and Obstetrics
Veterinary College and Research Institute, Tirunelveli
Tamil Nadu Veterinary and Animal Sciences University
Tirunelveli, Tamil Nadu, India

Chiezey Ngozi Pauline
National Animal Production Research Institute
Faculty of Veterinary Medicine
Ahmadu Bello University
Zaria, Kaduna, Nigeria

Chitra D. Chauhan
Department of Veterinary Medicine
College of Veterinary Science and Animal Husbandry
Kamdhenu University
Sardarkrushinagar, Gujarat, India

Deepak Ningwal
Department of Veterinary Gynaecology and Obstetrics
College of Veterinary Science and Animal Husbandry
Nanaji Deshmukh Veterinary Science University
Madhya Pradesh, India

Gitesh Saini
Department of Veterinary Gynaecology and Obstetrics
College of Veterinary Science, Rampura Phul
Guru Angad Dev Veterinary and Animal Sciences University,
Bathinda, Punjab, India

Gowdaiahnadoddi K. Chetan Kumar
Department of Veterinary Medicine
Veterinary College
Bangalore, Karnataka, India

Gurram S. Haritha
Department of Veterinary Clinical Complex
College of Veterinary Science (SVVU), Garividi
Vizianagaram District, Andhra Pradesh, India

Harshad H. Panchasara
Livestock Research Station
College of Veterinary Science and Animal Husbandry
Kamdhenu University
Sardarkrushinagar, Gujarat, India

Jitendra P. Singh
Department of Veterinary Medicine
College of Veterinary Science and Animal Husbandry
Acharya Narendra Deva University of Agriculture and Technology
Kumarganj, Ayodhya, Uttar Pradesh, India

Kabir Alam
Department of Veterinary Gynaecology and Obstetrics
College of Veterinary Science and Animal Husbandry
Acharya Narendra Deva University of Agriculture and Technology
Ayodhya, Uttar Pradesh, India

Kalyaan Udumalpet Sampathkumar
Department of Veterinary Gynaecology and Obstetrics
Madras Veterinary College
Tamil Nadu Veterinary and Animal Sciences University
Chennai, Tamil Nadu, India

Kanika Tiwari
Department of Veterinary Pharmacy and Toxicology
College of Veterinary and Animal Sciences
Govind Ballabh Pant University of Agriculture and Technology
Pantnagar, Uttarakhand, India

Manoj Kumar Ahirwar
Department of Veterinary Surgery and Radiology
College of Veterinary Science and Animal Husbandry
Nanaji Deshmukh Veterinary Science University
Jabalpur, Madhya Pradesh, India

Mojetoluwa S. Afolabi
Department of Biological Sciences
Alabama A&M University
Normal, Alabama, USA

Monica Gunasekar
Department of Clinics
Madras Veterinary College
Chennai, Tamil Nadu, India

Morteza Taravat
Department of Clinical Science
Faculty of Veterinary Medicine
University of Tabriz
Tabriz, East Azerbaijan, Iran

Nasrul I. Shaikh
All Vet Diagnostic Solutions India
New Delhi, Delhi, India

Nathaniel Ogunkunle
Department of Food and Animal Science
Alabama A&M University
Normal, Alabama, USA

Naveen Swaroop Murikipudi
Department of Veterinary Biochemistry
Sri Venkateswara Veterinary University
Tirupati, Andhrapradesh, India

Neeti Lakhani
Department of Animal Nutrition
College of Veterinary Science, Rampura Phul
Guru Angad Dev Veterinary and Animal Sciences University
Bathinda, Punjab, India

Pradeep Nag Beladakere Subramanyam
Department of Animal Sciences
University of Missouri
Columbia, Missouri, USA

Prakash M. Chauhan
Department of Veterinary Clinics
College of Veterinary Science and Animal Husbandry
Kamdhenu University
Sardarkrushinagar, Gujarat, India

Pramod Kumar
Department of Veterinary Physiology and Biochemistry
College of Veterinary Science and Animal Husbandry
Acharya Narendra Deva University of Agriculture and Technology, Kumarganj, Ayodhya
Uttar Pradesh, India

Pranav Anjaria
College of Veterinary Science and Animal Husbandry
Kamdhenu University
Anand, Gujarat, India

Rajesh Kumar
Department of Veterinary Gynaecology and Obstetrics
College of Veterinary Science and Animal Husbandry
Acharya Narendra Deva University of Agriculture and Technology
Ayodhya, Uttar Pradesh, India

Rajesh Kumar
Department of Veterinary Surgery and Radiology
Bihar Veterinary College
Patna, Bihar, India

Ramasamy Rajkumar
Department of Veterinary Gynaecology and Obstetrics
Veterinary College and Research Institute
Tamil Nadu Veterinary and Animal Sciences University
Salem, Tamil Nadu, India

R.S. Sethi
College of Dairy Science and Technology
Guru Angad Dev Veterinary and Animal Sciences University
Ludhiana, Punjab, India

Randhir Singh
Department of Veterinary Surgery and Radiology
College of Veterinary Science and Animal Husbandry
Nanaji Deshmukh Veterinary Science University
Jabalpur, Madhya Pradesh, India

Ravi Shankar Kumar Mandal
Department of Veterinary Medicine
Bihar Veterinary College
Bihar Animal Sciences University
Patna, Bihar, India

Rayal S. Sagar
Department of Veterinary Medicine
Veterinary College
Bangalore, Karnataka, India

Reza Asadpour
Department of Clinical Science
Faculty of Veterinary Medicine
University of Tabriz
Tabriz, East Azerbaijan, Iran

Sabarinathan Akambaram
Veterinary Clinical Complex
Veterinary College and Research Institute, Tirunelveli
Tamil Nadu Veterinary and Animal Sciences University
Tirunelveli, Tamil Nadu, India

Sakhahari Daund Sushant
Department of Veterinary Gynaecology and Obstetrics
College of Veterinary Science and Animal Husbandry
Acharya Narendra Deva University of Agriculture and Technology
Ayodhya, Uttar Pradesh, India

Sakthivel Manokaran
Department of Veterinary Gynaecology and Obstetrics
Veterinary College and Research Institute
Tamil Nadu Veterinary and Animal Sciences University
Salem, Tamil Nadu, India

Samuel Uchenna Felix
National Animal Production Research Institute
Faculty of Veterinary Medicine
Ahmadu Bello University
Zaria, Kaduna, Nigeria;

Department of Food and Animal Science
Alabama A&M University
Normal, Alabama, USA

Sanjeev Kumar
Department of Veterinary Pathology
Bihar Veterinary College
Patna, Bihar, India

Sarath Thulasiraman
Department of Veterinary Gynaecology and Obstetrics
Veterinary Clinical Complex
Veterinary College and Research Institute
Tamil Nadu Veterinary and Animal Sciences University
Salem, Tamil Nadu, India

Sarita Devi
Department of Veterinary Medicine
College of Veterinary Science and Animal Husbandry
Kamdhenu University
Sardarkrushinagar, Gujarat, India

Satyavrat Singh
Department of Veterinary Medicine
College of Veterinary Science and Animal Husbandry
Acharya Narendra Deva University of Agriculture and Technology, Kumarganj
Ayodhya, Uttar Pradesh, India

Sengodan Raja
Department of Veterinary Gynecology and Obstetrics
Veterinary College and Research Institute, Orathnadu
Tamil Nadu Veterinary and Animal Sciences University
Thanjavur, Tamil Nadu, India

Shanmugasundaram Murugesan
Department of Veterinary Clinical Medicine
Veterinary College and Research Institute, Namakkal
Tamil Nadu Veterinary and Animal Sciences University
Namakkal, Tamil Nadu, India

Shivangi Udainiya
Veterinary Polytechnic Bhopal
Nanaji Deshmukh Veterinary Science University
Bhopal, Madhya Pradesh, India

Shubhamitra Chaudhuri
Department of Veterinary Clinical Complex
West Bengal University of Animal Fishery Sciences
Kolkata, West Bengal, India

Somu Yogeshpriya
Department of Veterinary Medicine
Veterinary College and Research Institute, Orathanadu
Thanjavur, Tamil Nadu, India

Sonam Bhatt
Department of Veterinary Medicine
Bihar Veterinary College, Bihar Animal Sciences University
Patna, Bihar, India

Sowmiya Lakshmanan
Department of Veterinary Public Health and Epidemiology
Veterinary College and Research Institute, Orathanadu
Thanjavur, Tamil Nadu, India

Srujan Racharla
Department of Veterinary Medicine
College of Veterinary and Animal Science
Govind Ballabh Pant University of Agriculture and Technology, Pantnagar, India

Subir Singh
Department of Medicine and Public Health
Agriculture and Forestry University
Rampur, Nepal

Subramaniam Sivaraman
Department of Clinics
Veterinary College and Research Institute, Namakkal
Tamil Nadu Veterinary and Animal Sciences University
Namakkal, Tamil Nadu, India

Suman Biswas
Department of Avian Science
West Bengal University of Animal Fishery Sciences
Kolkata, West Bengal, India

Suman K. Singh
Department of Veterinary Surgery, Medicine
Epidemiology and Public Health
Paklihawa Campus
Institute of Agriculture and Animal Science
Tribhuvan University, Kathmandu, Nepal

Suresh Kamineni
Veterinary Clinical Medicine
Sri Venkateswara Veterinary University
Tirupati, Andhrapradesh, India

Suryakant S. Parikh
Veterinary Gynaecology and Obstetrics
Cattle Breeding Farm
Kamdhenu University
Junagadh, Gujarat, India

Tanmoy Rana
Department of Veterinary Clinical Complex
West Bengal University of Animal & Fishery Sciences
Kolkata, West Bengal, India

Tapas K. Patbandha
Livestock Production and Management
Polytechnic in Animal Husbandry
College of Veterinary Science and Animal Husbandry
Kamdhenu University
Junagadh, Gujarat, India

Usmanu Danfodiyo
University Sokoto
Sokoto, Nigeria

Varun Asediya
M.B. Veterinary College
Rajasthan University of Veterinary and Animal Sciences
Bikaner, Dungarpur, Rajasthan, India

Vasantha Seshu Kumari Injarapu
Department of Veterinary Physiology
Sri Venkateswara Veterinary University
Tirupati, Andhrapradesh, India

Vivek Kumar Singh
Veterinary Clinical Complex
Bihar Veterinary College
Bihar Animal Sciences University
Patna, Bihar, India

Yakubu Mariam
Department of Food and Animal Science
Alabama A&M University
Normal, Alabama, USA

Preface

With its huge annual milk production, dairy farming is one of the most important areas of the agricultural sector worldwide. A considerably large amount of milk production was procured from dairy cattle. Cattle farming is the most significant branch of the animal production industry as it produces a constant income. Milk has a considerably high nutrient content. It is enriched in key vitamins and minerals needed to keep the body healthy, such as those for bone health. Dairy is one of the most important sources of calcium that human beings have in their diet. A major challenge for dairy farmers, managers, and veterinarians is monitoring a dairy cow and its health during the periparturient period. Parturition is one of the most significant critical stages of the reproductive cycle and is a period with a significant death rate and the potential for severe debilitating injury to newborn calves. In contrast, the future efficiency of reproduction and milk yield can be affected during this time. Therefore, major efforts should be undertaken to minimize health problems that generally arise during the periparturient period. Keeping cows healthy is one of the most important steps in monitoring good fertility and an efficient milk yield. In addition, healthy cows produce more milk, rebreed sooner, and have lower culling rates than their unhealthy herd mates. The main value of this reference book is to describe disorders related to the periparturient period and the development of new prevention strategies. This book addresses the definition of metabolic diseases, metabolic disorders, production diseases, and transition cow diseases. This book aids in the pathogenesis of diseases, diagnosis, treatment, and management of periparturient disorders in cattle. This book enhances our understanding of the etiology and pathogenesis of periparturient diseases in transition cattle. The basic version is beneficial as a reference book for doctor of veterinary medicine (DVM) students as well as veterinary technicians, researchers, farm managers, and academicians in veterinary medicine and animal sciences to systematically develop their knowledge about these disorders. This book solves various aspects of periparturient disorders in the cow including evaluating the etiology and pathogenesis, diagnostic approach, and treatment of periparturient diseases. This book is especially intended for animal nutritionists, academics, industrialists, progressive farm owners, researchers, veterinarians, and DVM graduate students with a special interest in dairy cattle health, and management. The book is designed to be engaging by providing color figures, line figures, and tables. The book also provides useful information about the application of various biological systems involving genomics, transcriptomics, proteomics, and metabolomics for understanding the pathomechanisms and early diagnosis using specific biomarkers of periparturient disease in cattle. I hope that this book provides new paradigms to stimulate further research in clarifying the pathomechanisms and causality of periparturient diseases of cattle as well as developing new preventive strategies for reducing the incidence rates of these diseases in the future. I expect that the reader will find this book interesting, containing up-to-date information about periparturient diseases and will utilize this knowledge in their research and teaching the new generation.

Dr. Tanmoy Rana
Department of Veterinary Clinical Complex
West Bengal University of Animal & Fishery Sciences
Kolkata, West Bengal, India

Acknowledgment

I would like to express my sincere gratitude to all those who contributed to this manuscript within the stipulated time. I am also extremely grateful to the Dean of the Faculty of Veterinary and Animal Sciences, and Hon'ble Vice Chancellor, West Bengal University of Animal and Fishery Sciences, Kolkata, India for providing me the opportunity to edit this book. I would also like to convey my warmest thanks to the departmental colleagues who energized my editing of the book. I want to thank Dr. Rituparna Bose, Editor, Health Sciences and Veterinary Medicines, Advanced Content Research and Learning; Bhavya Boopathi, Managing Editor, Health Professions and Veterinary Medicine; Susan Engelken, Editorial Program Coordinator; Selvakumar Gunakundru, Content Refinement Specialist; Baskaran; Keerthana, Support Service Administrator; Wiley; Dr. Ada Hagan, Alliance SciComm and Consulting, Owner; and others for their continual guidance and support during the preparation of this book. I also acknowledge the contributions of the many precious veterinary practitioners, researchers, and academicians whose works are cited profusely throughout the text of this book. This book is dedicated to veterinary students, researchers, academicians, farm managers, veterinary practitioners, and progressive farmers. I hope it will be a very useful resource. Lastly, I would like to convey my sincere thanks to my family who sacrificed a lot in giving me the time to edit this book.

Dr. Tanmoy Rana
Department of Veterinary Clinical Complex
West Bengal University of Animal & Fishery Sciences
Kolkata, West Bengal, India

1

Introduction to Periparturient Diseases of Cattle

Ambica Gadige[1], *Srujan Racharla*[2], *Aruna Maramulla*[3], *and Tanmoy Rana*[4]

[1] Department of Veterinary Medicine, College of Veterinary Science, Rajendranagar, Hyderabad, Telangana, India
[2] Department of Veterinary Medicine, College of Veterinary and Animal Science, Govind Ballabh Pant University of Agriculture and Technology, Pantnagar, India
[3] Department of Veterinary Clinical Complex, College of Veterinary Science, Mamnoor, Warangal, Telangana, India
[4] Department of Veterinary Clinical Complex, West Bengal University of Animal & Fishery Sciences, Kolkata, West Bengal, India

1.1 Introduction

The term "periparturient" arises from the word "parturition" and the prefix "peri," which literally but vaguely means "around." The periparturient period in cattle refers to the 2 to 3 weeks pre- and postpartum and is a transitional period characterized by changes in endocrine status of the animal for lactogenesis and parturition. It is also characterized by changes in tissue metabolism, nutrient utilization, and disruptions in immune system functions (Kimura et al. 2006; Borsberry and Dobson, 1989).

The periparturient or transition period starts 4 weeks before and ends 4 weeks after calving and is marked by a significantly increased risk of disease. This duration primarily involves a series of adjustments to meet the demands of lactation, a process referred to as "homeorhetic". Homeorhetic processes entail long-term physiological adaptations to changing states, such as transitioning from a nonlactating to a lactating state or from a nonruminant to a ruminant state. These processes encompass a combined series of metabolic changes that enable animals to adapt to the challenges of their altered state.

Disruptions in homeorhetic changes often result in homeostasis disorders, which leads to conditions like hypocalcemia, downer-cow syndrome, hypomagnesemia, ketosis, udder edema, abomasal displacement, metritis, and poor fertility, all of which are interconnected. The shifts in endocrine function and metabolism that accompany calving as well as the onset of lactation make the transition period inherently challenging for vets.

Despite these complexities, the potential to enhance subsequent production, health, and reproduction has spurred research into the nutritional management of periparturient cows. In broad terms, the goal for the transition cow is to minimize the risk of metabolic disorders related to macro-mineral metabolism, such as calcium (Ca), magnesium (Mg), or phosphorus (P) deficiencies, and to avoid imbalances of sodium (Na) and potassium (K). The aim is also to prevent lipid metabolism issues that stem from insufficient energy intake during the dry period and early lactation as well as to maintain proper rumen function amid dietary changes and support an effective immune response (Akers et al. 1979).

Many cows affected by these periparturient diseases are over conditioned, which increases their vulnerability to conditions like milk fever, ketosis, digestive disorders, retained fetal membranes, metritis, mastitis, and foot problems. The morbidity (50–90%) and mortality (60%) rates can be high in affected herds (Grunes 1973).

Periparturient, production, and metabolic diseases are most important in dairy cows and pregnant ewes, compared to other domestic farm animals for whom a sporadic incidence is noticed. The higher susceptibility to disease during the periparturient period is attributed to the extremely high turnover of fluids, salts, and soluble organic materials during the early part of lactation. Because of this rapid rate of exchange in water, sodium, calcium, magnesium, chlorides, and phosphates, a sudden change in their excretion or secretion (in milk or by other routes) or a sudden variation in their intake because of changes in ingestion, digestion, or absorption, may cause abrupt, damaging changes in the internal environment of the animal. It is the volume of change in intake and secretion as well as the rapidity with which they can occur that affects the

Periparturient Diseases of Cattle, First Edition. Edited by Tanmoy Rana.

metabolic stability of the cow. In addition, if the continued nutritional demands of pregnancy are exacerbated by an inadequate diet in the dry period, the incidence of metabolic disease will increase.

One of the major challenges faced by dairy farmers and veterinarians is the maintenance of a cow's health during the periparturient period. The incidence of these diseases is an important source of economic loss to the dairy industry. Studies have verified that the incidence of metabolic and production-related diseases including milk fever, mastitis, fatty liver disease, ketosis, metritis, hypomagnesemia, and abomasal displacements is highest during the periparturient period, and complications from dystocia and retained placentas commonly occur (Markusfeld 1987).

The initiating factor occurs before parturition, mainly during the dry period for most of these diseases. This is because pregnant heifers and cows in dry period are the most neglected animals on a farm due to poor housing and feeding conditions. This often results in decreased milk yield, poor reproductive efficiency, and increased periparturient disorders. Cows with high production are always at risk of problems in the early lactation period or periparturient period. As lactation is an extremely intensive metabolic process, high yielding cows may face severe metabolic disturbances around the period of parturition and lactation. The etiological factors can be hormone, metabolite, or nutrition based, which may lead to a metabolic imbalance in the animal. These imbalances, if prolonged, may result in extreme periparturient disorders that are detrimental to animal production and health.

Nutritional management in the early dry period is important for maintaining the health and productivity of cows in the transition period (Dann et al. 2006) as dry matter intake tends to decrease by more than 30% in the last 3 weeks of gestation (Hayirli et al. 2002). The incidence of metabolic diseases can be reduced by increasing dry matter intake and minimizing the period of a negative energy balance after calving (Roche et al. 2000).

Nutritional and sanitation requirements of the periparturient cow are understood better. Unfortunately, management and environmental conditions change constantly, and new problems develop as rapidly as old problems are solved. There is difficulty determining what a "normal" cow might be in a "normal" environment (Mather and Melancon 1981). Seasonal calving is often used in grazing dairy farms to maximize pasture nutrient utilization and avoid temporary environmental constraints, such as heat stress, during early lactation and the breeding period. In this type of dairy production system, reproductive efficiency is essential to obtain a concentrated calving season on a yearly basis. Cows must become pregnant in a short and preestablished period of time that in many cases uses a calendar day to begin and end it for all cows.

When concerned with breed susceptibility to periparturient diseases, between species and individuals, susceptibility varies according to the internal metabolism and quantity of milk production. Likewise, variation in the susceptibility between groups is due to variations in genetic (or) management factors. However, among all the breeds of dairy cattle, Jersey cows are high milk yielders and are found to be at high risk of developing periparturient diseases. Similarly, Guernsey's breed is reported to be more susceptible to ketosis (Radostits et al. 2006).

Several conditions such as milk fever, ketosis, injuries to the birth canal, nerve paralysis, mastitis, and metritis occur at a higher frequency during the periparturient period in cattle (Goff and Horst 1997). These conditions account for up to 8% of all diseases in dairy cattle (Markusfeld 1987) and cause substantial losses to the dairy industry in terms of increased generation interval, loss of genetic pool, increased deaths, reduced productivity of the animals, and the cost of treatment (Erb et al. 1985). To be successful and remain competitive, milk producers must minimize losses from infertility. Factors that affect fertility include both herd-level management and individual cow factors. In this case, clinical reproductive diseases cause short-term problems and milk yield losses as well as have long-term, harmful effects on fertility (Roche et al. 2000). Moreover, cows that present with periparturient diseases are more susceptible to developing other diseases (Williams et al. 2007); thus, a healthy passage through the transition period is essential for proper reproductive efficiency in dairy cows. Assessing the impact of gynecological diseases on the overall level of reproductive processes has been well documented in European dairy cattle in temperate climates (Gilbert 2011). A great number of these studies were carried out in herds with two milkings per day, without the use of recombinant bovine somatotropin (rBST), throughout lactation and at latitudes where the heat load is not a serious hurdle for dairy operations. The dramatic increase in nutritional demands at the onset of lactation, coupled with the concurrent appetite suppression near calving, leads to extreme metabolic stress. Excessive mobilization of adipose tissue occurs to meet the nutritional demands of lactation and results in elevated concentrations of non-esterified fatty acids (NEFA) and ketones, such as β-hydroxybutyric acid (BHBA), in the circulation. Extensive evidence has shown that elevated NEFA and BHBA can alter immune functions, which contributes to immune suppression (Ingvartsen and Moyes 2015). During the periparturient period, cattle suffer from oxidative stress, which refers to the accumulation of reactive oxygen species (ROS) when their production exceeds the neutralizing capacity of antioxidant mechanisms, and it has been identified as a significant underlying factor of periparturient immunosuppression.

Metabolic diseases are associated with significant economic losses due to a significant decrease in milk yield and impaired reproductive performance in animals (Wang et al. 2021). Attention to detail and an understanding of reproduction, metabolism, digestive functions, milk secretion, and all aspects of husbandry are essential. To be successful, producers must minimize reproductive failure because reproductive performance affects the quantity of milk produced per cow per day of herd life, the number of potential replacements needed to maintain a constant herd size, and the longevity of the cow in the herd. In practice, this translates into well-designed programs for herd health, milking, feeding, and reproductive management that minimize involuntary culling problems in cows by maintaining healthy, profitable cows.

The periparturient period is associated with multiple changes including hormonal changes, moving from a nonlactating to lactating state, and a major drop in feed intake. For these reasons, the serum levels of major macro minerals and glucose frequently change during this period (DeGaris and Lean 2008). Metabolic diseases are associated with low concentrations of these components in the blood. Moreover, subclinical forms of mineral deficiencies have been incriminated in decreasing production levels and decreased feed efficiency, which can cause huge losses to dairy farmers (Bacic et al. 2007). In this regard, metabolic profiling, which refers to the analysis of blood biochemical constituents, and monitoring parameters like milk production, urinalysis, and rectal temperature, are important tools for detecting metabolic disorders in dairy cattle before any clinical manifestations appear.

During the periparturient period, cattle are prone to disorders or diseases like milk fever, ketosis, post-parturient hypomagnesemia, post-parturient hypophosphatemia, ruminal acidosis, laminitis, fatty liver, fatty cow syndrome, hypokalemia, abomasal displacement (left side, right, or anterior), abomasal torsion, udder edema, mastitis, metritis, retention of the placenta, and pyometra.

Milk fever, or hypocalcemia, is the major periparturient disease in adult, lactating, dairy cattle during the third parity and older. It commonly occurs during the first 48 hours after parturition and less frequently, just before and even several weeks before parturition. It develops due to a decrease in the ionized calcium concentration in the body fluids and is characterized by generalized muscular weakness that results in sternal recumbency with a lateral deviation of the head and neck (Figure 1.1), anorexia, ruminal atony, scanty feces, and if not treated, it can lead to circulatory collapse and death (Radostits et al. 2006).

Ketosis in ruminants, particularly in cattle, is unique as it is as a primary metabolic disorder or syndrome distinct from any other recognized disease; it is characterized by abnormally high levels of acetone bodies in the blood and urine of cows displaying ketosis symptoms (Sjollema and Van Der Zande). Ketosis is commonly reported in fat, high producing cows 7–10 days after calving and is characterized by rapid weight loss, loss of appetite, dry feces, decreased milk production, and in many cases, nervous disturbances. Ketosis most commonly affects cows after their third to sixth calving, particularly when they are stabled. Repeated attacks could occur following subsequent calvings (Hutyra and Marek).

Post-parturient hemoglobinuria (PPH) is a common issue in lactating dairy cattle that primarily affects highly productive animals, it is characterized by intravascular hemolysis, anemia, and hemoglobinuria. This condition is most commonly observed in cattle during their third to sixth lactation periods, and the highest risk periods are during late pregnancy through early lactation and from calving up to 1 month post parturition, most cases occur 2 to 4 weeks postpartum. Hemoglobinuria is more frequent in buffaloes compared to crossbred cows in their third lactation, with the highest incidence occurring during the winter season. While the exact cause of PPH remains unknown, it has been linked to potential factors such as phosphorus depletion or hypophosphatemia, copper deficiency, and certain hemolyzing substances found in specific feeds. The disease carries economic losses including treatment costs, decreased milk production, and high mortality rates.

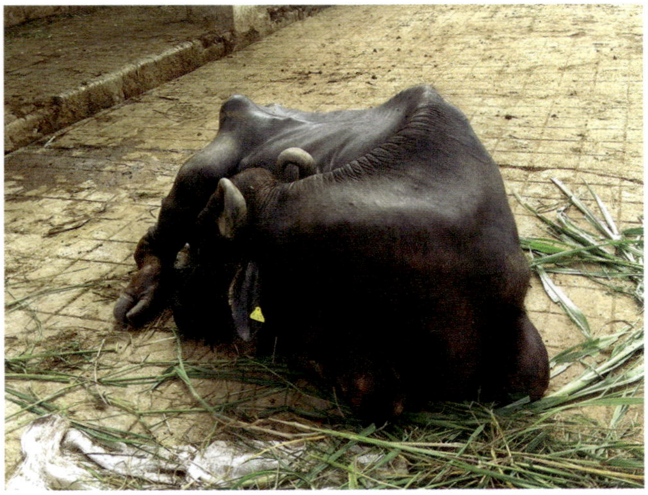

Figure 1.1 Milk fever in cattle.

Post-parturient hypomagnesemia, or low blood magnesium levels, is a condition more common in cattle with a clinical presentation that ranges from acute with sudden death to subacute and chronic with varying symptoms.

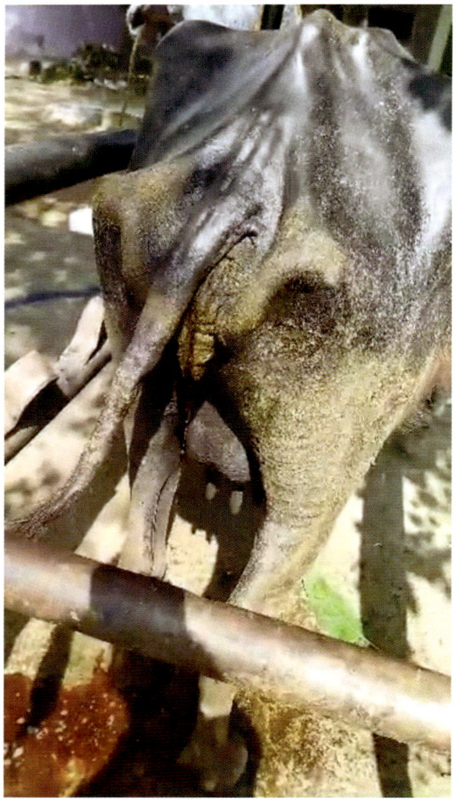

Figure 1.2 Post-parturient hypophosphatemia in cattle.

Occurrence is influenced by several factors including nutrition, lactation, and environmental conditions. The disease is characterized by hyperexcitability, incoordination, nervousness, seizures, and death. Prophylactic measures are important for prevention and involve soil and forage assessment as well as dietary supplementation with magnesium sources. Treatment options include intravenous, subcutaneous, or oral administration of magnesium-containing solutions (Figure 1.2).

Another condition is "downer cow complex," which encompasses various peripartum diseases in dairy cows that are often interconnected. Its incidence has risen due to drastic changes in management practices, in particular, the shift from individual cow care to group-focused approaches. The group feeding of dry and lactating cows has led to the overfeeding of dry cows, which makes them more susceptible to metabolic and infectious diseases, calving issues, and reduced fertility. These conditions are referred to by several names, including "downers," "alert downers," "atypical milk fever," "creeper cows," and "fat cow syndrome" (FCS). Complications that result from parturient hypocalcemia (milk fever) often involve muscle, tendon, or nerve injuries.

Over conditioned, dry cows may experience the entire FCS, which includes foot abscesses, parturient hypocalcemia, retained placentas, metritis, ketosis, abomasal displacement, diarrhea, and mastitis. Such cases have a poor prognosis, even with extensive treatment. The prevention of FCS in a herd can be challenging and requires months of proper management to improve the physical condition of over conditioned cows. Factors like low milk production, extended calving intervals, feeding excessive concentrates after peak lactation or during the dry period, and free-choice access to corn silage or high quality hay contribute to the development of FCS. Protein underfeeding or an early reduction in milk production combined with corn silage can also lead to energy over consumption and over conditioning in cows.

Hypokalemia in periparturient cattle is a commonly noticed disorder often associated with conditions such as left-displaced abomasa (LDA), right-displaced abomasa (RDA), abomasal volvulus (AV), abomasal impaction, clinical mastitis, retained placentas, and hepatic lipidosis. Severe hypokalemia in cows leads to decreased smooth muscle tone in the gastrointestinal tract, signs of depression, and profound skeletal muscle weakness that sometimes results in recumbency. The rise in severe hypokalemia cases may be attributed to factors like increased milk yield and the administration of multiple isoflupredone acetate doses to treat ketosis. The incidence of hypokalemia is common in lactating cows compared to beef cattle and is likely due to the higher incidence of LDA, RDA, and AV in dairy cows, conditions that cause alkalemia by sequestering chloride in the gastrointestinal tract, which decreases dietary chloride intake and causes potassium loss in the milk of lactating dairy cows. Hypokalemia can also occur in cattle with metabolic alkalosis or hyperglycemia due to a shift of potassium from extracellular to intracellular spaces. To develop effective treatment protocols for hypokalemic lactating dairy cows, a thorough understanding of the mechanisms that lead to hypokalemia is necessary.

Dairy cows experience moderate to severe fatty liver upon calving, which is associated with health issues that include mastitis, displaced abomasa, retained placentas, metritis, poor reproductive performance, immune suppression, ketosis, and production losses. Fatty liver occurs when the liver synthesizes triglycerides faster than they are removed through hydrolysis or secretion via very low-density lipoproteins (VLDLs). Ruminants have an unusually slow rate of hepatic VLDL secretion, possibly due to limited essential nutrients for lipoprotein assembly. Attempts to supplement these nutrients have not been successful. Microsomal triglyceride transfer protein (MTP) is essential for VLDL assembly. It consists of a larger and a smaller subunit. Hepatic MTP may be a key factor in determining the rate of VLDL secretion and the severity of fatty liver in dairy cows. Nutritional manipulation, such as increasing energy consumption at calving, adjusting dietary carbohydrate content, or supplementing with propylene glycol, can reduce fat mobilization from adipose tissue and hepatic triglyceride concentration. In vitro studies have shown that increasing fatty acid concentrations in media or the presence of insulin and glucagon can impact bovine hepatocyte metabolism.

References

Akers, R.M., Bauman, D.E., Capuco, A.V., and Tucker, H.A. (1979). Inhibition of periparturient prolactin secretion effects on bovine mamlnary gland function. *Federation Proceedings* 38 (3 Part 1): 1025.

Bacic, G., Karadjole, T., Macesic, N., and Karadjole, M. (2007). A brief review of etiology and nutritional prevention of metabolic disorders in dairy cattle. *Veterinary Archives* 77 (6): 567–577.

Borsberry, S. and Dobson, H. (1989). Periparturient diseases and their effect on reproductive performance in five dairy herd. *The Veterinary Record* 124 (9): 217–219. https://doi.org/10.1136/vr.124.9.217.

Dann, H., Litherland, N., Underwood, J. et al. (2006). Diets during far-off and close-up dry periods affect periparturient metabolism and lactation in multiparous cows. *Journal of Dairy Science* 89 (9): 3563–3577.

DeGaris, P.J. and Lean, I.J. (2008). Milk fever in dairy cows: a review of pathophysiology and control principles. *Veterinary Journal* 176 (1): 58–69.

Erb, H.N., Smith, R.D., Oltenacu, P.A. et al. (1985). Path model of reproductive disorders and performance, milk fever, mastitis, milk yield, and culling in Holstein cows. *Journal of Dairy Science* 68: 3337–3349.

Gilbert, R.O. (2011). The effects of metritis on the establishment of pregnancy in cattle. *Reproduction, Fertility and Development* 24: 252–257.

Goff, J.P. and Horst, R.L. (1997). Physiological changes at parturition and their relationship to metabolic disorders. *Journal of Dairy Science* 80: 1260–1268.

Hayirli, A., Grummer, R., Nordheim, E., and Crump, P. (2002). Animal and dietary factors affecting feed intake during the prefresh transition period in Holsteins. *Journal of Dairy Science* 85 (12): 3430–3443.

Ingvartsen, K.L. and Moyes, K.M. (2015). Factors contributing to immunosuppression in the dairy cow during the periparturient period. *The Japanese Journal of Veterinary Research* 63 (1): S15–S24.

Kimura, K., Reinhardt, T.A., and Goff, J.P. (2006). Parturition and hypocalcaemia blunt calcium signals in immune cells of dairy cattle. *Journal of Dairy Science* 89: 2588–2595.

Markusfeld, O. (1987). Periparturient traits in seven high yielding dairy herds. Incidence rates, association with parity and inter-relationships among traits. *Journal of Dairy Science* 70: 158–166.

Mather, E.C. and Melancon, J.J. (1981). The periparturient cow - a pivotal entity in dairy production. *Journal of Dairy Science* 64 (6): 1422–1430.

Radostits, O.M., Gay, C.C., Hinchcliff, K.W., and Constable, P.D. (2006). *Veterinary Medicine - a Textbook of the Diseases of Cattle, Horses, Sheep, Pigs and Goats*, 10e, 1613–1626.

Roche, J.F., Mackey, D., and Diskin, M.D. (2000). Reproductive management of postpartum cows. *Animal Reproduction Science* 60–61: 703–712.

Wang, N., Zhou, C., Basang, W. et al. (2021). Mechanisms by which mastitis affects reproduction in dairy cow: a review. *Reproduction in Domestic Animals* 56 (9): 1165–1175. https://doi.org/10.1111/rda.13953.

Williams, E.J., Fischer, D.P., Noakes, D.E. et al. (2007). The relationship between uterine pathogen growth density and ovarian function in the postpartum dairy cow. *Theriogenology* 68: 549–559.

2

Nutrition, Immune Function, and Health

Samuel U. Felix[1,2], *Chiezey N. Pauline*[1], *Yakubu Mariam*[2], *and Allam Lushaikyaa*[3]

[1] *National Animal Production Research Institute/Faculty of Veterinary Medicine, Ahmadu Bello University, Zaria, Kaduna, Nigeria*
[2] *Department of Food and Animal Science, Alabama A&M University, Normal, Alabama, USA*
[3] *Faculty of Veterinary Medicine, Ahmadu Bello University, Zaria, Kaduna, Nigeria*

2.1 Introduction

The dairy industry undergoes constant changes. Historically, animals have been chosen for their high milk production to enhance competitiveness (Bórawski et al. 2020). For instance, in Denmark, the average milk yield per cow annually surged from 6693 kg in 1989 to 8983 kg in 2009, marking a yearly growth of 1.5% and a remarkable 50% increase over 27 years. Nevertheless, it is important to note that there is considerable variability in milk yield among individual cows. A case in point is "Lucy," a cow that set a world record in 1998 by producing over 34 000 kg of milk in just 365 days to demonstrate the substantial potential of dairy cows (Kelly et al. 2020).

Coupled with increases in production per cow over the past few decades, there has been a major structural development in the dairy industry in Denmark (Ingvartsen and Moyes 2013). While the total national milk production has remained relatively stable over the past two decades, significant changes have occurred in the dairy industry due to the European Union quota system. Between 1989 and 2009, the number of dairy cows in the industry decreased from 769 000 to 563 000. However, the most striking change has been in the number of dairy farms, which plummeted from 21 500 to 4300 during the same period. Consequently, there has been a substantial shift in the average herd size, which increased from 36 cows per farm in 1989 to 131 cows per farm in 2009. This means that by 2009 farmers were tasked with overseeing 3.7 times as many cows as they did in 1989 (Jansik and Irz 2015).

The significant rise in milk production and the substantial structural changes within the dairy industry have led to significant alterations in how dairy cows are housed, fed, and managed (LeBlanc et al. 2006). There has been a marked enhancement in the quality of roughage, an increased proportion of concentrates, and a more balanced diet composition tailored to meet the dietary requirements of the typical modern dairy cow (Paura et al. 2023).

Earlier literature has argued that physiological imbalance (PI) and reduced immune competence are more significant risk factors for disease in dairy cows than milk yield alone (Kehrli et al. 2006; Mukhopadhyay et al. 2023). Mulligan and Doherty (2008), explored critical phases such as the transition period in cows and its impact on health and immune function, the intricate relationship between the endocrine and immune systems (Ingvartsen and Boisclair 2001; Vangroenweghe et al. 2005), the connection between nutrition and immune function (Kehrli et al. 2006), as well as PI and disease prevention in periparturient cows (Ingvartsen 2006). This work attempts to explore disease prevention and the well-being of herbivores with a primary focus on dairy cows.

2.2 Periparturient Period

The modern dairy cow is kept and selected for the purpose of producing milk and offspring and is consequently managed to secure a mammary tissue matrix capable of delivering a large milk output (Ponnampalam et al. 2022). This management involves, for example, drying off dairy cows before calving, and thus, the decisions on dry period length, reduction in

Periparturient Diseases of Cattle, First Edition. Edited by Tanmoy Rana.

feeding, and the cessation of milking and feeding during the dry period that may impact production, reproduction, and health (Mukherjee et al. 2023). In a recent comprehensive review by Pezeshki et al. (2010), the potential impacts of managing the length of the dry period on mammary gland biology and defense mechanisms were examined. This review underscored the importance of integrating mammary gland biology and defense mechanisms in studies that investigate alterations in dry period lengths. This integration has the potential to enhance disease resistance and animal welfare.

The periparturient period, which encompasses the last 1 to 2 months of gestation and the initial months post delivery, poses significant challenges for dairy cattle. Specifically, the transition period, which spans from 3 weeks before to 3 weeks after parturition, is marked by profound metabolic and host defense changes that render the animals more susceptible to disease. This period can be particularly demanding for mammals and may pose threats to both their health and welfare if the challenges they face surpass their coping mechanisms. During both the periparturient and transition periods, there is an increased incidence of diseases that include metabolic disorders, like fatty liver and ketosis, as well as infectious and noninfectious ailments such as milk fever, retained placentas, metritis, left-displaced abomasa, lameness, and clinical mastitis (Ingvartsen 2006).

Early lactation in mammals involves the mobilization of substantial nutrient reserves, especially lipids from adipose tissue, to support lactation. This mobilization of lipids is a normal physiological adaptation during critical states like the periparturient period. However, excessive mobilization has been associated with an elevated risk of diseases (Rico and Razzaghi 2023).

In a review of 11 epidemiological and 14 genetic studies, Ingvartsen et al. (2003) found limited evidence to suggest that high yielding cows are at an increased risk of dystocia, retained placentas, metritis, periparturient paresis, and left-displaced abomasa. While there was no clear phenotypical relationship between milk yield and the risk of ketosis and lameness, the selection for higher milk yield is likely to raise the risk of these diseases during lactation. Notably, mastitis was the only disease that exhibited a clear correlation between milk yield and the risk of infection. Ingvartsen et al. (2003) proposed that the rapid acceleration in milk yield might induce physiological stress that subsequently leads to health issues.

Subsequent studies have supported these findings, revealing that milk yield acceleration is most pronounced around calving and suggesting that cows with high milk yield acceleration tend to face elevated levels of stress and risk. Consequently, acceleration in milk yield is regarded as an indicator of the risk for health and reproductive problems (Hansen et al. 2006).

The nutrient demand increases quite dramatically during late pregnancy and particularly in early lactation. In late pregnancy, the nutrient demand increases as a result of fetal development, which specifically increases glucose and amino acids. The substantial milk yield acceleration, particularly seen in the last week prepartum and in the first 2 weeks of lactation, reflects the dramatic increase in nutrient demand at the onset of lactation. A cow with a milk yield of 50 kg secretes 2 kg of milk fat daily, 1.6 kg of milk protein, 2.5 kg of lactose, 65 g of calcium (Ca), 50 g of phosphorous (P), and 8 g of magnesium (Mg), all of which increase the demand for energy, protein, and minerals. The nutrient requirement in late pregnancy, particularly for lactation, calls for the coordination of physiological processes in different tissues that result in metabolic changes in an attempt to ensure that cows reach their maximum genetic potential for milk yield.

Consequently, this review will address the metabolic adaptations of periparturient animals with a specific focus on the changes in the concentration of nutrients/metabolites considered relevant for the immune function. We believe that these metabolic adaptations play a key role with regards to immune function and will discuss how immune competence and risk of disease can be improved through nutrition and management.

2.3 Physiological Imbalance

An inadequately coordinated regulation and thereby the adaptation to changed physiological states will lead to PI – a situation where the homeorhetic and homeostatic mechanisms are insufficient for the animal to function optimally. PI in cows has been defined as cows whose parameters deviate from the norm and who consequently have an increased risk of developing production diseases (clinical or subclinical) as well as reduced production and/or reproduction (Ingvartsen 2006). A prominent example of PI is excessive mobilization due to over conditioning or malnutrition, in some cases for extended periods, in early lactation. In the case of excessive mobilization, the rates of lipogenesis are very low, whereas lipolysis is very high, which results in high plasma concentrations of non-esterified fatty acids (NEFAs) and glycerol. Interlinked with these increased NEFAs is a reduced dry matter intake (Ingvartsen and Andersen 2000; Allen et al. 2009) and consequently, a low plasma concentration of glucose and increased ketogenesis with resultant increased levels of ketone bodies (Drackley et al. 2006; Ingvartsen 2006). The metabolic changes linked to excessive mobilization can also be secondary to diseases, for example, displaced abomasa and stress and pain due to lameness (Ingvartsen 2006). The above example also illustrates that generally, more metabolic parameters are affected in the case of excessive mobilization or disease, stress, or pain. Consequently, it is probably relevant to consider PI an index on the basis of several metabolic parameters, for example, NEFAs, glucose, and ketone bodies, that is, β-hydroxybutyrate (BHBA). In the following section, the focus will be on the effect of nutrition and different metabolic parameters on the immune system (Gross 2022).

2.4 General Aspects of the Immune Response

The immune system, or host defense system, consists of a variety of cells and molecules that are capable of specifically (specific immunity) or nonspecifically (innate immunity) recognizing and eliminating invading foreign microorganisms (Figure 2.1). The innate, or nonspecific, immunity is rapidly activated and serves as the primary immune defense in the initial stages of an infection. The innate immunity is provided by phagocytes, such as polymorphonuclear neutrophils (PMNs) and resident macrophages as well as mammary epithelial cells. Macrophages (i) detect and recognize nonspecific foreign pathogens; (ii) produce cytokines, that is, interleukin (IL)-1b, IL-6, and tumor necrosis factor-α (TNF-α) that initiate the innate and specific immune responses as well as recruit PMNs to the site of infection; (iii) phagocytose and kill invading pathogens; and (iv) are the bridge between the innate and specific immune responses through antigen presentation via the major histocompatibility complex (MHC) class II to T cells. After initiation of the inflammatory response, PMNs become the predominant cell type observed during an infection. PMNs migrate from the blood to the location of the invading organism by a process called chemotaxis. Once at the site of infection, PMNs and resident macrophages phagocytose, that is, engulf, and kill invading microorganisms. Once a microorganism is engulfed, a burst of oxidative metabolism called a respiratory burst occurs in activated phagocytes via the activation of a membrane-associated NADPH-linked oxidase that catalyzes the reduction of oxygen to superoxide anion, a reactive oxygen metabolite that is extremely toxic to ingested bacteria. After the respiratory burst, the digested contents of the microorganism are expelled by exocytosis (Parija 2023).

If the infection persists, the specific immune system becomes activated. Specific immunity consists of antibodies, macrophages (antigen-presenting cells), and T and B lymphocytes that recognize specific microorganisms. The T cells can be subdivided into T-helper and T-cytotoxic lymphocytes. The T-helper cells produce cytokines, such as IL-2 and interferon (IFN)-γ, which are crucial for an effective cell-mediated immune response. The cytotoxic T cells recognize and eliminate cells infected with an antigen, and old or damaged immune cells that, if present, can increase susceptibility to infections.

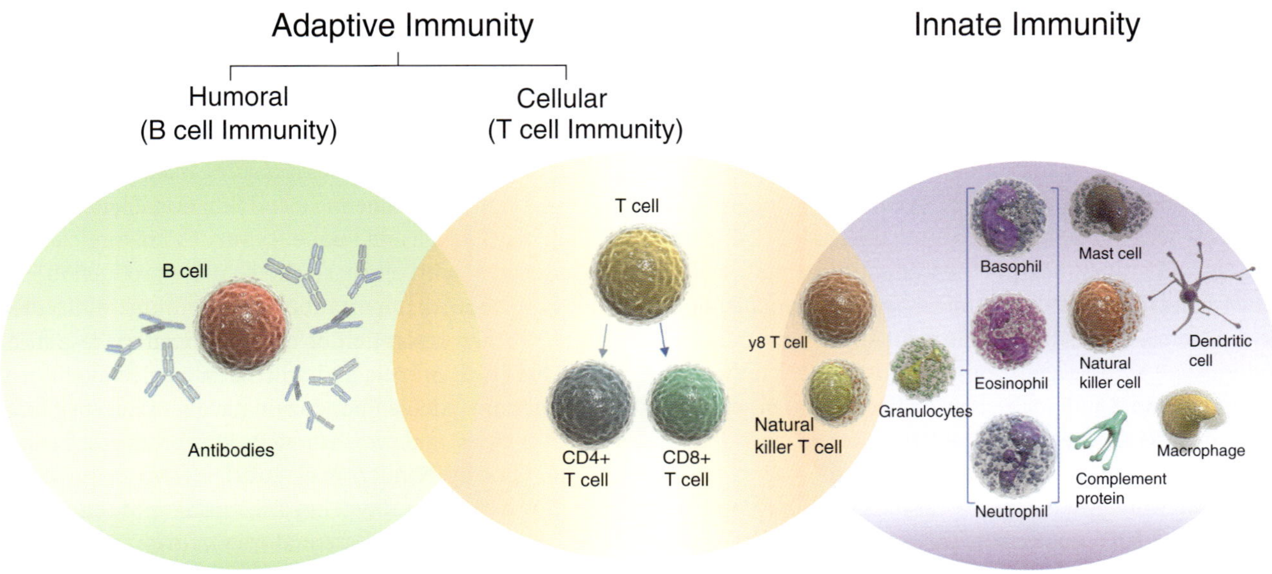

Figure 2.1 Adaptive and innate immunity.

The B lymphocytes differentiate into plasma cells that produce antibodies or immunoglobulins (Igs), that is, IgG1, IgG2, and IgM, or memory cells. Both innate and specific immunity have a broad diversity of mechanisms. Their interaction enables the body to recognize and discriminate between foreign substances and the host's own molecules (Mohanraju et al. 2022).

2.4.1 Innate Immunity

In cattle, like in many other animals, the first line of defense is represented by physical barriers and mechanisms that include skin and mucosal membranes as well as the elimination of invading microorganisms by coughing, sneezing, vomiting, and diarrhea (Figure 2.1). Besides forming mechanical barriers of the respiratory (RespT), gastrointestinal (GIT), and urogenitary tracts, epithelial cells secrete a number of antimicrobial factors, including antimicrobial peptides (AMPs) and defensins, and thus play an important role in the innate immune response. The other known critical cellular components of the innate immune system in cattle include neutrophils, natural killer (NK) cells, dendritic cells (DCs), γδT cells, mucosa-associated invariant T cells (MAITs), macrophages, and granulocytes. While the majority of information on their development and function comes from human and mouse studies, the available data for cattle were derived from studies on mastitis, tuberculosis, bovine viral diarrhea virus (BVDV), foot-and-mouth disease virus (FMDV), bovine herpesvirus-1 (BHV-1), and bovine respiratory syncytial virus (BRSV) (Upadhyay 2023). Unique to cattle, newborn calves have unusually high numbers of circulating γδT cells (up to 60% of the lymphocyte pool), and γδT cells of ruminants express the WC-1 antigen whose function is unknown (it may act as a microbial/pathogen pattern recognition [PPR] receptor). This can be a compensatory response that balances out the immaturity of neutrophil, macrophage, and DC functions in neonatal calves.

These diverse immune cell subsets are equipped with PPR molecules that interact with pathogen-associated molecular patterns (PAMPs) during the initial stages of the immune response. The best characterized PPRs are Toll-like receptors (TLRs). Ten TLRs with diverse and sometimes overlapping PAMP affinities have been confirmed in cattle. TLR-1 recognizes triacyl lipopeptide of mycobacteria; TLR-2, the peptidoglycans of gram-positive organisms and lipoarabinomannan of mycobacteria and zymosan of fungi; TLR-3, double-stranded (ds)RNA; TLR-4, lipopolysaccharide (LPS); TLR-5, flagellin; TLR-6, the diacyl-lipopeptides of mycoplasmas; TLR-7 and -8, single-stranded (ss)RNA; TLR-9, CpG; while TLR-10 function and affinity have not yet been fully assessed. Prior to binding to TLR-4, LPS, a bacterial component of *Histophilus somni*, *Mannheimia haemolytica*, and *Pasteurella multocida*, interacts with LPS-binding protein, soluble CD14, and the TLR-4 cofactor MD2. TLR-4 also recognizes and binds the F protein of BRSV. In addition to TLR-3, TLR-7–9, BHV-1, parainfluenza virus type 3 (PIV-3), BRSV, and BVDV can recognize and interact with cytosolic viral pathogen recognition receptors, retinoic acid–induced gene-I (RIG-I), and melanoma differentiation-associated gene (MDA)-5. These interactions lead to TLR-independent activation of NF-κB (nuclear factor κ-light-chain-enhancer of activated B cells) as well as interferon regulatory factor (IRF)-3 and -7 via Cardif, also known as the mitochondrial antiviral signaling adapter (MAVS), interferon-β promoter stimulator (IPS-1), and virus-inducing signaling adapter (VISA). Upon activation of the local effector cells (endothelial cells, epithelial cells, macrophages, and DCs) of the innate immune system by inflammatory cytokines (IL-1, TNF-α, and IL-6), they produce a number of cytokines and chemokines that attract the migration of neutrophils and monocytes into the affected area. They, in turn, signal to recruit to dendritic, NK, T, and B cells. In contrast, IL-4, IL-10, and IL-17 actively promote the resolution of the inflammatory cascade (Tufail et al. 2023).

Bovine mast cells are a heterogenous group of cells in the mucosa, skin, mammary glands, and other organs that play a pivotal role in allergic and inflammatory responses by secreting biologically active substances including histamine, leukotrienes, platelet-activating factors (PAFs), and prostaglandins. While the immunohistochemical and functional heterogeneity of mast cells in bovines is poorly characterized, it is known that their distribution and frequency vary by anatomical site, with age and animal health. The evaluation of mast cell functions associated with chymase and tryptase production has further confirmed their anatomical compartmentalization. Oxylipids are another important class of immune molecules derived from cellular lipids that regulate the onset, magnitude, duration, and resolution of the inflammatory response. Oxylipids are synthesized from polyunsaturated fatty acids (PUFAs; n-6 [ω-6] linoleic and arachidonic acids or the n-3 eicosapentaenoic and docosahexaenoic acids). These fatty acid substrates are oxidized nonenzymatically by reactive oxygen species (ROS) or enzymatically by different cyclooxygenases, lipoxygenases, and cytochrome P450 to produce a variety of oxylipids including prostaglandins, thromboxanes, leukotrienes, and lipoxins (Sanders et al. 2022).

Natural antibodies (NAbs) are an important humoral component of innate immunity. They are mostly IgM (and some IgG and IgA) Abs produced without antigenic stimulation by B1-B cells that play an essential role in primary immune response. A high proportion of NAbs bind to PAMPs with relatively low affinity. Complement activation by the classical pathway is one of the most important NAb functions.

Complement is another significant mechanism of innate immune defense. It consists of a group of proteins (C1–C9) present in serum in an inactive form that are activated by antigen–Ab complexes (classical pathway), by some carbohydrates (lectin pathway), or by a variety of surfaces that are not protected by natural inhibitors (alternative pathway). The classical pathway is initiated by the activation of C1 and the alternative pathway by the C3 through an enzyme cascade. The coating of bacteria- or virus-infected cells with fragments of the components C3 and C4 leads to their ingestion by phagocytic cells that possess receptors for these opsonins. Apart from its direct antimicrobial effects, complement maintains Igs in soluble form by limiting the formation of harmful immune complexes and Ig precipitation (Dyall et al. 2022).

2.4.2 Adaptive Immune Response

Bovine plasma cells produce at least five heavy chain classes (IgM IgG, IgA, IgD, and IgE), with three IgG subclasses (IgG1, IgG2, and IgG3), two IgM subclasses (IgM1 and IgM2), and two light chain types (λ and κ). While the functions of IgM, IgA, IgG1, and IgG2 molecules are well-studied, those of IgG3 and IgD have not been evaluated in depth due to their later discovery. In contrast to many other animals, cattle express a limited number of variable Ig gene segments, and it is thought that Ig diversity is achieved via frequent recombination and endogenous mutations in the complementarity-determining region (CDR)3. Additionally, an unusually long CDR3 results in "microfolds" that allow bovine Igs to bind antigens that would otherwise be inaccessible. Immunoglobulin functions include neutralizing antibody, complement activation, Fc receptor-mediated phagocytosis, and Ab-dependent cellular cytotoxicity. Differences exist between cattle breeds in relation to immunoglobulin quantities. IgG1 and IgG2 are highly important, with IgG1 being the most abundant in cow colostrum. IgG is important for virus and toxin neutralization as well as bacterial agglutination and opsonization. In cattle, IgG1 is known to be a less potent opsonin than IgG2. IgM is a pentameric molecule important for bacterial agglutination, complement fixation, and opsonization that is generally restricted to intravascular spaces because of its size. IgA is predominant in many secretions but present in low quantities in bovine serum. It is important for antiviral defense in the upper RespT and GIT. Although methods to analyze the clonal composition of T cells have been used extensively to better understand the mechanisms of T-cell responses in humans and mice, this knowledge is more limited for bovine T cells. The antigen specificity of $CD4^+$ and $CD8^+$ T cells is determined by the αβT cell receptor, which binds to peptides in association with MHC class II and class I molecules, respectively. Most $CD4^+$ T lymphocytes function to promote cell-mediated immunity and Ab production, while certain $CD4^+$ T lymphocytes can lyse appropriately sensitized target cells. Most $CD8^+$ T lymphocytes function as effector cells of direct target-cell lysis and are known as classical cytotoxic T lymphocytes (CTLs), but some may function as nonlytic suppressor cells. Major αβT cell subsets found in other species were also identified in cattle, including: T-killer ($CD8^+$), T-helper ($CD4^+$; Th1, Th2, and Th17) and T-regulatory ($CD4^+$ or $CD8^+$; $CD25^+$) cells, and their functions have been studied in relation to some infections and post-vaccine immune responses. Earlier data suggest that cytokine-mediated regulation of Th1/Th2 cell responses in bovids may be more complex and distinct from that observed in mice. Specifically, parasite-specific bovine Th cells produce IL-4 and IFN-γ, while IL-2 and IL-10 expression are not restricted to IFN-γ or IL-4 producing cells, respectively. Also, IL-4/IL-10 and IL-12 do not selectively exert their suppressive or stimulatory effects on Th1-like cells. Nevertheless, some studies demonstrated that the development and maintenance of a Th1 IFN-γ response can be associated with greater control of some infections (*Mycoplasma bovis*). Besides their critical role in shaping B-cell responses, several studies emphasize the importance of bovine T-cell responses that contribute to the clearance of infections (for example, *Cryptosporidium parvum*) in the absence of humoral/Ig responses. Of interest, memory $CD4^+$, $CD8^+$, and γδT cells are detected in calves in the presence of maternal Abs, even in the absence of an active Ab response (Table 2.1).

2.4.3 Mucosal Immune System

The mucosa includes four distinct major components: (i) microbiome, (ii) mucous layer, (iii) mucosal epithelial barrier, and (iv) immune cells of the mucosa-associated lymphoid tissues (MALT; lamina propria [LP], Peyer's patches [PPs] in the gut, and diffuse mucosal lymphocytes; Figure 2.2). The microbiome is critical for the immune development of young calves as well as the immune defense and health maintenance in cattle of all ages. While the role of the rumen in mucosal immunity has not been yet clarified, it is established that bacterial richness and diversity were the highest in the rumen compared to all other gut sections (Chase 2022).

Bile acids (BAs) in the small intestine represent another important mechanism of intestinal defense and the gut microbiota plays a role in their metabolism. BAs inactivate enveloped viruses and some enteropathogenic bacteria;

Table 2.1 Structures and properties of antibodies.

Name	Properties	Structure
IgA	Found in mucous, saliva, tears, and breast milk. Protects against pathogens.	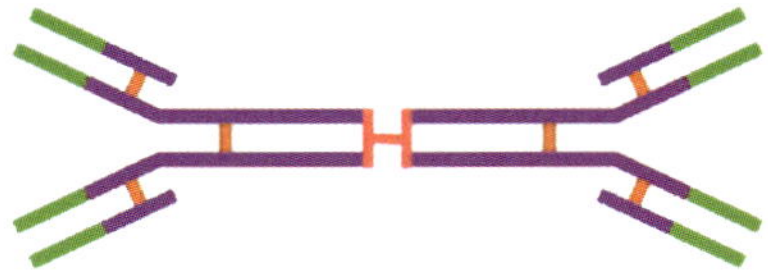
IgD	Part of the B-cell receptor. Activates basophils and mast cells.	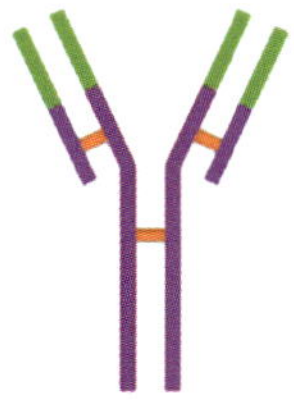
IgE	Protects against parasitic worms. Responsible for allergic reactions.	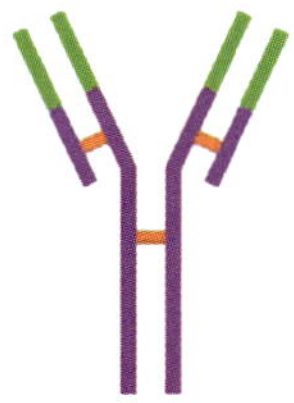
IgG	Secreted by plasma cells in the blood. Able to cross the placenta into the fetus.	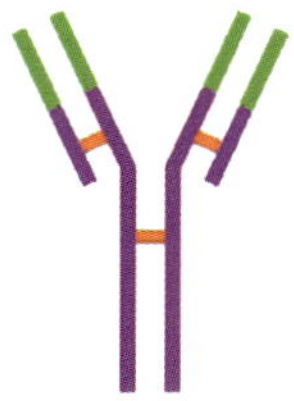
IgM	May be attached to the surface of a B cell or secreted into the blood. Responsible for the early stages of immunity.	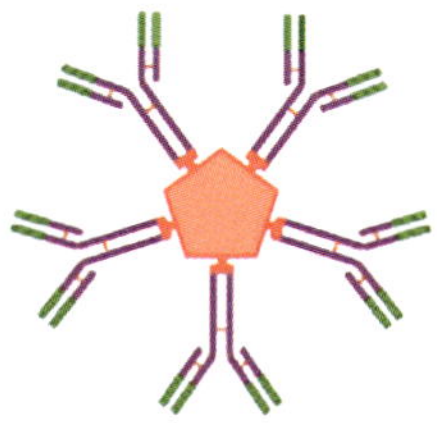

however, enterococci and *Bacteroides* spp. can degrade them, while commensal bacteria metabolize BAs in the colon. The mucous barrier consists of mucous and mucins (secreted by Goblet cells), AMPs (defensins, regenerating protein [Reg]-III, lactoferricin), and IgG and secretory IgA (transported from the LP). Epithelial cells (ECs; enterocytes in the gut and ciliated ECs in the lung) line the GIT, reproductive tract (RepT), urinary (UT), and RespT and express tight junction proteins that form the mucosal epithelium (ME). If the tight junctions break down, the epithelium becomes leaky, which leads to systemic inflammation. This condition is best known as "leaky gut" but can be observed in the RepT and RespT. Besides providing mechanical segregation, ME functions include secretion and absorption (in the gut), fetal development (in the uterus), oxygen exchange and clearance of foreign substances and pathogens (in the RespT), and the innate immune response. Bovine ECs express the whole repertoire of TLRs. Based on luminal stimuli, ECs can produce pro-inflammatory (IL-1α, IL-8, and TNF-α) or regulatory cytokines (IL-10 and transforming growth factor [TGF]-β). The microbial components stimulate ME to produce serum amyloid α, which stimulates DCs to activate other important mucosal Treg cells, Th17 cells that produce high amounts of IL-17A and IL-6 as well as moderate amounts of IL-22 and IFN-γ. The latter are critical for mucosal protection and repair as well as for defensin production (e.g. Reg-IIIg and Reg-IIIb).

While the information regarding rumen-associated lymphoid tissues is limited, rumen fluid leukocyte populations (including monocytes, T, and B cells) are likely to play a significant role in the regulation of cattle immune and

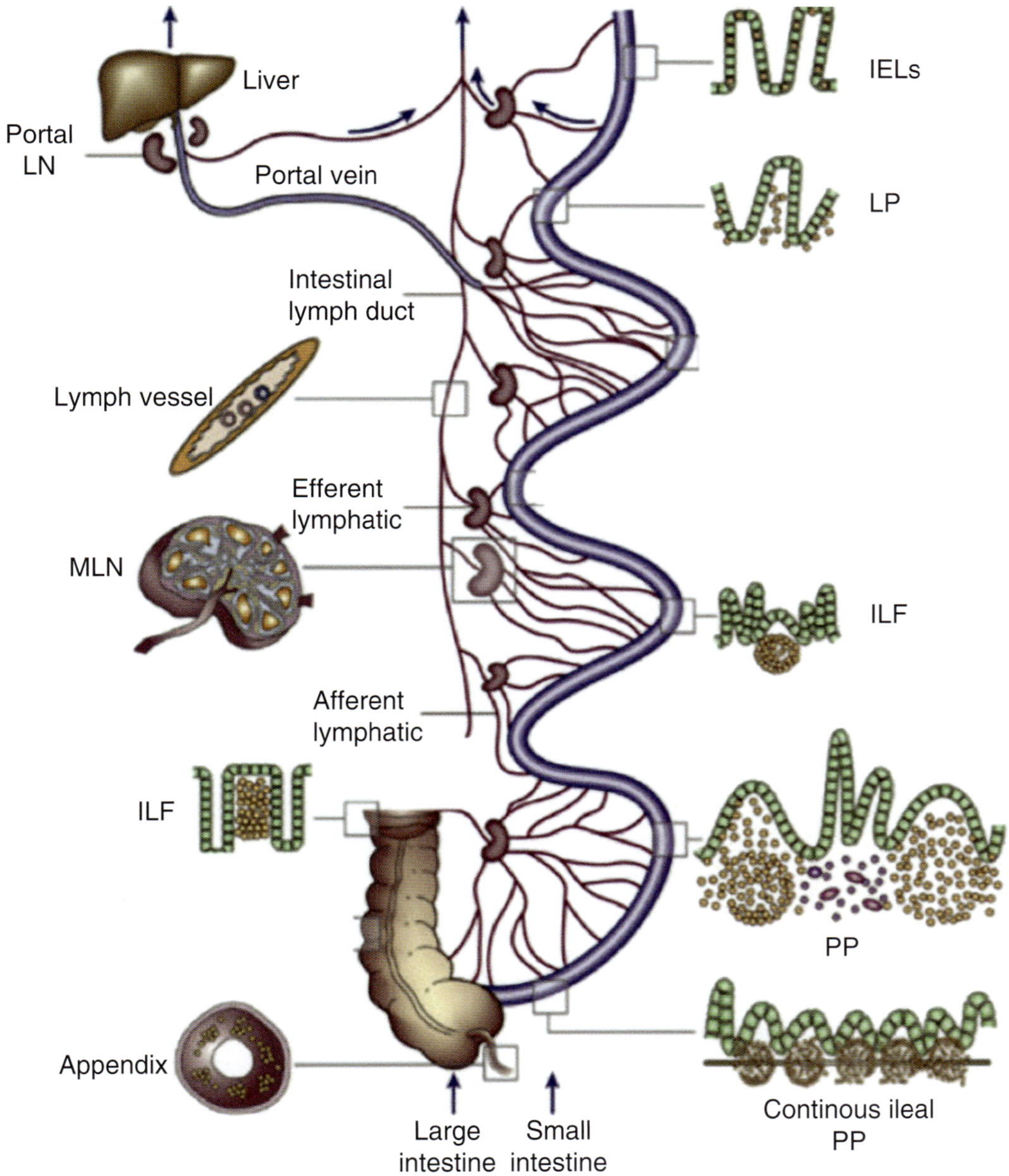

Figure 2.2 Gut immunology.

biochemical parameters. So, CD45 gene expression in rumen fluids (indicative of leukocyte infiltration) is negatively correlated with ruminal pH, while the frequencies of B cells (as well as total IgG and IgM numbers) are negatively affected by ruminal pH and high concentrations of volatile fatty acids. Additionally, rumen health disorders (e.g. subacute ruminal acidosis) were shown to cause ruminal dysbiosis, breaching the epithelial barrier and leading to inflammation (Xu, et al. 2022).

Organized MALT – the induction site of mucosal immunity – is widely distributed in mucosa throughout the body, which allows for antigen sampling from mucosal surfaces. It is composed of gut-associated lymphoid tissues (GALT), bronchus-associated lymphoid tissues (BALT), nasal (nasopharynx)-associated lymphoid tissues (NALT), and lymphoid tissues in the RepT, UT, mammary gland(s), lacrimal glands, and salivary glands. These lymphocyte aggregates or follicles [also known as lymphoid follicles (LF) or PP in the gut] of B cells, T cells, DCs, and macrophages antigen-presenting cells (APCs) are covered by specialized ECs called dome or M cells (found in BALT, GALT, and in the uterus). The GALT is the largest lymphoid organ and the largest body surface that comes in contact with a great diversity of food and microbial antigens. The M cells (present in MALT) pinocytose antigens and transport them across the ME where they are processed by APCs and presented to T and B lymphocytes. Then, antigen-stimulated mature T cells and B cells act together to produce IgA. Some of them express special molecules in their membranes (homing receptors) and leave the submucosal lymphoid tissue to enter the bloodstream; they can further exit the bloodstream through high endothelial venules and translocate to LP. Ultimately, this local stimulation results in memory T and B cells that can migrate to nearby and distant mucosal and other tissues, which is known as the "common mucosal immune system." A part of this "common mucosal immune system" – the bovine entero-mammary link (or gut-mammary axis) is critical for neonatal calf survival and health. This endogenous entero-mammary pathway not only allows lymphocytes to traffic to the mammary gland but also transports some bacterial components during lactation in the cow (2023).

2.4.4 Systemic Immunity

While the mucosal immune responses are more important for the clearance of most pathogens (especially enteric and respiratory), for a number of viral and bacterial agents associated with systemic, chronic, or lymphoid organ infections, protective immunity and pathogen clearance are unachievable without a robust systemic immune response (Smith et al. 2021).

These pathogens include (but are not limited to): *Staphylococcus aureus*, FMDV, BRSV, *Haemophilus somnus*, and *M. bovis*. Studies of immune responses to these pathogens have identified some commonalities as well as distinct systemic responses. IgG1 and IgG2 Ab responses are predominant in serum, in contrast to IgA in various mucosa, as well as potent and balanced $CD4^{+}$ and $CD8^{+}$ T-cell and IFN type-I responses in systemic immune organs and blood, were associated with improved protection. Another pathogen common in cattle, *Leptospira interrogans,* enters the hosts through chafed skin or mucosa and is then disseminated through the blood, potentially leading to renal infection. At disease onset, symptoms are nonspecific, which leads to it being underdiagnosed and poorly controlled by vaccines. Intraperitoneal priming with a TLR-2/NOD-2 (nucleotide oligomerization domain 2) agonist was shown to induce a sustained, protective, systemic innate immune response characterized by enhanced pro-inflammatory cytokine, chemokine, and nitric oxide production by macrophages independent of B and T cells. While most recent data suggest the importance of the systemic immune responses in some infections, it is also evident that tissue-specific immune responses may play important roles specific to each pathogen that require further evaluation (Rahman et al. 2020).

2.4.5 Immune System and Nutrition

Dairy cow nutritional status and the metabolism of specific nutrients are critical for adequate immune and other cell functions (Figure 2.3). The effects of nutrition may be direct through nutrients or indirect via metabolites. A majority of health problems in dairy cattle occur around parturition due to the hormonal shifts and the need for adaptation to the increased nutrient demands of lactation, which results in a negative energy balance (NEB). Diet-associated uncontrolled inflammation is considered a major contributing factor to several metabolic diseases common in dairy cattle, including mastitis, retained placentas, metritis, displaced abomasa, and ketosis. Previous studies demonstrated that over- or undernourished cows were more susceptible to various infectious diseases compared to those with adequate nutritional status in the periparturient period. Somewhat conflicting evidence of the associations between transient dietary restrictions, neutrophil function reduction, and various inflammatory diseases in postpartum dairy cows is discussed by Sordillo. The provision of appropriate antioxidants including ω-3 PUFA, conjugated linoleic acid, and vitamin D promotes anti-inflammatory responses (Alghamdi et al. 2022). Deficiencies in certain micronutrients (vitamins and trace elements) are associated with an increased incidence of mastitis, retained placentas, and metritis. The immunomodulatory and antioxidant effects of various macro- and micronutrients influence the incidence of health disorders in dairy cattle. These immunological and metabolic disturbances in lactating cows and dairy calf feeding practices may result in suboptimal nutrition and immune protection of neonatal calves (Lal et al. 2022).

2.5 Nutrition and the Immune System

Nutrition plays a pivotal role in the immune response, and nutrients can influence several, if not all, aspects of the immune response. This section discusses the complex relationships between metabolic status and immune function as well as how these complex interactions increase the risk of disease during early lactation (Kang et al. 2021). A special

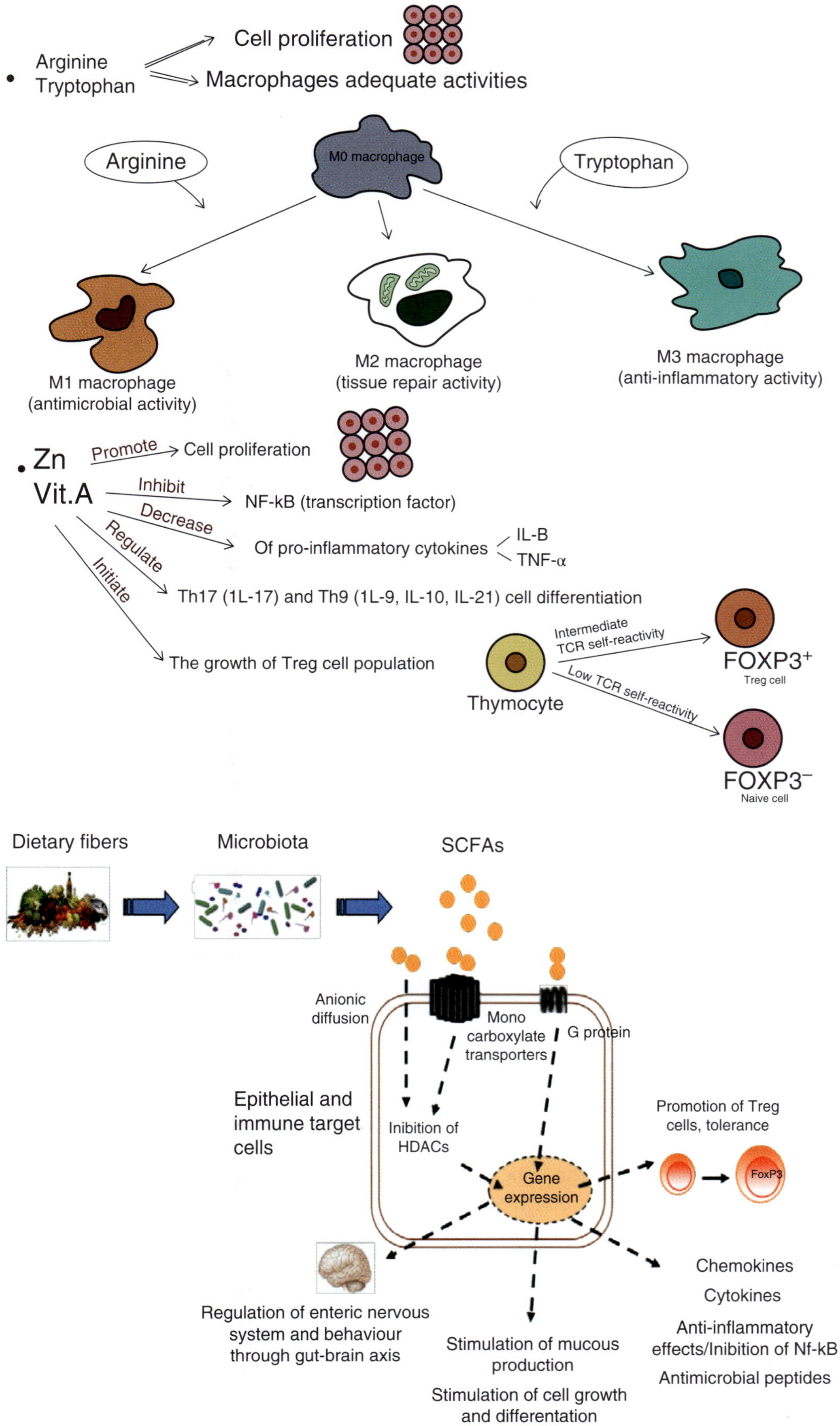

Figure 2.3 Immune system and nutrition.

focus will be placed on the major energetic fuels currently known to be used by immune cells (i.e. glucose, NEFA, BHBA, and glutamine [Gln]) and how certain metabolic states, such as PI or the degree of NEB, contribute to immunosuppression during the periparturient period. Gln, ketone bodies, fatty acids, glucose, and energy balance have an effect on the immune function of leukocytes, for example PMNs, macrophages, and lymphocytes. First, we will review the current literature regarding nutrient uptake and utilization by immune cells to better understand the mechanisms that relate nutrition and immunity (Bisinotto et al. 2018). To our knowledge, the metabolism and fates of energetic fuels in bovine leukocytes have not been characterized and most studies have used human, murine, or rodent models. Studies of the fuel use of ^{14}C-labeled glucose, amino acids, fatty acids and ketones by activated murine macrophages and PMNs have indicated that: (i) only 5% of glucose is completely oxidized via the Krebs cycle, and the rest is either directed toward the pentose phosphate pathway for the generation of NADPH as an electron donor during respiratory burst or is converted to lactate; (ii) Gln is the preferred amino acid utilized by phagocytes, with 74% of Gln being completely oxidized; (iii) fatty acids are primarily incorporated into cellular lipids that include triacylglycerols (79%), phospholipids (18%), and cholesterol esters (3%); and (iv) ketone bodies, such as acetoacetate and BHBA, are not utilized as an energy source by phagocytes (Wagner et al. 2023).

2.5.1 Glutamine (Gln)

Glutamine is considered a functional amino acid due to its multiple roles in various physiological processes. It serves as a precursor for several essential functions:

- **DNA and RNA synthesis:** Gln contributes to the synthesis of purines and pyrimidines, which are building blocks for DNA and RNA, making it vital for genetic material production.
- **NADPH production:** Gln is involved in generating NADPH, which is necessary for the production of superoxide by phagocytes, a crucial component of the immune response.
- **Energy production:** Gln can be oxidized to provide energy, which supports various cellular processes.
- **Nitric oxide generation:** Macrophages utilize Gln to produce nitric oxide, a signaling molecule important in immune responses.

In rodent and human models, Gln plays a significant role in the synthesis of cytokines like IL-1b and IL-6 in macrophages and monocytes as well as in processes such as phagocytosis and the production of reactive oxygen intermediates. Lymphocytes primarily use Gln for cell division and lactate production. Notably, lymphocytes have a high rate of Gln utilization that often exceeds requirements by more than 100-fold due to their rapid cell division, which is not observed in terminally differentiated cells like PMNs and macrophages. During infections, the plasma concentration of Gln decreases because it is taken up and utilized by immunological tissues and cells. Similarly, during the periparturient period in cows, plasma Gln levels also decrease, driven by the substantial metabolic demands for Gln in processes like gluconeogenesis, milk protein synthesis, and tissue growth, particularly in the intestine and mammary gland. Increasing the circulating supply of Gln to periparturient cows may have potential benefits of enhancing immune function and reducing the risk of mastitis during early lactation. Abomasal infusions of Gln during the first 21 days of milk production have been shown to elevate plasma Gln levels and increase the abundance of $CD4^+$ T cells. However, this treatment did not significantly impact T lymphocyte proliferation, the abundance of $CD8^+$ T cells, or the secretion of IFN-γ. To better understand the effects of an increased supply of circulating Gln on the immune response, further studies are needed. These studies could lead to the development of new management strategies aimed at improving the immune response and reducing the risk of mastitis in cows during the early lactation phase.

2.5.2 Glucose

Glucose is required by phagocytic cells (i.e. macrophages and PMNs) for proliferation, survival, and differentiation, and glucose is the preferred metabolic fuel during inflammation for activated PMNs, macrophages, and lymphocytes rather than fatty acids, amino acids, or ketone bodies (Ingvartsen and Moyes 2013). For example, the glucose uptake in murine PMNs and peritoneal macrophages increased after stimulation with LPS in vitro (Cortellino and Longo 2023). Studies have shown that the inhibition of glucose uptake decreased phagocytic capabilities and increased the risk of infection in murine macrophages. The cellular uptake of glucose in phagocytic cells is facilitated via the noninsulin dependent glucose transporter and evidence indicates that the glucose uptake may be restricted solely to the GLUT1 (glucose transporter 1) isoform in phagocytes. Interestingly, Moyes et al. (2009) observed that an intramammary challenge with *Streptococcus uberis* did not alter dry matter intake in cows during mid-lactation, whereas serum insulin and glucose concentrations increased after the challenge. Increases in serum glucose after intramammary infection may be associated with either enhanced hepatic gluconeogenesis or reduced uptake of glucose by peripheral tissues, thereby increasing the glucose availability for phagocytic cells during infection. An efficient glucose uptake by immune cells is critical for maintaining cellular functions and eliciting an optimal host response against invading microorganisms. Like Gln, serum glucose concentrations are lowest in cows during early lactation, and low glucose availability may limit the immune function and increase the risk of infection for cows during early lactation (Gross 2023).

2.5.3 Ketones

Cows experiencing subclinical ketosis (with BHBA levels exceeding 1000 or 1200 mmol/l) in the first 1 to 2 weeks after calving face a higher risk of diseases such as metritis (as noted by Zhang et al. 2023) and an increased occurrence and severity of mastitis. Numerous studies have identified potential mechanisms linked to the impairment of cellular immune function due to elevated ketone concentrations in the bloodstream (Titlestad et al. 2023). These mechanisms include a reduction in chemotactic capabilities and respiratory burst activity in bovine blood PMNs when supplemented with BHBA in vitro. Additionally, Sartorelli et al. (1999) observed an inhibition of superoxide anion production in bovine PMNs, with minimal effects from acetoacetate, which suggests that only the ketone body BHBA may hinder immune function during the transition and postpartum periods. This inhibitory effect of BHBA may be partly attributed to the fact that leukocyte migration relies on glucose, and these cells cannot utilize ketones as an additional energy source.

Concerning specific immunity, in vitro studies have demonstrated that BHBA incubation reduces blastogenesis, mitogenic responses, and inhibits IgM secretion and proliferation in bovine blood lymphocytes. Therefore, higher circulating BHBA levels in cows experiencing subclinical or clinical ketosis may compromise immune function and increase the risk of mastitis and other infectious diseases during early lactation.

Elevated circulating NEFA concentrations in cows during the periparturient period have been associated with an increased risk of diseases such as hepatic lipidosis, left displacement of the abomasum, retained placentas, and mastitis. The effects of NEFA on immune function, particularly saturated (SFA), unsaturated (UFA), and polyunsaturated (PUFA) fatty acids, are complex and not well understood. NEFA can have both immunostimulatory and immunosuppressive effects on cellular function and may act as ligands for TLRs, primarily on resident macrophages.

In cows, Lacetera et al. (2004) reported that higher NEFA concentrations (1.0 mM) suppressed DNA synthesis, IgM secretion, and IFN-γ production in blood monocytes when compared to lower NEFA concentrations in vitro (0.0625 and 0.125 mM). Several studies have also shown that NEFAs alter the oxidative burst, apoptosis, and necrosis of PMNs and macrophages in vitro, which potentially leads to cell and tissue damage during early lactation. The type of NEFA, whether SFA, UFA, or PUFA, has been shown to affect the immune response, with SFAs decreasing macrophage phagocytic capability and PUFAs inhibiting antigen presentation to lymphocytes, among other effects.

However, some studies have reported immunostimulatory effects of NEFA. For instance, UFAs have been shown to increase macrophage phagocytosis, and eicosapentaenoic acid (EPA) and docosahexaenoic acid (DHA; n-3 PUFA) can enhance the production of certain cytokines and lymphocyte proliferation in vitro. The specific NEFA profile in circulation may have varying effects on immune cell function. The relationship between NEFAs and the immune response is not fully understood and more research is needed.

Energy balance plays a crucial role in these interactions. Research has explored the relationship between individual metabolites that characterize NEB (NEFA, BHBA, and glucose) and postpartum immunosuppression in vitro. However, most in vivo studies have focused on the effects of individual metabolites associated with severe NEB rather than energy balance alone.

Dietary-induced NEB models have been used to investigate the mechanisms that link energy status with immune function during early lactation. These models, often employed in later lactation cows, may not accurately represent the more severe NEB observed during early lactation. Large-scale epidemiological studies provide stronger evidence of the links between the circulating metabolites that characterize NEB and the immune response, particularly mastitis risk, in dairy cows during the peripartum period. Indices based on multiple blood metabolites may better predict disease risk than calculated energy balance or individual metabolites.

Recent advances in immunology, functional genomics, proteomics, and metabolomics have shed light on the mechanistic links between metabolic status, an NEB, and the immune response. However, these relationships remain complex and require further investigation to develop effective management practices for cows during the transition period.

2.6 Conclusion

A majority of health problems in the dairy cow occur around parturition and relate to the difficulty adapting to the nutritional needs for lactation. Complex relationships between metabolic status and immune function exist and potentially influence the risk of disease. Physiological parameters show major individual differences, and some cows experience PI in the periparturient period as a consequence of inadequate adaptation to lactation. This imbalance may decrease immune function and increase the risk for disease as metabolites and nutrients, for example, Gln, glucose, BHBA, and NEFAs, can influence several important aspects of the immune response and potentially disease resistance. It is argued that implementing feeding strategies to avoid PI may improve the immune response and thereby disease resistance and health.

References

Alghamdi, M., Gutierrez, J., and Komarnytsky, S. (2022). Essential minerals and metabolic adaptation of immune cells. *Nutrients* 15 (1): 123.

Allen, M.S., Bradford, B.J., and Oba, M. (2009). Board-invited review: The hepatic oxidation theory of the control of feed intake and its application to ruminants. *Journal of animal science* 87 (10): 3317–3334.

Bisinotto, R.S., Greco, L.F., Ribeiro, E.S. et al. (2018). Influences of nutrition and metabolism on fertility of dairy cows. *Animal Reproduction (AR)* 9 (3): 260–272.

Bórawski, P., Pawlewicz, A., Parzonko, A. et al. (2020). Factors shaping cow's milk production in the EU. *Sustainability* 12 (1): 420.

Chase, C.C. (2022). Acceptable young calf vaccination strategies – what, when, and how? *Veterinary Clinics: Food Animal Practice* 38 (1): 17–37.

Cortellino, S. and Longo, V.D. (2023). Metabolites and immune response in tumor microenvironments. *Cancers* 15 (15): 3898.

Drackley, J.K., Donkin, S.S., and Reynolds, C.K. (2006). Major advances in fundamental dairy cattle nutrition. *Journal of Dairy Science* 89 (4): 1324–1336.

Dyall, S.C., Balas, L., Bazan, N.G. et al. (2022). Polyunsaturated fatty acids and fatty acid-derived lipid mediators: recent advances in the understanding of their biosynthesis, structures, and functions. *Progress in Lipid Research* 86: 101165.

Gross, J.J. (2022). Limiting factors for milk production in dairy cows: perspectives from physiology and nutrition. *Journal of Animal Science* 100 (3): skac044.

Gross, J.J. (2023). Dairy cow physiology and production limits. *Animal Frontiers: The Review Magazine of Animal Agriculture* 13 (3): 44.

Hansen, J.V., Friggens, N.C., and Højsgaard, S. (2006). The influence of breed and parity on milk yield, and milk yield acceleration curves. *Livestock Science* 104 (1–2): 53–62.

Ingvartsen, K.L. (2006). Feeding-and management-related diseases in the transition cow: Physiological adaptations around calving and strategies to reduce feeding-related diseases. *Animal feed science and technology* 126 (3–4): 175–213.

Ingvartsen, K.L. and Andersen, J.B. (2000). Integration of metabolism and intake regulation: a review focusing on periparturient animals. *Journal of dairy science* 83 (7): 1573–1597.

Ingvartsen, K.L. and Boisclair, Y.R. (2001). Leptin and the regulation of food intake, energy homeostasis and immunity with special focus on periparturient ruminants. *Domestic Animal Endocrinology* 21 (4): 215–250.

Ingvartsen, K.L. and Moyes, K. (2013). Nutrition, immune function and health of dairy cattle. *Animal* 7 (s1): 112–122.

Ingvartsen, K.L., Dewhurst, R.J., and Friggens, N.C. (2003). On the relationship between lactational performance and health: is it yield or metabolic imbalance that cause production diseases in dairy cattle? *A position paper. Livestock production science* 83 (2-3): 277–308.

Jansik, C. and Irz, X. (2015). Competitiveness of dairy farms in northern Europe: a cross-country analysis. *Agricultural and Food Science* 24 (3): 206–218.

Kang, C.M., Chiang, B.L., and Wang, L.C. (2021). Maternal nutritional status and development of atopic dermatitis in their offspring. *Clinical Reviews in Allergy & Immunology* 61: 128–155.

Kehrli, M.E., Neill, J.D., Burvenich, C. et al. (2006). Energy and protein effects on the immune system. Ruminant physiology. In: *Digestion, Metabolism and Impact of Nutrition on Gene Expression, Immunology and Stress*, 455–471.

Kelly, P., Shalloo, L., Wallace, M., and Dillon, P. (2020). The Irish dairy industry – recent history and strategy, current state and future challenges. *International Journal of Dairy Technology* 73 (2): 309–323.

Lacetera, N., Cockburn, I.M., and Henderson, R. (2004). Do firms change capabilities by hiring new people? A study of the adoption of science-based drug discovery. In: *Business Strategy Over the Industry Lifecycle*, 133–159. Emerald Group Publishing Limited.

Lal, M.K., Sharma, E., Tiwari, R.K. et al. (2022). Nutrient-mediated perception and signalling in human metabolism: a perspective of nutrigenomics. *International Journal of Molecular Sciences* 23 (19): 11305.

LeBlanc, S.J., Lissemore, K.D., Kelton, D.F. et al. (2006). Major advances in disease prevention in dairy cattle. *Journal of Dairy Science* 89 (4): 1267–1279.

Mohanraju, P., Saha, C., van Baarlen, P. et al. (2022). Alternative functions of CRISPR–Cas systems in the evolutionary arms race. *Nature Reviews Microbiology* 20 (6): 351–364.

Moyes, L.H., Leitch, E.F., McKee, R.F. et al. (2009). Preoperative systemic inflammation predicts postoperative infectious complications in patients undergoing curative resection for colorectal cancer. *British journal of cancer* 100 (8): 1236–1239.

Mukherjee, J., Das, P.K., and Banerjee, D. (2023). Lactation physiology. In: *Textbook of Veterinary Physiology* (ed. P.K. Das, V. Sejian, J. Mukherjee, and D. Banerjee), 639–674. Singapore: Springer Nature Singapore.

Mukhopadhyay, C.S., Choudhary, R.K., Panwar, H., and Malik, Y.S. (ed.) (2023). *Biotechnological Interventions Augmenting Livestock Health and Production*. Springer Nature.

Mulligan, F.J. and Doherty, M.L. (2008). Production diseases of the transition cow. *The Veterinary Journal* 176 (1): 3–9.

Parija, S.C. (2023). Immune response. In: *Textbook of Microbiology and Immunology*, 211–226. Singapore: Springer Nature Singapore.

Paura, L., Berzina, L., Degola, L. et al. (2023). Trends in milk yield productivity and emissions from the dairy sector in Latvia. *Agronomy Research* 20: https://doi.org/10.15159/ar.23.047.

Pezeshki, A., Capuco, A.V., De Spiegeleer, B. et al. (2010). An integrated view on how the management of the dry period length of lactating cows could affect mammary biology and defence. *Journal of animal physiology and animal nutrition* 94 (5): e7–e30.

Ponnampalam, E.N., Kiani, A., Santhiravel, S. et al. (2022). The importance of dietary antioxidants on oxidative stress, meat and milk production, and their preservative aspects in farm animals: antioxidant action, animal health, and product quality – invited review. *Animals* 12 (23): 3279.

Rahman, M.T., Sobur, M.A., Islam, M.S. et al. (2020). Zoonotic diseases: etiology, impact, and control. *Microorganisms* 8 (9): 1405. https://doi.org/10.3390/microorganisms8091405. PMID: 32932606; PMCID: PMC7563794.

Rico, D.E. and Razzaghi, A. (2023). Animal board invited review: the contribution of adipose stores to milk fat: implications on optimal nutritional strategies to increase milk fat synthesis in dairy cows. *Animal* 17 (4): 100735. https://doi.org/10.1016/j.animal.2023.100735.

Sanders, A.E., Weatherspoon, E.D., Ehrmann, B.M. et al. (2022). Circulating Omega-6 and Omega-3 polyunsaturated fatty acids in painful temporomandibular disorder and low back pain. *The Journal of Pain* 23 (10): 1724–1736.

Sartorelli, V., Puri, P.L., Hamamori, Y. et al. (1999). Acetylation of MyoD directed by PCAF is necessary for the execution of the muscle program. *Molecular cell* 4 (5): 725–734.

Smith, N., Goncalves, P., Charbit, B. et al. (2021). Distinct systemic and mucosal immune responses during acute SARS-CoV-2 infection. *Nature Immunology* 22: 1428–1439. https://doi.org/10.1038/s41590-021-01028-7.

Titlestad, I., Watne, L.O., Caplan, G.A. et al. (2023). Impaired glucose utilization in the brain of patients with delirium following hip fracture. *Brain* awad296. https://doi.org/10.1093/brain/awad296.

Tufail, T., Rasheed, Y., Ain, H.B.U. et al. (2023). A review of current evidence on food allergies during pregnancy. *Food Science & Nutrition* 11 (8): 4432–4443.

Upadhyay, R.K. (2023). Mucosal membranes, their interactions to microbial infections and immune susceptibility in human hosts. *European Journal of Biological Research* 13 (1): 41–70.

Vangroenweghe, F., Lamote, I., and Burvenich, C. (2005). Physiology of the periparturient period and its relation to severity of clinical mastitis. *Domestic animal endocrinology* 29 (2): 283–293.

Wagner, L.A., Fritsche, D., Gross, J.J. et al. (2023). Effects of different nutrient supply on metabolism and mammary immune response to an LPS challenge in early lactation of dairy cows. *Journal of Dairy Science* 106 (4): 2948–2962.

Xu, R., Shandilya, U.K., Yiannikouris, A., and Karrow, N.A. (2022). Ochratoxin A and citrinin differentially modulate bovine mammary epithelial cell permeability and innate immune function. *Toxins* 14 (9): 640.

Zhang, M.Q., Heirbaut, S., Jing, X.P. et al. (2023). Transition cow clusters with distinctive antioxidant ability and their relation to performance and metabolic status in early lactation. *Journal of Dairy Science* 106 (8): 5723–5739.

3

Metabolic Profile Tests

Ankit S. Prajapati[1], *Abhinav Suthar*[2], *Prakash M. Chauhan*[2], *and Harshad H. Panchasara*[3]

[1] Veterinary Clinical Complex (Medicine), College of Veterinary Science and Animal Husbandry, Kamdhenu University, Sardarkrushinagar, Gujarat, India
[2] Department of Veterinary Clinics, College of Veterinary Science and Animal Husbandry, Kamdhenu University, Sardarkrushinagar, Gujarat, India
[3] Livestock Research Station, College of Veterinary Science and Animal Husbandry, Kamdhenu University, Sardarkrushinagar, Gujarat, India

3.1 Introduction

Cattle are the backbone of livestock farming and one of the most commonly reared animals for several reasons. Many conditions affect their health, production, and reproduction efficiency throughout life. Metabolic diseases are one of the most critical conditions responsible for reducing milk production (Prajapati et al. 2023). The rural dairy and meat industry thrives on healthy and productive livestock, which is, in turn, responsible for self-employment, the empowerment of women, and a sustainable rural economy, apart from providing food and nutritional security to society at large. The combined stress of high production and modern intensive husbandry has markedly increased the incidence of production diseases in dairy animals. Production-associated diseases cause a significant dent in the dairy sector's economy, and the clinical diagnosis and therapeutic management of metabolic and deficiency diseases are tedious for veterinary clinicians.

Moreover, metabolic disorders are neglected in veterinary medicine textbooks. Over the past several decades, livestock has undergone an intensive genetic selection, and modern husbandry practices augment productivity at a level where multiple metabolic systems are broken. Production diseases are now considered the gateway of most livestock disease. Hence, the definition of production disease has expanded to include metabolic and nutritional diseases as well as diseases of an infectious or genetic nature. The metabolic profile test is intended to provide a balance between "input," in terms of nutrients absorbed from the gastrointestinal tract, and "output," in terms of the nutritional requirements to maintain pregnancy and lactation.

3.2 Metabolic Profile

Metabolic profile testing is an excellent tool for detecting the most common early lactation disorders. The term "metabolic profile" refers to the analysis of milk and blood biochemical parameters to assess and prevent metabolic and nutritional disorders in dairy herds (Kuczynska et al. 2021). The metabolic profiling of particular animals and herds is currently needed in the diagnostic process for screening and supporting the herd disease process (Bhadauria et al. 2020). The Compton metabolic profile test (CMPT) was designed by Payne et al. (1970) to monitor the metabolic health of the herd. The CMPT is a traditional approach for the metabolic profiling of representative samples from the herd. The main objective of the CMPT is to indicate whether a herd is sensitive to production disease (Rowlands and Manston 1976). The CMPT can indicate the primary cause in herds with a high incidence of production diseases (Payne et al. 1970). The test was designed to monitor the metabolic health of cows in dairy herds in relation to farming, nutrition, milk production, and disease incidence as well as to assist in diagnosing metabolic problems. To overcome this problem, the mini Compton metabolic profile (MCMP) was developed by Blowey (1972). The MCMP is a modified test that measures fewer parameters to evaluate the health status of a herd. The cost of the test is also lower (Blowey 1975). Blood metabolites have a direct impact on the milk

Periparturient Diseases of Cattle, First Edition. Edited by Tanmoy Rana.

production of dairy animals. The assessment is conducted to evaluate the adequacy of protein and energy intake as well as optimize nutrition for maximum production (Blowey et al. 1973).

The periparturient period, particularly the postpartum period, is the most vulnerable period for metabolic sicknesses in dairy cattle. About 75% of the diseases in dairy cows classically occur within the first month after calving (LeBlanc et al. 2006). The periparturient period, or transition period, generally extends from 3 weeks before parturition through 3 weeks after parturition (Aleri et al. 2016). The imbalance between dietary input and production output is the precipitating factor. The conversion of nutrients into milk depends on the capacity of the animals, i.e. throughput. When significant changes occur in the throughput, it gives rise to production diseases. The urge to obtain more milk in the form of production without considering the individual's health status often causes production-related metabolic disorders. A balanced ration and an ideal management system prevent such conditions in the dairy herd.

A metabolic profile is a series of specific analytic tests run in combination and used as a diagnostic aid (Puppel and Kuczynska 2016). The traditional approach to metabolic profiling was the CMPT, in which a representative sampling of individuals was collected and analyses performed. With the CMPT, a mean value for an individual was determined and compared to some reference value. The problem with this approach is the cost and a lack of sensitivity. In the CMPT, seven animals are considered the minimum sample size from three predefined groups of dairy animals, i.e. dry (30 days before calving), early lactation (between 10 and 20 days of lactation), and mid-lactation (50–120 days of lactation) for a statistically significant interpretation (Figure 3.1). Cows should be selected randomly but within the typical stage of lactation. Cows with extreme performance should be avoided. Cows with other abnormal conditions should also not be included in the test because it affects the interpretation of the test.

Sample collection and handling are essential to expect fruitful diagnostic information. The jugular or coccygeal vein is preferred to collect blood with minimal stress. Vacuum tubes are commonly selected for blood collection, and the chances of contamination are also lower. Blood samples from the mammary gland are not appropriate due to the loss of nutrients in the mammary gland. Blood glucose, hemoglobin, packed cell volume (PCV), and blood urea nitrogen should be analyzed from the blood. From serum, phosphorus, calcium, magnesium, potassium, sodium, copper, iron, total protein, and albumin should be estimated. These values correctly diagnosed malnutrition as the cause of periparturient diseases (Kida 2002). In contrast, the MCMP estimates the PCV, hemoglobin, red blood cells (RBCs), white blood cells (WBCs), albumin, glucose, and blood urea nitrogen (Prajapati et al. 2023).

The sampling time relative to feeding and feeding management may also influence the metabolite concentration. As the diet of a ruminant changes, the characteristics of rumen activity require changes. Blood samples for metabolic profiles should not be collected until 2 weeks after a major change in activity and the animals have had time to adapt. Minor changes, such as an increase in the quantity of an existing component, do not require a wait longer than 7–10 days. There can be changes in blood biochemical values associated with feeding. These are most noticeable in cows that receive their entire concentrate ration at milking time. In such cases, wait 2 hours after milking before taking a blood sample. In circumstances where most of the concentrated input is mixed with the forage and is available for most of a 24-hour day, the timing of tests in relation to feeding is less critical.

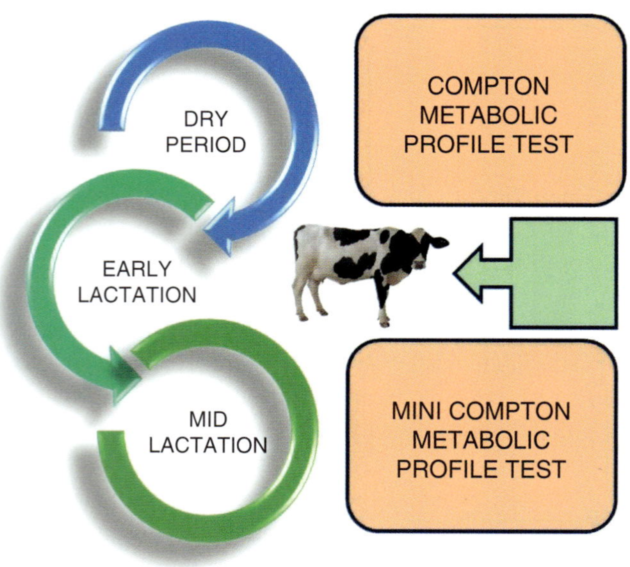

Figure 3.1 Schematic diagram of metabolic profiling in cattle. *Source:* Ankit Prajapati.

The primary components of any feed are carbohydrates, protein, and fat. These are required for the normal physiological function of the body. Carbohydrates are the main basis of energy for animals. Energy balance is a crucial nutritional factor that impacts animal health, lactation, and reproductive performance.

Glucose is a universal fuel for cellular energy metabolism and biological synthesis pathways in animals (Cankaya et al. 2007). In dairy cattle, dietary carbohydrates provide a significant energy source for maintenance, growth, and milk production. Animal cells require glucose for oxidative and nonoxidative adenosine triphosphate (ATP) production and for anabolic reactions that produce vital sugars (Noziere et al. 2010). Blood glucose has greater potential as an indicator of carbohydrate status and dietary starch content than as an energy balance indicator. Several factors, including stress, affect glucose metabolism during the periparturient period and reduce milk production (Wheelock et al. 2010) (Figure 3.2). In a negative energy balance state, non-esterified fatty acids (NEFAs) are produced and are considered a sensitive indicator for the energy status of dry cows in the last month of gestation (Hubner et al. 2022). Generally, circulating NEFAs are absorbed and metabolized for energy by the liver and other tissues. Higher NEFA production is associated with a higher risk of postpartum diseases, poorer reproductive performance, and lower milk production. After NEFA, β-hydroxybutyrate (BHBA) is the most commonly used parameter to measure the energy status (Prajapati et al. 2023). Other conditions, like placental retention, also interfere with NEFA and BHBA values (Nogalski et al. 2012). Serum glucose is an essential factor that modulates reproduction, and lower glucose levels are responsible for decreased fertility rates (Yadav et al. 1995).

Cows experiencing subclinical endometritis or puerperal metritis in the periparturient period had decreased dry matter intake with higher NEFA and BHBA levels, all indicators of a prolonged negative energy balance in the periparturient period (Huzzey et al. 2007; Sakowski et al. 2012).

Many hematologic changes are observed during the transition of reproductive stages. Immediately postpartum, there was increased production of RBCs above the reference limits. Blood tests for hemoglobin and RBCs are necessary during the peripartum period due to the changes that occur during this period and the increased incidence of diseases during this phase. In this sense, evaluating an erythrogram helps assess animal health, especially for detecting anemias of various etiologies. Drastic physiological changes, such as those that occur in the peripartum period, may significantly influence various hematologic measures (Paiano et al. 2020). A reduction in hemoglobin affects milk production as a whole and the overall health of cattle. Hemoglobin actively involves oxygen transportation, and a low level might interfere with a reduction in oxygen-carrying capacity, which ultimately invites other complications. Increased RBCs and hemoglobin concentration at parturition indicate hemoconcentration, which probably occurs because of increased physical effort during parturition and decreased water intake. These parameters are mostly neglected and not extensively documented.

A PCV (hematocrit) evaluates the proportion of blood composed of RBCs. This measurement indicates the viscosity or thickness of the blood, and it depends on the size and number of RBCs in a blood sample. The PCV is often evaluated as part of a complete blood count that includes measuring RBCs, WBCs, platelets, and hemoglobin (Turkson and Ganyo 2015). Blood and fluid loss during parturition affects and decreases the PCV level, which should be monitored by metabolic profiling (Pohler et al. 2020). An acute loss of 20–25% of the blood volume will result in marked clinical signs of anemia, including tachycardia and maniacal behavior. The PCV is only a helpful tool to monitor acute blood loss after intravascular equilibration with other fluid compartments. An acute, developing PCV of 15% or less may require a transfusion. Chronic anemia with a PCV of 7–12% can be tolerated without a transfusion if the animal is not stressed and no further decline in erythrocyte mass occurs (Hunt and Wood 1999).

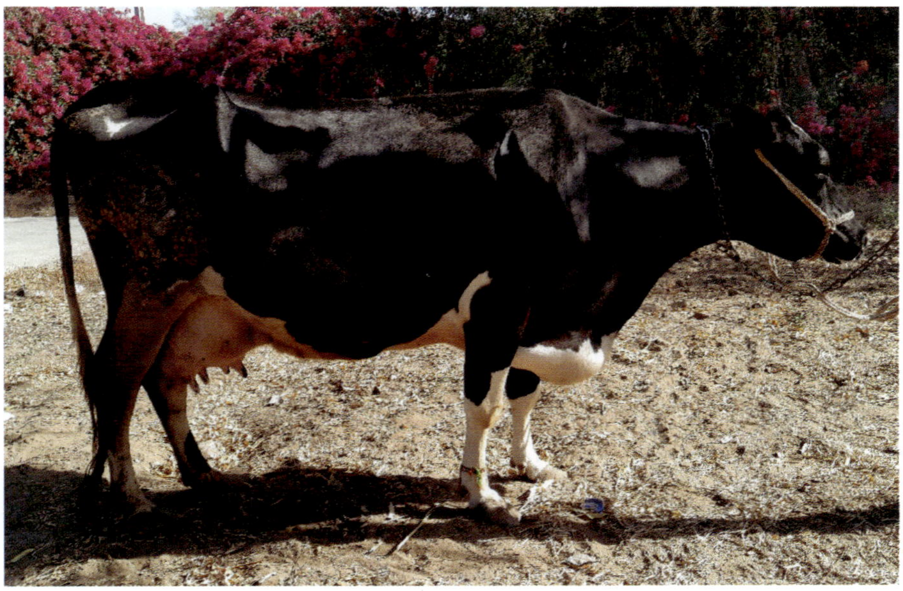

Figure 3.2 Cattle suffering from ketosis. *Source:* Ankit Prajapati.

Biochemical components play a significant role in the maintenance of normal physiology. Therefore, optimum blood biochemical components are essential for the normal function of the reproductive system as well as other systems in the body (Barson et al. 2019). Blood urea nitrogen reveals the functional status of kidneys in animals. Waste and toxic products are not filtered out in disturbed homeostasis and instead accumulate in the circulation. Increased nitrogenous waste products also interfere with the normal functioning of other organs and lead to a reduction in the health status of cattle.

Many parameters influence urea nitrogen concentrations, including dietary protein intake and rumen degradability, dietary amino acid composition, protein intake relative to requirements, liver and kidney function, and muscle tissue breakdown. Increased plasma urea concentrations indicate increased ammonia detoxification in the liver, whereas an increase in total blood protein concentrations indicates intestinal protein absorption (Law et al. 2009). The metabolic burden in liver function is often associated with abomasal displacements, ketosis, mastitis, parturient paresis, placental retention, and endometritis, often in postpartum cows (Andjelic et al. 2022).

Cattle need phosphorus for almost every vital body function including bone and muscle building, fat metabolization, milk production, and feed intake (Peterson et al. 2005). Phosphorus deficiency and hypophosphatemia are believed to be associated with muscle function disturbances in dairy cows, particularly around parturition (Grunberg et al. 2019). Hypophosphatemia is a condition caused by decreased phosphorus levels in the blood. Phosphorus also helps in the maintenance of calcium levels. Proper nutritional management during the dry period is required to prevent metabolic disorders during parturition and potentially increase milk yield during early lactation, especially during the heat of summer.

Calcium is a critical ion that plays a vital role in metabolic profiling. During the periparturient period, dairy cows suffer marked immune suppression and moderate to severe hypocalcemia. Around the parturition period, the demands for calcium increase; these increased demands can result in subclinical or clinical hypocalcemia (Figure 3.3). Periparturient cows also experience significant immune suppression (Kimura et al. 2006). Calcium estimation is crucial for estimating the level at and around the lactation period. The differing metabolites in cows with milk fever reflect the pathological features of a negative energy balance and fat mobilization, which suggests that milk fever is associated with altered energy metabolism (Sun et al. 2014). Calcium levels decrease in blood and cytosol during calving, which limits nerve impulse transmission, muscle contraction, and immune cell activity. In the nervous system, calcium participates in the conduction of stimuli. The muscular system decreases contractions, which causes alterations in the smooth muscle, uterus, and mammary glands. In the uterus, uterine fluids and waste are retained with bacterial complications. In the immune system, the function of neutrophils is essential, and it manifests as a decrease in cells engaged in phagocytosis, which predisposes the animal to mastitis and metritis.

Magnesium is a mineral that is an essential cofactor for more than 300 enzymes. Magnesium supplementation in farm animals and human nutrition is recommended to avoid deficiency and ensure adequate growth and health maintenance. Magnesium supplementation above the estimated minimum requirements is the best practice to improve farm animals'

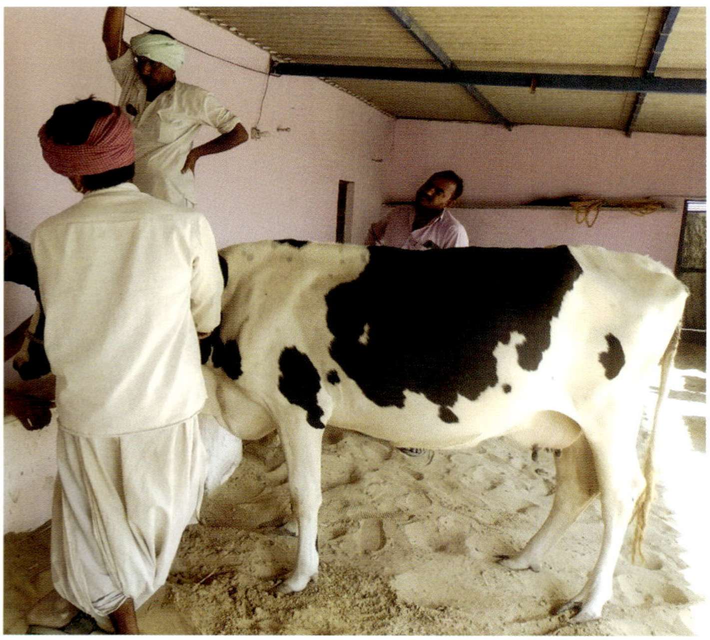

Figure 3.3 Cattle suffering from hypocalcemia. *Source:* Ankit Prajapati.

performances and food product quality since the enactment of farm animals has grown in recent decades (Pinotti et al. 2021). Magnesium supplementation remarkably improves feed digestibility and reproduction and shortens the service period (Gaal et al. 2004). An insufficient absorption of magnesium in ruminants leads to magnesium deficiency, which manifests in clinical signs such as tetany or paresis (Schonewille 2013). Magnesium absorption decreases after parturition, so that must be compensated for by providing it in adequate amounts (Schonewille et al. 2008).

Potassium is essential for animal life. Potassium is involved in many body functions and is required for proper muscle development. Adequate potassium is also crucial for good heart function. The recommended daily allowance of potassium varies depending on the species, stage of growth, and levels of other dietary minerals (West et al. 1987).

Sodium is an essential element for animals. Dairy cows routinely expel sodium from the body in urine, feces, saliva, and milk, which must be replaced. Maintaining an animal's water balance as well as nerve and muscle function is essential. Polyuria, polydipsia, salt hunger, pica, weight loss, and decreased milk production are clinical signs of cattle with low sodium levels (Whitlock et al. 1975). Sodium intoxication in cattle affects the gastrointestinal and central nervous systems. Reported clinical symptoms include diarrhea, anorexia, abdominal pain, excitement, ataxia, tremors, seizures, recumbency, opisthotonos, coma, and death (Romano et al. 2021).

Copper, an essential trace element for animals, is a required cofactor for hundreds of enzymatic reactions involved in RBC production, energy manufacturing, hormone formation, collagen synthesis, and protection against oxidative damage (Lopez-Alonso and Miranda 2020). Copper supplementation in ruminants deserves special attention because of the narrow margin between deficiency and toxicity, which ruminants are susceptible to.

Iron is one of the critical micronutrients in the bodies of cattle. The largest amounts of iron in the body are incorporated into proteins, mainly hemoglobin and myoglobin. This element participates in several biochemical processes, including blood production, oxygen transport, energy metabolism, and immune functions. Iron deficiency can result in so-called iron-deficiency anemia, mostly in young calves, due to low iron content in the dam's milk and the high demand for this element by calves (Wysocka et al. 2020).

Protein is involved in many processes in cattle and is required for muscle development (Alberghina et al. 2011). Immunity against different agents is also formed against protein parts. Albumin is a negative acute phase protein (APP), and its concentration falls gradually during infectious and inflammatory diseases (Kaneko et al. 2008). The functions of APPs are varied but generally relate to the defense of the animal from pathological damage and the restoration of homeostasis; the level of APPs rises in response to inflammation and is associated with fatty liver in dairy cows (Katoh and Nakagawa 1999). Serum albumin levels have been shown to decrease as the severity of fatty liver increases; however, serum levels alone are not an adequate diagnostic tool as albumin may be impacted by inflammation of the liver and other causes of liver disease (Lager and Jordan 2012). Albumin was found to be associated with postpartum disease and can be used to predict disease risk in closeup and fresh periods. The total protein and albumin concentrations at puerperium were significantly lower compared with the dry period and at day 60 of lactation (Prodanovic et al. 2012).

Different parameters surrounding the periparturient period need to be evaluated to know their status inside the body, and mean values can predict the herd's health. Metabolic profiling can help increase the profit from cattle farming.

References

Alberghina, D., Giannetto, C., Vazzana, I. et al. (2011). Reference intervals for total protein concentration, serum protein fractions, and albumin/globulin ratios in clinically healthy dairy cows. *Journal of Veterinary Diagnostic Investigation: Official Publication of The American Association of Veterinary Laboratory Diagnosticians, Inc.* 23 (1): 111–114.

Aleri, J.W., Hine, B.C., Pyman, M.F. et al. (2016). Periparturient immunosuppression and strategies to improve dairy cow health during the periparturient period. *Research in Veterinary Science* 108: 8–17.

Andjelic, B., Djokovic, R., Cincovic, M. et al. (2022). Relationships between milk and blood biochemical parameters and metabolic status in dairy cows during lactation. *Metabolites* 12 (8): 733.

Barson, R.K., Padder, S., Sayam, A.S.M. et al. (2019). Serum glucose, urea nitrogen, cholesterol, and total proteins in crossbred repeat breeder and normally cyclic cows. *Journal of Advanced Veterinary and Animal Research* 6 (1): 82–85.

Bhadauria, P., Lathwal, S.S., Jadoun, Y.S., and Gupta, R. (2020). Metabolic profiling of normal and lame Karan fries cows and its association with lameness during transition period. *Journal of Animal Research* 10 (3): 375–382.

Blowey, R.W. (1972). Metabolic profiles-some aspects of their interpretation and use in the field. In: *The Veterinary Annual 1973, Fourteenth Year* (ed. C.S.G. Grunsell and F.W.G. Hill), 21–30. Bristol: John Wright.

Blowey, R.W. (1975). A practical application of metabolic profiles. *The Veterinary Record* 97 (17): 324–327.

Blowey, R.W., Wood, D.W., and Davis, J.R. (1973). A nutritional monitoring system for dairy herds based on blood glucose, urea and albumin levels. *Veterinary Record* 92: 691–696.

Cankaya, M., Hernandez, A.M., Ciftci, M. et al. (2007). An analysis of expression patterns of genes encoding proteins with catalytic activities. *BMC Genomics* 8: 232.

Gaal, K.K., Safar, O., Gulyas, L., and Stadler, P. (2004). Magnesium in animal nutrition. *Journal of the American College of Nutrition* 23 (6): 754S–757S.

Grunberg, W., Scherpenisse, P., Cohrs, I. et al. (2019). Phosphorus content of muscle tissue and muscle function in dairy cows fed a phosphorus-deficient diet during the transition period. *Journal of Dairy Science* 102 (5): 4072–4093.

Hubner, A., Canisso, I.F., Peixoto, P.M. et al. (2022). Characterization of metabolic profile, health, milk production, and reproductive outcomes of dairy cows diagnosed with concurrent hyperketonemia and hypoglycemia. *Journal of Dairy Science* 105 (11): 9054–9069.

Hunt, E. and Wood, B. (1999). Use of blood and blood products. *The Veterinary Clinics of North America. Food Animal Practice* 15 (3): 641–662.

Huzzey, J.M., Veira, D.M., Weary, D.M., and von Keyserlingk, M.A. (2007). Prepartum behavior and dry matter intake identify dairy cows at risk for metritis. *Journal of Dairy Science* 90 (7): 3220–3233.

Kaneko, J.J., Harvey, J.W., and Bruss, M.L. (2008). *Clinical Biochemistry of Domestic Animals*, 6e. San Diego, CA: Academic Press.

Katoh, N. and Nakagawa, H. (1999). Detection of haptoglobin in the high-density lipoprotein and the very high-density lipoprotein fractions from sera of calves with experimental pneumonia and cows with naturally occurring fatty liver. *The Journal of Veterinary Medical Science* 61 (2): 119–124.

Kida, K. (2002). The metabolic profile test: its practicability in assessing feeding management and periparturient diseases in high yielding commercial dairy herds. *The Journal of Veterinary Medical Science* 64 (7): 557–563.

Kimura, K., Reinhardt, T.A., and Goff, J.P. (2006). Parturition and hypocalcemia blunts calcium signals in immune cells of dairy cattle. *Journal of Dairy Science* 89 (7): 2588–2595.

Kuczynska, B., Puppel, K., Gołębiewski, M. et al. (2021). Metabolic profile according to the parity and stage of lactation of high-performance Holstein-Friesian cows. *Animal Bioscience* 34 (4): 575–583.

Lager, K. and Jordan, E. (2012). The metabolic profile for the modern transition dairy cow. *Proceedings of the Mid-South Ruminant Nutrition Conference*, Grapevine, Texas, USA (26 April 2012), 9–16. Champaign, Illinois, USA: Texas Animal Nutrition Council.

Law, R.A., Young, F.J., Patterson, D.C. et al. (2009). Effect of dietary protein content on animal production and blood metabolites of dairy cows during lactation. *Journal of Dairy Science* 92 (3): 1001–1012.

LeBlanc, S.J., Lissemore, K.D., Kelton, D.F. et al. (2006). Major advances in disease prevention in dairy cattle. *Journal of Dairy Science* 89 (4): 1267–1279.

Lopez-Alonso, M. and Miranda, M. (2020). Copper supplementation, a challenge in cattle. *Animals: An Open Access Journal from MDPI* 10 (10): 1890.

Nogalski, Z., Wronski, M., Lewandowska, B., and Pogorzelska, P. (2012). Changes in the blood indicators and body condition of high yielding Holstein cows with retained placenta and ketosis. *Acta Veterinaria* 81: 359–364.

Noziere, P., Ortigues-Marty, I., Loncke, C., and Sauvant, D. (2010). Carbohydrate quantitative digestion and absorption in ruminants: from feed starch and fibre to nutrients available for tissues. *Animal: An International Journal of Animal Bioscience* 4 (7): 1057–1074.

Paiano, R.B., Birgel, D.B., and Birgel Junior, E.H. (2020). Influence of peripartum on the erythrogram of Holstein dairy cows. *Journal of the South African Veterinary Association* 91 (0): e1–e6.

Payne, J.M., Dew, S.M., Manston, R., and Faulks, M. (1970). The use of a metabolic profile test in dairy herds. *The Veterinary Record* 87 (6): 150–158.

Peterson, A.B., Orth, M.W., Goff, J.P., and Beede, D.K. (2005). Periparturient responses of multiparous Holstein cows fed different dietary phosphorus concentrations prepartum. *Journal of Dairy Science* 88 (10): 3582–3594.

Pinotti, L., Manoni, M., Ferrari, L. et al. (2021). The contribution of dietary magnesium in farm animals and human nutrition. *Nutrients* 13 (2): 509.

Pohler, K.G., Reese, S.T., Franco, G.A. et al. (2020). New approaches to diagnose and target reproductive failure in cattle. *Animal Reproduction* 17 (3): e20200057.

Prajapati, A., Panchasara, H., Suthar, A. et al. (2023). Evaluation of health status of Kankrej cattle using mini compton metabolic profile test and correlation with production status. *The Indian Journal of Animal Sciences* 93 (3): 276–278.

Prodanovic, R., Sladojevi, C., Kirovski, D. et al. (2012). Use of metabolic profiles and body condition scoring for the assessment of energy status of dairy cows. *Biotechnol Animal Husbandry* 28: 25–32.

Puppel, K. and Kuczynska, B. (2016). Metabolic profiles of cow's blood; a review. *Journal of the Science of Food and Agriculture* 96 (13): 4321–4328.

Romano, M.C., Higgs, G.E., Helm, M.N. et al. (2021). Sodium distribution in the bovine brain. *Journal of Veterinary Diagnostic Investigation: Official Publication of The American Association of Veterinary Laboratory Diagnosticians, Inc* 33 (2): 384–387.

Rowlands, G.J. and Manston, R. (1976). The potential uses of metabolic profiles in the management and selection of cattle for milk and beef production. *Livestock Production Science* 3 (3): 1976.

Sakowski, T., Kuczynska, B., Puppel, K. et al. (2012). Relationships between physiological indicators in blood, and their yield, as well as chemical composition of milk obtained from organic dairy cows. *Journal of the Science of Food and Agriculture* 92 (14): 2905–2912.

Schonewille, J.T. (2013). Magnesium in dairy cow nutrition: an overview. *Plant and Soil* 368: 167–178.

Schonewille, J.T., Everts, H., Jittakhot, S., and Beynen, A.C. (2008). Quantitative prediction of magnesium absorption in dairy cows. *Journal of Dairy Science* 91 (1): 271–278.

Sun, Y., Xu, C., Li, C. et al. (2014). Characterization of the serum metabolic profile of dairy cows with milk fever using 1H-NMR spectroscopy. *The Veterinary Quarterly* 34 (3): 159–163.

Turkson, P.K. and Ganyo, E.Y. (2015). Relationship between haemoglobin concentration and packed cell volume in cattle blood samples. *The Onderstepoort Journal of Veterinary Research* 82 (1): 863.

West, J.W., Coppock, C.E., Milam, K.Z. et al. (1987). Potassium carbonate as a potassium source and dietary buffer for lactating Holstein cows during hot weather. *Journal of Dairy Science* 70 (2): 309–320.

Wheelock, J.B., Rhoads, R.P., Vanbaale, M.J. et al. (2010). Effects of heat stress on energetic metabolism in lactating Holstein cows. *Journal of Dairy Science* 93 (2): 644–655.

Whitlock, R.H., Kessler, M.J., and Tasker, J.B. (1975). Salt (sodium) deficiency in dairy cattle: polyuria and polydipsia as prominent clinical features. *The Cornell Veterinarian* 65 (4): 512–526.

Wysocka, D., Snarska, A., and Sobiech, P. (2020). Iron in cattle health. *Journal of Elementology* 25 (3): 1175–1185.

Yadav, N.K., Lohan, J.S., Singh, B., and Chand, D. (1995). Studies on some serum constituents in anoestrous buffaloes. *Indian Journal of Animal Research* 29 (1): 85–88.

4

The Behavior of Cattle During and After Parturition

Aminu M. Galadima

Usmanu Danfodiyo University Sokoto, Sokoto, Nigeria

4.1 Introduction

4.1.1 Importance of Studying Cattle Behavior During Calving

The study of cattle behavior during calving is of paramount importance for several reasons. First, understanding the behavioral patterns exhibited by cattle during this crucial period allows farmers and caretakers to anticipate and provide appropriate support and care. By recognizing the signs of impending calving and understanding the stages of labor, interventions can be implemented, if necessary, to ensure the health and well-being of both the cow and the calf. Additionally, studying the behavior of cattle during calving sheds light on the natural instincts and maternal behaviors displayed by the cows. This knowledge helps to create an environment that supports and promotes these natural behaviors, which leads to reduced stress and improved welfare for the animals. Furthermore, understanding the communication and recognition cues between the cow and the newborn calf aids in strengthening the bond between them, which fosters a nurturing and protective environment. By studying cattle behavior during calving, we gain insights into the complex dynamics that contribute to successful calving outcomes, which enables better management practices and ultimately, improves the overall health and productivity of the herd.

Calving is a critical period for cattle as it is the onset of lactation and when cows are at their highest risk of developing various health complications. In addition to health issues, cow behavior during and after calving has significant implications for calf survival, welfare, and productivity.

These behaviors enable the cow to form a connection with her calf, protect and provide it with nourishment, and eventually, break this bond during weaning. Various farming techniques have emphasized different maternal behaviors, with some being viewed as advantageous while others are considered a hindrance. In large-scale farming operations, such as beef cattle production, the mother cow bears the primary responsibility of raising her newborn, and issues, such as cross licking, that interfere with the bonding process still pose a significant practical challenge.

This chapter will discuss the behavior of cattle during and after calving as well as the factors that influence it.

4.2 Precalving Behavior

Precalving behavior refers to the specific behaviors exhibited by cows in the period leading up to giving birth. Understanding and recognizing these behaviors is crucial for effective management and preparation for the calving process.

During this stage, cows may display the following:

1) Nesting and seeking isolation
2) Signs of impending calving
3) Physical changes and discomfort

Periparturient Diseases of Cattle, First Edition. Edited by Tanmoy Rana.

4.2.1 Nesting and Seeking Isolation

During the calving process, cows often exhibit a natural instinct to isolate themselves from the rest of the herd. This behavior, known as self-isolation, serves several important purposes for the cow and her calf. This section explores the reasons behind this behavior and its significance in dairy cow management.

Cows prefer to use a secluded area for calving and begin to use this area more in the first hour before calving. After calving, cows that become ill continue to use the secluded area more than healthy cows (Proudfoot et al. 2014).

In the pasture, cows separate themselves from the herd during calving, opting to give birth in a dry area with the presence of trees or bushes for cover (Lidfors et al. 1994). Like other species that tend to hide their young, calves spend the initial days of their lives concealed in brush or tree cover, typically in the vicinity of where they were born, while their mother grazes in close proximity (Vitale et al. 1986).

4.2.1.1 Importance of Self-isolation

Self-isolation during calving offers several advantages for both the cow and the calf. First, it provides a quiet and secure environment that minimizes external stressors. This calm setting allows the cow to focus on calving, which reduces anxiety and promotes a smoother delivery. Additionally, self-isolation ensures the safety of the newborn calf by preventing interference from other herd members and reducing the risk of accidental injuries. The secluded environment also facilitates the establishment of the cow–calf bond by enabling the cow to care for and protect her offspring without distractions.

On many commercial dairy farms, cows are given little opportunity to isolate when calving or ill. The management and housing of cows at calving and during illness are highly variable; cows are typically either housed in group pens or individual maternity or hospital pens. Individual pens are often in highly trafficked areas, which allows producers to more easily monitor ill and calving cows (Proudfoot et al. 2014).

4.2.2 Signs of Impending Calving

Parturition in a pregnant cow, also known as calving, is a critical event in animal agriculture. As with human childbirth, the cow's body undergoes a series of preparatory events that lead up to the delivery of the newborn calf. The preparatory period usually begins about 2 weeks before the expected due date and is characterized by a series of physiological changes in the cow's body. During this period, the cow's body prepares for calving by softening and thinning the cervix, initiating uterine contractions, and positioning the fetus for delivery.

As the preparatory period progresses, the pregnant cow may begin to exhibit prodromal external signs of parturition. These signs may include restlessness, pawing at the ground, tail raising, and increased vocalization. Additionally, the cow may show a decrease in appetite, and there may be a noticeable drop in milk production. These signs are often indicative of impending calving and can serve as an important warning for livestock producers (Larson and Watt 2020).

4.2.3 Physical Changes and Discomfort

Physical changes and discomfort during calving are natural occurrences that cows experience as they give birth to their calves. These changes are important indicators of labor progression and can help farmers and caretakers provide appropriate support and intervention when necessary.

In cattle, the relaxation of the broad pelvic ligaments is considered the best individual sign of impending parturition (Strey et al. 2011; Shah et al. 2006). As calving approaches, the ligaments around the cow's tailhead loosen, which allows for the pelvic canal to widen and facilitate the passage of the calf during delivery. This relaxation may cause the tailhead to become more prominent and the hips to appear wider.

There is also a gradual increase in the natural inflammation of the udder (mammogenesis); the udder becomes larger and firmer due to the growth of glandular tissue and the accumulation of colostrum, which creates internal pressure. Some cows may begin to leak colostrum several hours before giving birth due to both internal pressure and the release of oxytocin. In some cases, excessive inflammation close to calving can lead to the rupture of blood vessels, which causes colostrum to change from a yellowish color to reddish or brown due to the presence of oxidative hemoglobin. Blood clots may also be present during the first milking (João Simões 2021).

External physical changes also occur, specifically in the udder (breasts and nipples), vulva, and rump (pelvic ligaments and base of the tail). The growth of lobuloalveolar tissue in the mammary gland, known as mammogenesis, is controlled by various hormones during pregnancy (João Simões 2021).

Recognizing these physical changes and signs of discomfort is crucial for providing appropriate care and support to the cow during calving. Farmers and caretakers can monitor the progression of labor, offer a calm and comfortable calving environment, and intervene if complications arise to ensure the well-being and successful delivery of both the cow and the calf.

4.3 Labor and Parturition (Delivery)

Labor and delivery, also known as calving, is a critical stage in the reproductive cycle of cattle. It marks the culmination of the gestation period and the beginning of a new life. Understanding the process of labor and delivery is essential for farmers, veterinarians, and caretakers involved in cattle management.

During labor the cow goes through a series of physiological changes and behavioral cues that signify the impending birth of her calf. These changes include the relaxation of pelvic ligaments, the onset of uterine contractions, and the release of hormones that initiate the birthing process. Recognizing these signs and monitoring the progression of labor allows for timely interventions and assistance, if needed.

The delivery itself involves the expulsion of the calf from the cow's uterus. It is a complex and dynamic process that requires coordination between the cow's contractions and the positioning of the calf for a successful birth. The cow utilizes her maternal instincts, such as vigorous straining and pushing, to help expel the calf safely into the world.

Successful labor and delivery depend on multiple factors, including the health and condition of the cow, the size and positioning of the calf, and the environmental conditions in which calving takes place. Proper management practices, such as providing clean and comfortable calving areas, regular monitoring, and timely veterinary assistance, contribute to favorable outcomes and the well-being of both the cow and the calf.

Here, we will delve into the various aspects of labor and delivery in cattle, exploring the stages of labor, the behavioral and physiological changes exhibited by cows, and the importance of proper management practices during this critical period. By gaining a deeper understanding of labor and delivery in cattle, we can enhance our ability to support and promote successful calving outcomes, which ensures the health and productivity of our herds.

4.3.1 Stages of Labor

The calving process is divided into three stages (Noakes et al. 2009; (US) NAHMS 2010), and under normal conditions (eutocia), it progresses gradually from one stage to the next.

- **Stage I (dilatation phase):** Marked by the opening of the cervix (ligaments and joints of the pelvic bone) and contractions of the uterus. While there may be differences in behavioral signs between cows and first-calving heifers, stage I is characterized by specific behaviors. These behaviors include sniffing the ground for scent cues, engaging in nest building–like behavior, self-grooming by licking various parts of their bodies (such as back and hindlimbs), vocalizing, passing feces, and displaying restlessness through activities like walking, standing up, and lying down as well as raising their tails (Wehrend et al. 2006; Miedema et al. 2011). The average duration of the first stage is about 2.5 hours but it can last more than 6 hours, especially in primiparous cows. For stillborn calves, the time interval from the onset of labor until calving is completed is approximately twice as long as for live-born calves (Berglund et al. 1987). Some of these behavioral signs such as tail raising, restlessness, and vocalization extend into stage II of labor. Stage I ends with a fully dilated cervix (Noakes et al. 2009; (US) NAHMS 2010).
- **Stage II (expulsion phase):** This is identified by the emergence of the amniotic sac (AS) outside the vulva. During this phase, visible contractions in the abdomen become noticeable, and the calf gradually advances through the birth canal, starting with the feet, which are followed by the nose and head. The average duration of the second stage is approximately 30–70 minutes, again taking a little longer in the case of primiparous cows (Figure 4.1). At the onset of this stage, the fetus reaches and enters the cranial end of the birth canal. The dam is usually lying down. The slight protrusion of the AS through the vulva is considered a clinical indicator of the onset of this stage. While the AS remains intact, which minimizes thermal and tactile stressors for the fetus, and the umbilical cord is free from obliteration or compression,

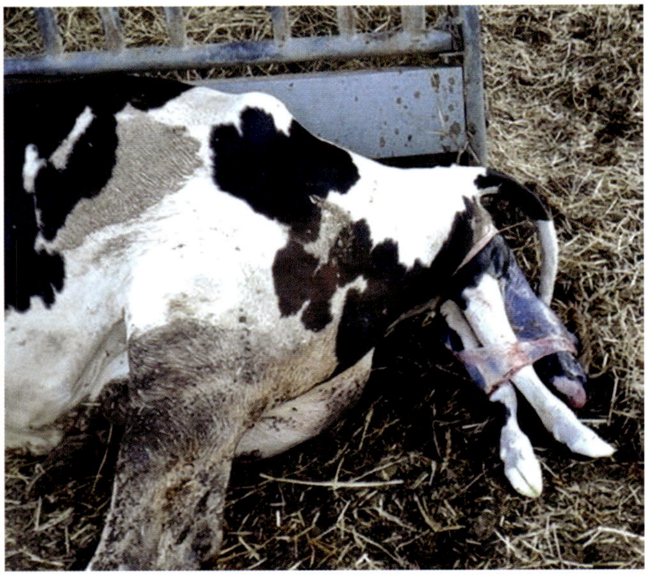

Figure 4.1 Video box of stage II of labor.

which maintains the normal blood fetal partial pressures of O_2 (pO_2) and CO_2 (pCO_2), the fetus is in a favorable environment even if other environmental stressors persist (João Simões 2021). Stage II concludes when the calf is fully delivered (Noakes et al. 2009; (US) NAHMS 2010).

- **Stage III (placental expulsion phase):** The process of expelling the fetal membranes, referred to as stage III, involves the passage of these membranes within the first 24 hours after birth (Kelton et al. 1998; LeBlanc 2008). In the expulsion phase, when observing multiparous cows, it was observed that they would lie down when the abdominal contractions began and continue to remain in a recumbent position until the birth occurred. This stage usually occurs within the first 6 hours after fetus delivery. However, in some cases, a retained placenta may be defined only if it does not occur within 12 or even 24 hours after the expulsion of the fetus. The continued contractions of the uterine muscles, stimulated by oxytocin, along with abdominal contractions, play a mechanical role in separating the cotyledons and expelling the placental membranes. The presence of these membranes within the cervical canal can potentially slow the closure of the cervix in the subsequent days. However, it is the local biochemical effects that are believed to be crucial for the normal expulsion of the placenta, and cases of placenta retention due to uterine inertia are rare. The third stage of labor concludes with the expulsion of the placenta, followed by the process of uterine involution and the discharge of lochia during the early postpartum period (João Simões 2021).

4.3.2 Maternal Instinct During Calving

Occasionally, there are instances when a cow or heifer shows reluctance in assuming the role of a mother to her newborn calf. Most hesitant mothers change their attitude within a day or so and become nurturing and attentive. However, a small number of these individuals may have an underlying hormonal deficiency that persists and leads to recurring reluctance in mothering their calves after subsequent calvings. While many improve over time and become more accepting, there are some cows that remain just as stubborn with their fifth calf as they were with their first (Thomas 2015).

4.3.2.1 Hormones Are the Driving Force

Experience also plays a role in this matter, as older cows typically exhibit greater consistency in their mothering behavior and possess a stronger maternal drive compared to heifers. However, it is important to note that we often attribute too much significance to experience alone. According to Dr. Joseph Stookey, a Professor Emeritus of Large Animal Clinical Sciences in the Western College of Veterinary Medicine at the University of Saskatchewan, the cow's receptiveness and desire for a newborn calf are most pronounced when she gives birth.

Hormones play a crucial role in initiating and driving what we perceive as maternal behavior in cows. According to Dr. Stookey, hormones are responsible for most aspects of maternal behavior. He explains that some cows develop an interest in any newborn calf up to a week before their own calving. Their hormone levels are already elevated, making them receptive to any new calf, even if it is not their own.

On the other hand, there are cows that experience inadequate hormone profiles or levels after calving, which leads to a lack of interest in their own calf. This is commonly observed in first-calf heifers, cows that require assistance during calving, or those that undergo a cesarean section. If a cow undergoes a challenging experience during calving or is subjected to significant stress or pain, it can affect the overall hormonal balance. Additionally, certain medications administered during a cesarean section may impact the cow's hormone levels and maternal behavior.

Dr. Stookey emphasizes that factors such as stress, pain, and the use of certain drugs can influence the cow's hormone profile and override the natural maternal instincts. It is important to consider these factors when evaluating a cow's behavior toward her newborn calf (Thomas 2015).

4.4 Nurturing the Newborn

After the labor and delivery process, the critical task of nurturing the newborn calf begins. Cows and heifers instinctively exhibit maternal behaviors that promote the well-being and growth of their offspring. These nurturing behaviors include licking and cleaning the calf to stimulate circulation and remove birth fluids, encouraging the calf to stand and nurse, and providing warmth and protection.

Immediately following birth, calves engage in head shaking, snuffling, and sneezing to remove amniotic fluid from their air passageways (Selman et al. 1970). The mother vigorously licks the calf to remove amniotic fluid (Edwards 1983), establish the cow–calf bond (reviewed by von Keyserlingk and Weary 2007), and stimulate urination and defecation (Edwards 1983). Licking soon after birth is seen in wild ungulates, such as free-ranging reindeer (*Rangifer tarandus* Linnaeus) and wild Plains bison (*Bison bison*) (Espmark 1971; Lott and Galland 1985). When permitted, cows in loose-housing barns begin licking their calf on average (Illmann and Špinka 1993) 5–7 minutes after parturition (Lidfors et al. 1994). Young ungulates typically spend most of the first hour after parturition being licked; for example, one study showed that Friesian calves born in individual pens were licked 30–50% of the time during their first hour of life (Edwards and Broom 1982), and Danish Holstein calves born indoors have recently been reported to be licked for the first 40 minutes after birth (Jensen et al. 2019).

4.4.1 Cow–calf Bond

The bond between a cow and her calf is a remarkable and essential aspect of their natural behavior and survival. It is a unique and nurturing relationship that begins at birth and strengthens over time (Zilkha et al. 2016). This bond plays a crucial role in the emotional well-being and development of both the cow and the calf.

In most mammalian species, the mother plays a crucial role in caring for and providing social contact to the young. During the initial months of life, the mother not only fulfills the basic needs of feeding and care but also imparts important information about the physical and social environment to her offspring (Mandujano-Camacho 2010; Mora-Medina et al. 2018). The bond formed at birth, facilitated through a learning process called "imprinting," is essential for the survival of the young as it enables them to recognize and identify their mother (Yamaguchi et al. 2012), and is fundamental for the survival of the young.

A bonded mother exhibits evident maternal behavior, such as suckling, and displays negative responses, such as increased vocalizations and activity, when separated from her offspring. These responses tend to diminish upon reunion (Solano et al. 2007; Sirovnik et al. 2020). Similarly, bonded offspring demonstrate affiliative behavior toward their mother and experience distress when separated from her (Sirovnik et al. 2020) (Figure 4.2).

This bonding period, known as the "sensitive period," is a critical stage that relies on early exposure to sensory stimuli (sight, touch, smell, and hearing) naturally exchanged between the mother and the environment during the neonatal phase (Mandujano-Camacho 2010; Mora-Medina et al. 2018; Yamaguchi et al. 2012). Any disruption or interference during this sensitive period, whether due to human intervention or other external factors, can lead to inaccurate imprinting and affect the bond between mother and offspring. This, in turn, may result in reproductive, social, or behavioral disturbances in the young and could even lead to the mother rejecting her offspring (Madigan et al. 2006). Furthermore, the imprinted bond with the mother can influence sensory preferences in adult animals, including feeding, maternal behaviors, and sexual preferences (Fillion and Blass 1986; Shah et al. 2002). An extreme example of this phenomenon was observed in small ruminants, where rams raised by goats or goats raised by sheep displayed a preference for sexual partners of the species that raised them, rather than their own species, as adults (Kendrick et al. 1998).

The presence of potential predators at the calving site is mentioned as a factor that can interfere with the establishment of the cow–calf bond. (Orihuela and Galina 2021) (Figure 4.3).

Understanding and respecting the cow–calf bond is crucial for ethical and sustainable farming practices. Recognizing the emotional needs of both the cow and calf promotes animal welfare and supports a healthier and more natural rearing environment. It also highlights the intricate social dynamics within the animal kingdom, which reminds us of the importance of compassion and empathy in our interactions with all living beings.

4.4.2 Encouraging Standing and Suckling

4.4.2.1 Standing

Wild ungulates possess a precocious nature, with numerous young individuals demonstrating the ability to stand and walk shortly after being born. This enables them to promptly engage in nursing and acquire nourishment soon after their birth.

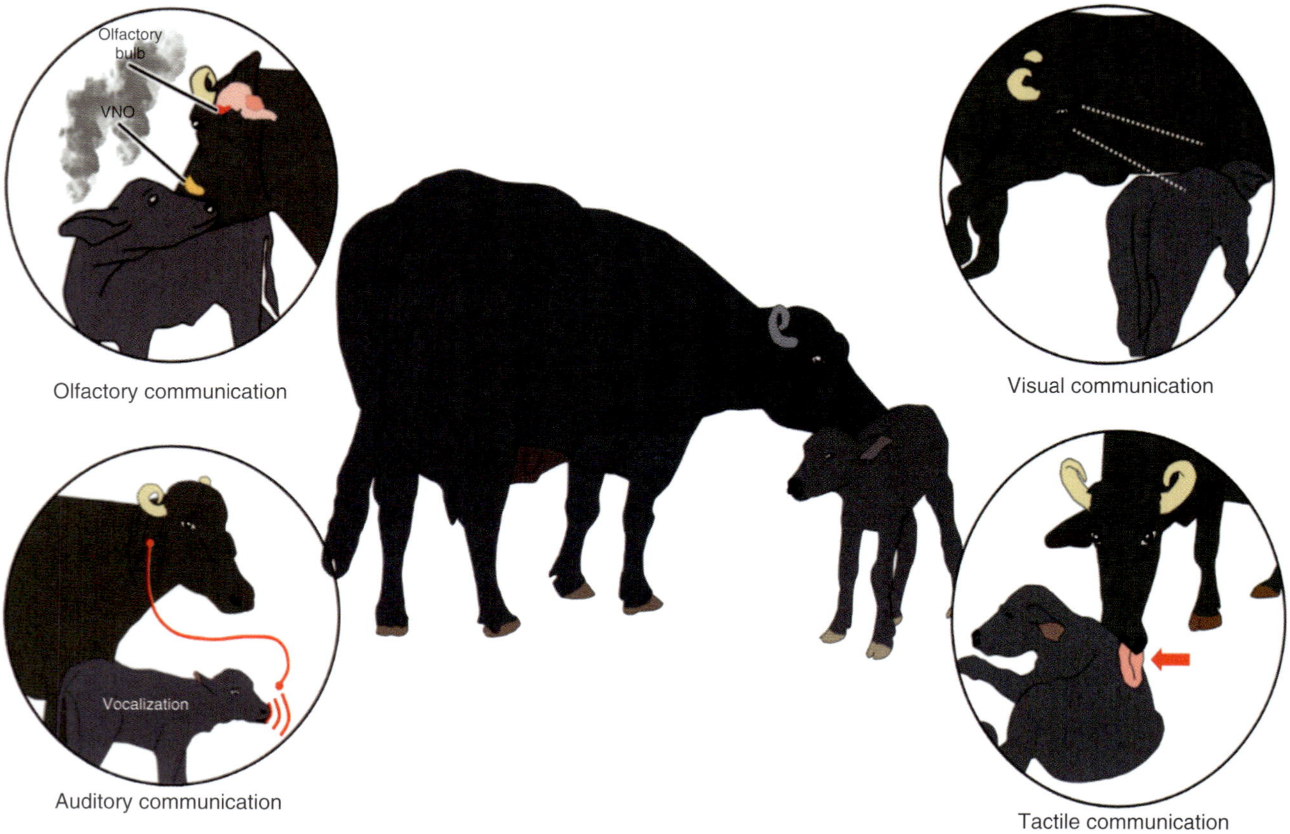

Figure 4.2 Senses and site of action in the brain during the imprinting process (VNO = vomeronasal organ).

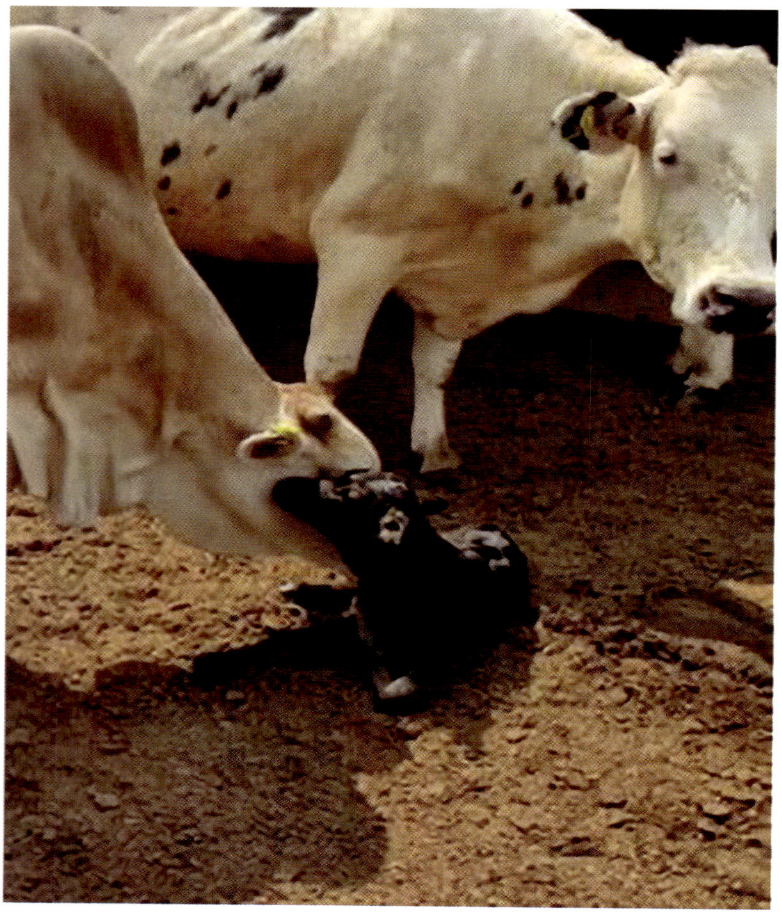

Figure 4.3 The cow–calf bond.

(Geist 1974). Wild Plains bison calves in the United States were observed to attempt standing approximately 3 minutes after birth and on average, required only 11 minutes to successfully stand (Lott and Galland 1985). Water buffalo calves (*Bubalus bubalis*) in Australia made their first attempts to stand just 10 minutes after being born, and they were able to stand successfully within 50 minutes of birth (Illmann and Špinka 1993; DG 1979). Similarly, reindeer calves in Sweden displayed their innate ability to stand shortly after birth, with their initial attempts occurring within 5–29 minutes after birth and successful standing achieved within 10–40 minutes of birth (Espmark 1971). Dairy calves born indoors seem to behave similarly to their wild counterparts in this respect. Calves attempt to stand on average 17 minutes after birth and successfully stand after an average of (Lidfors et al. 1994) 37–58 minutes (Selman et al. 1970). Calves from dystocia births may have reduced vitality that possibly causes a reduced motivation to stand (reviewed by Fischer et al. 2018). Calves with primiparous mothers have been reported to take longer (Selman et al. 1970) and spend less time standing during their first 6 hours of life than calves from multiparous cows (Edwards and Broom 1982). While studies have indicated that the time taken for a calf to stand within the first 6 hours of life is not influenced by the amount of licking received from the mother, it is worth noting that certain first-time mothers in individual indoor pens may not engage in licking behavior toward their calves. Additionally, some primiparous cows may display fear or anxiety toward their calf, which can potentially impact the time it takes for the calf to stand (Edwards and Broom 1982).

4.4.2.2 Suckling

The absorption of immunoglobulins from colostrum is most efficient immediately after birth, and this ability may decline within 6 hours post birth (Fischer et al. 2018; Espmark 1971). Therefore, the importance of early standing and quick suckling is evident in ungulate species. On average, wild ungulates take less than 90 minutes to initiate suckling (reindeer: an average of 82 minutes (Espmark 1971); wild Plains bison: an average of 32 minutes (Lott and Galland 1985)). In dairy cattle born indoors, the newborn will often nuzzle different parts of the cow's body before finally locating the teat (Lidfors et al. 1994; Edwards and Broom 1982). In cow–calf pairs housed separately from the group indoors, beef calves suckled their mothers on average 81 minutes after birth (Selman et al. 1970). In contrast, although 9 of the 11 dairy calves observed in a loose-housing barn contacted their mother's udder, only 4 (36%) of the calves successfully suckled within 3 hours of birth (Lidfors et al. 1994). Age of the cow may play a role in suckling success; 61% (17 out of 28) and 89% (25 out of 28) of Friesian calves from first lactation mothers suckled within 2 and 6 hours of birth, unlike calves from multiparous mothers, where only 15% (8 out of 54) and 54% (29 out of 54) suckled within 2 and 6 hours, respectively (Edwards and Broom 1979). These differences may be because the older Friesian cows had pendulous udders that limited the calf's ability to suckle (Edwards and Broom 1979). One study classified udder shape as either "good" (optimal for suckling) or "poor" and found that calves spent 17 minutes teat seeking before suckling from a "good" udder compared to 40 minutes for calves trying to suckle from a "poor" udder (Selman et al. 1970). As research in cow–calf systems continue to burgeon, different methods to ensure adequate suckling and colostrum intake should be described (Whalin et al. 2021).

4.5 Protective Behavior of the Mother

In beef cattle, the maternal behavior of the cow is essential for the proper development of the newborn calf. Maternal–offspring bonding plays a crucial role in maternal behavior, and a significant aspect of this bonding is the mother's aggressive defense of her calf. However, when human intervention is involved, excessively protective cows can pose a risk of injury to either the caretaker or the calf. Dealing with aggressive cows adds additional challenges to the tasks of identification and record keeping (Buddenberg et al. 1986). As a prey species, a crucial aspect of maternal behavior is being defensive, as the calf requires constant care and protection from predators and potentially aggressive individuals within the same species during the initial weeks of life (Lent 1974). While maternal defense behaviors are essential and beneficial in natural settings, cows that exhibit overly protective responses toward their calves in agricultural production systems can pose a risk by potentially threatening or attacking handlers during initial handling. These extreme reactions increase the likelihood of accidents on the farm by endangering the well-being of both handlers and animals and even jeopardizing the welfare of the calves, which leads to physical harm or potential abandonment (Turner et al. 2013; Buddenberg et al. 1986).

Our study observed two distinct categories of maternal behavior: "protective-attentive mothers" and "protective-aggressive mothers." The former were cows that remained vigilant and attentive during the handling of their calves without posing any threat or displaying aggression toward the handlers. On the other hand, the latter were cows that exhibited both attentiveness and hostility, displaying threatening or attacking behavior during handling of their calves (Vicentini et al. 2022). The expression and intensity of maternal defense can be influenced by various individual factors, including temperament, body condition, offspring sex, and vitality as well as previous experience and parity (Fairbanks 1996; Orihuela and Galina 2021; Edwards and Broom 1982; Pires et al. 2020; Pitts et al. 2020; Stěhulová et al. 2013). Previous studies on Taurine cattle have also shown that multiparous cows tend to be more protective than primiparous cows when their calves are handled (Hoppe et al. 2008; Buddenberg et al. 1986; Geburt et al. 2015).

References

(US) National Animal Health Monitoring System (2010). Dairy 2007: Heifer Calf Health and Management Practices on US Dairy Operations, 2007. Fort Collins (CO): US Department of Agriculture, Animal and Plant Health Inspection Service, Veterinary Services, Center for Epidemiology and Animal Health. *Report No. 550.0110.*

Berglund, B., Philipsson, J., and Danell, Ö. (1987). External signs of preparation for calving and course of parturition in Swedish dairy cattle breeds. *Animal Reproduction Science* 15 (1–2): 61–79.

Buddenberg, B.J., Brown, C.J., Johnson, Z.B., and Honea, R.S. (1986). Maternal behavior of beef cows at parturition. *Journal of Animal Science* 1 (62): 42–46.

DG, T. (1979). The water Buffalo, *Bubalus Bubalis*, in Australia: reproductive and parent-offspring behaviour. *Wildlife Research* 6 (3): 265–287.

Edwards, S.A. (1983). The behaviour of dairy cows and their newborn calves in individual or group housing. *Applied Animal Ethology* 10: 191–198.

Edwards, S.A. and Broom, D.M. (1979). The period between birth and first suckling in dairy calves. *Research in Veterinary Science* 26 (2): 255–256.

Edwards, S.A. and Broom, D.M. (1982). Behavioural interactions of dairy cows with their newborn calves and the effects of parity. *Animal Behaviour* 30 (2): 525–535.

Espmark, Y. (1971). Mother-young relationship and ontogeny of behaviour in reindeer (*Rangifer tarandus* L.). *Zeitschrift für Tierpsychologie* 29 (1): 42–81.

Fairbanks, L. .A. (1996). Individual differences in maternal style: causes and consequences for mothers and offspring. In: *Advances in the Study of Behavior* (ed. J.S.S.C. Rosenblatt), 579–611. Academic Press.

Fillion, T.J. and Blass, E.M. (1986). Infantile experience with suckling odors determines adult sexual behavior in male rats. *Science* 231 (4739): 729–731.

Fischer, A.J., Song, Y., He, Z. et al. (2018). Effect of delaying colostrum feeding on passive transfer and intestinal bacterial colonization in neonatal male Holstein calves. *Journal of Dairy Science* 101 (4): 3099–3109.

Geburt, K., Friedrich, M., Piechotta, M. et al. (2015). Validity of physiological biomarkers for maternal behavior in cows – a comparison of beef and dairy cattle. *Physiology and Behavior* 139: 361–368.

Geist, V.W.F. and Walther F. ed. (1974). Behaviour of ungulates and its relation to management. *Symposium on the Behavior of Ungulates and Its Relation to Management,* Calgary, Alberta, Canada (2–5 November 1971). Morges, Switzerland: IUCN Publications.

Hoppe, S., Brandt, H.R., Erhardt, G., and Gauly, M. (2008). Maternal protective behaviour of German Angus and Simmental beef cattle after parturition and its relation to production traits. *Applied Animal Behaviour Science* 114 (3–4): 297–306.

Illmann, G. and Špinka, M. (1993). Maternal behaviour of dairy heifers and sucking of their newborn calves in group housing. *Applied Animal Behaviour Science* 36 (2–3): 91–98.

Jensen, M.B., Herskin, M.S., and Rørvang, M.V. (2019). Secluded maternity areas for parturient dairy cows offer protection from herd members. *Journal of Dairy Science* 102 (6): 5492–5500.

João Simões, G.S. (2021). *Calving Management and New Born Care*, 1e. Springer Cham.

Kelton, D.F., Lissemore, K.D., and Martin, R.E. (1998). Recommendations for recording and calculating the incidence of selected clinical diseases of dairy cattle. 81 (9): 2502–2509.

Kendrick, K.M., Hinton, M.R., Atkins, K. et al. (1998). Mothers determine sexual preferences. *Nature* 395 (6699): 229–230.

Larson, R.L. and Watt, T.J. (2020). Parturition and periparturient diseases. In: *Large Animal Internal Medicine*, 6e (ed. B.P. Smith, D.C. Van Metre, and N. Pusterla).

LeBlanc, S.J. (2008). Postpartum uterine disease and dairy herd reproductive performance: a review. *Veterinary Journal* 176 (1): 102–114.

Lent, P.C. (1974). Mother-infant relationships in ungulates. In: *The Behaviour of Ungulates and Its Relation to Management*, vol. 1, 14–55. Morges: IUCN Publications.

Lidfors, L.M., Moran, D., Jung, J. et al. (1994). Behaviour at calving and choice of calving place in cattle kept in different environments. *Applied Animal Behaviour Science* 42 (1): 11–28.

Lott, D.F. and Galland, J.C. (1985). Parturition in American bison: precocity and systematic variation in cow isolation. *Zeitschrift für Tierpsychologie* 69 (1): 66–71.

Madigan, S., Bakermans-Kranenburg, M.J., Van Ijzendoorn, M.H. et al. (2006). Unresolved states of mind, anomalous parental behavior, and disorganized attachment: a review and meta-analysis of a transmission gap. *Attachment & Human Development* 8 (2): 89–111.

Mandujano-Camacho, H. (2010). Ecología y sociobiología de la impronta: Perspectivas para su estudio en los Crocodylia. *Ciencia y* 14: 49–54.

Miedema, H.M., Cockram, M.S., Dwyer, C.M., and Macrae, A.I. (2011). Behavioural predictors of the start of normal and dystocic calving in dairy cows and heifers. *Applied Animal Behaviour Science* 132 (1–2): 14–19.

Mora-Medina, P., Orihuela, A., Arch-Tirado, E. et al. (2018). Metabolic changes during brief periods of ewe–lamb separation at different ages. *Animal Production Science* 58: 1297–1306.

Noakes, D., Parkinson, T., and England, G. (2009). Dystocia and other disorders associated with parturition. In: *Veterinary Reproduction and Obstetrics*, 9e (ed. D.E. Noakes, T.J. Parkinson, and G.C.W. England), 207–305. Edinburgh; New York: Saunders.

Orihuela, A. and Galina, C.S. (2021). The effect of maternal behavior around calving on reproduction and wellbeing of zebu type cows and calves. *Animals Science* 11 (11): 3164.

Pires, B.V., Freitas, L.A.D., Silva, G.V.D. et al. (2020). Maternal-offspring behavior of Guzerat beef cattle. *Pesquisa Agropecuária Brasileira* 55: e01504.

Pitts, A.D., Weary, D.M., Fraser, D. et al. (2020). Alternative housing for sows and litters. Part 5. Individual differences in the maternal behaviour of sows. *Applied Animal Behaviour Science* 76 (4): 291–306.

Proudfoot, K.L., Weary, D.M., and von Keyserlingk, M.A.G. (2014). Dairy cows seek isolation at calving and when ill. *Journal of Dairy Science* 97 (5): 2731–2739.

Selman, I.E., McEwan, A.D., and Fisher, E.W. (1970). Studies on natural suckling in cattle during the first eight hours post partum II. Behavioural studies (calves). *Animal Behaviour* 18: 284–289.

Shah, A., Oxley, G., Lovic, V., and Fleming, A.S. (2002). Effects of preweaning exposure to novel maternal odors on maternal responsiveness and selectivity in adulthood. *Developmental Psychobiology* 41 (3): 187–196.

Shah, K.D., Nakao, T., and Kubota, H. (2006). Plasma estrone sulphate (E1S) and estradiol-17β (E2β) profiles during pregnancy and their relationship with the relaxation of sacro sciatic ligament, and prediction of calving time in Holstein–Friesian cattle. *Animal Reproduction Science* 95 (1–2): 38–53.

Sirovnik, J., Varth, K., de Oliveira, D. et al. (2020). Methodological terminology and definitions for research and discussion of cow-calf contact systems. *The Journal of Dairy Research* 87 (s1): 108–114.

Solano, J., Orihuela, A., Galina, C.S., and Aguirre, V. (2007). A note on behavioral responses to brief cow-calf separation and Reunion in cattle (Bos indicus). *Journal of Veterinary Behavior* 2: 10–14.

Stěhulová, I., Špinka, M., Šárová, R. et al. (2013). Maternal behaviour in beef cows is individually consistent and sensitive to cow body condition, calf sex and weight. *Applied Animal Behaviour Science* 144 (3–4): 89–97.

Strey, D., Sauter-Louis, C., Braunert, A. et al. (2011). Establishment of a standard operating procedure for predicting the time of calving in cattle. *Journal of Veterinary Science* 12 (2): 177–185.

Thomas, H.S. (2015). Motherly instinct. *Hereford World*. https://hereford.org/static/files/0115_MaternalBehavior.pdf (accessed 29 December 2023).

Turner, S.P., Jack, M.C., and Lawrence, A.B. (2013). Precalving temperament and maternal defensiveness are independent traits but precalving fear may impact calf growth. *Journal of Animal Science* 91 (1): 4417–4425.

Vicentini, R.R., El Faro, L., Ujita, A. et al. (2022). Is maternal defensiveness of Gyr cows (Bos taurus indicus) related to parity and cows' behaviors during the peripartum period? *PLoS One* 17 (9): e0274392.

Vitale, A.F., Tenucci, M., Papini, M., and Lovari, S. (1986). Social behavior of the calves of semi-wild Maremma cattle, Bos primigenius taurus. *Applied Animal Behaviour Science* 16 (3): 217–231.

Von Keyserlingk, M.A.G. and Weary, D.M. (2007). Maternal behavior in cattle. *Hormones and Behavior* 52 (1): 106–113.

Wehrend, A., Hofmann, E., Failing, K., and Bostedt, H. (2006). Behaviour during the first stage of labour in cattle: influence of parity and dystocia. *Applied Animal Behaviour Science* 100 (3–4): 164–170.

Whalin, L., Weary, D.M., and von Keyserlingk, M.A.G. (2021). Understanding behavioural development of calves in natural settings to inform calf management. *Animals* 11 (8): 24–46.

Yamaguchi, S., Aoki, N., Kitajima, T. et al. (2012). Thyroid hormone determines the start of the sensitive period of imprinting and primes later learning. *Nature Communications* 3: 1081.

Zilkha, N., Sofer, Y., Beny, Y., and Kimchi, T. (2016). From classic ethology to modern neuroethology: overcoming the three biases in social behavior research. *Current Opinion in Neurobiology* 38: 96–108.

5

Rumen Acidosis

Shivangi Udainiya[1], Amita Tiwari[2], Manoj K. Ahirwar[3], and Apoorva Mishra[3]

[1] *Veterinary Polytechnic Bhopal, Nanaji Deshmukh Veterinary Science University, Bhopal, Madhya Pradesh, India*
[2] *Department of Veterinary Medicine, College of Veterinary Science and Animal Husbandry, Nanaji Deshmukh Veterinary Science University, Jabalpur, Madhya Pradesh, India*
[3]*Department of Veterinary Surgery and Radiology, College of Veterinary Science and Animal Husbandry, Nanaji Deshmukh Veterinary Science University, Jabalpur, Madhya Pradesh, India*

5.1 Introduction

The main constraints that hinder the productivity of the livestock sector in most countries are diseases, poor nutrition, breeding policies, and management. Ruminal acidosis is a metabolic disorder that occurs due to feeding errors in ruminants that may manifest in acute, subacute, and chronic forms. The rapid fermentation of carbohydrates alters ruminal function through the proliferation of acid-resistant bacteria and an increase in the production of volatile fatty acids and lactate, which cause a sharp drop in ruminal pH. It is characterized by severe dehydration, diarrhea, ruminal stasis, toxemia, recumbency, and a high mortality.

The functional health of the rumen is an essential requirement for productive behavior that encompasses livestock health and animal welfare (Vuuren et al. 2012). Most health problems encountered in cattle are rumen related, and among rumen disorders, ruminal acidosis is a fairly common affection in ruminants that occurs for many reasons, such as change in feed, feeding habits, poor managemental practices, etc. Ruminal acidosis is a common metabolic disorder that occurs due to the abrupt feeding of a large amount of a highly fermentable diet that leads to changes in the rumen pH (<6). The damage of the pH reduction to the ruminal mucosa allows fluid from the bloodstream to enter the rumen, which causes severe dehydration (Aschenbach and Gabel 2000) and worsens metabolic acidosis (Braun et al. 1992).

Ruminal acidosis in the case of feedlot cattle has gained special attention because of its economic importance. In fact, digestive disorders, including ruminal acidosis, are second only to respiratory diseases in depressing animal performance and production efficiency. Clinically, this disorder can have mild to severe manifestations that may even lead to death (Figure 5.1).

A diagnosis can be made primarily based on clinical observations such as ruminal movement, temperature, pulse, respiration rate, heart rate, and rumen fluid analysis. In ruminal acidosis, the pH of rumen liquor is less than 5.2, the color is milky gray or brown, the consistency is watery, the methylene blue reduction time (MBRT) and sedimentation activity time are increased, and rumen protozoal motility is decreased (Petrovski 2017).

The treatment of ruminal acidosis depends upon its severity. It is primarily focused on addressing the plasma volume deficit, correcting acid–base disturbances, and restoring a normal rumen microenvironment. The intravenous administration of sodium bicarbonate has been a mainstay in the treatment of lactic acidosis (Warner and Vaziri 1981). However, the aggressive use of this therapeutic modality can lead to serious complications.

Ruminants have a complex system for acid–base regulation. Increasing levels of dietary fiber can increase the buffering capacity of the rumen due to the stimulation of saliva production (Kohn and Dunlop 1998). However, in situations where high levels of concentrates are required, the use of pH buffer additives becomes necessary (Erdman 1988). Recent approaches for the treatment of ruminal acidosis are based on the use of dietary buffers. The most common buffer in the livestock industry is sodium bicarbonate.

Periparturient Diseases of Cattle, First Edition. Edited by Tanmoy Rana.

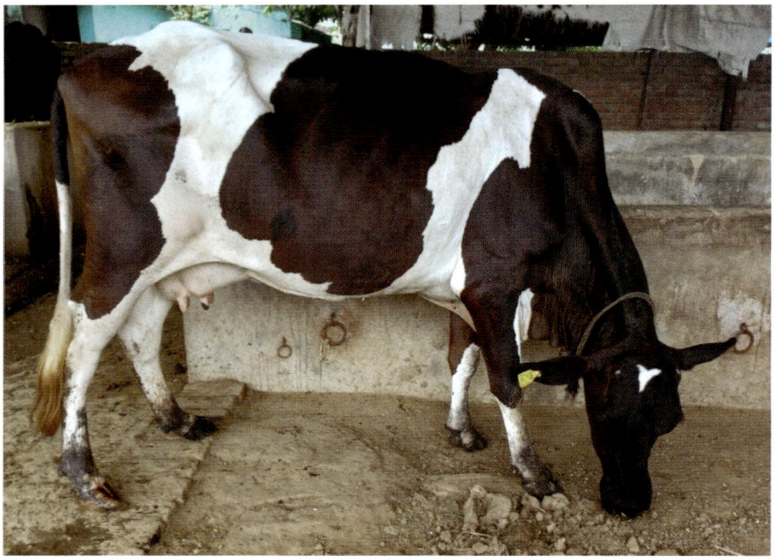

Figure 5.1 A cow affected with chronic rumen acidosis.

5.2 Etiopathogenesis

Rumen acidosis can be defined as a fermentation disorder in the rumen characterized by a lower than normal ruminal pH, but it reflects an imbalance between the microbial production, microbial utilization, and ruminal absorption of volatile fatty acids (VFAs) (Castillo et al. 2012). To maintain a neutral pH, the absorption of VFAs occurs by removing unionized acids and exchanging ionized VFAs for bicarbonate (HCO_3^-) during the absorption process. Consequently, a reduced rate of VFA absorption causes the ruminal pH to drop for two reasons: (i) ruminal VFAs accumulate and (ii) bicarbonate input from the blood stream is decreased (Owens et al. 1998). Based on different factors, like ruminal pH threshold, the predominant acid (VFA or lactic), and ruminal population bacteria, ruminal acidosis can be classified into two forms: acute and subacute acidosis.

Based on the degree of pH ruminal decrease, health disorders that result from acidogenic diets are classified as acute acidosis and subacute ruminal acidosis (SARA). Acute ruminal acidosis is a metabolic state defined by the decrease of blood pH and bicarbonate (Hernandez et al. 2014), the ruminal pH is less than 5.0 and the animals have depression, loss of appetite, reduced rumination, diarrhea, and dehydration (Laskoski et al. 2014); in these animals, microbial metabolism and food digestion are also affected, inflammatory processes occur, and milk fat decreases.

SARA is a common health and production problem occuring in ruminants with a low ruminal pH from a low fiber diet (Zhao et al. 2011). SARA is defined as a drop in rumen pH from 5.5 to 5.0 that is maintained for 111–180 minutes within a 24-hour period (Castillo-Lopez et al. 2014). SARA is a state of temporary disruption to the rumen that amends fermentation patterns; however, the intensity and duration are not sufficient to cause immediate clinical signs (Maulfair et al. 2013). The low ruminal pH characteristic of SARA may primarily be due to changes in the buffering capacities of carbonic acid and VFAs.

Another consequence of the reduction in pH is the decrease in digestible organic matter ingested and VFA production, which may be part of the rumen ecosystem self-regulatory mechanisms against ruminal acidosis. SARA is a pH-dependent disorder as well as the result of changes in the secondary microbial population and the type of diet fed (Calsamiglia et al. 2012).

5.2.1 Changes in Rumen Bacteria

Ruminal acidosis increases the growth rates of all bacteria in the rumen, which results in an increase in total VFA production and a decrease in ruminal pH. It is likely that the provision of increased substrates for microbial production, e.g. ammonia and peptides, will favor bacterial growth rather than VFA production. When large amounts of starch are added to the diet, the growth of *Streptococcus bovis* is no longer restricted by a lack of this energy source, and this population grows faster than other species of rumen bacteria. *S. bovis* produces lactic acid, an acid 10 times stronger than acetic, propionic, or butyric acid, whose accumulation eventually exceeds the buffering capacity of rumen fluid. Glucose produced from the breakdown of starch and other carbohydrates is converted to fructose 1,6-diphosphate. Russell and Hino (1985) found that fructose 1,6-diphosphate has a positive feedback on the conversion of pyruvate to lactate by activating lactate dehydrogenase. Fructose 1,6-diphosphate is also converted to triose phosphate in increasing concentrations. Triose phosphate acts to inhibit pyruvate formate-lyase. The net effect of these changes is a switch from predominantly acetate and formate production to lactate production (Russell and Hino 1985). Rumen lactate accumulates in two isomers: D-lactate, which is produced in lower amounts than L-lactate, whose absorption is greater than D-lactate; an increase of D-lactate ruminal absorption to the blood system can exhaust the buffering capacity of HCO_3^- and produce a generalized acidosis (Harmon et al. 1985). The ruminal microbiome is determined by the type of feed ingested by the ruminant, and rumen bacteria (*Ruminococcus*) predominate at pH 6.8 in cellulolytic diets. However, increasing concentrate in the diet and reducing the forage modifies the microbial population, changes the ruminal pH (5.5 and 6.5), and increases amylolytic bacteria such as *S. bovis* (Lean et al. 2007).

5.2.2 Changes to Rumen Motility

When VFA concentrations increase, there is also an initial decrease in reticuloruminal motility on receptors in the rumen wall. According to Crichlow and Chaplin (1985), the decrease in ruminal motility is independent of a decrease in rumen or systemic pH and occurs when venous blood concentrations are normal. A decrease in motility leads to a decrease in rumination and saliva production. Saliva contains high concentrations of bicarbonate ions and is an important buffering mechanism for the rumen.

5.2.3 Changes in Rumen pH and Lactic Acid Absorption

A decrease in bicarbonate and increase in lactic acid concentrations in the rumen further decreases ruminal pH. When ruminal pH is maintained above 5.5, equilibrium exists between producers and utilizers of lactic acid such that lactic acid does not accumulate in the rumen (Nocek 1997). When the pH is less than 5.5, no cellulolytic and relatively few saccharolytic bacteria – including *Prevotella ruminicola*, a significant producer of VFAs – survive. In contrast, *S. bovis* multiplies until ruminal pH is less than 5.0, a pH that allows an increase in *Lactobacillus* growth. Both of these bacterial species produce D- and L-lactic acid. D-lactate and L-lactate are absorbed across the rumen wall and depress blood pH. As L-lactate is metabolized more rapidly than D-lactate, the metabolic acidosis is due in large part to the accumulation of the latter (Bolton and Pass 1988). The lowered pH creates a ruminal environment hostile to protozoa and fungi, and both these populations fall precipitously. Chemical damage to the surface epithelium of the rumen mucosa occurs, which results in the adherence of debris and penetration by particulate matter from the rumen. Bacterial and mycotic organisms begin to invade the rumen wall, which causes ruminitis. Rumen papillae are damaged and can slough from the rumen wall (Lee et al. 1982). Absorption patterns change and endotoxins and histamine are released in the acute stages of the disease process (Mullenax et al. 1966).

5.2.4 Acidosis and Diarrhea

As lactate passes from the abomasum into the intestinal tract it creates an osmotic gradient. The resultant increase in fluid in the lumen is responsible for the profuse diarrhea and subsequent dehydration seen in clinical acidosis.

5.2.5 Morbidity and Case-fatality Rates

Usually, outbreaks of this disease occur in cattle herds kept on grain farms and in feedlots. Depending on the species of grain, the total amount eaten, and the previous experience of the animals, the morbidity will vary from 10% to 50%. The case-fatality rate may be up to 90% in untreated cases, whereas in treated cases it may still reach 30–40% (Constable et al. 2017).

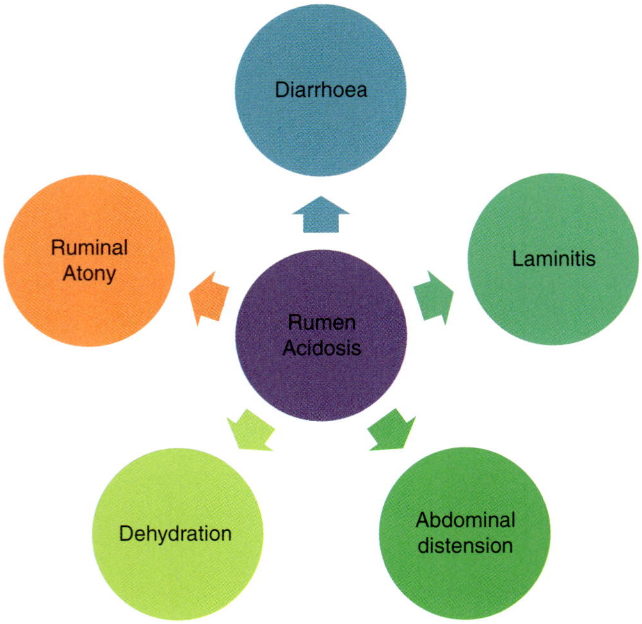

Figure 5.2 A clinical picture of rumen acidosis.

5.3 Clinical Signs

The clinical signs of ruminal acidosis usually reflect the severity of the case and are frequently not recognized or are too subtle for milder cases of ruminal acidosis, particularly as their onset can have a time lag after a predisposing event (Nordlund and Garrett 1994). As the pH of rumen intake severely decreases toward pH 5.0, the amplitude and frequency of rumen contractions progressively decrease until reaching rumen stasis. Three mechanisms may be responsible for ruminal atony after acidification of the rumen: (i) the effect of hydrogen ions on receptors in the gastrointestinal system, (ii) central inhibition by acid absorption, and (iii) inhibition by amines or absorbed toxins (Huber 1976). Ruminal atony manifests as a poor appetite because if the rumen is not functioning then degradation and nutrient absorption through the ruminal epithelium do not occur and animals stop eating (González et al. 2012). In acute acidosis, the rumen epithelium alters its function and structure; with diets high in grains, the rumen papillae show a large detachment of the corneum stratum and the adhesion of cells is affected, causing the appearance of large gaps between cells across the layer (Steel et al. 2009). As the ruminal epithelium is damaged, an inflammatory process that causes pain in ruminants begins and manifests as the clenching of teeth, loss of appetite, and ruminal atony. Pharmacologically active amines have been detected within the rumen intake from animals with acidosis, such as histamine that comes from histidine decarboxylation when the rumen intake approaches a of pH 5.0 or less (Huber 1976). Histamine release in the rumen and its absorption into the circulatory system allow these compounds to reach the extremities where they cause inflammatory reactions such as laminitis, which causes pain when moving. Another consequence of ruminal acidosis is that the fluid balance is affected. Animals that develop ruminal acidosis may experience diarrhea and dehydration with consequent fluid loss and an increase in the hematocrit, which decreases the elasticity of the skin. The rumen fluid becomes hypertonic compared to plasma, therefore water is absorbed from the blood system into the rumen and the water lost from the body and blood enters the rumen (Huber 1976). Fluid loss through feces is high during diarrhea and occurs when rumen motility is inhibited, which suggests a net movement of body water toward the intestines (Figure 5.2).

5.4 Diagnosis

A diagnosis can be made primarily based on clinical observations such as ruminal movement, temperature, pulse, respiration rate, heart rate, and rumen fluid analysis. In ruminal acidosis, the pH of rumen liquor is less than 5.2, its color is milky gray or brown, its consistency is watery, both MBRT and sedimentation activity time are increased, and rumen protozoal motility is decreased (Petrovski 2017). The clinical signs of ruminal acidosis usually reflect the severity of the case and are frequently not recognized or are too subtle in milder cases of ruminal acidosis as their onset can have a time lag after a predisposing event (Nordlund and Garrett 1994). The occurrence of milder ruminal acidosis is often a herd problem and is difficult to diagnose in individuals. In the case of a single animal affected with ruminal acidosis, a physical examination should be performed that includes the measurement of heart rate, respiration rate, rate of rumen contractions, and body temperature. The locomotion, body condition, perineal staining, fecal consistency, and rumen fill should also be scored (Bramley et al. 2012). Further, demeanor, dehydration, and sites of pain should be assessed. Samples of rumen fluid should be taken; we prefer to use stomach tube methods. Cattle with rumen perturbations consistent with subacute acidosis may present with a range of clinical and subclinical signs that include: diarrhea, poor body condition, a dull and lethargic demeanor, dehydration, a lack of rumen fill, lameness, weak rumen contractions, depression in milk fat, and inappetence.

For acute acidosis: Ruminal distension, diarrhea (often with grain in the feces and a sickly, sweet smell), abdominal pain, tachycardia, tachypnea, staggering, recumbency, coma, a marked decline in milk yield, and death may occur (Oetzel 2000). The speed of progression for clinical signs may depend on the severity of rumen perturbation, but death can occur within 12–24 hours in peracute cases (Dirksen 1970).

For chronic cases: Lameness with poverty lines, evidence of disseminated infections (especially hepatic and pulmonary), sporadic nosebleeds, and declines in milk production and weight loss may occur. The key considerations in diagnosing acute cases of acidosis are a history of: (i) access to sugars – sources of which include forage beets, turnips, cereals that are frosted (e.g. oats, wheats), sugar, fruit, and molasses – and (ii) access to rapidly fermentable starch, grains have the following order of increasing risk for acidosis: wheat, triticale, barley, oats, maize, and sorghum (Opatpatanakit et al. 1994).

Laminitis occurs in acute, subclinical, and chronic forms that are associated with varying degrees of ruminal acidosis severity (Figure 5.3). The association between acidosis and laminitis appears to be associated with altered hemodynamics of the peripheral microvasculature. Vasoactive substances are released during the decline of rumen pH as well as bacteriolysis and tissue degradation (Figure 5.3). These substances cause vasoconstriction and dilatation, which injure the microvasculature of the corium. Ischemia causes a reduction in the oxygen and nutrients that reach the extremities of the corium and cell swelling. Ischemia causes physical degradation of junctures between tissues that are structurally critical for locomotion, and cell swelling within an enclosed noncompliant structure such as the hoof can further decrease blood flow within the digit. The insidious rotation of the distal phalanx (pedal bone) can result in permanent anatomic change (Constable et al. 2017).

5.4.1 Confirmation of Diagnosis

Samples of rumen fluids consistent with acute acidosis have a low pH, i.e. less than 5, and changes in the rumen fluid that include a milky white appearance, the presence of grain (if grain overload is the cause), and a sickly sweet smell.

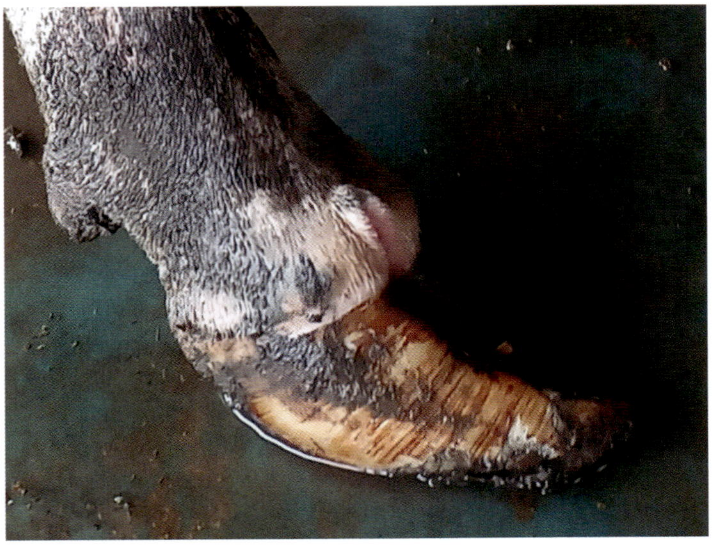

Figure 5.3 A hoof with chronic laminitis in a cow affected with rumen acidosis.

5.4.2 Parameters of the Study

History: A complete history of the animal should be recorded, including the ingestion of a large amount of grains or fermented feed, age, breed, sex, and duration of illness.

Clinical examination: Animals should be clinically examined for the presence of symptoms like a distended abdomen, diarrhea, dehydration, anorexia, laminitis, etc.

Body temperature (°F): The rectal temperature of the animal should be recorded using a clinical thermometer. Variation in the temperature of the affected animal may be due to mild dehydration resulting from diarrhea, in the case of ruminal acidosis.

Pulse rate: In cases of ruminal acidosis, the pulse rate is usually increased. The increase in the pulse rate might be due to the toxic effects of lactic acid that have accumulated in the body and a reduced plasma volume due to dehydration (Tufani et al. 2013).

Respiratory rate (per minute): An increased respiration rate in an acidosis-affected animal might be due to the stimulation of the respiratory center caused by an increased carbon dioxide tension of the blood and decreased blood pH (Ullah et al. 2013).

Ruminal motility (per minute): Ruminal motility should be recorded by palpating the left flank of the animal, and ruminal contractions should be recorded per minute. A complete cessation or decrease in ruminal motility in ruminal acidosis may result due to muscular atony from the depression of sympathetic and sympathomimetic ganglion (Rahman et al. 2014).

5.4.3 Sample Collection

5.4.3.1 Collection of Rumen Fluid

Three techniques for rumen fluid collection may be used to determine the ruminal pH.

5.4.3.2 Rumen Cannula

The collection of ruminal contents from cattle with an indwelling ruminal cannula remains the preferred method for determining ruminal pH. However, practical limitations, including the need to regularly clean and monitor rumen cannula sites, limit their use in commercial situations. Some large dairy herds have rumen-cannulated cows to provide a ready monitor of rumen function and provide fluid for transfaunation, although this is not common practice in Australia.

5.4.3.3 Rumenocentesis

The collection of ruminal fluid using percutaneous needle aspiration is a more practical method for determining ruminal pH. Rumen fluid is collected using a 14-gauge, 1.5-inch (about 4 cm) disposable needle attached to a 30-ml eccentric syringe. A 2×2 cm area is shaved on the left paralumbar fossa approximately one hand length ventral to the lumbar spinal transverse processes and one hand width caudal to the last rib, avoiding the major muscle masses. This area is surgically prepared, a local anesthetic injected, and the sampling needle is inserted firmly through into the rumen. A minimum of 4 ml should be obtained from most animals using this procedure.

5.4.3.4 Rumen Stomach Tube

A stomach tube suited to collecting ruminal fluid can be constructed using a 3.5-m long, 19-mm diameter, plastic-reinforced garden hose attached to an equine stomach pump. The other end should be riveted to a 10–15 cm length of copper pipe with multiple holes drilled along all sides. This reduces the risk of blockages with ingesta. Samples of ruminal fluid taken by stomach tube have a higher pH than those obtained through a rumen cannula (Erdman 1988), either as a result of salivary contamination or sampling in the fiber mat of the rumen. Therefore, ruminal pH samples collected by stomach tube should be interpreted with caution. This method will be more specific but less sensitive for the detection of acidosis. The rumen fluid collected from the stomach tube should be examined for evidence of saliva contamination before measuring pH and the samples discarded if contaminated. The most accurate field test for ruminal pH is rumenocentesis.

Rumen fluid examination: It should be conducted by physical, chemical, and microscopic examinations of ruminal fluid as per the method described by Petrovski (2017).

- **Physical characteristics**
  - Color: The color should be assessed by visual inspection after placing the ruminal fluid in a glass tube. The color of admixtures (e.g. large feed particles) should be ignored. Due to the prolonged stasis of rumen that occurs in ruminal acidosis, the rumen fluid changes to a milky gray or greenish black color (Constable et al. 2017).

- Consistency: Rumen fluid consistency should be assessed by slowly turning a glass tube half filled with rumen fluid 45–60° to the left and right from an upright position. The watery consistency of rumen fluid in a ruminal acidosis–affected animal might be due to the passage of fluid from vascular bed into the rumen because of the increased osmolarity of ruminal content (Ram et al. 2007).
- Sedimentation activity time (SAT): This test should be carried out on a fresh sample (less than 2 hours old) in a test tube. The assessment is based on the time required for the sedimentation of the fine particles and flotation of the coarser particles to occur. A prolonged SAT of rumen fluid may occur due to the depletion of normal ruminal microbiota and infusoria in the acidotic animal.

- **Chemical characteristics**
  - Rumen fluid pH: Rumen fluid pH should be measured using a digital pH meter. It should be measured within a few minutes of collection (Figure 5.4). A decrease in the pH of the ruminal fluid in the affected animal may be due to increased production of VFAs like acetic acid, propionic acid, and butyric acid. The decrease in rumen pH favors the growth of streptococci with a decline in the number of normal gram-negative bacteria and protozoa, which further aggravates the process of lactic acid production (Ullah et al. 2013).
  - MBRT: This test should be conducted shortly after the collection of ruminal fluid by mixing 0.5 ml of 0.04% methylene blue with 10 ml of rumen fluid in a plain tube. The time for decolorization from blue to normal should be measured in minutes. An increased MBRT might be due to the presence of inactive microbiota during ruminal acidosis, which takes more than 15 minutes to reduce methylene blue, whereas in the presence of normal active rumen microbiota, it is reduced within 3 minutes (Sharma et al. 2009).
  - Cellulose digestion test: The test should be conducted by mixing 10 ml of rumen fluid with 0.3 ml of 16% glucose in a test tube. Then a pure cellulose thread, weighted by a glass bead, is immersed in the mixture and incubated at 39 °C. The time for the bead to drop to the bottom of the test tube should be recorded. The reason for prolonged or absent cellulose thread digestion in an acidotic animal might be due to the fact that destruction of the normal microbiota (cellulolytic bacteria) of the rumen and a shift in their pattern from gram-negative to gram-positive nature. This indicates a gross inactivity of rumen microbes that results in a disturbance of the normal digestive process (Ram et al. 2007).

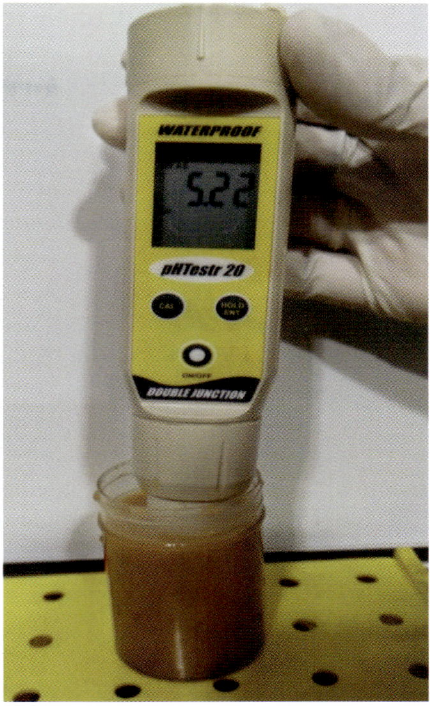

Figure 5.4 Measurement of rumen fluid pH using a digital pH meter.

- **Microscopic examination**
  - Rumen fluid protozoa: The activity and number of rumen fluid protozoa should be assessed as per the method described by Petrovski (2017). A drop of fresh rumen fluid should be placed on a microscope slide and viewed under a low power objective. The assessment should be completed by counting the number of protozoa present per field and the protozoa that enter a single microscopic field within 30 seconds. The absence of rumen protozoa in a ruminal acidosis–affected animal might be attributed to the fact that normal protozoa in the rumen could be destroyed by the changed rumen ecosystem (Figure 5.5), i.e. an increase in lactate and lactate-producing gram-positive bacteria causes an increasingly abnormal fermentation process in the rumen (Tambe et al. 2017). The predominantly gram-negative bacterial microbiota of the rumen is replaced by a gram-positive one.

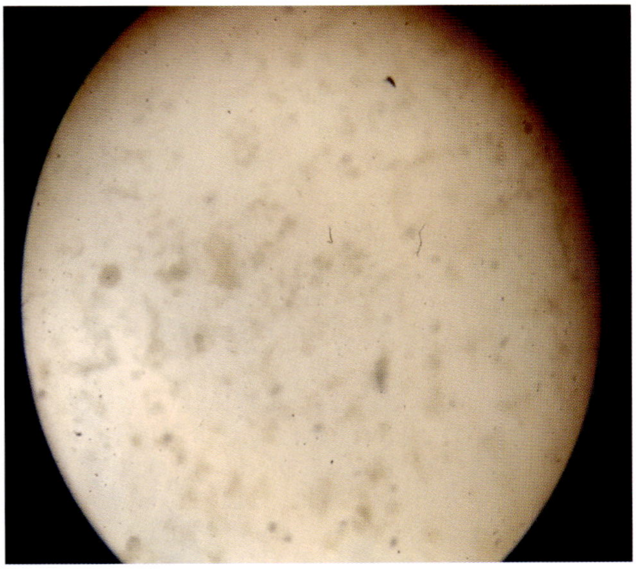

Figure 5.5 Microscopic image devoid of rumen protozoa in the rumen fluid of a ruminal acidosis–affected cow.

5.5 Therapeutic Approach Toward Ruminal Acidosis

In an outbreak, some animals will not require any treatment, whereas severely affected cases will need a rumenotomy. For those that are not severely affected, it is often difficult to decide whether to treat them only medically with alkalinizing agents orally and systemically or to do a rumenotomy. Each case must be examined clinically, and the most appropriate treatment selected. The degree of mental depression, muscular strength, degree of dehydration, heart rate, body temperature, and rumen pH are clinical parameters that can be used to assess severity and determine the treatment most likely to be successful.

The treatment of ruminal acidosis mainly depends upon its severity. It is primarily focused on addressing the plasma volume deficit, correcting acid–base disturbances, and restoring a normal rumen microenvironment.

In the case of clinical acidosis, treatment can be difficult, and chances of success depend on the severity of the case. Individual cattle can be treated successfully, however, if a significant proportion of the herd is involved, a triage approach is critical. While in severe cases (dehydration > 8%, collapsed and subnormal temperature, static rumen, and evidence of diarrhea) treatment can be unrewarding, time consuming, and expensive. These cases should only be treated when economic value determines that the attempt is warranted (RAGFAR 2007).

Sodium bicarbonate at 1 g/kg body weight (BW) dissolved in 10 l of water given via stomach tube, followed by 0.5 g/kg BW of sodium bicarbonate dissolved in 5 l of water given by stomach tube every 6 hours for an additional two to three treatments are mainstays in the treatment of ruminal acidosis. Sodium bicarbonate results in the release of carbon dioxide (CO_2) from the solution and eventually, from the rumen via belching, which directly neutralizes the ruminal acidity (Kohn and Dunlap 1998). It can increase the osmolarity, water consumption, production of saliva, and therefore, increases the dilution rate of VFAs in the rumen (Gastaldello et al. 2013). However, 0.5 g/kg BW of magnesium hydroxide suspended in 5 l of water given via stomach tube only once, after the first sodium bicarbonate, is also very effective. Other symptomatic and supportive therapy includes the use of anti-inflammatories such as flunixin meglumine at 1 mg/kg BW intravenously every 8 hours for a maximum of three treatments (other alternate anti-inflammatories are fine, e.g. ketoprofen). Thiamine at 10 mg/kg BW given by intramuscular injection every 24 hours for three treatments is also helpful because the abnormal growth of thiaminase-producing bacteria inside the rumen causes thiamine deficiency. Thiamine aids lactic acid metabolism and thus prevents further systemic lactic acidosis (Tufani et al. 2013). Procaine penicillin G at 12 mg/kg BW given by intramuscular injection twice daily for 3 days is also an option. To counteract histamine released due to ruminitis as well as to reduce histamine levels in the rumen and blood (Ram et al. 2007), 1 ml/50 kg BW of chlorpheniramine maleate can be given by intramuscular injection every 8 hours for four treatments. Sometimes 250 ml calcium borogluconate (either straight or 4 : 1) subcutaneously is also used. Offering clover or legume and oat hay with monitoring and the re-introduction of grain in the feed may also be helpful.

In severe cases, instigate and maintain the treatments outlined above and inject 7500 mg of procaine penicillin G into the rumen via the left paralumbar fossa. The intraruminal administration of procaine penicillin G might be helpful in reducing the pathogenic ruminal bacteria population and restoring the normal rumen microbiota (Constable et al. 2017). Administer 2 l of hypertonic saline slowly intravenously and 5–7 l of 5% sodium bicarbonate solution intravenously over approximately 30 minutes. Sometimes a further 150 ml/kg BW of isotonic (1.3%) sodium bicarbonate solution may need to be administered intravenously over the next 12 hours. At times the condition is so serious that a rumenotomy is needed to evacuate the rumen and replace the rumen contents with at least 12 l of contents obtained by stomach tube from one or several other cows (RAGFAR 2007).

5.6 Preventive Approach Toward Ruminal Acidosis

Prevent accidental access to grain. Perform gradual introductions to high level grain diets in feedlots. Total mixed rations that contain chopped roughage and grain help ensure a controlled intake of carbohydrates. Use careful feeding management of dairy cattle during late pregnancy and early lactation. The use of ionophores in feed alter rumen metabolism and can potentially control ruminal acidosis. For preventing the occurrence of ruminal acidosis there are some points on which we need to focus, and these are described in this section.

5.6.1 Diet Form, Formulation, and Function

Diets formulated as partial mixed rations were safer, despite a higher nonfibrous carbohydrate (NFC) content than diets that were component-fed. Sugars in the diet should be controlled based on Golder 2014. We suggest the following guidelines for total mixed rations (TMR) based on Golder (2014) for a maximum total NFC of 40–42%, 22–24% starch, and 8% sugar, based on not exceeding approximately 0.35% of the BW for sugar intake. It is very likely that not all sugars will have the same effect on the rumen (Plaizier et al. 2018), and it is very evident that not all grains (Lean et al. 2013) or starches have the same effect on rumen function. Further, the form of processing the concentrate components in the diet will influence function.

5.6.2 Total Mixed Rations

One of the safest procedures is to feed a milled mixed ration that consists of 50–60% roughage and 40–50% grain as the starting ration for 7–10 days and monitor the response. If results are satisfactory, decrease the level of roughage by 10% every 2–4 days, down to 10–15% roughage with the remainder grain and a vitamin–mineral–salt supplement. The use of roughage-grain mixtures ensures that cattle do not engorge themselves on grain, and adaptation can occur in about 21 days (Constable et al. 2017).

5.6.3 Buffers and Neutralizing Agents

Buffering agent requirements in the diet are based on the buffer capacity of the saliva secreted, buffer capacity of the food, and diet acidity (Erdman 1988). Buffer substance supplementation can be a way to limit the adverse effects of ruminal acidosis and can be added in whole rations from 0.5% to 2.5%. The following compounds have been used: sodium bicarbonate, disodium carbonate, magnesium oxide, potassium carbonate, and anhydrous limestone (Gastaldello et al. 2013). In dairy cows, a meta-analysis of 40 publications with several buffer substances was conducted: sodium bicarbonate, disodium carbonate, magnesium oxide, potassium monoanhydro carbonate, monosodium carbonate, and magnesium oxide; the dry matter intake was improved in 0.15 kg/d, milk production 0.52 kg/d, and fat percentage 0.15%. The addition of sodium bicarbonate results in the release of CO_2 from the solution and eventually, from the rumen via belching. This process directly neutralizes ruminal acidity. The extent to which the process proceeds depends on the partial pressure of CO_2 in the gas phase, the pH, and a constant (7.74), according to the Henderson–Hasselbalch equation: $pH = 7.74 + \log[(HCO_3^-)/CO_2 \text{ pressure in atmospheres}]$ (Kohn and Dunlap 1998). Sodium bicarbonate can increase the osmolarity, water consumption, saliva production, and therefore, the dilution rate of VFAs in the rumen and the passage rate of the liquid phase (Gastaldello et al. 2013).

5.6.3.1 Antibiotics

While these are subject to regulatory change, there is strong evidence that some antibiotics can control the risk of acidosis (Lean et al. 2014). Tylosin has been widely used in finishing diets for the US beef industry. Virginiamycin is effective at controlling acidosis, and tylosin, in combination with monensin, is also effective. It appears that combinations of monensin and bambermycin are also effective at favorably modifying rumen function. Both of the latter are nonhuman-class therapeutical agents.

5.6.3.2 Ionophores

Ionophores, particularly monensin and lasalocid, are widely used in beef and dairy production. There is evidence of a more sustained appetite (Lunn et al. 2005) and increased production of propionate from lactate – a ruminal adaptation that sequesters hydrogen ions in safer ruminal pools – when monensin is fed in diets that may cause acidosis. Monensin appears to be very effective at controlling acidosis risk when fed with tylosin or virginiamycin. Nagaraja et al. (1981) investigated the use of lasalocid to control lactic acidosis induced using finely ground corn or glucose. The use of lasalocid equaled or exceeded the reduction in lactic acid production observed for monensin (Nagaraja et al. 1981). Both monensin and lasalocid prevented acute lactic acidosis in a study by Nagaraja et al. (1981); however, both products were included in the diet at concentrations of 1.30 ppm, and the above concentrations were recommended. Nagaraja et al. (1982) found that 0.33, 0.65, and 1.30 ppm of lasalocid were effective at reducing lactic acid concentrations and increasing pH compared to control cattle with induced lactic acidosis (using glucose at 12.5 g/kg). More studies would be useful to evaluate the effect of lasalocid on rumen acidosis.

5.6.3.3 Yeasts

There is increasing evidence that yeasts and yeast cultures may have a role in stabilizing rumen function. Actions that have been identified with live yeasts include small increases in rumen pH, reductions in lactic acid, enhanced fiber digestion, alterations in immune function, and small increases in VFA production. These actions are modest in magnitude but may synergize with other strategies to control the risk of acidosis. Li et al. (2016) found that a *Saccharomyces cerevisiae* fermentation product stabilized rumen pH, and Bach et al. (2018) demonstrated changes in immune markers in the epithelium and rumen due to live yeast. Weight gains and average daily gain improvements have been identified in beef cattle fed hydrolyzed yeast, and reductions in severe liver abscess incidence were also noted with autolyzed yeast (Ran et al. 2018). While these findings are encouraging, it is challenging to understand the differences between yeast-based products and the best application of these in the field.

5.6.3.4 Probiotics

There is also some evidence that probiotics may provide benefits in terms of acidosis control; however, there are challenges in this area as candidate agents such as *Megasphera elsdenii* have not provided clear and consistent benefits in studies to date. It seems likely that more studies will investigate the roles of other acidosis control agents in the future.

5.6.4 Vaccination Against Lactic Acidosis

Some preliminary research has investigated the immunization of cattle against lactic acid–producing bacteria, *S. bovis* and *Lactobacillus*. Immunization induced high levels of persistent saliva antibody responses against *S. bovis* and *Lactobacillus*, which reduced the risk of lactic acidosis in cattle.

References

Aschenbach, J.R. and Gabel, G. (2000). Effect and absorption of histamine in sheep rumen: significance of acidotic epithelial damage. *Journal of Animal Science* 78: 464–470.

Bach, A., Guasch, I., Elcoso, G. et al. (2018). Changes in gene expression in the rumen and colon epithelia during the dry period through lactation of dairy cows and effects of live yeast supplementation. *Journal of Dairy Science* 101: 2631–2640.

Bolton, J.R. and Pass, D.A. (1988). The alimentary tract. In: *Clinicopathologic Principles for Veterinary Medicine* (ed. W.F. Robinson and C.R.R. Huxtable), 99–121. Cambridge: Cambridge University Press.

Bramley, E., Lean, I.J., Fulkerson, W.J., and Costa, N.D. (2012). Feeding management and feeds on dairy farms in New South Wales and Victoria. *Animal Production Science* 52: 20–29.

Braun, U., Rih, T., and Schefer, U. (1992). Ruminal lactic acidosis in sheep and goats. *The Veterinary Record* 130 (16): 343–349.

Calsamiglia, S., Blanch, M., Ferret, A., and Moya, D. (2012). Is subacute acidosis a pH related problem? Causes and tools for its control. *Animal Feed Science and Technology* 172: 42–50.

Castillo, C., Hernandez, J., Pereira, V., and Benedito, J.L. (2012). Update about nutritional strategies in feedlot for preventing ruminal acidosis. In: *Advances in Zoology Research*, vol. 4 (ed. O.P. Jenkins), 1–84. New York, NY, USA: Nova Science Publishers.

Castillo-López, E., Wiese, B., Hendrick, S. et al. (2014). Incidence, prevalence, severity and risk factors for ruminal acidosis in feedlot steers during back grounding diet transition, and finishing. *Journal of Animal Science* 92: 3053–3063.

Constable, P.D., Hinchcliff, K.W., Done, S.H., and Grunberg, W. (2017). *Veterinary Medicine: A Textbook of the Diseases of Cattle, Horses, Sheep, Pigs and Goats*, 11e, 461–472. Missouri: Elsevier.

Crichlow, E.C. and Chaplin, R.K. (1985). Ruminal lactic acidosis: relationship of forestomach motility to nondissociated volatile fatty acids levels. *American Journal of Veterinary Research* 46 (9): 1908–1911.

Dirksen, G. (1970). Acidosis. Pages 612-625 in Proc. 3rd International Symposium on the Physiology of Digestion and Metabolism in the Ruminant. Oriel Press, Newcastle, England.

Erdman, R.A. (1988). Dietary buffering requirements of the lactating dairy cow: a review. *Journal of Dairy Science* 71: 3246–3266.

Gastaldello, A., Pires, A., Susin, I. et al. (2013). Limestone with different particle size and sodium bicarbonate to feedlot lambs fed high grain diets with or without monensin. *Small Ruminant Research* 114: 80–85.

Golder, H.M. (2014). Increased understandings of ruminal acidosis in dairy cattle. Doctoral dissertation. University of Sydney.

González, L., Manteca, X., Calsamiglia, S. et al. (2012). Ruminal acidosis in feedlot cattle: interplay between feed ingredients, rumen function and feeding behavior (a review). *Animal Feed Science and Technology* 172: 66–79.

Harmon, D.L., Britton, R.A., Prior, R.L., and Stock, R.A. (1985). Net portal absorption of lactate and volatile fatty acids in steers experiencing glucose-induced acidosis or fed a 70% concentrate diet ad libitum. *Journal of Animal Science* 60: 560–569.

Hernandez, J., Benedito, J.L., Abuelo, A., and Castello, C. (2014). Rumnal acidosis in feedlot: from aetiology to prevention. *The Scientific World Journal* 1: 1–8.

Huber, T.L. (1976). Physiological effects of acidosis on feedlot cattle. *Journal of Animal Science* 43 (4): 902–909.

Kohn, R. and Dunlap, T. (1998). Calculation of the buffering capacity of bicarbonate in the rumen an in vitro. *Journal of Animal Science* 76: 1702–1709.

Laskoski, L.M., Muraro, L.S., Santana Júnior, M.S. et al. (2014). Sodium bicarbonate as prevention of metabolic acidosis in sheep submitted to experimental ruminal acidosis. *Pesquisa Veterinaria Brasileira* 34: 822–826.

Lean, I., Annison, F., Bramley, E. et al. (2007). Ruminal acidosis-understandings, prevention and treatment. A review for veterinarians and nutritional professionals. *Australian Veterinary Association* 3: 46.

Lean, I.J., Golder, H.M., Black, J.L. et al. (2013). In vivo indices for predicting acidosis risk of grains in cattle: comparison with in vitro methods. *Journal of Animal Science* 91: 2823–2835.

Lean, I.J., Golder, H.M., and Hall, M.B. (2014). Feeding, evaluating, and controlling rumen function. *Veterinary Clinics of North America: Food Animal A* 30: 539–575.

Lee, G.J., McManus, W.R. et al. (1982). Changes in rumen fluid composition and in the rumen epithelium when wheat is introduced to the diet of sheep: the influence of wheat and Hay consumption. *Australian Journal of Agricultural Research* 33: 321–333.

Li, S., Yoon, I., Scott, M. et al. (2016). Impact of *Saccharomyces cerevisiae* fermentation product and subacute ruminal acidosis on production, inflammation, and fermentation in the rumen and hindgut of dairy cows. *Animal Feed Science and Technology* 211: 50–60.

Lunn, D., Mutsvangwa, T., Odongo, N. et al. (2005). Effect of monensin on meal frequency during sub-acute ruminal acidosis in dairy cows. *Canadian Journal of Animal Science* 85: 247–249.

Maulfair, D., Mcintyre, K., and Heinrichs, A. (2013). Subacute rumial acidosis and total mixed ration preference in lactating dairy cows. *Journal of Dairy Science* 96: 6610–6620.

Mullenax, C.H., Keeler, R.F. et al. (1966). Physiologic responses of ruminants to toxic factors extracted from rumen Bacteria and rumen fluid. *American Journal of Veterinary Research* 27: 857–868.

Nagaraja, T.G., Avery, T.B., Bartley, E.E. et al. (1981). Prevention of lactic acidosis in cattle by lasalocid or monensin. *Journal of Animal Science* 53: 206–216.

Nagaraja, T.G., Avery, T.B., Bartley, E.E. et al. (1982). Effect of lasalocid, monensin or thiopeptin on lactic acidosis in cattle. *Journal of Animal Science* 54: 649–658.

Nocek, J.E. (1997). Bovine acidosis: implications on laminitis. *Journal of Dairy Science* 80 (5): 1005–1028.

Nordlund, K.V. and Garrett, E.F. (1994). Rumenocentesis – a technique for collecting rumen fluid for the diagnosis of subacute rumen acidosis in dairy herds. *The Bovine Practitioners* 28: 109–112.

Oetzel, G.R. (2000). Clinical aspects of ruminal acidosis in dairy cattle. *Proceedings of the Thirty-Third Annual Conference, American Association of Bovine Practitioners*, Rapid City, South Dakota, USA (21–23 September 2000). Fort Collins, CO: Frontier Printers, Inc.

Opatpatanakit, Y., Kellaway, R., Lean, I. et al. (1994). Microbial fermentation of cereal grains in vitro. *Australian Journal of Agricultural Research* 45: 1247–1263.

Owens, F.N., Secrist, D.S., Hill, W.J., and Gill, D.R. (1998). Acidosis in cattle: a review. *Journal of Animal Science* 76 (1): 275–286.

Petrovski, K.R. (2017). Assessment of the rumen fluid of a bovine patient. *Journal of Dairy and Veterinary Sciences* 2: 1–7.

Plaizier, J.C., Derakhshani, H., Golder, H. et al. (2018). Invited review: enhancing gut health in dairy cows. *Animal* 12 (Suppl 2): s399–s418.

Rahman, M.D., Islam, M.S., Adam, G.O. et al. (2014). Prevalence of ruminal lactic acidosis and clinical assessment of four therapeutics in goats of Bangladesh. *Journal of Veterinary Clinics* 31 (3): 0–6.

Ram, P.K., Verma, S.P., Agarwal, A.K., and Jayachandra, C. (2007). Effect of severity of acidosis on ruminal activity in goats. *Indian Journal of Animal Research* 41: 256–260.

Ran, T., Shen, Y., Saleem, A.M. et al. (2018). Using ruminally protected and nonprotected active dried yeast as alternatives to antibiotics in finishing beef steers: growth performance, carcass traits, blood metabolites, and fecal Escherichia coli. *Journal of Animal Science* 96: 4385–4397.

Reference Advisory Group on Fermentative Acidosis of Ruminants (RAGFAR) (2007). *Ruminal Acidosis – Aetiopathogenesis, Prevention and Treatment. A Review for Veterinarians and Nutritional Professionals*. (ed. A. V. Association). Carlton, Vic. Australia: Blackwell Publishing Asia Pty. Ltd.

Russell, J.B. and Hino, T. (1985). Regulation of lactate production in *Streptococcus bovis*: a spiraling effect that contributes to rumen acidosis. *Journal of Dairy Science* 68: 1712–1721.

Sharma, M.C., Kumar, M., and Sharma, R.D. (2009). *Textbook of Clinical Veterinary Medicine*, 134–137. New Delhi: Indian Council of Agricultural Research.

Steel, M., Alzahal, O., Hook, D. et al. (2009). Ruminal acidosis and the rapid onset of ruminal parakeratosis in a mature dairy cow: a case report. *Acta Veterinaria Scandinavica* 51: 39.

Tambe, S.V., Padmaja, K., Nagaraj, P., and Reddy, A.G. (2017). Therapeutic studies of ruminal acidosis in goats. *The Pharma Innovation Journal* 6: 44–48.

Tufani, N.A., Makhdoomi, D.M., and Hafiz, A. (2013). Rumen acidosis in small ruminants and its therapeutic management. *Iranian Journal of Applied Animal Science* 3: 19–24.

Ullah, H.A., Khan, J.A., Khan, M.S. et al. (2013). Clinico-therapeutical trials of lactic acidosis in small ruminants. *Journal of Animal and Plant Sciences* 23 (1): 80–83.

Vuuren, A.D.V., Calsamiglia, S., and Udén, P. (2012). Rumen health: a 360° analysis. *Animal Feed Science Techniques* 172: 1–3.

Warner, A. and Vaziri, N.D. (1981). Treatment of lactic acidosis. *Southern Medical Journal* 74: 841–847.

Zhao, X., Zhang, T., Xu, M., and Yao, J. (2011). Effects of physically effective fiber on chewing activity, ruminal fermentation, and digestibility in goats. *Journal of Dairy Science* 89: 501–509.

6

Ketosis

Sarita Devi[1], Ankit S. Prajapati[1], Chitra D. Chauhan[1], and Rajesh Kumar[2]

[1] *Department of Veterinary Medicine, College of Veterinary Science and Animal Husbandry, Kamdhenu University, Sardarkrushinagar, Gujarat, India*
[2] *Department of Veterinary Gynaecology and Obstetrics, College of Veterinary Science and Animal Husbandry, Acharya Narendra Deva University of Agriculture and Technology, Ayodhya, Uttar Pradesh, India*

6.1 Introduction

In modern dairy production, as productivity rises, ketosis has emerged as a prevalent metabolic disease during the periparturient period (also called the transition period) (Figure 6.1). The 3 weeks before and 3 weeks following parturition comprise the transition period (Contreras and Sordillo 2011). Cows with higher milk production are more likely to suffer from ketosis (Januś and Borkowska 2013). While ketosis can affect cows of all parities, research and observation have indicated that the risk of ketosis tends to increase with increasing parity. Ketosis in dairy cows was first documented in the 1950s (Holmes 1950). Stinson identified ketosis as an issue for the first time between 1920 and 1930; it is also known as acetonemia or ketosis (Zhang et al. 2012). The impaired metabolism of carbohydrates and volatile fatty acids results in ketosis (Constable et al. 2016). Ketosis is characterized by elevated levels of ketone bodies in an affected cow's blood, urine, and milk. Ketones are a group of organic compounds that are intermediate metabolites of fat and include acetone (AC; formed because of spontaneous decarboxylation of acetoacetate), acetoacetic acid (ACAC; as anion-acetoacetate), and β-hydroxybutyric acid (BHBA; as anion-β-hydroxybutyrate). Lethargy, a drop in dry matter intake (DMI), decreased milk output and quality, and frequently, a sweet-smelling breath are the main clinical manifestations of ketosis (McArt et al. 2013).

6.1.1 Significance of Gluconeogenesis in Ruminants

Gluconeogenesis is continuously required for the regulation of energy metabolism in ruminants. In ruminants, 80% of the dietary carbohydrates are fermented by rumen microbes to short-chain volatile fatty acids, mainly acetate (70%), propionate (20%), and butyrate (10%). The rumen weighs between one-seventh and one-tenth of the animal's total weight and has an 80 l capacity. Rumen microbes include large, diversified communities of strictly anaerobic microorganisms, including bacteria, protozoa, and fungus. Propionate is the only volatile fatty acid among these three that majorly contributes to gluconeogenesis (Overton and Waldron 2004). Propionate production is favored by a high grain inclusion in an animal's diet (Herdt 2000). The diet's propionic acid enters the tricarboxylic acid (TCA) cycle and is then transformed into glucose via gluconeogenesis. Glucose is synthesized in the liver and renal cortex by the gluconeogenic pathway. Additionally, microbial amino acids and proteins, lactic acid, and glycerol are considered essential precursors for gluconeogenesis.

6.2 Pathogenesis

During the early lactation stage, cows experience increased energy requirements due to various factors. One of the primary reasons is the production and secretion of milk. A significant amount of energy is needed to support milk production and overall cow health. Additionally, the milk contains sugar, protein, and fat derived from the cows' body reserves. Effective

Periparturient Diseases of Cattle, First Edition. Edited by Tanmoy Rana.

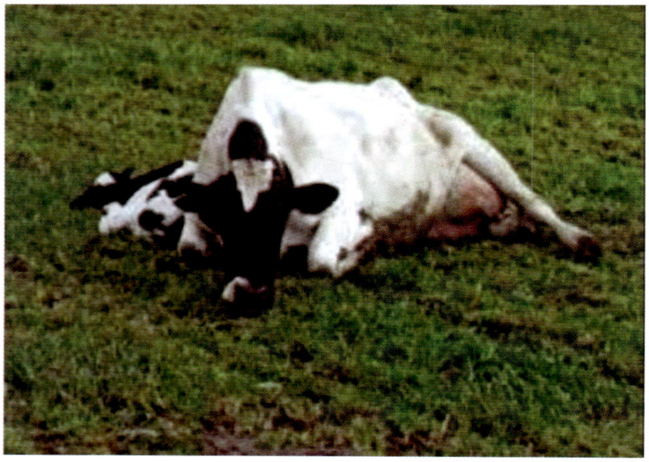

Figure 6.1 Ketosis in a crossbred cow. *Source:* Photo courtesy of Dr. Nasir Ali, Health Executive at Sharif Dairy Farm Private Limited, Chiniot, Punjab, Pakistan.

gluconeogenesis is crucial in high yielding dairy cows because it is the main mechanism for conferring a sufficient supply of glucose for the udder (Reynolds et al. 1998). Cow body systems continue to function normally if their diets are sufficient for drawing energy from a carbohydrate source and if hepatic glycogen reserves are also available. However, if the cow's diet is insufficient to maintain adequate blood glucose levels, it results in the depletion of hepatic glycogen reserves, and a condition arises called a negative energy balance (NEB).

In dairy cows, the peak of daily milk production is commonly observed at around 4–6 weeks of lactation. On the other hand, the peak in DMI often occurs later, typically between 9 and 11 weeks of lactation (Guliński 2021). Factors that contribute to the reduced feed intake during this period might be a reduced rumen capacity owing to increasing abdominal space requirements of the growing fetus in late pregnancy, hormonal changes associated with late pregnancy and parturition that affect the cow's appetite and feed intake, physiological stress due to various metabolic changes or adjustments, and secondary diseases like mastitis, metritis, etc. Cows need 0.5 kg of glucose daily to maintain their bodily functions and roughly 0.05 kg for every liter of milk they produce (Guliński 2021).

The cow breaks down body fat reserves to compensate for this shortage, which form ketone bodies. This process is known as ketogenesis and is the body's compensatory mechanism for low glucose availability. It causes the body to produce ketone bodies (BHBA, ACAC, and AC) as it utilizes stored fat as a substitute fuel source. Ketone bodies are formed when the liver rapidly metabolizes fatty acids into acetyl coenzyme A (acetyl-CoA). These ketone bodies are then released into the bloodstream and serve as an alternative energy source for various tissues, including the brain.

The body can process small quantities of these ketone bodies. But if hypoglycemia persists, the ketone body formation rate can exceed the utilization rate. Increased oxaloacetate extraction from the TCA cycle leads to an excess of acetyl-CoA, which causes the formation of more ketone bodies and leads to ketosis. The animal's body tries to compensate for hypoglycemia by speeding up the rate of fat metabolism in the liver through the production of acetyl-CoA (Chapinal et al. 2011).

Normally, acetyl-CoA enters the TCA cycle by combining with oxaloacetic acid/oxaloacetate (from the precursor propionate) and oxidizes itself. In ketosis, however, enough oxaloacetate is not formed due to depression of glucose metabolism. Hence, acetyl-CoA cannot enter the TCA cycle and is instead metabolized to acetoacetyl-CoA and subsequently to acetoacetate and BHBA (ketone bodies). Low blood glucose concentrations are associated with hypoinsulinemia, which subsequently triggers the mobilization of fatty acids from adipose tissue, thereby increasing ketone body formation (Zhang and Ametaj 2020).

The liver is the principal organ where ketone bodies are produced. The severity of ketosis is directly related to the level of glucose deficiency. The excessive fatty acids produced are re-esterified into triglycerides (TGs) for storage and inclusion into very low density lipoproteins (VLDL), which leads to fatty liver (Lyle 1983) and further compromises liver function and hence, gluconeogenesis. If the ketone bodies cannot be metabolized further by the liver they are passed into the blood and other tissues where they can be oxidized. There is no inability of the tissues, other than the liver, to oxidize either glucose or ketone bodies under those conditions.

6.3 Classification of Ketosis

Various clinical classifications have been used to describe ketosis in cattle. Some of the most commonly used classifications are described in this section.

6.3.1 Subclinical Ketosis (SCK)

Subclinical ketosis (SCK) in cows is characterized by elevated levels of circulating ketone bodies without noticeable clinical signs (Carrier et al. 2004; Melendez et al. 2006). SCK can occur in up to 60% of cows in a herd (Van der Drift et al. 2012). β-hydroxybutyrate (BHBA) levels in the blood, measured through diagnostic methods, are commonly used to identify SCK in dairy cattle. The specific thresholds for BHBA levels may vary slightly, depending on guidelines or research references. In healthy, nonketotic cows, plasma BHBA concentrations are typically less than 1000 μmol/l (Constable et al. 2016). SCK is generally defined as a blood BHBA concentration of 1.4 μmol/l or higher during early lactation (Duffield et al. 2009; Constable et al. 2016). However, some publications have reported thresholds between 1.2 and 1.4 μmol/l serum BHBA (Suthar et al. 2013; Raboisson et al. 2014), while others define SCK as a blood BHBA concentration of 1.2–2.9 mmol/l (Oetzel 2004).

Although the concentration of BHBA in milk is usually lower than in the blood of affected animals, it can still be a useful indicator of SCK. Milk cutoff values proposed in different studies range from 0.080 to 0.100 mmol/l (Ježek et al. 2017) and 0.05 to 0.09 mmol/l (Dirksen et al. 1995) in dairy cows. SCK is more common than clinical ketosis in dairy cows, and it can go unnoticed by farmers due to the absence of overt signs. The herd prevalence of SCK depends on the BHBA cutoff used and the method of herd selection. The regular monitoring of BHBA levels allows for early SCK diagnosis, which enables appropriate management interventions to prevent its progression into clinical ketosis. By monitoring ketone levels in the serum to identify cows at risk, farmers can make timely adjustments to their nutrition and management practices, which promotes better metabolic health in the herd and prevents the development of clinical ketosis (Figure 6.2).

6.3.2 Clinical Ketosis (CK)

Studies have shown that, in dairy cows, clinical ketosis generally occurs between 2 and 7 weeks after calving (Ospina et al. 2010). Clinical ketosis can occur in 2–15% of cows (Van der Drift et al. 2012). It is characterized by hyperketonemia, hypoglycemia, and the presence of various clinical symptoms that often include a reduced appetite, rapid weight loss, declining milk production, dry and hard feces with a dark "waxy" appearance, and sometimes apparent blindness in cattle (Zhang et al. 2012; Eddy 2008; Berge and Vertenten 2014). Affected cows may refuse to eat grain or concentrated feed but

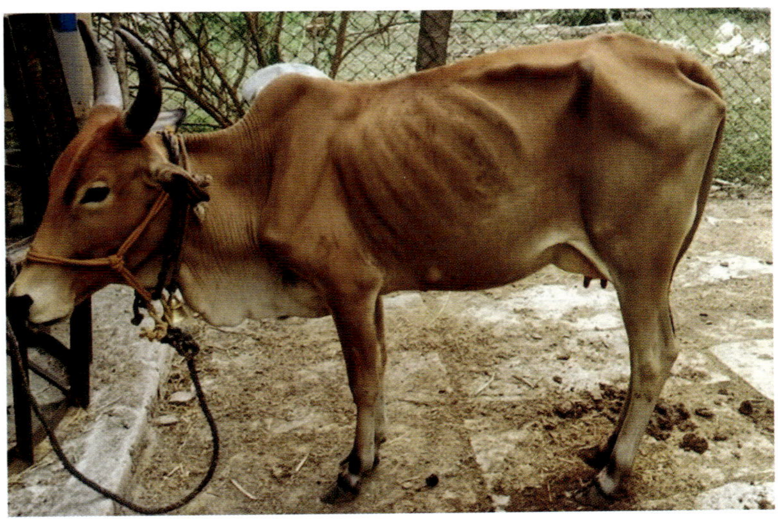

Figure 6.2 Nutritional ketosis in dairy cattle – a woody appearance and dry scant dung. *Source:* Photo courtesy of Dr. Induja P., Subject Matter Specialist, Indian Council of Agricultural Research-Krishi Vigyan Kendra, Coimbatore, Tamil Nadu, India.

continue to consume hay. The characteristic sweet smell of acetone, which results from the increased ketone bodies, can be detected on the breath and sometimes in the milk of affected animals. The diagnosis of clinical ketosis is typically confirmed by measuring the levels of BHBA in the blood. Blood sampling is considered the gold standard for diagnosis, and a concentration of BHBA above 2500 μmol/l is often used as a cutoff value (Radostits et al. 2006). A few authors have reported concentrations of BHBA in the blood that range between 2600 and 3000 μmol/l for clinical ketosis (Duffield 2000; Oetzel 2004). The concentration of individual ketone compounds in the blood of cows with ketosis was reported to be 1719 mmol/l for BHBA, 236 mmol/l for ACAC, and 356 mmol/l for AC (Enjalbert et al. 2001). However, milk samples can also be used to determine ketosis in cattle due to their convenience during regular milking procedures. A common cutoff value for BHBA concentration in milk is 100–200 μmol/l, with concentrations above this range indicating the presence of ketosis, even in subclinical cases (Ježek et al. 2017). Blood glucose levels drop to 20–40 mg/dl (hypoglycemia) from the normal 50 mg/dl range in ketotic animals (Radostits et al. 2006).

6.3.3 Primary Ketosis (Production Ketosis)

Primary ketosis, also known as "early lactation ketosis" or "type I ketosis," is a metabolic disorder that commonly occurs in dairy cows between 3 and 6 weeks postpartum (Holtenius and Holtenius 1996; Radostits et al. 2006). It is defined as type I ketosis because it is aligned with type I diabetes mellitus in humans (Zhang and Ametaj 2020). It is characterized by a shortage of glucose availability caused by underfeeding and an NEB. This triggers the activation of lipolysis and ketogenesis pathways in the cow's body (Zhang and Ametaj 2020). As a result, there is an increase in the production of ketone bodies, such as BHBA, ACAC, and AC. Concurrently, there is a decrease in insulin levels (hypoinsulinemia) due to chronic hypoglycemia. In primary ketosis, maximum stimulation of the gluconeogenesis pathway is due to the high energy requirements during the early lactation period that leads to most of the non-esterified fatty acids (NEFAs) released from the breakdown of fat being converted into ketone bodies rather than used for TG synthesis, which prevents significant accumulation of lipids in the liver (Herdt 2000).

6.3.4 Secondary Ketosis

Secondary or type II ketosis in dairy cattle occurs immediately after parturition. It is named type II because it resembles type II diabetes mellitus in humans (Zhang and Ametaj 2020). The primary cause of type II ketosis is a long period of reduced food intake or anorexia that often results from concurrent diseases such as fatty liver, abomasal displacement, traumatic reticulitis, metritis, mastitis, or other post-parturient conditions (Guliński 2021; Radostits et al. 2006; Holtenius and Holtenius 1996; Gordon et al. 2013). Some other factors that contribute to the development of type II ketosis include fluorosis in affected herds (Radostits et al. 2006) and occasional outbreaks associated with rations contaminated by substances such as lincomycin (9.5 ppm) (Rice et al. 1983).

Affected animals typically have an exaggerated body condition score (BCS; obesity) and have been overfed during the dry season. At the time of diagnosis, animals with type II ketosis exhibit hyperketonemia (lower than in type I ketosis), due to the excessive mobilization of adipose tissue, and hyperglycemia that cause the body to become resistant to insulin (Holtenius and Holtenius 1996; Zhang and Ametaj 2020). The excessive mobilization of adipose tissue produces large amounts of NEFAs. If the pathways of gluconeogenesis and ketogenesis are not adequately stimulated, NEFAs are re-esterified into TGs. Due to the limited capacity to export TGs to other tissues, a significant portion accumulates in the liver to result in hepatic steatosis (fatty liver) (Lei and Simões 2021).

6.3.5 Alimentary Ketosis

This condition is associated with consuming silage that contains excessive amounts of butyric acid, a type of fatty acid (Tveit et al. 1992). The accumulation of butyric acid in silage can be influenced by multiple factors, including the use of succulent material that is highly ketogenic, silage preparation with hay that is low in water-soluble carbohydrates, and chopping silage when it is too wet, which promotes the growth of bacteria (*Clostridium* spp.) that produce butyric acid (Radostits et al. 2006). Spoiled silage and toxic biogenic amines, like putrescine, found in silage can also contribute to ketosis development in cows (Radostits et al. 2006). It is important to note that butyric acid silage ketosis is often subclinical and may not exhibit obvious symptoms. However, it can increase the risk of developing production or primary ketosis, which are more severe forms of ketosis in cows.

6.3.6 Starvation Ketosis/Wasting Form/Chronic Ketosis

The wasting form of ketosis in cattle typically occurs in animals that are in poor body condition and are fed low quality feedstuffs or provided with inadequate nutrition. This condition is associated with a deficiency of propionate and protein in the diet and a limited capacity for gluconeogenesis from body reserves (Radostits et al. 2006). Chronic cases can also arise from inadequate treatment or returning treated animals to the same conditions that initially lead to the problem. In most instances, these animals will reduce or cease milk production, although in rare cases they may continue to lactate while becoming very thin.

6.3.7 Nervous Ketosis

The nervous form of ketosis, also known as mania puerperalis (Upadhyay et al. 2007), is a condition observed in cattle characterized by the sudden onset of neurological symptoms. The underlying mechanisms that contribute to nervous ketosis development are not fully elucidated, but various factors have been proposed as potential causes (Mcart et al. 2018). As a result, incidents of pure primary ketosis that lead to the nervous form of ketosis either go undetected or are improperly diagnosed or distinguished.

Nervous symptoms have been observed in a small percentage (about 10%) of primary bovine ketosis cases (Upadhyay et al. 2007; Foster 1988; Reddy et al. 2014; Patel and Patel 2017; Chahar and Chahar 2018). Blood glucose levels are reduced from normal, approximately 50 mg/dl, to 20–40 mg/dl (Radostits et al. 2006). The production of isopropyl alcohol (a breakdown product of ACAC in the rumen), the requirement of glucose for nervous tissue to maintain normal function, and lastly, the imbalanced ratio of ACAC to BHBA levels are proposed theories for nervous ketosis (Radostits et al. 2006; Reddy et al. 2014).

6.4 Clinical Signs

A cow during an early lactation period is suspected to be suffering from clinical ketosis based on a history of a sudden decrease in milk production over a period of 2–4 days, weight loss, and refusal to eat grain, followed by silage, and eventually, hay. The presence of an acetone odor on the breath or in the milk indicates ketosis. BHBA reduces the signaling of hypothalamic cells that are responsible for stimulating appetite. In addition to metabolic and clinical abnormalities, clinical ketosis can lead to complications and concurrent illnesses. Cows with ketosis are more susceptible to conditions such as mastitis, metritis, abomasal displacement, and poor reproductive performance.

Cows with wasting ketosis may appear dull with glazed eyes or exhibit "stargazing behavior" or "hangdog appearance." The coat may appear lusterless, and the feces may be firmer than usual. Parameters, such as temperature, heart rate, and respiratory rate, only deviate from normal if there are other concomitant conditions (Mcart et al. 2018). The ruminal movements become less frequent and weaker. The animal gives a woody appearance due to wasting and the disappearance of subcutaneous fat.

In the nervous form, signs are usually bizarre and begin quite suddenly. The nervous signs start suddenly and occur at short intervals that last for 1 or 2 hours and may occur at intervals of about 8–12 hours. The cow may lick itself or inanimate objects persistently, exhibit erratic aggressive behavior (aimless movements and wandering, vigorous licking of skin and inanimate objects), present abnormal head posture, depraved appetite, chewing movement with salivation, and even suffer from blindness. The animal manifests hyperesthetic behavior by bellowing, pinching, or stroking. Affected cows may injure themselves during the nervous episodes.

6.5 Diagnosis

Elevated levels of BHBA in the blood, along with increased concentrations of AC and ACAC in body fluids, indicate ketosis (Iwersen et al. 2009). Clinical signs in cows, including a decrease in appetite, weight loss, and decrease in milk production, are also diagnostic clues for ketosis. However, the signs of ketosis are often subtle, usually difficult to detect, and missed by farmers; subsequently, the true incidence of ketosis may be underdiagnosed. Therefore, the amount of ketone bodies present in the blood, milk, urine, and lymph indicates subclinical cases in cows (Biswal et al. 2016; Tetens et al. 2015). Through

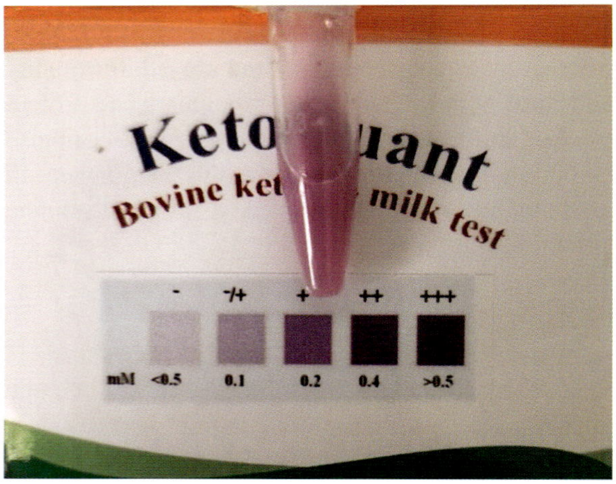

Figure 6.3 Positive cow-side milk test for the presence of ketone bodies. *Source:* Photo courtesy of Dr. Induja P., Subject Matter Specialist, Indian Council of Agricultural Research-Krishi Vigyan Kendra, Coimbatore, Tamil Nadu, India.

early detection, the cow can be treated in time to prevent a more severe course of disease (Sturm et al. 2020). Measuring the levels of blood BHBA is the gold-standard technique for diagnosing ketosis in animals (Djokovic et al. 2019). Compared to AC and ACAC, BHBA is more stable in the blood, which makes it a reliable marker for ketosis diagnosis (Duffield 2000). However, testing for plasma BHBA concentrations is not practical or cost-effective for routine analysis (Fønss and Munksgaard 2008; Pryce et al. 2016; Madreseh-Ghahfarokhi et al. 2018), so cow-side monitoring and the amount of ACAC or BHBA in milk and urine are used instead. Plasma BHBA concentrations in normal cows are less than 1000 µmol/l, those in SCK are larger than 1400 µmol/l, and those in clinical ketosis are frequently above 2500 µmol/l (Radostits et al. 2006; Djokovic et al. 2019; Mahrt et al. 2014).

On-farm screening tools can be valuable for diagnosing SCK cases in livestock (Enjalbert et al. 2001; Tatone et al. 2016). Farmers can proactively identify animals at risk of or experiencing SCK by regularly monitoring ketone levels using these screening tools (Figure 6.3). These tests are designed to detect and measure ketone bodies in various body fluids such as blood, milk, or urine. Handheld ketone meters are portable devices designed to measure the concentration of ketone bodies in blood or milk samples. They use test strips and provide quantitative results, which allow for a more accurate assessment of ketone levels. Milk test strips are designed to measure the concentration of BHBA specifically in milk and provide a quick, on-farm assessment of ketone levels. A strong correlation of 0.705 suggests a positive relationship between BHBA levels in milk and blood (Ježek et al. 2017). Ketone test strips or dipsticks are also available that specifically detect acetoacetate and acetone in the urine. Both milk and urine dipsticks are observations of color change and hence, provide a qualitative or semiquantitative indication of ketosis. Rothera's test is a qualitative chemical test commonly used to detect the presence of ketone bodies, specifically acetone and acetoacetate, in urine. The test involves a chemical reaction between the ketone bodies and reagents (sodium nitroprusside) that results in the formation of a purple ring (Figure 6.4) (Rothera 1908).

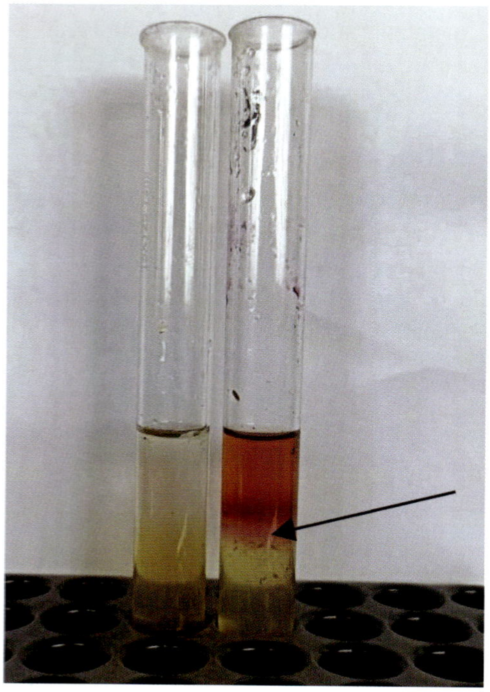

Figure 6.4 **Negative:** No ring formation. **Positive:** Formation of a purple ring (black arrow) in the tested sample.

Blood glucose measurements in affected animals provide effective insight into ketosis. The levels drop to 20–40 mg/dl from the normal range of 50 mg/dl (Radostits et al. 2006).

Studies have explored AC concentrations in cow breath as a noninvasive method for determining ketosis (Dobbelaar et al. 1996). However, it is not a common practice, partly because no sensors or tests are yet available for routine cow breath analysis (Küntzel et al. 2018). The principle behind this is that blood flow to capillaries in the lungs releases AC into the alveoli, which is then exhaled. Some studies have suggested that AC levels in breath increase earlier than BHBA levels in milk and ACAC levels in urine (Mottram et al. 1999; Mottram and Masson 2001; Van der Drift et al. 2012). In contrast, others have reported increased AC in the breath following the rise in BHBA in blood (Dobbelaar et al. 1996; Erp-van der Kooij et al. 2023). Some studies have reported breath AC concentrations in cows with ketosis to range from 2.3 to 20.0 ppm (Erp-van der Kooij et al. 2023) and 0 to 14 ppm (Dobbelaar et al. 1996). On the other hand, nonketotic cows were reported to have breath AC concentrations ranging from 0 to 2 ppm (Dobbelaar et al. 1996; Mottram et al. 1999).

Metabolomics is a rapidly evolving field of science that focuses on the detection, identification, and quantification of metabolites and small molecules (ketones, fatty acids, sugars, amino acids, nucleotides, organic acids, and many others) in various biological samples (Tran et al. 2012). By studying metabolite profiles, researchers can gain insight into the biochemical processes that occur within an organism, understand alterations in metabolic pathways associated with diseases, identify potential biomarkers, and discover new pathologies (Johnson et al. 2016).

Nuclear magnetic resonance (NMR) spectroscopy and mass spectrometry (MS) are two commonly used analytical techniques in metabolomics. These techniques are nondestructive, highly accurate, and reproducible, which make them valuable tools for metabolite detection and quantification (Zhang and Ametaj 2020). Studies regarding metabolomic investigations have demonstrated that cows with ketosis also have numerous additional altered metabolites (amino acids, carbohydrates, and fatty acids) in the same biofluids, in addition to higher blood and milk ketone bodies as measured by gas chromatography (GC)-MS, liquid chromatography (LC)-MS, and NMR (Tran et al. 2012; Klein et al. 2012; Sun et al. 2014; Li et al. 2014; Zhang et al. 2017a,b).

Additionally, elevated levels of folic acid and long-chain fatty acids in milk fat during the first 9 weeks of lactation (Geishauser et al. 2001) in cows with SCK as well as a fat–protein ratio greater than 1.5 in first-day teat milk is considered indicative of an insufficient energy supply in the cow's diet and can be a risk factor for ketosis (Heuer et al. 2001).

6.6 Economic Significance

Ketosis in livestock, particularly in dairy cows, can have high economic costs due to its high incidence, the prevalence of subclinical cases, and its associations with various concurrent health issues (displaced abomasa [DA], cystic ovaries, and mastitis) and production problems (Suthar et al. 2013; McArt et al. 2015; Berge and Vertenten 2014; Seifi et al. 2011; Probo et al. 2018).

The average cost of a single case of SCK, as stated by several authors, is €257 (Raboisson et al. 2015), €130 (Mostert et al. 2018), €150 (Steeneveld et al. 2020), $203 (McArt et al. 2015), and €21 per cow each year (Van Soest et al. 2019). On the other hand, the average cost of a single clinical ketosis case was reported to be €709 (Steeneveld et al. 2020) and $289 (Gohary et al. 2016). Moreover, the expenses of clinical ketosis and SCK at the herd level were calculated in the Netherlands and are reported to be, on average, €3613 and €7371 per year for default and high risk farms, respectively (Steeneveld et al. 2020).

6.7 Differential Diagnosis

The nervous form of ketosis in cattle should be differentiated from rabies, hypomagnesemia, listeriosis, plumbism, and bovine spongiform encephalopathy due to similarity in one or more clinical signs. The wasting form of ketosis must be differentiated from abomasal displacement, traumatic reticulitis, primary indigestion, diaphragmatic hernia, cystitis, and pyelonephritis (Radostits et al. 2006).

6.8 Treatment

Ketosis in dairy cattle is a metabolic disorder that can have severe consequences if not treated promptly. Several approaches have been used successfully to treat ketosis in dairy cattle. Early intervention is crucial for treating ketosis in dairy cattle to minimize losses (Enjalbert et al. 2001). In some rare cases, ketosis in dairy cattle may persist despite treatment and can lead to severe complications, including mortality. These cases are often secondary in nature and are because of an underlying primary disease or condition that hinders a satisfactory response to treatment. Treating bovine ketosis often involves increasing feed intake, using intravenous (IV) dextrose solutions, utilizing glucocorticoids, and giving oral propylene glycol (Gordon et al. 2017).

Offering highly palatable and energy-dense feeds, such as grains and high quality forages, can stimulate cows' appetites and help combat ketosis. Injecting 500 ml of a 50% glucose solution intravenously over a period of 2–3 hours or as needed has shown excellent results in severe cases of ketosis or when oral intake is compromised (Radostits et al. 2006). Close monitoring during the infusion is necessary to ensure a safe and appropriate response. The direct and rapid availability of glucose bypasses the need for digestion and absorption from the rumen. It suppresses the mobilization of fatty acids and reduces the level of NEFAs in the bloodstream, which is desirable as elevated NEFA concentrations are associated with ketosis.

Moreover, glucose infusion stimulates insulin secretion and inhibits glucagon release, which promotes glucose utilization and a shift toward a more anabolic state. Following the IV glucose infusion, a temporary increase in blood glucose levels, termed transitory hyperglycemia, typically lasts 2–2.5 hours. Relapses can occur unless therapy is repeated, which highlights the importance of ongoing monitoring and preventive measures. In cases where a prolonged response is needed, alternate methods, such as intraperitoneal injections of a 20% dextrose solution or subcutaneous injections of a 50% dextrose solution, can be considered. These methods provide extended glucose support, but strict hygiene protocols must be followed to minimize the risk of infection (Radostits et al. 2006).

Propylene glycol can be administered orally as a drench, which provides a convenient method of delivering the treatment without the need for frequent injections. The standard dosage for propylene glycol in cattle is 225 g, given twice a day for 2 days, followed by 110 g once daily for 2 days (Radostits et al. 2006). However, dosage adjustments may be made based on the severity of ketosis and the individual cow's response to treatment. Propylene glycol is directly absorbed from the rumen and raises citrate levels in mitochondria to inhibit the production of ketone bodies. Propylene glycol is converted to pyruvate and then to oxaloacetate via the enzyme pyruvate carboxylase, which promotes gluconeogenesis and increases glucose availability. Propylene glycol is preferred over substances such as propionate or glycerol for ketosis treatment because both propionate and glycerol have the potential to perpetuate and worsen the ketotic state by disrupting digestion and being metabolized into ketogenic acids in the rumen (Radostits et al. 2006). Propylene glycol offers a more direct route for glucose production without interfering with rumen fermentation.

Sodium propionate (110–225 g daily, by mouth), which is a form of propionic acid, can be administered orally or as a drench to cows with ketosis (Radostits et al. 2006) for the therapeutic management of ketosis. After absorption, propionic acid undergoes conversion to glucose through the process of gluconeogenesis in the liver. This helps replenish blood glucose levels and supports metabolic function in cows with ketosis. It is important to note that cattle may respond slowly to the oral administration of propionic acid. The response time can vary among individual cows. Close monitoring of the cow's condition and response to treatment is necessary to determine the effectiveness and the dosage needed.

Fructose can be used as an additional sugar source for treating ketosis. It is taken up by liver cells and undergoes enzymatic reactions to convert it into glucose, glycogen, lactate, or other metabolites. The metabolism of fructose in the liver is largely insulin independent. The aim is to provide a readily available energy source for the liver and support glucose production. Invert sugar, which is a combination of glucose and fructose, can be used to prolong the response in ketosis treatment. This mixture of sugars provides a variety of substrates that can be metabolized for energy. Xylitol, a sugar alcohol, has been used as an alternative sugar source in some cases of ketosis treatment. It can be converted to glucose in the liver, which provides an energy substrate. It is important to note that idiosyncratic reactions such as polypnea (rapid breathing), muscle tremors, weakness, or collapse can occur when administering these sugars (Radostits et al. 2006). Close observation and monitoring during treatment are necessary to detect any adverse reactions promptly.

Lactates, specifically calcium and sodium lactate (1 kg initially, followed by 0.5 kg for 7 days) as well as ammonium lactate (200 g for 5 days), have been used as glucogenic agents to treat ketosis in dairy cattle (Radostits et al. 2006). They are administered orally or as a drench to provide an exogenous supply of glucogenic precursors. However, compared to other treatments (like sodium propionate), calcium and sodium lactate have been reported to yield less satisfactory results in some cases. The reasons for this may include differences in the rate of lactate utilization, individual cow responses, and other factors that affect gluconeogenesis. Ammonium lactate is another form of lactate used in the treatment of ketosis. It is a source of gluconeogenic precursors and can be metabolized to glucose in the liver. Ammonium lactate has been used extensively and reported to yield good results when treating ketosis in dairy cattle.

Glucocorticoids, including dexamethasone, can be used to treat ketosis. They have anti-inflammatory properties and can enhance glucose metabolism by increasing hepatic gluconeogenesis. Glucocorticoids are typically administered under veterinary supervision and are more commonly used in refractory cases or when other treatment options have been exhausted. Glucocorticoids rapidly and effectively raise blood glucose levels over an extended period, typically 48–72 hours after administration. They increase glucose availability in the bloodstream by promoting gluconeogenesis in the liver.

Glucocorticoids reduce the synthesis of ketone bodies by inhibiting the breakdown of fatty acids and the subsequent production of acetyl-CoA. Temporary declines in milk yield may be observed after glucocorticoid administration but an overall health improvement and a decrease in BHBA concentrations can be seen (Marczuk et al. 2013). Glucocorticoids can be administered alone or in combination with glucose therapy or glucose precursors. It is essential to consider the potential side effects and physiological effects of glucocorticoids. The choice of glucocorticoid and administration route depends on the specific product and the cow's needs. Glucocorticoids such as dexamethasone (10 mg dexamethasone isonicotinate [2%]; 40 mg dexamethasone sodium phosphate), betamethasone (5 mg), and flumethasone (5 mg) are commonly used to treat ketosis in dairy cattle (Radostits et al. 2006). They are available in different formulations and can be administered through injections or other routes. After receiving a dexamethasone injection, plasma levels of both glucose and insulin dramatically rise 48 hours later (Jorritsma et al. 2004). Corticosteroids may initially cause a reduction in blood glucose levels and should not be used in cases of nervous ketosis. Isoflupredone acetate is a glucocorticoid commonly used in veterinary medicine, including the treatment of ketosis in dairy cattle. Prolonged or excessive use of glucocorticoids can lead to potassium depletion and associated health issues (Sielman et al. 1997). Profound hypokalemia can have significant consequences and may manifest as muscle weakness, abnormal heart rhythms, reduced feed intake, and a high case-fatality rate.

In cases of ketosis in dairy cattle, insulin therapy can be considered a treatment option, particularly in early onset instances of ketosis that do not respond to glucose or corticosteroid therapy. Insulin promotes hepatic gluconeogenesis, inhibits fatty acid metabolism, and facilitates cellular glucose uptake. Careful monitoring is required during insulin therapy to avoid complications such as hypoglycemia and other adverse effects. Insulin is usually administered with glucose or a glucocorticoid to support its action and optimize treatment efficacy. Protamine zinc insulin is a type of insulin formulation that can be used for subcutaneous administration in dairy cattle at a dose rate of 200–300 IU per animal every 24–48 hours as required (Radostits et al. 2006). It has a longer duration of action than regular insulin due to the inclusion of protamine and zinc, which helps prolong its release and action in the body.

Anabolic steroids have been used to treat acetonemia (ketosis) in dairy cattle, but their effectiveness and usage in this context can vary. Anabolic steroids are synthetic variations of testosterone that promote protein synthesis and tissue growth. They can have metabolic effects that may aid in the management of ketosis. Anabolic steroids, such as trenbolone acetate (as a single injection at doses of 60 and 120 mg in experimental conditions), have been reported to increase the levels of TCA cycle intermediates, particularly oxaloacetate, in the liver (Radostits et al. 2006). This can promote the complete oxidation of fatty acids and reduce the production of ketone bodies. Anabolic steroids in veterinary medicine are subject to regulations and restrictions, and their usage in dairy cattle may raise concerns about potential residues in milk or meat products, which affect food safety and public health. Anabolic steroids can have an appetite-stimulating effect that leads to increased feed intake. This increased appetite ensures a greater supply of glucogenic precursors necessary for gluconeogenesis and glucose production in the liver. Anabolic steroids do not directly increase blood sugar levels but primarily enhance metabolic processes in the liver and improve nutrient utilization, which indirectly contributes to better glucose regulation. Regarding recombinant bovine somatotrophin (rBST), it is a protein growth hormone that increases milk production in dairy cattle. While it is effective at treating severe ketosis and fat cow syndrome experimentally, its usage may also be subject to regulations and restrictions, and its use should be discussed with a veterinarian (Radostits et al. 2006). Contrary to corticosteroid or glucose therapy alone, a combination of corticosteroids and IV glucose therapy frequently improves the response to ketosis in cows (Shpigel et al. 1996).

Glucagon, despite being ketogenic, has significant gluconeogenic and glycogenolytic effects. Glucagon regulates blood glucose levels by stimulating the breakdown of glycogen (glycogenolysis) and promoting the production of glucose (gluconeogenesis) in the liver. The use of glucagon in the prevention and treatment of ketosis in cows has been considered due to the observed lower concentrations of glucagon in the blood during ketosis, which can contribute to metabolic imbalances. However, a limitation of using glucagon as a therapeutic agent is its relatively short physiological half-life and transient effects after a single injection. To overcome this limitation, various approaches have been explored to achieve sustained glucagon delivery (Hippen 2000). These include using controlled-release formulations or developing implantable devices that provide continuous and controlled release of glucagon over an extended period. Moreover, further studies are needed to evaluate the efficacy and safety of sustained glucagon delivery in curing and treating ketosis in cows.

There are reports of using miscellaneous treatments as adjunct therapies for ketosis in dairy cattle. These treatments include the administration of vitamin B12, cobalt, cysteamine (a biological precursor of coenzyme A, 750 mg IV in three doses at 1–3 day intervals), and sodium fumarate (Radostits et al. 2006). They are involved in various enzymatic reactions, including those related to glucose metabolism. Supplementing with vitamin B12 or cobalt can help support metabolic function and improve energy production in cows with ketosis. Sodium fumarate, a compound that can influence ruminal fermentation, improves the availability of nutrients, including glucose precursors, for energy production.

6.9 Prevention of Ketosis

The prevention of ketosis is integrally related to adequate cow nutrition, management of body condition, and the use of certain feed additives during the dry and lactating periods. Cows fed restricted/controlled energy diets throughout the dry season have a decreased chance of experiencing ketosis without affecting milk production (Mann et al. 2015). Here are a few important key points to prevent ketosis.

- Monitoring the BCS before calving is important to manage herd health (Gillund et al. 2001; Roche et al. 2013). Cows should ideally have a BCS of 2.5–3.0 to prevent excessive fat mobilization (Eddy 2008; Andrews 1998; Melendez et al. 2004). A higher BCS (> 3.25) before calving can lead to increased fat mobilization and ketosis risk (Busato et al. 2002; Gillund et al. 2001; Roche et al. 2013).
- When introducing concentrates during lactation, start with small quantities (1–2 kg/day) about 2 weeks before calving. Changes to the diet should be made gradually to allow for the adjustment of rumen microbiota.
- Forages that contain ketogenic substances, such as butyric acid, should be avoided in early lactation. Roughage should comprise at least 40% of the diet. The proper digestion of structural carbohydrates in roughage should be ensured by providing high quality forage with the proper ratio of its dry matter to the dry matter of concentrated feed, which in an adequately arranged ration should be approximately 1 : 1. Ensure adequate fermentation in the rumen with an appropriate amount of concentrated feed and limited starch fermentation (Guliński 2021). Access to a plentiful supply of long coarse fiber during the dry period promotes good rumen digestion (Moorby et al. 2002).
- Limit the basal diet for dry cows to 75–80% of nutrition standards and increase the amount of straw to prevent type II ketosis. This slows down the release of fat reserves after calving (Ranaraja et al. 2016).
- Shortening or eliminating the dry period can reduce the NEB after calving and prevent metabolic diseases associated with imbalanced energy levels like ketosis (Grummer 2008).
- Blood glucose estimations, testing for ketones in urine or milk, and routine monitoring can help detect SCK early enough for a timely treatment, generally in the second week of lactation (Geishauser et al. 2001).
- The daily use of sodium propionate (0.25 pounds for each cow) after calving can be preventive against ketosis by leading to higher blood sugar levels, lower blood ketone bodies, and increased milk production (Schultz 1958).
- During the last 2 weeks of pregnancy and the first few months of lactation, niacin feeding (6 g per head per day) raises the blood plasma glucose content and the rate of fat metabolism, which prevents the formation of ketone bodies, especially in over conditioned cows (Panda et al. 2017).
- Ionophores like monensin can alter rumen microbial populations, increase propionate production, and decrease acetate and butyrate production (Radostits et al. 2006). Monensin is a polyether antibiotic produced by *Streptomyces cinnamonensis* (Duffield et al. 2008a). Treatment with monensin reduced the likelihood of conditions such as mastitis, DAs, and ketosis (Duffield et al. 2008b). It can be administered as a slow-release capsule to cattle 2–4 weeks before calving. The capsule contains 32 g of monensin and releases approximately 335 mg daily for 95 days (Radostits et al. 2006).
- Administering oral glucose precursors (e.g. glycerine, propylene glycol, calcium, or sodium propionate) before and after calving can inhibit excessive fat reserve use, reduce free fatty acid concentrations, and raise TG and insulin levels, thus reducing the risk of ketosis and fatty liver syndrome (Guliński 2021; Grummer 2008).
- The administration of oral propylene glycol (300 ml) can effectively prevent ketosis and increase milk production (Madreseh-Ghahfarokhi et al. 2018). A dose of 1 l per day of propylene glycol as an oral drench for 9 days before parturition has also been shown efficacious (Studer et al. 1993). Propionic acid fed at 110 g daily for 6 weeks, commencing at calving, has yielded good results in reducing the incidence of clinical bovine ketosis and improving production. Still, it is not palatable and has the risk of reducing feed intake (Radostits et al. 2006).
- A specific drink composed of propylene glycol (230 ml), calcium propionate (450 g), rumen-protected choline (50 g) and methionine (25 g), yeast (50 g), and potassium chloride (170 g) can be used as a prophylactic measure (Marczuk et al. 2013).
- The supplementation of rumen-protected choline (Grummer 2008) and glucagon may prevent ketosis (Hippen 2000; Radostits et al. 2006). Cobalt-deficient areas should ensure adequate cobalt intake by spreading cobalt sulfate on pastures (Eddy 2008).

6.10 Genetic Control of Ketosis

Ketosis is a multifaceted trait with poor inheritance, which demonstrates the need for a more profound knowledge of the underlying genetic causes of this illness. Estimates for the heritability of clinical ketosis range from 0.02 to 0.16, and those for SCK range from 0.04 to 0.17 (Lee et al. 2016; Pryce et al. 2016). Research has focused on identifying polymorphic genes associated with ketosis susceptibility in dairy cows. By identifying genetic markers or variations associated with higher or lower susceptibility to ketosis, it may be possible to select animals less prone to developing the condition. Genetic analysis techniques, such as genome-wide association studies (GWAS), to identify genetic variants or markers associated with the condition have been employed by researchers. Six candidate genes that showed potential involvement in ketosis metabolism (Kroezen et al. 2018) and a few genes involved in lipid metabolism and the immune response associated with ketosis (Parker Gaddis et al. 2018) have been reported by employing GWAS. Reports on the identification of a novel region on bovine chromosome 20 (BTA 20) in Canadian dairy Holstein cattle (Nayeri et al. 2019) and a specific single nucleotide polymorphism (SNP; a molecular marker; rs109896020) on BTA 5 was found to be significantly associated with ketosis in dairy cattle (Klein et al. 2019) by employing GWAS.

Overall, searching for genetic markers associated with ketosis susceptibility is an important avenue of research. Still, it is essential to recognize the multifactorial nature of the condition and consider a holistic approach that combines genetic selection with appropriate nutritional and management practices to manage and prevent ketosis in livestock effectively.

References

Andrews, T. (1998). Ketosis and fatty liver in cattle. *In Practice* 20 (9): 509–513.

Berge, A.C. and Vertenten, G. (2014). A field study to determine the prevalence, dairy herd management systems, and fresh cow clinical conditions associated with ketosis in western European dairy herds. *Journal of Dairy Science* 97: 2145–2154.

Biswal, S., Nayak, D.C., and Sardar, K.K. (2016). Prevalence of ketosis in dairy cows in milk shed areas of Odisha state, India. *Veterinary World* 9: 1242–1247.

Busato, A., Faissler, D., Küpfer, U., and Blum, J.W. (2002). Body condition scores in dairy cows: associations with metabolic and endocrine changes in healthy dairy cows. *Journal of Veterinary Medicine Series A* 49: 455–460.

Carrier, J., Stewart, S., Godden, S. et al. (2004). Evaluation and use of three cowside tests for detection of subclinical ketosis in early postpartum cows. *Journal of Dairy Science* 87: 3725–3735.

Chahar, S.K. and Chahar, N.B. (2018). Management of nervous form of ketosis in buffalo: a case report. *Journal of Entomology and Zoology Studies* 6: 947–948.

Chapinal, N., Carson, M., Duffield, T.F. et al. (2011). The association of serum metabolites with clinical disease during the transition period. *Journal of Dairy Science* 94 (10): 4897–4903.

Constable, P.D., Hinchcliff, K.W., Done, S.H., and Grünberg, W. (2016). *Veterinary Medicine: A Textbook of the Diseases of Cattle, Horses, Sheep, Pigs and Goats*. Elsevier Health Sciences.

Contreras, G.A. and Sordillo, L.M. (2011). Lipid mobilization and inflammatory responses during the transition period of dairy cows. *Comparative Immunology, Microbiology and Infectious Diseases* 34: 281–289.

Dirksen, G., Breitner, W., and Berger, G. (1995). Diagnosis of ketosis: semi quantitative determination of beta-hydroxy-butyric acid in milk by means of a new test strip. *Tierärztliche Umschau* 50: 239–244.

Djokovic, R., Ilic, Z., Kurcubic, V. et al. (2019). Diagnosis of subclinical ketosis in dairy cows. *Biotechnology in Animal Husbandry* 35: 111–125.

Dobbelaar, P., Mottram, T., Nyabadza, C. et al. (1996). Detection of ketosis in dairy cows by analysis of exhaled breath. *Veterinary Quarterly* 18: 151–152.

Duffield, T. (2000). Subclinical ketosis in lactating dairy cattle. *Veterinary Clinics of North America: Food Animal Practice* 16: 231–253.

Duffield, T.F., Rabiee, A.R., and Lean, I.J. (2008a). A meta-analysis of the impact of monensin in lactating dairy cattle. Part 1. Metabolic effects. *Journal of Dairy Science* 91: 1334–1346.

Duffield, T.F., Rabiee, A.R., and Lean, I.J. (2008b). A meta-analysis of the impact of monensin in lactating dairy cattle. Part 3. Health and reproduction. *Journal of Dairy Science* 91: 2328–2341.

Duffield, T.F., Lissemore, K.D., McBride, B.W., and Leslie, K.E. (2009). Impact of hyperketonemia in early lactation dairy cows on health and production. *Journal of Dairy Science* 92: 571–580.

Eddy, R.G. (2008). Major metabolic disorders. In: *Bovine Medicine: Diseases and Husbandry of Cattle* (ed. A.H. Andrews, R.W. Blowey, H. Boyd, and R.G. Eddy), 781–803. UK: Blackwell Publishing Company.

Enjalbert, F., Nicot, M.C., Bayourthe, C., and Moncoulon, A.R. (2001). Ketone bodies in milk and blood of dairy cows: relationship between concentrations and utilization for detection of subclinical ketosis. *Journal of Dairy Science* 84: 583–589.

van Erp-van der Kooij, E., Derix, J., van Gorp, S. et al. (2023). Breath analysis for early detection of rising ketone bodies in postpartum dairy cows classified as at risk of ketosis. *Ruminants* 3: 39–54.

Fønss, A. and Munksgaard, L. (2008). Automatic blood sampling in dairy cows. *Computers and Electronics in Agriculture* 64: 27–33.

Foster, L.A. (1988). Clinical ketosis. *Veterinary Clinics of North America: Food Animal Practice* 4: 253–265.

Geishauser, T., Leslie, K., Kelton, D., and Duffield, T. (2001). Monitoring for subclinical ketosis in dairy herds. *Compendium* 23: S65–S71.

Geishauser, T., Leslie, D., Kelton, D., and Duffield, T. (2001). Monitoring for subclinical ketosis in dairy herds. *Compendium on Continuing Education for the Practicing Veterinarian* 23: 65–71.

Gillund, P., Reksen, O., Gröhn, Y.T., and Karlberg, K. (2001). Body condition related to ketosis and reproductive performance in Norwegian dairy cows. *Journal of Dairy Science* 84: 1390–1396.

Gohary, K., Overton, M.W., Von Massow, M. et al. (2016). The cost of a case of subclinical ketosis in Canadian dairy herds. *The Canadian Veterinary Journal* 57: 728–732.

Gordon, J.L., LeBlanc, S.J., and Duffield, T.F. (2013). Ketosis treatment in lactating dairy cattle. *Veterinary Clinics of North America: Food Animal Practice* 29: 433–445.

Gordon, J.L., Duffield, T.F., Herdt, T.H. et al. (2017). Effects of a combination butaphosphan and cyanocobalamin product and insulin on ketosis resolution and milk production. *Journal of Dairy Science* 100: 2954–2966.

Grummer, R.R. (2008). Nutritional and management strategies for the prevention of fatty liver in dairy cattle. *The Veterinary Journal* 176: 10–20.

Guliński, P. (2021). Ketone bodies–causes and effects of their increased presence in cows' body fluids: a review. *Veterinary World* 14: 1492–1503.

Herdt, T.H. (2000). Ruminant adaptation to negative energy balance: influences on the etiology of ketosis and fatty liver. *Veterinary Clinics of North America: Food Animal Practice* 16: 215–230.

Heuer, C., Schukken, Y.H., Jonker, L.J. et al. (2001). Effect of monensin on blood ketone bodies, incidenceand recurrence of disease and fertility in dairy cows. *Journal of Dairy Science* 84: 1085–1097.

Hippen, A.R. (2000). Glucagon as a potential therapy for ketosis and fatty liver. *Veterinary Clinics of North America: Food Animal Practice* 16: 267–282.

Holmes, J.R. (1950). Observations on the incidence of subclinical ketosis: in a dairy herd. *British Veterinary Journal* 106: 385–377.

Holtenius, P. and Holtenius, K. (1996). New aspects of ketone bodies in energy metabolism of dairy cows: a review. *Journal of Veterinary Medicine Series A* 43: 579–587.

Iwersen, M., Falkenberg, U., Voigtsberger, R. et al. (2009). Evaluation of an electronic cowside test to detect subclinical ketosis in dairy cows. *Journal of Dairy Science* 92: 2618–2624.

Januś, E. and Borkowska, D. (2013). Occurrence of ketone bodies in the urine of cows during the first three months after calving and their association with milk yield. *Archives Animal Breeding* 56: 581–588.

Ježek, J., Cincović, M.R., Nemec, M. et al. (2017). Beta-hydroxybutyrate in milk as screening test for subclinical ketosis in dairy cows. *Polish Journal of Veterinary Sciences* 20: 507–512.

Johnson, C.H., Ivanisevic, J., and Siuzdak, G. (2016). Metabolomics: beyond biomarkers and towards mechanisms. *Nature Reviews Molecular Cell Biology* 17: 451–459.

Jorritsma, R., Thanasak, J., Houweling, M. et al. (2004). Effects of a single dose of dexamethasone-21-isonicotinate on the metabolism of heifers in early lactation. *Veterinary Record* 155: 521–523.

Klein, M.S., Buttchereit, N., Miemczyk, S.P. et al. (2012). NMR metabolomic analysis of dairy cows reveals milk glycerophosphocholine to phosphocholine ratio as prognostic biomarker for risk of ketosis. *Journal of Proteome Research* 11 (2): 1373–1381.

Klein, S.L., Scheper, C., Brügemann, K. et al. (2019). Phenotypic relationships, genetic parameters, genome-wide associations, and identification of potential candidate genes for ketosis and fat-to-protein ratio in German Holstein cows. *Journal of Dairy Science* 102: 6276–6287.

Kroezen, V., Schenkel, F.S., Miglior, F. et al. (2018). Candidate gene association analyses for ketosis resistance in Holsteins. *Journal of Dairy Science* 101: 5240–5249.

Küntzel, A., Oertel, P., Trefz, P. et al. (2018). Animal science meets agricultural practice: preliminary results of an innovative technical approach for exhaled breath analysis in cattle under field conditions. *Berliner und MünchenerTierärztliche Wochenschrift* 131: 417–443.

Lee, S., Cho, K., Park, M. et al. (2016). Genetic parameters of milk β hydroxybutyric acid and acetone and their genetic association with milk production traits of Holstein cattle. *Asian-Australasian Journal of Animal Sciences* 29: 1530.

Lei, M.A.C. and Simões, J. (2021). Invited review: ketosis diagnosis and monitoring in high-producing dairy cows. *Dairy* 2: 303–325.

Li, Y., Xu, C., Xia, C. et al. (2014). Plasma metabolic profiling of dairy cows affected with clinical ketosis using LC/MS technology. *Veterinary Quarterly* 34: 152–158.

Lyle, R.R. (1983). *Glucose Kinetics and Hepatic Gluconeogenesis in Ketotic and Fasted Steers*. Iowa State University.

Madreseh-Ghahfarokhi, S., Dehghani-Samani, A., and Dehghani-Samani, A. (2018). Ketosis (acetonaemia) in dairy cattle farms: practical guide based on importance, diagnosis, prevention and treatments. *Journal of Dairy, Veterinary and Animal Research* 7: 299–302.

Mahrt, A., Burfeind, O., and Heuwieser, W. (2014). Effects of time and sampling location on concentrations of β-hydroxybutyric acid in dairy cows. *Journal of Dairy Science* 97: 291–298.

Mann, S., Yepes, F.A.L., Overton, T.R. et al. (2015). Dry period plane of energy: effects on feed intake, energy balance, milk production, and composition in transition dairy cows. *Journal of Dairy Science* 98: 3366–3382.

Marczuk, J., Kiczorowska, B., Kurek, Ł., and Brodzki, P. (2013). Advances in the diagnosis, therapy and prophylaxis of ketosis in dairy cattle [Postępy w Diagnostyce, Terapii i Profilaktyce Ketozy u Bydła Mlecznego (in Polish)]. *Magazyn Weterynaryjny* 12 (4): 953–962.

McArt, J.A., Nydam, D.V., Oetzel, G.R. et al. (2013). Elevated non-esterified fatty acids and β-hydroxybutyrate and their association with transition dairy cow performance. *The Veterinary Journal* 198: 560–570.

McArt, J.A.A., Nydam, D.V., and Overton, M.W. (2015). Hyperketonemia in early lactation dairy cattle: a deterministic estimate of component and total cost per case. *Journal of Dairy Science* 98: 2043–2054.

Mcart, J.A.A., Peek, S.F., and Divers, T.J. (2018). Metabolic diseases. In: *Rebhun's Diseases of Dairy Cattle*, 3e (ed. S.F. Peek and T.J. Divers), 713–736. Amsterdam: Elsevier.

Melendez, P., Donovan, G.A., Risco, C.A., and Goff, J.P. (2004). Plasma mineral and energy metabolite concentrations in dairy cows fed an anionic prepartum diet that did or did not have retained fetal membranes after parturition. *American Journal of Veterinary Research* 65: 1071–1076.

Melendez, P., Goff, J.P., Risco, C.A. et al. (2006). Incidence of subclinical ketosis in cows supplemented with a monensin controlled-release capsule in Holstein cattle, Florida, USA. *Preventive Veterinary Medicine* 73: 33–42.

Moorby, J.M., Dewhurst, R.J., Evans, R.T., and Fisher, W.J. (2002). Effects of level of concentrate feeding during the second gestation of Holstein-Friesian dairy cows. 2. Nitrogen balance and plasma metabolites. *Journal of Dairy Science* 85: 178–189.

Mostert, P.F., Bokkers, E.A.M., Van Middelaar, C.E. et al. (2018). Estimating the economic impact of subclinical ketosis in dairy cattle using a dynamic stochastic simulation model. *Animal* 12: 145–154.

Mottram, T.T. and Masson, L. (2001). Dumb animals and smart machines: the implications of modern milking systems for integrated management of dairy cows. *BSAP Occasional Publication* 28: 77–84.

Mottram, T.T., Dobbelaar, P., Schukken, Y.H. et al. (1999). An experiment to determine the feasibility of automatically detecting hyperketonaemia in dairy cows. *Livestock Production Science* 61: 7–11.

Nayeri, S., Schenkell, F., Fleming, A. et al. (2019). Genome-wide association analysis for β-hydroxybutyrate concentration in milk in Holstein dairy cattle. *BMC Genetics* 20: 1–17.

Oetzel, G.R. (2004). Monitoring and testing dairy herds for metabolic disease. *Veterinary Clinics of North America: Food Animal Practice* 20: 651–674.

Ospina, P.A., Nydam, D.V., Stokol, T., and Overton, T.R. (2010). Associations of elevated nonesterified fatty acids and β-hydroxybutyrate concentrations with early lactation reproductive performance and milk production in transition dairy cattle in the northeastern United States. *Journal of Dairy Science* 93: 1596–1603.

Overton, T.R. and Waldron, M.R. (2004). Nutritional management of transition dairy cows: strategies to optimize metabolic health. *Journal of Dairy Science* 87: E105–E119.

Panda, S., Panda, N., Panigrahy, K.K. et al. (2017). Role of niacin supplementation in dairy cattle: a review. *Asian Journal of Dairy and Food Research* 36: 93–99.

Parker Gaddis, K.L., Megonigal, J.H. Jr., Clay, J.S., and Wolfe, C.W. (2018). Genome-wide association study for ketosis in US Jerseys using producer-recorded data. *Journal of Dairy Science* 101: 413–424.

Patel, B.R. and Patel, J.S. (2017). Clinico-therapeutic management of nervous ketosis in Jaffarabadi buffalo (*Bubalus bubalis*). *Buffalo Bulletin* 36: 547–550.

Probo, M., Pascottini, O.B., LeBlanc, S. et al. (2018). Association between metabolic diseases and the culling risk of high-yielding dairy cows in a transition management facility using survival and decision tree analysis. *Journal of Dairy Science* 101: 9419–9429.

Pryce, J.E., Gaddis, K.P., Koeck, A. et al. (2016). Invited review: opportunities for genetic improvement of metabolic diseases. *Journal of Dairy Science* 99: 6855–6873.

Raboisson, D., Mounié, M., and Maigné, É. (2014). Diseases, reproductive performance, and changes in milk production associated with subclinical ketosis in dairy cows: a meta-analysis and review. *Journal of Dairy Science* 97: 7547–7563.

Raboisson, D., Mounie, M., Khenifar, E., and Maigne, E. (2015). The economic impact of subclinical ketosis at the farm level: tackling the challenge of over-estimation due to multiple interactions. *Preventive Veterinary Medicine* 122: 417–425.

Radostits, O.M., Gay, C.C., Hinchcliff, K.W., and Constable, P.D. (2006). *Veterinary Medicine. A Textbook of the Diseases of Cattle, Horses, Sheep, Pigs, and Goats*, 10e. Philadelphia, USA: Saunders Elsevier.

Ranaraja, U., Cho, K.H., Park, M.N. et al. (2016). Impact of environmental factors on milk β-hydroxybutyric acid and acetone levels in Holstein cattle associated with production traits. *Korean Journal of Agricultural Science* 43: 394–400.

Reddy, B.S., Reddy, B.S.S., Reddy, Y.P., and Vennkatasivakumar, R. (2014). Nervous form of ketosis in cows and its treatment. *International Journal of Biological Research* 2: 143–144.

Reynolds, C.K., Huntington, G.B., Tyrrell, H.F., and Reynolds, P.J. (1998). Net portal-drained visceral and hepatic metabolism of glucose, L-lactate, and nitrogenous compounds in lactating Holstein cows. *Journal of Dairy Science* 71: 1803–1812.

Rice, D.A., McMurray, C.H., and Davidson, J.F. (1983). Ketosis in dairy cows caused by low levels of lincomycin in concentrate feed. *Veterinary Record* 113: 495–496.

Roche, J.R., Kay, J.K., Friggens, N.C. et al. (2013). Assessing and managing body condition score for the prevention of metabolic disease in dairy cows. *Veterinary Clinics of North America: Food Animal Practice* 29: 323–336.

Rothera, A.C.H. (1908). Note on the sodium nitro-prusside reaction for acetone. *The Journal of Physiology* 37: 491–494.

Schultz, L.H. (1958). Use of sodium propionate in the prevention of ketosis in dairy cattle. *Journal of Dairy Science* 41 (1): 160–168.

Seifi, H.A., LeBlanc, S.J., Leslie, K.E., and Duffield, T.F. (2011). Metabolic predictors of post-partum disease and culling risk in dairy cattle. *The Veterinary Journal* 188: 216–220.

Shpigel, N.Y., Chen, R., Avidar, Y., and Bogin, E. (1996). Use of corticosteroids alone or combined with glucose to treat ketosis in dairy cows. *Journal of the American Veterinary Medical Association* 208: 1702–1704.

Sielman, E.S., Sweeney, R.W., and Whitlock, R.H. (1997). Hypokalemia syndrome in dairy cows: TO cases (1992–1996). *Journal of the American Veterinary Medical Association* 210: 240–243.

Steeneveld, W., Amuta, P., van Soest, F.J. et al. (2020). Estimating the combined costs of clinical and subclinical ketosis in dairy cows. *PLoS One* 15: e0230448.

Studer, V.A., Grummer, R.R., Bertics, S.J., and Reynolds, C.K. (1993). Effect of prepartum propylene glycol administration on periparturient fatty liver in dairy cows. *Journal of Dairy Science* 76: 2931–2939.

Sturm, V., Efrosinin, D., Oehlschuster, M. et al. (2020). Combination of sensor data and health monitoring for early detection of subclinical ketosis in dairy cows. *Sensors* 20: 1484.

Sun, L.W., Zhang, H.Y., Wu, L. et al. (2014). ^{1}H-Nuclear magnetic resonance-based plasma metabolic profiling of dairy cows with clinical and subclinical ketosis. *Journal of Dairy Science* 97: 1552–1562.

Suthar, V.S., Canelas-Raposo, J., Deniz, A., and Heuwieser, W. (2013). Prevalence of subclinical ketosis and relationships with postpartum diseases in European dairy cows. *Journal of Dairy Science* 96: 2925–2938.

Tatone, E.H., Gordon, J.L., Hubbs, J. et al. (2016). A systematic review and meta-analysis of the diagnostic accuracy of point-of-care tests for the detection of hyperketonemia in dairy cows. *Preventive Veterinary Medicine* 130: 18–32.

Tetens, J., Heuer, C., Heyer, I. et al. (2015). Polymorphisms within the APOBR gene are highly associated with milk levels of prognostic ketosis biomarkers in dairy cows. *Physiological Genomics* 47: 129–137.

Tran, H., McConville, M., and Loukopoulos, P. (2012). Metabolomics in the study of spontaneous animal diseases. *Journal of Veterinary Diagnostic Investigation* 32: 635–647.

Tveit, B., Lingaas, F., Svendsen, M., and Sjaastad, O.V. (1992). Etiology of acetonemia in Norwegian cattle. 1. Effect of ketogenic silage, season, energy level, and genetic factors. *Journal of Dairy Science* 75: 2421–2432.

Upadhyay, S.R., Sharma, N., and Pandey, V. (2007). Nervous ketosis in buffalo-a case report. *Intas Polivet* 8: 404–406.

Van der Drift, S.G.A., Houweling, M., Schonewille, J.T. et al. (2012). Protein and fat mobilization and associations with serum β-hydroxybutyrate concentrations in dairy cows. *Journal of Dairy Science* 95: 4911–4920.

Van der Drift, S.G.A., Jorritsma, R., Schonewille, J.T. et al. (2012). Routine detection of hyperketonemia in dairy cows using Fourier transform infrared spectroscopy analysis of β-hydroxybutyrate and acetone in milk in combination with test-day information. *Journal of Dairy Science* 95: 4886–4898.

Van Soest, F.J.S., Mourits, M.C.M., Blanco-Penedo, I. et al. (2019). Farm-specific failure costs of production disorders in European organic dairy herds. *Preventive Veterinary Medicine* 168: 19–29.

Zhang, G. and Ametaj, B.N. (2020). Ketosis an old story under a new approach. *Dairy* 1: 42–60.

Zhang, Z., Liu, G., Wang, H. et al. (2012). Detection of subclinical ketosis in dairy cows. *Pakistan Veterinary Journal* 32: 156–160.

Zhang, G., Dervishi, E., Dunn, S.M. et al. (2017a). Metabotyping reveals distinct metabolic alterations in ketotic cows and identifies early predictive serum biomarkers for the risk of disease. *Metabolomics* 13: 1–15.

Zhang, G., Dervishi, E., Mandal, R. et al. (2017b). Metallotyping of ketotic dairy cows reveals major alterations preceding, associating, and following the disease occurrence. *Metabolomics* 13: 1–16.

7

Parturient Paresis (Milk Fever)

Naveen S. Murikipudi[1], *Vasantha Seshu Kumari Injarapu*[2], *Suresh Kamineni*[3], *and Rajesh Kumar*[4]

[1] *Department of Veterinary Biochemistry, Sri Venkateswara Veterinary University, Tirupati, Andhra Pradesh, India*
[2] *Department of Veterinary Physiology, Sri Venkateswara Veterinary University, Tirupati, Andhra Pradesh, India*
[3] *Veterinary Clinical Medicine, Sri Venkateswara Veterinary University, Tirupati, Andhra Pradesh, India*
[4] *Department of Veterinary Gynecology, Acharya Narendra Deva University of Agriculture and Technology, Ayodhya, Uttar Pradesh, India*

7.1 Introduction

Milk production has steadily increased in terms of both average production per animal and total annual milk production. The total global milk production is 544 million metric tons (www.stastica.com), and milk production has increased by 5.29% over the previous year.

World milk production in 2022 was forecast at around 930 million tonnes, up by 0.6% from 2021 (www.fao.org). This tremendous increase in milk yield has had a great impact on the metabolic capacities of dairy cows, which results in metabolic diseases (Seifi 2011). These are manifestations of the animal's ability to cope with the metabolic demands of high milk production.

The management of dairy animals is crucial during the transitional period as the animals, particularly high yielders, are subjected to higher production stress, which leads to the onset of metabolic diseases post calving.

The transition period, which includes 3 weeks prior to calving and 3 weeks post calving, is the most susceptible phase in the life cycle of a dairy animal. As the physiology of the animal changes from nonlactating to lactating during the periparturient period, there are a series of changes that alter the metabolism of the animal as an adaptation to the new physiological state. During this phase, if the animal is under nutritional stress it results in disruption of homeostasis and makes the animal susceptible to various metabolic disorders like milk fever, hypocalcemia, downer-cow syndrome, hypomagnesemia, ketosis, udder edema, abomasal displacement, metritis, and poor fertility, all of which are correlated with each other (Seifi and Kia 2017).

One such macro-mineral metabolic disease that affects transition dairy cows and is of prime significance is milk fever or clinical hypocalcemia, which is characterized by abnormally low blood calcium ($Ca \leq 2.0$ mmol/l) (LeBlanc et al. 2006).

Hypocalcemia, also known as milk fever or parturient paresis, is a common metabolic disorder that affects cows around the time of calving. It occurs when there is a sudden drop in blood calcium levels, which leads to muscle weakness and other symptoms. These symptoms include (Figure 7.1):

- **General weakness:** Affected cows may display weakness, depression, and have difficulty standing or walking.
- **Muscle tremors:** Tremors, particularly in the hindlimbs, are commonly observed.
- **Reduced appetite:** Cows with hypocalcemia often have a decreased appetite and may show signs of ruminal stasis.
- **Decreased milk production:** A drop in milk production or even complete cessation of milk flow may occur.
- **Cold extremities:** The ears, tail, and limbs may feel cool to the touch due to poor circulation.
- **Dilated pupils:** Cows with hypocalcemia may exhibit dilated pupils.

Periparturient Diseases of Cattle, First Edition. Edited by Tanmoy Rana.

(a)

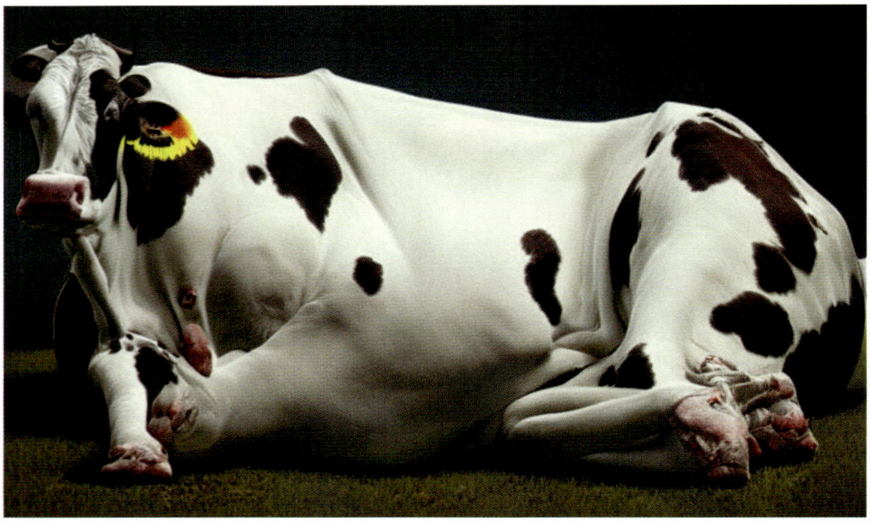

(b)

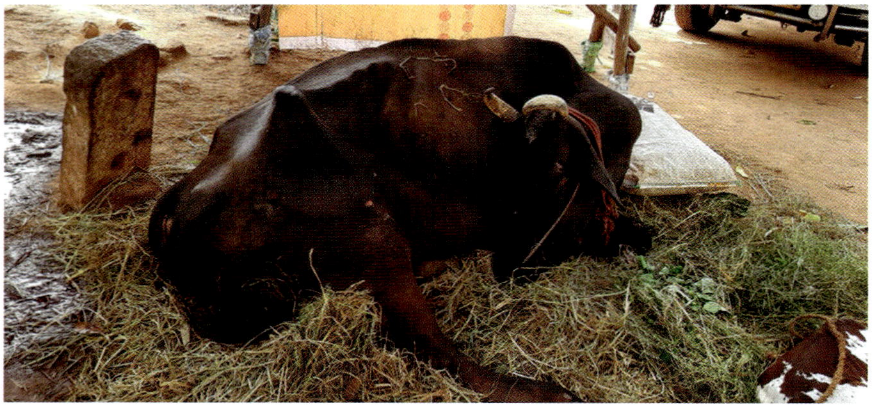

Figure 7.1 (a) A hypocalcemic cow showing symptoms like muscle tremors, weakness, reduced milk yield, and cold extremities. (b) A hypocalcemic buffalo spotted at the Department of Veterinary Clinical Complex, Veterinary College and Research Institute, Orathanadu, Thanjavur, Tamil Nadu, India. *Source:* Picture courtesy of Dr. M. Saravanan.

7.2 Predisposing Factors

The nutritional stress during the transitional period disrupts calcium (Ca) homeostasis and makes the animal susceptible to milk fever (Seifi and Kia 2017). Calcium homeostasis in the body is coordinated by parathormone, calcitonin, and vitamin D that coordinate the minute-to-minute regulation of blood calcium, which thus, is not affected by dietary calcium (Whitaker 2000). Blood Ca in the adult cow ranges between 8.5 and 10 mg/dl (Goff 2004). About 50% of blood Ca is bound to plasma proteins like albumin, less than 10% is in mineral complexes with inorganic phosphates, and the remaining is ionized, which is the biologically active form important for immediate metabolic function (Thrall et al. 2004; Seifi and Kia 2017). The role of each hormone in relation to Ca regulation is discussed in this section.

7.2.1 Parathormone

Hypocalcemia is detected within minutes by the calcium-sensing receptor (CaSR) of the parathyroid gland, which induces immediate parathyroid hormone (PTH) release (Kumar and Thompson 2011) to stimulate osteoclastogenesis via interaction with the OPG-RANKL-RANK signaling system (Ben-awadh et al. 2014). PTH also stimulates the expression and activity of 1α-hydroxylase (CYP27B1), which is located in the mitochondria of the proximal convoluted tubule and converts 25-hydroxy vitamin D_3 [$25(OH)D_3$] to the most biologically active vitamin D metabolite, $1,25(OH)_2D_3$ (Fraser and Kodicek 1973).

7.2.2 Vitamin D

The $1,25(OH)_2D_3$ hormone is a potent calciotropic agent that increases serum Ca within a few hours of injection (Vieira-Neto et al. 2017). It also stimulates intestinal and renal resorption of Ca (Dusso et al. 2005). The vitamin limits its own synthesis by inhibiting CYP27B1 and stimulating 24-hydroxylase (CYP24A1), an enzyme that initiates the inactivation and clearance of both $25(OH)D_3$ and $1,25(OH)_2D_3$ through hydroxylation at position 24 (Beckman and DeLuca 2002; Wilkens et al. 2020). A bone-derived phosphatonin, fibroblast growth factor 23 (Saji et al. 2010), interacts with PTH expression and vitamin D metabolism to decrease plasma concentrations of $1,25(OH)_2D_3$ (Krajisnik et al. 2007). 7-Dehydrocholesterol in the skin or dietary ergosterol is converted to 25-hydroxy-cholecalciferol, which is the major circulating form that undergoes hydroxylation in the liver and then in the kidney to form $1,25(OH)_2D_3$, as explained in Figure 7.2.

Absorption of Ca from the intestine is influenced by the dietary levels of Ca under the control of $1,25(OH)_2D_3$ and Ca mobilization from bone. As total dietary Ca intake increases, the efficiency of intestinal absorption and Ca mobilization from bone decrease (Ramberg 1984). Vitamin D circulates in blood, primarily bound to vitamin D–binding protein (DBP), while less than 5% circulates in a free state (El-Samad et al. 2002). The free form of $1,25(OH)_2D_3$ enters the target cell and binds with the vitamin D receptor (VDR). The complex is phosphorylated and combines with a nuclear accessory factor, retinoic acid-X receptor (RXR), to form a heterodimer, VDR–RXR (Haussler et al. 1995). This binds to vitamin D response elements (VDRE5) present in the promoter region of $1,25(OH)_2D_3$-dependent genes. Altered expression of these genes results in the expression of biological effects like bone remodeling, intestinal calcium and phosphorus (P) resorption, PTH suppression, and catabolism of $1,25(OH)_2D_3$ by 24-hydroxylase (Haussler et al. 1995).

7.2.3 Calcitonin

Calcitonin is secreted from the parafollicular, or C cells, of the thyroid gland in response to elevated plasma Ca. Although its main action is the inhibition of bone resorption during hypercalcemia (Hoff et al. 2002), its potential role in the development of hypocalcemia has not received much consideration due to conflicting research results. Shappell et al. (1987) found lower calcitonin concentrations in multiparous, hypocalcemic cows, whereas no differences were reported by Bandzaite et al. (2005). These discrepancies might occur because alterations in calcitonin could be both a cause and consequence of hypocalcemia. Interestingly, it has recently been demonstrated that, in contrast to dairy cows experiencing low grade subclinical hypocalcemia (plasma Ca between 1.88 and 2.13 mmol/l), plasma calcitonin is transiently increased in dairy cows developing severe SCH, which is defined as blood Ca concentrations between 1.50 and 1.85 mmol/l at calving (Rodríguez et al. 2017). A rise in calcitonin could interfere with PTH-mediated bone resorption and thus induce hypocalcemia.

7.2.4 Interaction of PTH and Vitamin D to Maintain Eucalcemia

Elevated blood Ca concentrations stimulate the release of calcitonin, while lowered blood Ca stimulates the release of PTH from the parathyroid glands. PTH increases the mobilization of Ca from bone and is involved in regulating the final hydroxylation of 25-hydroxy-cholecalciferol [$25(OH)D_3$] to $1,25(OH)_2D_3$ in the kidney. The active metabolite of vitamin D increases the intestinal absorption of Ca and its resorption from bone (DeGaris and Lean 2008). The normal periparturient cow

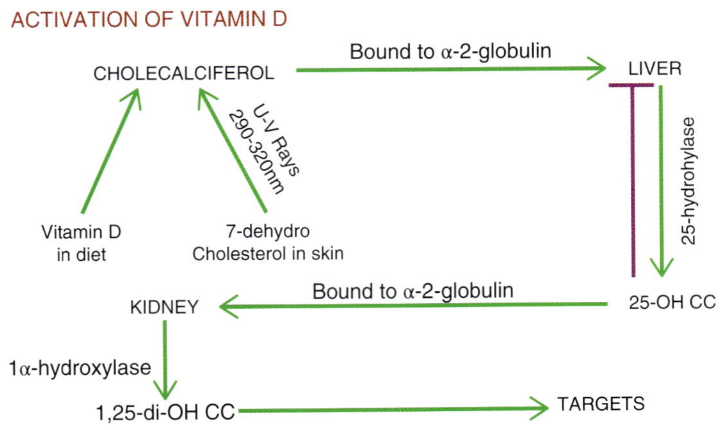

Figure 7.2 Flow diagram depicting the activation of vitamin D (1,25 dihydroxy-cholecalciferol). (1,25-di-OH CC = 1,25-dihydroxy-cholecalciferol; 25-OH CC = 25-hydroxy-cholecalciferol)

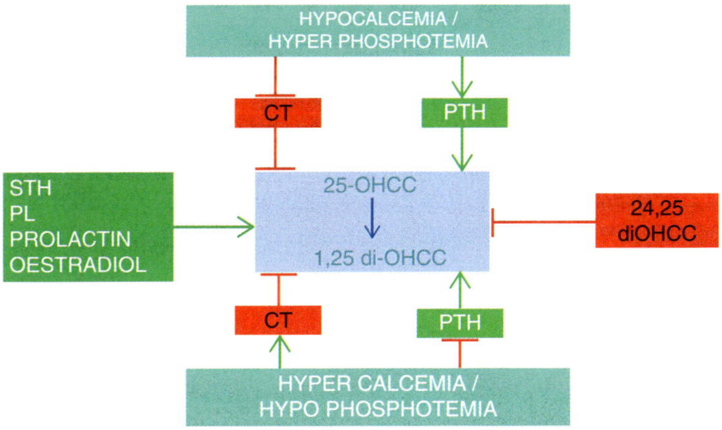

Figure 7.3 Flow diagram depicting the cross talk of hormones in the regulation of calcium homeostasis. (1,25 di-OHCC = 1,25-dihydroxy-cholecalciferol; 24,25 diOHCC = 24,25-dihydroxy-cholecalciferol; 25-OHCC = 25-hydroxy-cholecalciferol; CT = calcitonin; PL = Placental Lactogen; PTH = parathyroid hormone; STH =)

responds to decreased plasma Ca concentrations by increasing PTH and subsequently, 1,25$(OH)_2D_3$ concentrations. The result is increased intestinal absorption of Ca, increased resorption of Ca from bone, and increased renal tubular reabsorption of Ca. The cow is, however, limited in its capacity to respond to increased metabolic demands by (i) the rate at which increased absorption may occur from the intestine and (ii) the rate at which Ca may be mobilized from the bones. The availability of dietary Ca to the intestine gradually changes, even if more dietary Ca is supplied, due to the buffering action of the rumen, which acts as a reservoir for Ca (Ramberg Jr 1972). It has been suggested that hormonal insufficiencies, a lack of response of PTH, or low 1,25$(OH)_2D_3$ may be important in the pathogenesis of hypocalcemia. A flow diagram depicts the various hormonal interactions in Figure 7.3.

Diets deficient in Ca before calving have been associated with higher plasma levels of 1,25$(OH)_2D_3$ (Green et al. 1981). 24,25-Dihydroxy-cholecalciferol was elevated in paretic cows (Barton et al. 1984). A high PTH and 1,25$(OH)_2D_3$ in higher concentrations were reported in cows with milk fever (DeGaris and Lean 2008). Various forms of vitamin D_3 have been used in pharmacological doses before calving to prevent milk fever in cows. 1-α-Hydroxy-cholecalciferol and 1,25$(OH)_2D_3$, metabolites of vitamin D have hypercalcemic effects through increased Ca intestinal absorption (Goff et al. 1988) and bone resorption (Littledike and Horst 1982). However, low Ca in pre- and post-calving diets could also impact the success of vitamin D_3 supplementation (Goff et al. 1988). Persistent hypercalcemia and the metastatic calcification of body tissues are risks of vitamin D_3-metabolite toxicity, which is a point of concern (Littledike and Horst 1982).

7.2.5 Metabolic Alkalosis

Cows with metabolic alkalosis are more likely to experience subclinical hypocalcemia and milk fever (Hibbs 1950). The sensitivity of the cow to PTH is blunted by metabolic alkalosis (Goff et al. 1988; Hibbs 1950). Metabolic alkalosis alters the function of the PTH receptor, which makes the tissues less responsive to PTH. Ineffective bone canaliculi-fluid Ca utilization, also known as osteocytic osteolysis, and the activation of osteoclastic bone resorption are both prevented by the lack of a PTH response by bone tissue, which lowers glomerular filtration and Ca reabsorption by the kidneys as well. Furthermore, the kidneys are unable to change 25$(OH)D_3$ into 1,25$(OH)_2D_3$. Consequently, increased intestinal absorption of dietary Ca fails to bring blood Ca to normal.

7.2.6 Dietary Ions

Diets high in cations (potassium [K^+], sodium [Na^+], Ca^+, and magnesium [Mg^+]) and low in anions (chloride [Cl^-], sulfate [SO_4^-], and phosphate [PO_4^-]) lead to metabolic alkalosis, which is mostly the result of this imbalance. Simply put, when animals are fed these diets, there is an imbalance in the electrical charge of their body fluids because more positively charged cations enter the blood than negatively charged anions. A positive charge in the form of a hydrogen ion (H^+) must be removed from the blood compartment to electro neutralize this highly cationic, positively charged blood. Adding readily absorbable anions to the diet increases the total negative charges in the blood, which allows more H^+ to exist and the blood pH decreases as it becomes more acidic.

7.2.7 Hypo- and Hypermagnesemia

Low serum Mg can produce hypocalcemia due to enhanced PTH resistance. This happens when the serum Mg level falls below 0.8 mEq/l (1 mg/dl or 0.4 mmol/l). PTH secretion can be reduced in severe hypomagnesemia. Although severe hypermagnesemia is uncommon, it can produce hypocalcemia by inhibiting PTH secretion via the decreased sensitivity of CaSRs (Jacob et al. 2021).

7.2.8 Drugs

Bisphosphonates and denosumab both block osteoclastic bone resorption, which can result in severe hypocalcemia in some circumstances. Hypocalcemia is more prevalent in patients treated with these medicines if they also have a vitamin D deficit. Animals being treated with these drugs should have their Ca and vitamin D levels evaluated, and low levels should be rectified before starting treatment. Cinacalcet is a calcimimetic drug that operates by activating the CaSR and thereby lowering PTH secretion. It is used to treat both primary and secondary hyperparathyroidism. Hypocalcemia can result from the decrease in PTH secretion. Cisplatin, a chemotherapy medication, can potentially produce hypocalcemia via hypomagnesemia. Foscarnet can cause hypocalcemia by forming complexes with ionized Ca and lowering ionized Ca levels (Liamis et al. 2009)

7.2.9 Pseudohypocalcemia

Because serum Ca is often associated to blood proteins, most notably albumin, low albumin conditions can result in an artificially low total serum calcium level. It is recommended to adjust the blood calcium level by adding 0.8 mg/dl for every 1-g decrease in serum albumin below the normal range (4 g/dl) as ionized Ca levels are often normal in these circumstances. Illustrated in Figure 7.4.

7.3 Failure of Regulatory Mechanisms: The Key Factor in Hypocalcemia

7.3.1 Role of Calcium

Calcium homeostasis is precisely regulated as it is involved in many fundamental biological processes in the body, both intra- and extracellularly, such as bone mineralization, muscle contractility, nerve impulse transmission, blood clotting, hormone regulation as a second messenger, etc. Even small disturbances in Ca homeostasis detrimentally affect muscle, endocrine, and immune function, thereby depicting the negative effects of hypocalcemia on the health and production of dairy cows (Wilkens et al. 2020). In view of its significance, it is important for Ca levels to be precisely regulated within a narrow range (Goff 2004). Extracellular Ca is involved in the excitability of neurons and muscle cells (Han et al. 2015). It is crucial for the excitation–contraction coupling in smooth muscle cells. Indeed, the role of Ca in smooth muscle function likely explains the negative effects of hypocalcemia on contractility and motility of the gastrointestinal (GI) and

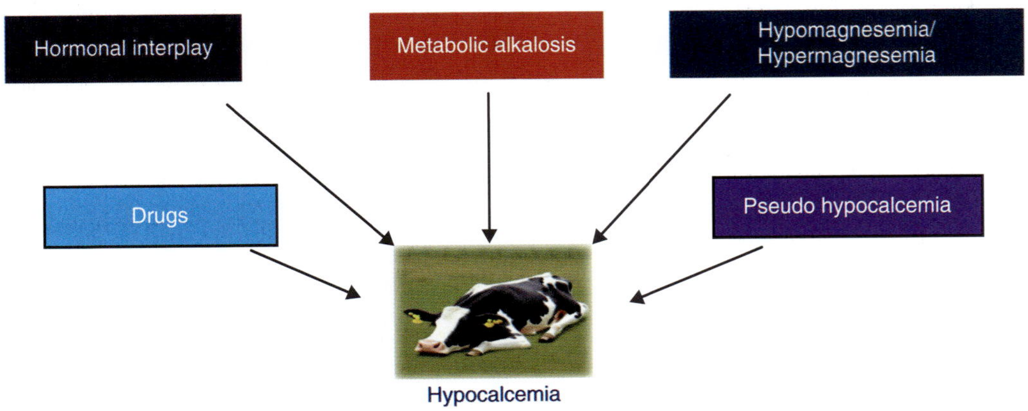

Figure 7.4 Etiology of hypocalcemia.

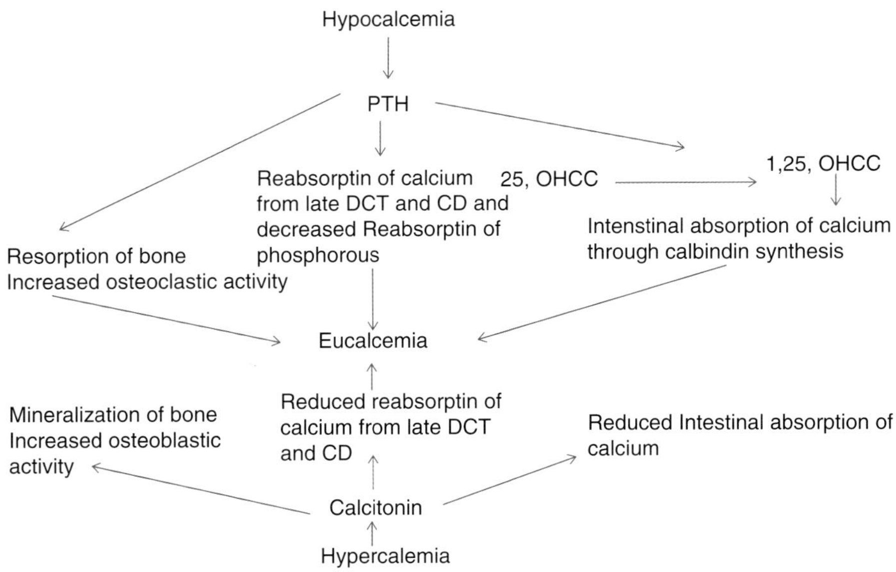

Figure 7.5 Flow chart showing the interaction of calcium-regulating hormones through their targeted actions on bone, kidney, and intestine. (1,25,OHCC = 1,25-dihydroxy-cholecalciferol; 25,OHCC = 25-hydroxy-cholecalciferol; CD = collecting duct; DCT = distal convoluted tubules; PTH = parathyroid hormone)

reproductive tracts (Heppelmann et al. 2015; Wilkens et al. 2020). The role of Ca as a second messenger also has significant implications for the endocrine and immune functions of periparturient cows that are key contributors to diseases and disorders post parturition. Many hormone and immune cell extracellular receptors act through the inositol–trisphosphate–intracellular Ca signaling pathway (Martinez et al. 2014). When blood Ca levels drop below the normal range (typically less than 8.5 mg/dl or 2.12 mmol/l), the body activates compensatory mechanisms to restore Ca balance. Some of the key mechanisms involved in calcium regulatory process, also depicted in Figure 7.5., include:

- **Bones:** Bone is the primary target that buffers Ca regulation. Hypocalcemia stimulates PTH release, which increases osteoclastic activity and thereby induces bone resorption to maintain eucalcemia. Contrarily, hypercalcemia stimulates calcitonin release, which increases osteoblastic activity and thereby increases the deposition of Ca salts in the bone.
- **Kidneys:** When blood Ca levels are low, under the influence of PTH, the kidneys reabsorb calcium from the renal filtrate back into the bloodstream, which minimizes Ca loss through urine.
- **Intestines:** Vitamin D, primarily in its active form, plays a vital role in Ca homeostasis. Low blood Ca levels stimulate the conversion of inactive vitamin D (calcidiol) to its active form (calcitriol) in the kidneys with the help of PTH. Calcitriol enhances the intestinal absorption of dietary Ca through calbindin synthesis.
- **CaSRs:** Specialized receptors located on parathyroid cells, kidneys, and other tissues detect changes in blood calcium levels.

7.4 Deleterious Effects of Milk Fever

On an average, 5–10% of dairy cows succumb to milk fever (LeBlanc et al. 2006), while 30–50% have been affected with subclinical hypocalcemia on the day of calving (Reinhardt et al. 2011). Both are predisposing factors for the onset of mastitis, retained placenta, endometritis, slower uterine involution, delayed first ovulation after calving, ketosis, displaced abomasum, and reduced gastrointestinal motility (Seifi and Kia 2017) as shown in Figure 7.6. The effects of hypocalcemia during lactation are more significant than at parturition as the loss of blood Ca to milk may exceed 50 g/d. Circulating blood Ca reserves are limited, however; the increasing demand is met through increased absorption from the rumen/intestines and mobilization from bone. Fifty percent of circulating blood Ca reserves may be drained from an animal before a hypocalcemia crisis is precipitated.

7.5 Preventive Measures/Strategies

Many strategies have been tested to mitigate postpartum hypocalcemia, such as the use of vitamin D treatments, enteral and parenteral Ca supplementation, and the manipulation of dietary Ca and negative dietary cation–anion difference diet, as shown in Figure 7.7. The concept of a low blood Ca environment before calving, which essentially begins a preadaptation of the cow to hypocalcemia, is the widely adapted strategy.

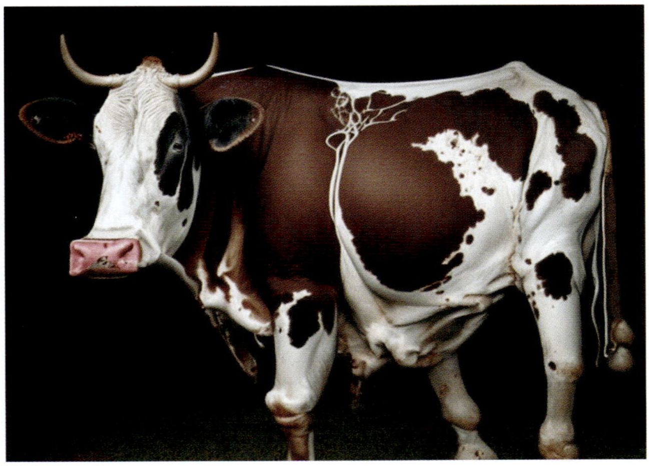

Figure 7.6 Deleterious effects on a hypocalcemic cow with a retained placenta, endometritis, slower uterine involution, delayed first ovulation after calving, ketosis, displaced abomasum, and reduced gastrointestinal motility.

- A low Ca diet through the inclusion of Ca binders in the prepartum diet is mediated through administration of zeolite A, a synthetic sodium–aluminum silicate. Zeolite A binds Ca, P, and Mg in the rumen to create a diet low in Ca (Thilsing et al. 2006).
- Feeding acidogenic diets prepartum to induce a compensated metabolic acidosis is another proven strategy against hypocalcemia (Santos et al. 2019).
- Supplementing 25(OH)D_3 to achieve superphysiological serum 25(OH)D concentrations in the periparturient period has improved the health and performance of dairy cows. Subcutaneous or intravenous administration of Ca and the oral administration of Ca boluses postpartum provide animals with an immediate Ca source to return to eucalcemia.
- The feeding of acidifying rations by anionic salt supplementation and low calcium rations during the last weeks of pregnancy as well as the prepartum administration of vitamin D, vitamin D metabolites, and analogs are other strategies. Other less specific control measures include management practices like controlling peripartum dietary Mg levels, body condition, peripartum carbohydrate intake, shortening of the dry period, prepartum milking, and reduced milking in early lactation (Thilsing-Hansen et al. 2002).
- Calcium propionate is less injurious to tissues and is not acidogenic. It has the added benefit of supplying propionate, a gluconeogenic precursor (Pehrson et al. 1998). For best control of hypocalcemia, a dose is given at calving and again 24 hours later. Larger or more frequent dosing can be toxic.

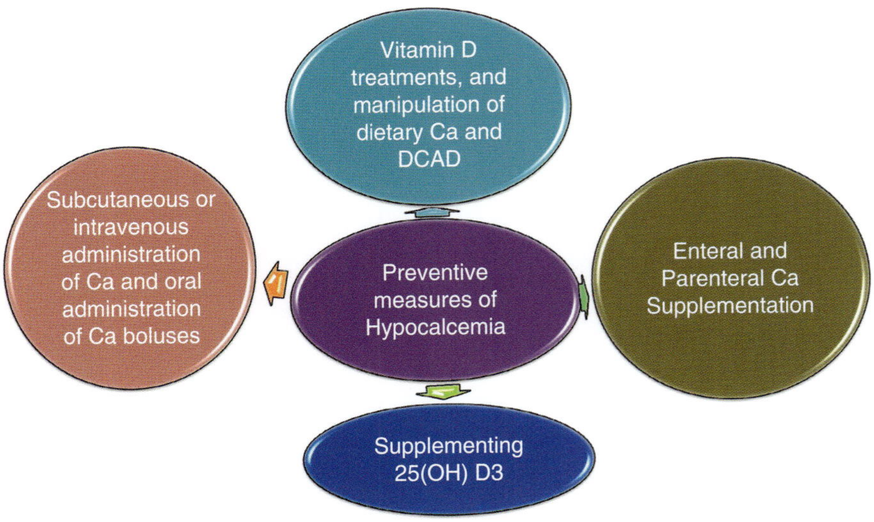

Figure 7.7 Preventive strategies to mitigate hypocalcemia. (25(OH)D3 = 25-hydroxy vitamin D_3; Ca = calcium; DCAD = dietary cation–anion difference)

Table 7.1 The approximate requirement of Ca and P (g/animal) based on body weight and age of the animal.

Dairy cattle, kg body weight and function	Calcium, g/animal	Phosphorous, g/animal	Vitamin D
Growing heifers (large breeds)			300 IU/kg dry matter
159	15	12	
300	24	18	
400	26	20	
Growing heifers (small breeds)			
100	9	7	
200	15	11	
300	19	14	
Growing bulls (large breeds)	27	20	
300	27	20	
400	30	23	
500	30	23	
Maintenance of mature lactating cows			
400	17	13	
500	20	15	
600	22	17	
Maintenance and pregnancy			
400	23	18	
500	29	22	
600	34	26	
Milk production	Add 2–3 g calcium and 1.7–2.4 g phosphorous to the maintenance requirement for each kg of milk produced.		

7.6 Conclusion

Clinical and subclinical hypocalcemia have great economic impact on the dairy industry as they induce potential health risks to transitional cows. Milk fever directly and indirectly affects the productive life span of the dairy animal through health problems, complications of parturition, loss of milk production, low fertility, and culling. Therefore, the economic losses due to clinical and subclinical hypocalcemia are tremendous. Good dry cow management, appropriate nutrition, feeding anionic diets to primiparous cows, and herd-based monitoring of hypocalcemia are a few management strategies that will result in substantial production, reproduction, and health of the animals.

References

(India) Department of Animal Husbandry and Dairying. (2023). Basic Animal Husbandry Statistics - 2022. New Delhi: Government of India, Ministry of Fisheries, Animal Husbandry and Dairying. https://dahd.nic.in/schemes/programmes/animal-husbandry-statistics (accessed 19 February 2024).

Bandzaite, V., Klimiene, I., Spakauskas, V., and Matusevicius, A. (2005). Interaction between the levels of hormones and minerals in sera of healthy and sick cows. *Polish Journal of Veterinary Sciences* 8 (4): 269–274.

Barton, B.A., Hodnett, D.W., Jorgensen, N.A., and DeLuca, H.F. (1984). 24, 25-Dihydroxyvitamin D3 administration increases incidence of parturient paresis. *Journal of Dairy Science* 67 (6): 1236–1239.

Beckman, M.J. and DeLuca, H.F. (2002). Regulation of renal vitamin D receptor is an important determinant of 1α,25-dihydroxyvitamin D3 levels in vivo. *Archives of Biochemistry and Biophysics* 401: 44–52. https://doi.org/10.1016/S0003-9861(02)00010-3.

Ben-awadh, A.N., Delgado-Calle, J., Tu, X. et al. (2014). Parathyroid hormone receptor signaling induces bone resorption in the adult skeleton by directly regulating the RANKL gene in osteocytes. *Endocrinology* 155 (8): 2797–2809.

DeGaris, P.J. and Lean, I.J. (2008). Milk fever in dairy cows: a review of pathophysiology and control principles. *The Veterinary Journal* 176 (1): 58–69.

Dusso, A.S., Brown, A.J., and Slatopolsky, E. (2005). Vitamin D. *American Journal of Physiology. Renal Physiology* 289: F8–F28.

El-Samad, H., Goff, J.P., and Khammash, M. (2002). Calcium homeostasis and parturient hypocalcemia: an integral feedback perspective. *Journal of Theoretical Biology* 214 (1): 17–29.

Fraser, D.R. and Kodicek, E. (1973). Regulation of 25-hydroxycholecalciferol-1-hydroxylase activity in kidney by parathyroid hormone. *Nature: New Biology* 241: 163–166. https://doi.org/10.1038/newbio241163a0.

Goff, J.P. (2004). Macromineral disorders of the transition cow. *Veterinary Clinics of North America: Food Animal Practice* 20 (3): 471–494.

Goff, J.P., Horst, R.L., Beitz, D.C., and Littledike, E.T. (1988). Use of 24-F-1, 25-dihydroxyvitamin D3 to prevent parturient paresis in dairy cows. *Journal of Dairy Science* 71: 1211–1219.

Green, H.B., Horst, R.L., Beitz, D.C., and Littledike, E.T. (1981). Vitamin D metabolites in plasma of cows fed a prepartum low-calcium diet for prevention of parturient hypocalcemia. *Journal of Dairy Science* 64 (2): 217–226.

Han, P., Trinidad, B.J., and Shi, J. (2015). Hypocalcemia-induced seizure: demystifying the calcium paradox. *ASN Neuro* 7 (2): 1759091415578050.

Haussler, M.R., Jurutka, P.W., Hsieh, J.C. et al. (1995). New understanding of the molecular mechanism of receptor-mediated genomic actions of the vitamin D hormone. *Bone* 17 (2): S33–S38.

Heppelmann, M., Krach, K., Krueger, L. et al. (2015). The effect of metritis and subclinical hypocalcemia on uterine involution in dairy cows evaluated by sonomicrometry. *Journal of Reproduction and Development* 61 (6): 565–569.

Hibbs, J.W. (1950). Milk fever (parturient paresis) in dairy cows – a review. *Journal of Dairy Science* 33 (10): 758–789.

Hoff, A.O., Catala-Lehnen, P., Thomas, P.M. et al. (2002). Increased bone mass is an unexpected phenotype associated with deletion of the calcitonin gene. *The Journal of Clinical Investigation* 110 (12): 1849–1857.

Jacob, J., Raghothama, S., Subramanyam, K., and Johny, D. (2021). Hypomagnesaemia causing functional hypoparathyroidism in rheumatic mitral stenosis leading to sudden cardiac arrest in a young woman. *BML Case Reports* 19: 1.

Krajisnik, T., Björklund, P., Marsell, R. et al. (2007). Fibroblast growth factor-23 regulates parathyroid hormone and 1α-hydroxylase expression in cultured bovine parathyroid cells. *The Journal of Endocrinology* 195: 125–131. https://doi.org/10.1677/JOE-07-0267.

Kumar, R. and Thompson, J.R. (2011). The regulation of parathyroid hormone secretion and synthesis. *Journal of the American Society of Nephrology* 22: 216–224. https://doi.org/10.1681/ASN.2010020186.

LeBlanc, S.J., Lissemore, K.D., Kelton, D.F. et al. (2006). Major advances in disease prevention in dairy cattle. *Journal of Dairy Science* 89 (4): 1267–1279.

Liamis, G., Milionis, H.J., and Elisaf, M. (2009). A review of drug-induced hypocalcemia. *Journal of Bone and Mineral Metabolism* 27 (6): 635–642.

Littledike, E.T. and Horst, R.L. (1982). Vitamin D3 toxicity in dairy cows. *Journal of Dairy Science* 65: 749–759.

Martinez, N., Sinedino, L.D.P., Bisinotto, R.S. et al. (2014). Effect of induced subclinical hypocalcemia on physiological responses and neutrophil function in dairy cows. *Journal of Dairy Science* 97 (2): 874–887.

Pehrson, B., Svensson, C., and Jonsson, M. (1998). A comparative study of the effectiveness of calcium propionate and calcium chloride for the prevention of parturient paresis in dairy cows. *Journal of Dairy Science* 81 (7): 2011–2016.

Ramberg Jr, C. F. (1972). Kinetics of hypocalcemia in cows fed high or low calcium diets. Oak Ridge, TN: Office of Scientific and Technical Information, Department of Energy (US). *Report Nos.: COO-3400-12; CONF-720858-1.*

Reinhardt, T.A., Lippolis, J.D., McCluskey, B.J. et al. (2011). Prevalence of subclinical hypocalcemia in dairy herds. *The Veterinary Journal* 188 (1): 122–124.

Rodríguez, E.M., Arís, A., and Bach, A. (2017). Associations between subclinical hypocalcemia and postparturient diseases in dairy cows. *Journal of Dairy Science* 100 (9): 7427–7434.

Saji, F., Shigematsu, T., Sakaguchi, T. et al. (2010). Fibroblast growth factor 23 production in bone is directly regulated by 1α,25-dihydroxyvitamin D, but not PTH. *American Journal of Physiology. Renal Physiology* 299: F1212–F1217. https://doi.org/10.1152/ajprenal.00169.2010.

Santos, J.E.P., Lean, I.J., Golder, H., and Block, E. (2019). Meta-analysis of the effects of prepartum dietary cation-anion difference on performance and health of dairy cows. *Journal of Dairy Science* 102: 2134–2154. https://doi.org/10.3168/jds.2018-14628.

Seifi, H.A. (2011). Production diseases in dairy herds: monitoring transition cows. In: *Dairy Cows: Nutrition, Fertility and Milk Production* (ed. R.E. Marek), 99–121. New York: Nova Science Publishers, Inc.

Seifi, H.A. and Kia, S. (2017). Subclinical hypocalcemia in dairy cows: pathophysiology, consequences and monitoring. *Iranian Journal of Veterinary Science and Technology* 9 (2): 1–15.

Shappell, N.W., Herbein, J.H., Deftos, L.J., and Aiello, R.J. (1987). Effects of dietary calcium and age on parathyroid hormone, calcitonin and serum and milk minerals in the periparturient dairy cow. *The Journal of Nutrition* 117 (1): 201–207.

Thilsing, T., Jorgensen, R.J., and Poulsen, H.D. (2006). In vitro binding capacity of zeolite A to calcium, phosphorus and magnesium in rumen fluid as influenced by changes in pH. *Journal of Veterinary Medicine. A, Physiology, Pathology, Clinical Medicine* 53: 57–64. https://doi.org/10.1111/j.1439-0442.2006.00798.x.

Thilsing-Hansen, T., Jørgensen, R.J., and Østergaard, S. (2002). Milk fever control principles: a review. *Acta Veterinaria Scandinavica* 43 (1): 1–19.

Thrall, M.A., Baker, D.C., Compbell, T.W. et al. (2004). *Veterinary Hematology and Clinical Chemistry*, 77. United State of America: Lippincott Williams and Wilkins.

Vieira-Neto, A., Lima, I.R.P., Lopes, F. Jr. et al. (2017). Use of calcitriol to maintain postpartum blood calcium and improve immune function in dairy cows. *Journal of Dairy Science* 100: 5805–5823. https://doi.org/10.3168/jds.2016-12506.

Whitaker, D.A. (2000). Use and interpretation of metabolic profiles. In: *The Health of Dairy Cattle* (ed. A.H. Andrews), 89–107. Oxford: Blackwell Science.

Wilkens, M.R., Nelson, C.D., Hernandez, L.L., and McArt, J.A. (2020). Symposium review: transition cow calcium homeostasis—health effects of hypocalcemia and strategies for prevention. *Journal of Dairy Science* 103 (3): 2909–2927.

8

Cystic Ovarian Disease

Arunmozhi Narayanaswamy[1], *Chhavi Gupta*[2], *Pradeep Nag Beladakere Subramanyam*[3], *and Sarath Thulasiraman*[4]

[1] Veterinary Clinical Complex, Veterinary College and Research Institute, Tamil Nadu Veterinary and Animal Sciences University, Orathanadu, Thanjavur, Tamil Nadu, India
[2] Department of Veterinary Gynaecology and Obstetrics, Veterinary College and Research Institute, Tamil Nadu Veterinary and Animal Sciences University, Tirunelveli, Tamil Nadu, India
[3] Department of Animal Sciences, University of Missouri, Columbia, Missouri, USA
[4] Veterinary Clinical Complex, Veterinary College and Research Institute, Tamil Nadu Veterinary and Animal Sciences University, Salem, Tamil Nadu, India

8.1 Introduction

Reproduction in a herd is considered economical when a calf is produced every year from a cow, this ensures maximum production. In the recent past, artificial insemination was extensively used for genetic improvement; upgrading the genetic makeup of cattle on the Indian subcontinent was mainly based on production parameters like milk production and feed efficiency. An increase in milk production over certain limits results in the reduction of reproductive efficiency. The increased production can also result in ovulatory abnormalities, predominantly ovarian cysts (OCs), which result in reduced fertility. Cystic ovarian disease was first observed in the early twentieth century and was recognized as one of the most important economical diseases of cattle (Jeengar et al. 2014).

OCs were defined as a fluid-filled or hard structures of 2.5 cm or more in diameter that persist on the ovarian surface for 10 or more days (Roberts 1971; Youngquist and Threlfall 2007). This condition was synonymous with adrenal virilism, nymphomania, cystic ovarian degeneration, cystic ovaries, and OCs (Garverick 1997). In the recent past, modifications have been considered to this definition as all animals exhibiting the disease did not fall under the disease definition. Silvia et al. (2002) defined a cystic ovary as having follicle-like structures with a minimum diameter of 17 mm that persist for more than 6 days in the absence of a corpus luteum and interfere with ovarian cyclicity. Recently, an ovarian cyst was defined as anovulatory follicles (< 2 cm) on one or both ovaries that fail to regress yet maintain growth and steroidogenesis, persist for more than 10 days, and interfere with normal ovarian cyclicity in the absence of a corpus luteum (Vanholder et al. 2006).

8.1.1 Is it Cystic Ovarian Disease, Cystic Ovarian Follicles, or Ovarian Cysts?

Cysts are often diagnosed in the absence of clear clinical signs and often go unnoticed; therefore, the term "cystic ovarian disease" is a misnomer and "cystic ovarian follicle (COF)" could be used as it does not implicate a disease condition (Vanholder et al. 2006). Additionally, nonsteroidogenic cysts coexist with the corpus luteum and will not interfere with the estrous cycle. Vanholder et al. (2006) opined that "ovarian cysts" could be the appropriate term as it describes an ovarian disorder characterized by abnormal ovarian cavity structures that have failed to ovulate (anovulation) or regress. Considering this aspect, recent studies define COF differently, all of which may indicate OCs.

Periparturient Diseases of Cattle, First Edition. Edited by Tanmoy Rana.

8.2 Incidence

The incidence of OCs in cattle varies among different breeds; overall, in dairy cattle, it varies from 2.7% to 30%; in the Guernsey breed it was reported to be 20% and 6% in Holsteins. A few studies reported that the peak incidence occurs between 14 and 40 days postpartum, while a few studies reported between 16 and 50 days after calving, with the highest occurrence between 30 and 40 days after calving. Rigorous selection pressure for milk production has been attributed as a cause for the increase in ovarian cyst incidence by 1.5% per 500 kg milk yield increase. The condition incurs a huge economical loss to the dairy industry as it increases the calving-to-conception and intercalving intervals (Mimoune et al. 2021).

8.3 Classification of Ovarian Cysts

OCs could be classified as follicular cysts (FCs), luteal cysts (LCs), and cystic corpus lutea based on macroscopic observations. Among these, a cystic corpus luteum is nonpathological and contains an antrum within the corpus luteum. Further, Wills (2012) identified three types of cysts in dairy cattle, viz. (i) large thin-walled anovulatory FCs, characterized by low progesterone (P4) and high estradiol secretion; (ii) thick-walled anovulatory LCs, characterized by prolonged and elevated P4 secretion; and (iii) FCs that luteinize (Mimoune et al. 2021).

FCs have been defined as one or more anovulatory follicular structures (diameter > 25 mm) that persist for 10 or more days in the absence of a functional corpus luteum and are accompanied by either nymphomania or continuous or frequent estrus. LCs are anovulatory follicles over 2.5 cm in diameter that are partially luteinized, persist for a prolonged period, and are characterized by anestrus (Cairoli et al. 2002). FCs initially continue to produce estrogen in the absence of other follicles greater than 5 mm; after a variable period of time, estrogen production may cease and luteinization of the follicular cyst will occur (Farin et al. 1992).

8.4 Etiopathogenesis

The exact mechanisms involved in the pathogenesis of OCs in dairy cattle are not fully understood. The most accepted hypothesis that explains OC formation is that the release of luteinizing hormone (LH) by the hypothalamic–pituitary–gonadal (HPG) axis is altered. The disease has multifactorial etiology including genetic, phenotypic, and environmental factors (Cattaneo et al. 2014) and is depicted in Figure 8.1.

8.4.1 Hypothalamic–pituitary Dysfunction

Alteration of the HPG axis is a widely accepted hypothesis that explains the formation of a cyst. The preovulatory LH surge may either be absent, of an insufficient magnitude, or may not synchronize with the maturation of the dominant follicle, which leads to the failure of maturation and the formation of a cyst. The aberrant release of LH is neither due to reduced gonadotropin-releasing hormone (GnRH) concentration nor due to reduced GnRH receptors but might be due to altered feedback mechanisms of estrogen on the HPG axis that lead to aberrant LH release (Gümen and Wiltbank 2002, Zaied et al. 1980).

Recently, kisspeptin has been regarded as a mediator of GnRH release in the hypothalamus, and kisspeptin plays a crucial role in controlling gonadotropin secretions and ovulation. Kisspeptin interacts with neurokinin B and dynorphin neuropeptides to control GnRH release. Further, the kisspeptin level is regulated by various factors including nutritional status and stress. The stress to an animal might inhibit kisspeptin and lead to altered GnRH or LH secretion, especially during lactation, which may cause anovulation (Yeo and Colledge 2018).

8.4.2 Ovarian/Follicular Dysfunction

An LH surge is a complex multistep process that involves multiple genes acting synchronously to lead to the ovulation of the dominant follicle. Follicular dysfunction may lead to alterations in the HPG axis that cause alterations in LH and follicle-stimulating hormone (FSH) receptor expression, which then may lead to the failure of ovulation and predispose the animal to OCs. Additionally, impaired steroidogenesis in the dominant follicle may also be involved in cystic ovarian degeneration (Calder et al. 2001).

After all, the dominant follicle must elicit the feedback mechanism via estrogen to initiate the LH surge at the right time. Estrogen-active cystic animals show a higher expression of 3β-hydroxysteroid dehydrogenase mRNA, a steroidogenic

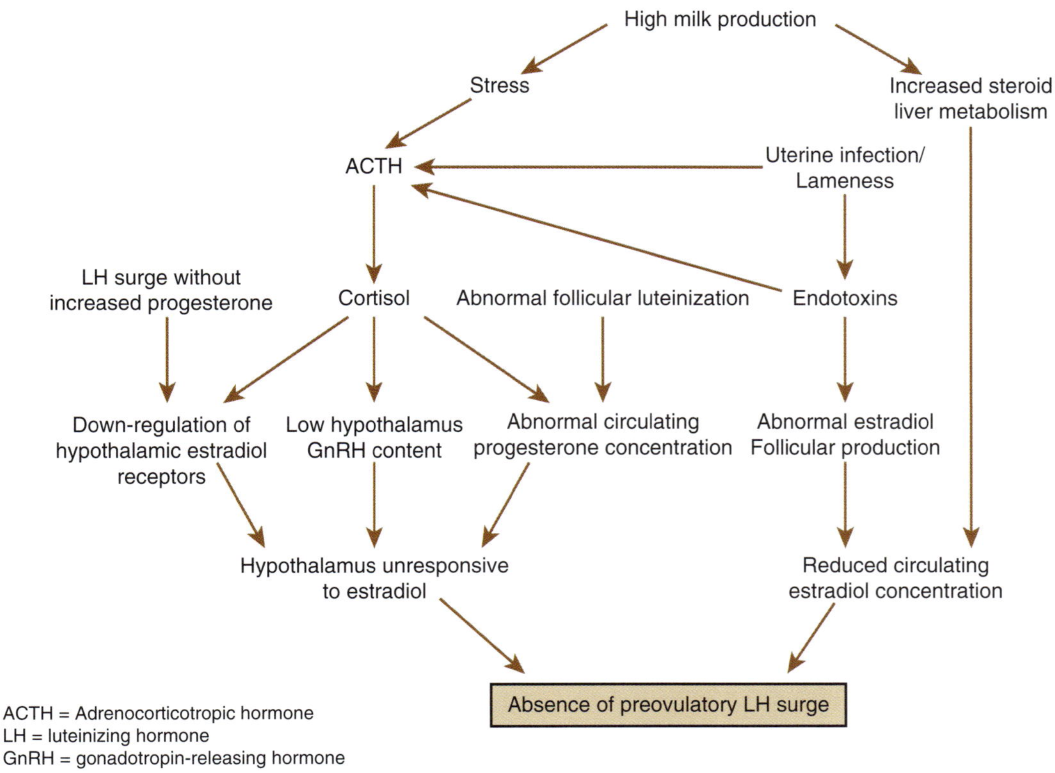

Figure 8.1 The etiopathogenesis of ovarian cysts in cattle involves the absence of the preovulatory luteinizing hormone surge that results from a disturbance in the positive feedback effect of estradiol on the hypothalamus. This disturbance is caused by hypothalamic unresponsiveness or by reduced circulating estradiol concentration. (ACTH = adrenocorticotropic hormone; LH = luteinizing hormone; GnRH = gonadotropin-releasing hormone)

enzyme, and have increased estradiol concentrations during follicular dominance. Further, a decrease in cell proliferation and an increase in apoptosis of the granulosa and theca interna cell layers may also lead to the formation of a follicular cyst (Rosenfeld et al. 1999).

Matrix metalloproteinases (MMP) will be secreted in an inactive form, i.e. pro-MMPs, that will be converted into MMPs upon an LH surge and are involved in follicle wall remodeling and rupture. During ovulation, animals with OCs have been shown to express higher concentrations of pro-MMP-2 and pro-MMP-9 in the follicular fluid compared to normal animals. This indicates that an insufficient or aberrant LH surge affects the conversion of inactive to active forms and results in the failure of follicular wall remodeling that causes retention of the follicle as an ovarian cyst (Imai et al. 2003).

8.5 Predisposing Factors for Ovarian Cyst Formation

- Most prevalent in high production dairy cows (30–60 days after calving).
- Common in closely confined and stabled animals.
- Occurs more often during winter months than in summer and fall months.
- Commonly observed between the second and fifth parturitions.
- Intake of estrogen-containing forages.
- Increased stress at calving.
- Metabolic diseases.
- Excess negative energy balance.
- Hereditary.
- High protein diet.
- Uterine infection.
- Postpartum complications.

8.6 Clinical Signs and Symptoms

8.6.1 Follicular Cysts (FCs)

- **Nymphomania**
  - Frequent, irregular, prolonged, or continuous signs of estrus.
  - Often nervous, restless, and bellow frequently.
  - Frequently attempt to ride other cows but refuse to stand to be ridden.
  - Aggravated homosexual characteristics (bullers).
- **Sterility hump**
  - Excess relaxation of the pelvic ligament leads to tipping of the pelvis and elevation of the tail head.
  - Often swollen vulva.
- **Adrenal virilism**
  - Commonly observed in chronic follicular cyst cases.
  - Exhibit a muscular behavior and appearance.
  - Increased level of 17β-keto steroids in the urine from the adrenal gland.
  - Masculinization of head and neck (steer-like appearance) (Figures 8.2 and 8.3).

8.6.2 Luteal Cysts (LCs)

- Prolonged anestrus.
- Erratic changes in milk production.

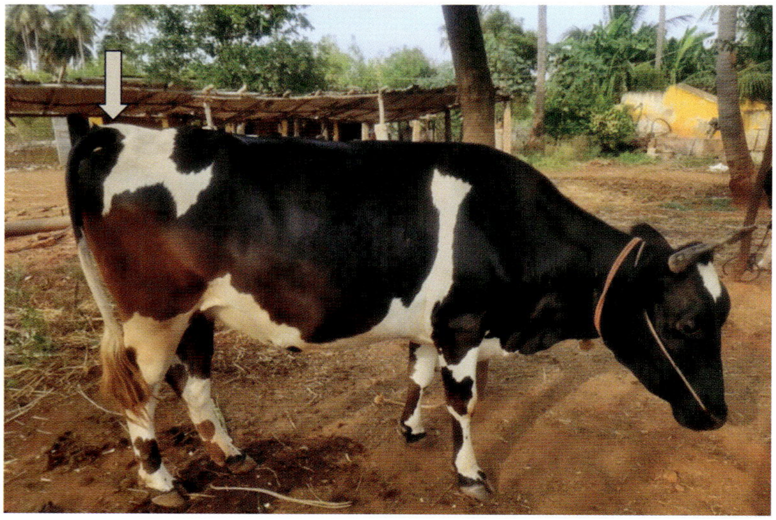

Figure 8.2 Sterility hump: a raised tail and the sinking of croup muscles.

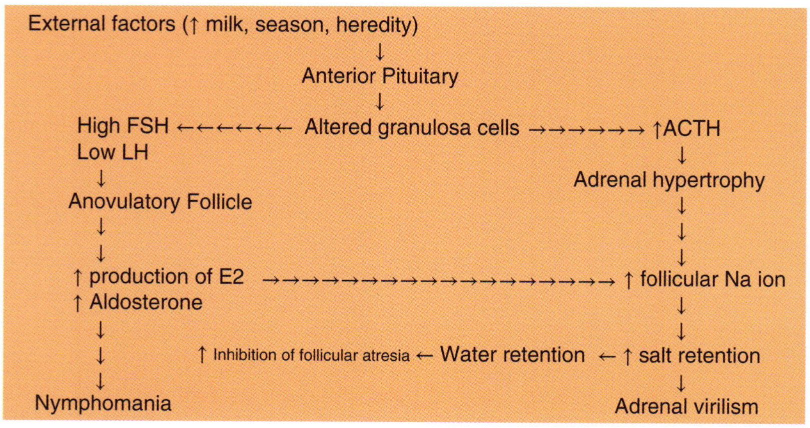

Figure 8.3 Pathophysiology of chronic follicular cysts in dairy cows. (FSH = follicle-stimulating hormone; LH = luteinizing hormone; ACTH = adrenocorticotropic hormone; E2 = estradiol; Na = sodium)

- Rough, dry hair coat.
- Nervous tension.
- Disturbed feeding and rumination.
- Progressive emaciation.

8.7 Diagnosis of Ovarian Cysts in Cattle

8.7.1 Rectal Examination

- **Follicular cyst:** FCs are single or multiple thin-walled, fluid-filled, distended, fluctuating structures within an enlarged ovary. They are often accompanied by a turgid and edematous uterus as well as voluminous thin or flocculating cervico-vaginal discharge (Coleman 2008).
- **Luteal cyst:** LCs are single thick-walled cysts that are firmer to palpate than FCs, although they are not as strong as the corpus luteum with a flaccid uterus and constricted cervix.

The transrectal palpation is the most frequently used method, although it does not allow for precise differentiation between FCs and LCs, and studies have shown that an accurate diagnosis is only possible in 50% of cases (Coleman 2008).

8.7.2 Transrectal Ultrasonography

- **Follicular cyst**: On an ultrasound, the FC is diagnosed as singular or multiple, anechoic, fluid-filled cavities with a diameter greater than 1.7 cm and a wall thickness more than 3 mm in the absence of a hypoechoic corpus luteum (CL) (Douthwaite and Dobson 2000) (Figures 8.4 and 8.5).
- **Luteal cyst**: On the other hand, an LC is diagnosed as a single, irregular, anechoic, fluid-filled structure with hypoechoic borders of a diameter greater than 2.5 mm and a wall thickness greater than 3 mm in the absence of a hypoechoic CL (Douthwaite and Dobson 2000).

Using these criteria, a correct diagnosis is possible in about 85% of cases. Therefore, an ultrasound examination is much more accurate at diagnosing the types of OCs than manual palpation due to its ability to detect luteal structures. Further, when an ultrasound is combined with an analysis of circulating P4 levels, the diagnosis accuracy improves to 92% for FCs and 82% for LCs (Douthwaite and Dobson 2000).

8.7.3 Progesterone Estimation

FCs are typically associated with a P4 plasma concentration of less than 1 ng/ml. However, some researchers suggest that concentrations varying from 0.5 to 5 ng/ml have been used as a maximum in cases of FCs. On the other hand, LCs are

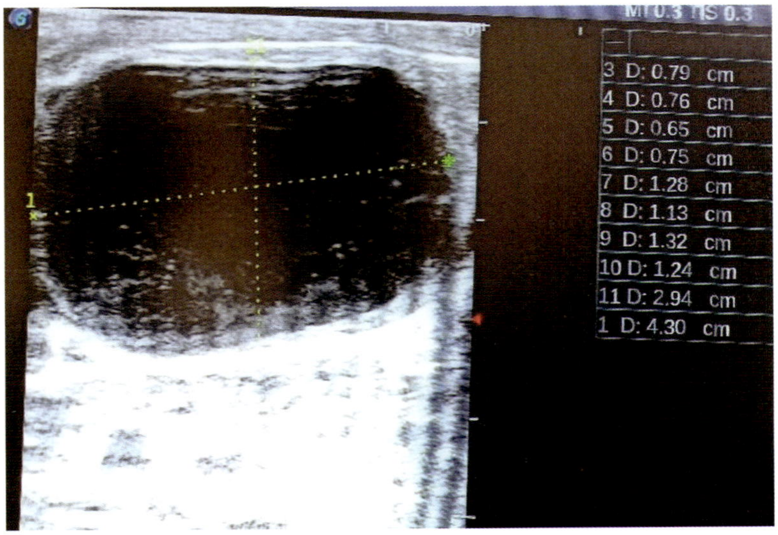

Figure 8.4 An ultrasonographic image of a follicular cyst that measures 3.62 cm in diameter (2.94 × 4.30 cm).

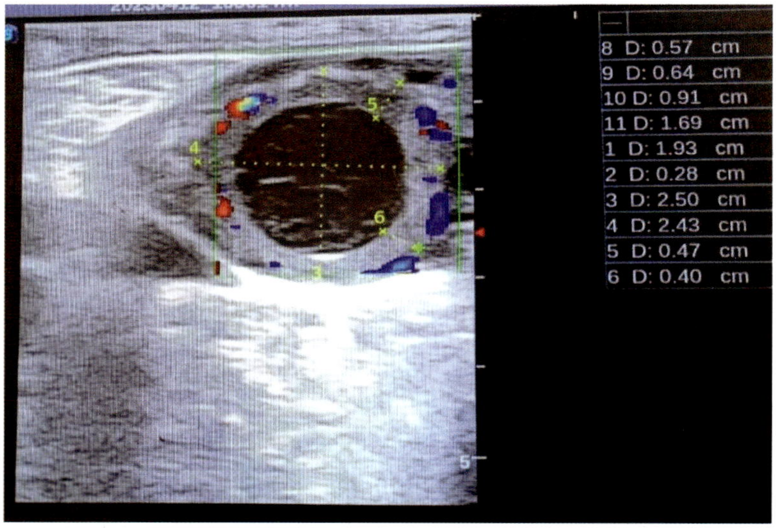

Figure 8.5 An ultrasonographic image of a luteal cyst with a 0.43-mm wall thickness (the average of 0.47 and 0.40 mm).

accompanied by a minimum plasma concentration greater than 1 ng/ml. However, P4 concentrations from 0 ng/ml (plasma) up to 10 ng/ml (milk) have been used in the case of LCs (Santos et al. 2009).

Thus, an accurate diagnosis of the OC type requires a combination of diagnostic approaches such as transrectal palpation, transrectal ultrasonography, and plasma P4 profiles (Mimoune et al. 2021).

8.7.3.1 Histopathology of the Uterus

In some cases, the uterus has multiple, small, anechoic, cystic structures due to endometrial hyperplasia that is commonly described as a "Swiss cheese appearance."

8.8 Treatment

8.8.1 Hormonal Treatment

8.8.1.1 hCG (Human Chorionic Gonadotropin)

Human chorionic gonadotropin is the drug of choice for FCs since it has predominantly LH-like action.

- **Dose:** 1500–3000 IU total dose/animal, intravenous (IV) or intramuscular (IM).
- **Mechanism of action:** A protein hormone with luteotropic effects that induces the luteinization of FCs or other follicles present; therefore, endogenous or exogenous prostaglandin (PG)F2α causes luteolysis and a new cycle begins (Roberts 1971).
- **Disadvantage:** Very expensive and antigenic, this protein can cause anaphylactic shock or a refractory state in cows.
- **Success rate:** In response to hCG, 58–86% of cows develop luteal tissue.

8.8.1.2 GnRH

GnRH is an effective treatment for FCs as it will initiate the secretion of LH from the anterior pituitary.

- **Dose:** Buserelin acetate at 20 µg total dose/animal, IM.
- **Mechanism of action:** GnRH causes an immediate increase in LH secretion and luteinization of the cyst. The ovulation of a cyst does not occur, but other follicles present at the time of treatment may ovulate. After luteinization, the elevated levels of P4 restore the hypothalamic response to the positive feedback of estradiol, and normal cyclic ovarian activity is restored after the release of endogenous $PGF_{2}\alpha$ and regression of the OC (Probo et al. 2011).
- **Advantage:** Since it is less antigenic and less expensive than hCG, GnRH is the most effective conventional treatment for OCs in cattle.
- **Success rate:** The percentage of cows that resume cyclicity is between 72% and 85%. The interval between treatment and first estrus is 19–23 days, and the rate of conception at first estrus ranges from 46% to 58% (Peter 2004).

8.8.1.3 PGF2α and Hormonal Associations

PGF2α is the most effective treatment for LCs. Cows with OCs at a low P4 concentration that did not respond to treatment with PGF2α alone had a high percentage of cyst turnover compared to those with a high P4 level (White and Erb 1980).

- **Dose:** Cloprostenol sodium at 500 µg total dose/animal or dinoprost at 25 mg total dose/animal, IM.
- **Mechanism of action:** Recent studies report that simultaneous treatment with PGF2α and GnRH analogs resulted in early estrus re-establishment in cows with LCs (50% of cows were in estrus). Cows with FCs responded more to GnRH and PGF2α in combination on days 0 and 7, respectively, compared to the administration of GnRH alone (López-Gatius and López-Bejar 2002).
- **Advantages:** This treatment is beneficial since the differentiation between FCs and LCs is difficult.

8.8.1.4 Progestogens

- **Dose:** Intravaginal implants (controlled intravaginal device release [CIDR]; progesterone-releasing intravaginal device [PRID]) for 9–12 days.
- **Mechanism of action:** Progesterone reduces the frequency of LH pulses for 9–12 days, so LH remains stored in the pituitary, and upon implant removal, GnRH stimulates LH discharge, which subsequently induces ovulation (Arunmozhi et al. 2016). Further, P4 restores the response of the hypothalamus to the positive feedback effect of estradiol, and estrus is followed by ovulation within 7 days of implant removal (Douthwaite and Dobson 2000).
- **Advantage:** Progesterone reduces the risk of OC persistence.
- **Success rate:** Estrus rates ranging from 82% to 100% and conception rates at first estrus ranging from 18% to 28% have been reported after P4 treatment. Further, treating OCs with the CIDR implant, followed by PGF2α upon removal, ensured good reproductive performances (Iwakuma et al. 2008).

8.8.2 Nonhormonal Treatment: OC Manual Rupture and Puncture

1) **Manual rupture:** In 1874, manual cyst rupture was used for the first time in Germany by Zschokke and successfully treated approximately 45% of OCs. Subsequently, studies have shown that this procedure can lead to trauma and bleeding that causes adhesions and contributes to reduced fertility, although it is not expensive (Roberts 1971).
2) **Ultrasound-guided transvaginal aspiration of FCs:** The nonresponsive ovarian cystic follicles can be aspirated by ultrasound-guided transvaginal aspiration (Pugazharasi et al. 2020). Upon aspiration, first estrus and gestation were observed at 34 and 55 days, respectively. The simultaneous injection of GnRH has also been suggested and, when followed by PGF2α on day 7, led to 100% and 68.8% estrus and conception rates, respectively. This method is expensive and noninvasive for animals (Cruz et al. 2004) (Figures 8.6 and 8.7).
3) **Transgluteal aspiration of FCs:** This method is also applicable for nonresponsive OCs. The cyst is aspirated through the transgluteal muscle, this technique further reduces the damage of the birth canal and ovarian stroma. This method has the same success rate as above, while being less expensive and noninvasive.

8.9 Prevention

Strategies to reduce OC incidence should focus on reducing diseases and stress as well as optimizing food intake during dry-off and postpartum periods.

1) Balanced diet.
2) Administration of antioxidants (β-carotenes, selenium) may be the most effective way to eliminate or reduce the harmful effects of this stress (Folnožić et al. 2019).
3) Regular assessment of the body condition score makes it possible to check the evolution and duration of the negative energy balance.
4) In order to restore ovarian activity as quickly as possible and to reduce the incidence of OCs, an injection of GnRH 10–15 days postpartum can be administered (Noseir et al. 2013).

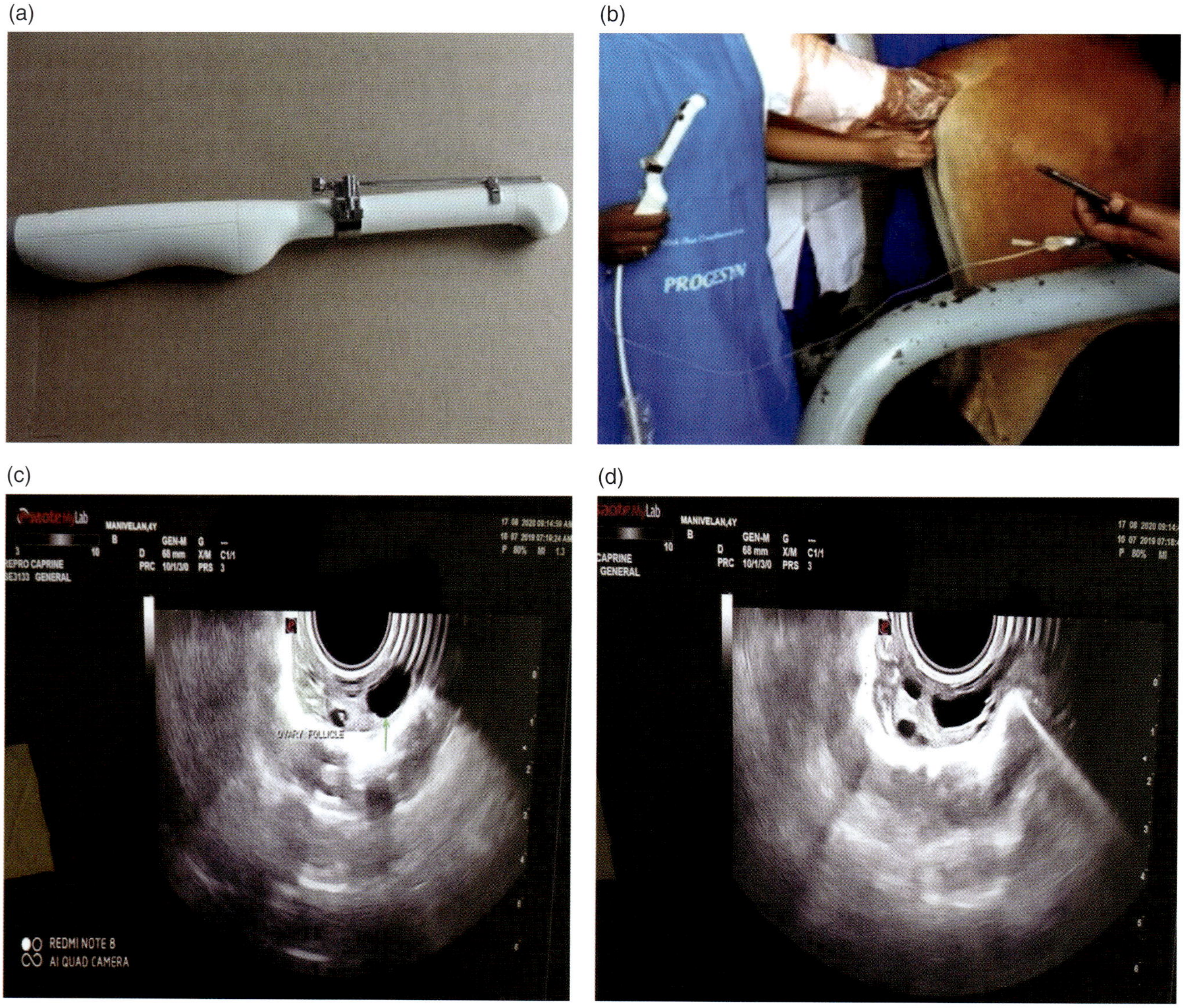

Figure 8.6 Ultrasound-guided transvaginal follicular aspiration. (a) The probe used for transvaginal aspiration along with the provision for insertion of the needle. (b) Image showing the transvaginal aspiration procedure. (c and d) The ultrasound image before and during follicular aspiration.

8.10 Conclusion

- OCs (follicular or luteal) in dairy cattle could be defined as anovulatory ovarian structures (i) with a cavity diameter greater than 20 mm in the absence of a CL, (ii) characterized by a combination of signs and symptoms of hormonal disorder and ovarian dysfunction, and (iii) in which the interaction of several genetic and environmental factors determine the heterogeneous, clinical, and biochemical phenotype.
- Therapeutic approaches should be targeted to restore the ovarian function and to improve pregnancy rates.

We do not know all the aspects that relate to the pathogenesis of OCs. The study of neuroendocrine feedback at the level of Kiss1 neurons with regards to OC formation might help elucidate this in more detail.

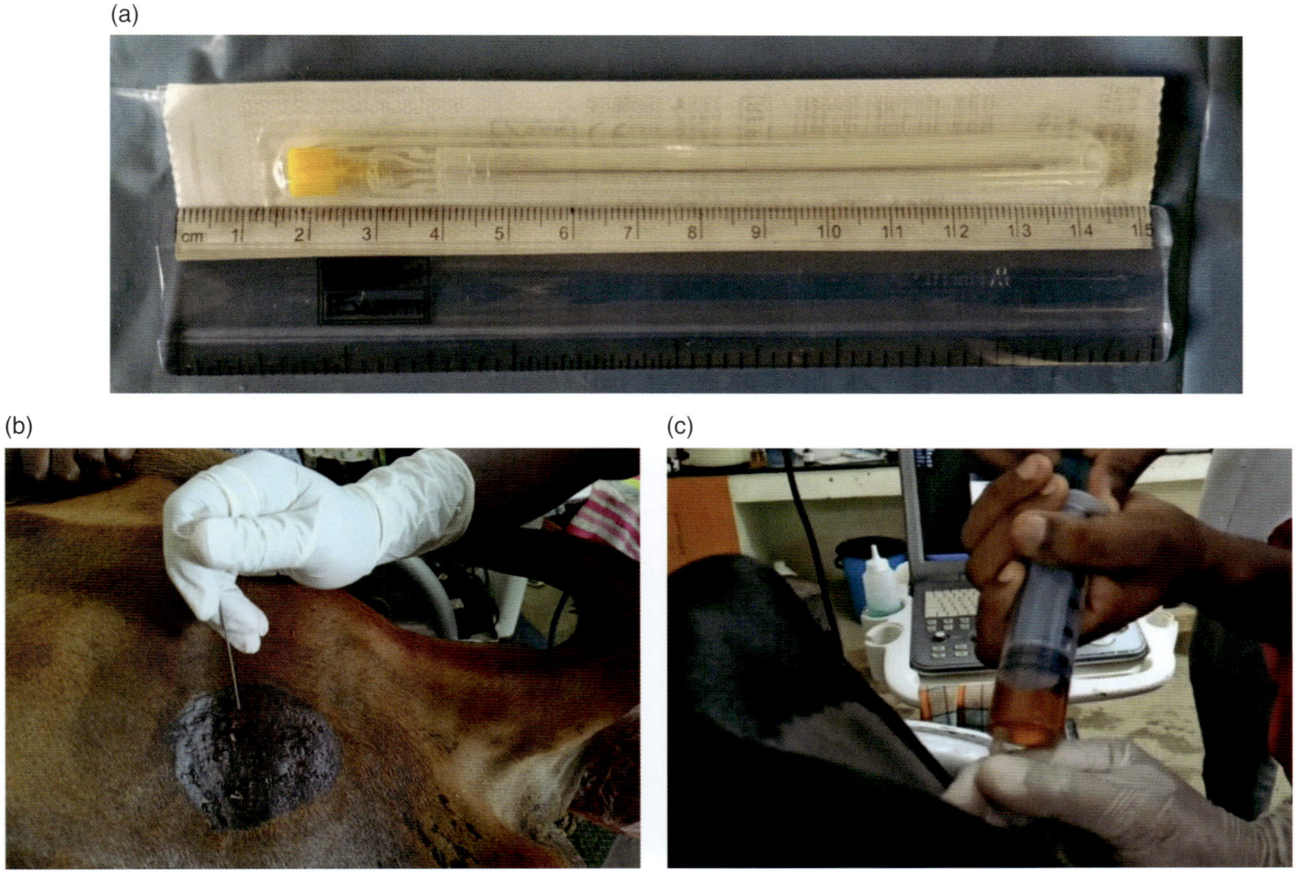

Figure 8.7 Transgluteal follicular aspiration using a spinal needle. (a) The spinal needle used for transgluteal follicular aspiration. (b) Insertion of the spinal needle for follicular aspiration. (c) The aspiration of follicular fluid through a transgluteal approach.

References

Arunmozhi, N., Rachel Jemimah, E., Sarath, T. et al. (2016). Fertility enhancement using P-24 and fixed time artificial insemination (FTAI) protocol in repeat breeder buffaloes. *The Indian Journal of Animal Sciences* 86 (2): 172–173.

Cairoli, F., Vigo, D., Battochio, M. et al. (2002). 17β-estradiol, progesterone and testosterone concentrations in cystic fluids and response to GnRH treatment after emptying of ovarian cysts in dairy cattle. *Reproduction in Domestic Animals* 37: 294–298.

Calder, M.S., Manikkam, M., Salfen, B.E. et al. (2001). Dominant bovine ovarian follicular cysts express increased levels of messenger RNAs for luteinizing hormone receptor and 3β-hydroxysteroid dehydrogenase Δ4,Δ5 isomerase compared to normal dominant follicles. *Biology of Reproduction* 65: 471–476.

Cattaneo, L., Signorini, M., Bertoli, J. et al. (2014). Epidemiological description of cystic ovarian disease in Argentine dairy herds: risk factors and effects on the reproductive performance of lactating cows. *Reproduction in Domestic Animals* 49: 1028–1033.

Coleman, D.A. (2008). *Cystic Ovarian Disease*. Dairy Integrated Reproductive Management, West Virginia University.

Cruz, C.E.F., Combellini, L.G., and Driemeier, D. (2004). Simple procedure for emptying longterm ovarian cysts in cattle. *The Veterinary Record* 155: 599–601.

Douthwaite, R. and Dobson, H. (2000). Comparison of different methods of diagnosis of cystic ovarian disease in cattle and an assessment of its treatment with a progesterone-releasing intravaginal device. *The Veterinary Record* 147: 355–359.

Farin, P.W., Youngquist, R.S., Parfet, J.R. et al. (1992). Diagnosis of luteal and follicular ovarian cysts by palpation per rectum and linear-array ultrasonography in dairy cows. *Journal of the American Veterinary Medical Association* 200: 1085–1089.

Folnožić, I., Đuričić, D., Žura Žaja, I. et al. (2019). Influence of dietary clinoptilolite on blood serum mineral profile in dairy cows. *Veterinarski Arhiv* 89: 447–462.

Garverick, H.A. (1997). Ovarian follicular cysts in dairy cows. *Journal of Dairy Science* 80: 995–1004.

Gümen, A. and Wiltbank, M.C. (2002). An alteration in the hypothalamic action of estradiol due to lack of progesterone exposure can cause follicular cysts in cattle. *Biology of Reproduction* 66: 1689–1695.

Imai, K., Amy Khandoker, M., Yonai, M. et al. (2003). Matrix metalloproteinases-2 and -9 activities in bovine follicular fluid of different-sized follicles: relationship to intrafollicular inhibin and steroid concentrations. *Domestic Animal Endocrinology* 24: 171–183.

Iwakuma, A., Suzuki, Y., Haneishi, T. et al. (2008). Efficacy of intravaginal progesterone administration combined with prostaglandin (F2 alpha) for cystic ovarian disease in Japanese Black cows. *The Journal of Veterinary Medical Science* 70: 1077–1083.

Jeengar, K., Chaudhary, V., Kumar, A. et al. (2014). Ovarian cysts in dairy cows: old and new concepts for definition, diagnosis and therapy. *Animal Reproduction* 11 (2): 63–73.

López-Gatius, F. and López-Bejar, M. (2002). Reproductive performance of dairy cows with ovarian cysts after different GnRH and cloprostenol treatments. *Theriogenology* 58: 1337–1348.

Mimoune, N., Azzouz, M.Y., Khelef, D., and Kaidi, R. (2021). Ovarian cysts in cattle: a review. *Veterinarska Stanica* 52 (5): 587–603.

Noseir, W.M.B., Metwally, K.K., and Shaker, N.N. (2013). Using double dose of GnRH for reducing incidence of cystic ovaries in cows. *Alexandria Journal of Veterinary Sciences* 39: 124–132.

Peter, A.T. (2004). An update on cystic ovarian degeneration in cattle. *Reproduction in Domestic Animals* 39: 1–7.

Probo, M., Comin, A., Mollo, A. et al. (2011). Reproductive performance of dairy cows with luteal or follicular ovarian cysts after treatment with buserelin. *Animal Reproduction Science* 127: 135–139.

Pugazharasi, C., Sarath, T., Arunmozhi, N. et al. (2020). Ultrasound guided transvaginal follicular aspiration technique for chronic follicular cyst in a Holstein Friesian crossbred cow. *Indian Journal of Veterinary and Animal Sciences Research* 49 (3): 66–69.

Roberts, S.J. (1971). *Veterinary Obstetrics and Genital Diseases*. Ann Arbor, MI: Edward Brothers Inc.

Rosenfeld, C.S., Yuan, X., Manikkam, M. et al. (1999). Cloning, sequencing, and localization of bovine estrogen receptor-β within the ovarian follicle. *Biology of Reproduction* 60: 691–697.

Santos, R.M., Démetrio, D.G.B., and Vasconcelos, J.L.M. (2009). Cisto ovarianoemvacas de leite: incidência, resposta à aplicação de GnRH e desempenhoreprodutivo. *Arquivo Brasileiro de Medicina Veterinária e Zootecnia* 61: 3.

Silvia, W.J., Hatler, T.B., and Nugent, A.M. (2002). Ovarian follicular cysts in dairy cows: an abnormality in folliculogenesis. *Domestic Animal Endocrinology* 23: 167–177.

Vanholder, T., Opsomer, G., and de Kruif, A. (2006). Aetiology and pathogenesis of cystic ovarian follicles in dairy cattle: a review. *Reproduction, Nutrition, Development* 46: 105–119.

White, M.E. and Erb, H. (1980). Treatment of ovarian cysts in dairy cattle. A decision analysis. *The Cornell Veterinarian* 70: 247–257.

Wills, J.R. (2012). Diagnosis and mechanisms of bovine ovarian cysts. PhD thesis, University of Nottingham. http://eprints.nottinghamac.uk/12674/3/Chapter_1. Literature Review. (accessed May 27, 2019).

Yeo, S.H. and Colledge, W.H. (2018). The role of Kiss1 neurons as integrators of endocrine, metabolic, and environmental factors in the hypothalamic-pituitary-gonadal axis. *Frontiers in Endocrinology* 9: 188.

Youngquist, R.S. and Threlfall, W.R. (2007). Ovarian follicular cysts. In: *Current Therapy in Large Animal Theriogenology* (ed. R.S. Youngquist and W.R. Threlfall), 379–383. St. Louis, MO: Saunders Elsevier.

Zaied, A.A., Garverick, H.A., Bierschwal, C.J. et al. (1980). Effect of ovarian activity and endogenous reproductive hormones on GnRH induced ovarian cycles in postpartum dairy cows. *Journal of Animal Science* 50: 508–513.

9

Retained Fetal Membranes: A Review

Sarath Thulasiraman[1], *Monica Gunasekar*[2], *Pradeep Nag Beladakere Subramanyam*[3], *and Arunmozhi Narayanasamy*[4]

[1] *Veterinary Clinical Complex, Veterinary College and Research Institute, Salem, Tamil Nadu Veterinary and Animal Sciences University, Attur, Tamil Nadu, India*
[2] *Department of Clinics, Madras Veterinary College, Chennai, Tamil Nadu, India*
[3] *Division of Animal Sciences, University of Missouri, Columbia, Missouri, USA*
[4] *Teaching Veterinary Clinical Complex, Veterinary College and Research Institute, Orathanadu, Thanjavur, Tamil Nadu Veterinary and Animal Sciences University, Chennai, Tamil Nadu, India*

9.1 Introduction

Retained fetal membranes (RFMs) in dairy cows refer to a situation where the fetal membranes are not expelled within 12–24 hours after calving (Fourichon et al. 2000). The occurrence of RFMs typically ranges from 3% to 12% in normal calving instances (Eiler 1997). Several factors increase the risk of RFMs, including abortion, difficult birth, multiple fetuses, concurrent illnesses, age, diet, seasonal influences, and the length of gestation. Despite the implication of numerous factors, the exact cause of RFMs remains unclear (Noakes et al. 2003). A common consequence of an RFM is postpartum metritis, which is characterized by an elevated body temperature for up to 10 days after birth that is accompanied by a foul-smelling, pus-filled, vaginal discharge. This condition is often linked to a delayed uterine involution (Sheldon and Dobson 2004). This chapter discusses various aspects of this disease.

9.2 Prevalence

The prevalence of RFMs could vary depending on several attributes like age, breed, calving, and sex of the fetus. The highest incidence of RFMs is reported between 6 and 7 years of age. Crossbred Jersey cows had the highest prevalence of RFM followed by crossbred Holstein–Friesian (HF) cows and Zebu cows. Early calves (two to three calvings) show a higher incidence of RFMs, and thereafter decrease steadily. Higher milk yield during second and third lactation might be due to increased calcium drainage in the milk leading to uterine atony. A higher prevalence of RFMs was observed for female fetuses compared to males, which might be due to a shorter gestational length. Parturition abnormalities like abortion, still birth, and twinning have been reported to cause a higher incidence of RFMs (Ahmed et al. 1999).

9.3 Predisposing Factors for RFMs

The primary factor for the normal shedding of fetal membranes after parturition is the timely breakdown of the cotyledon–caruncle complex, i.e. cotyledon proteolysis (dehiscence) and decreasing adhesiveness (viscosity) of the cotyledon–caruncle interface fluids rather than myometrial contraction. Any discrepancies in the cotyledon–caruncle detaching mechanisms result in the retention of fetal membranes.

Periparturient Diseases of Cattle, First Edition. Edited by Tanmoy Rana.

9.3.1 Damage to the Uterus

Trauma induced to the uterus while handling dystocia during obstetrical maneuvers including forced extraction, fetotomy, and cesarean section leads to the release of heparin from mast cells at the site of trauma. This heparin inhibits the secretion of collagenase, which aids in decreasing the adhesiveness between cotyledon and caruncle. Furthermore, insults caused to the muscle of the uterus due to dystocia will hinder the contracting power of uterus, thus hampering the expulsion of fetal membranes.

9.3.2 Hormonal Imbalance

Physiologically, just prior to parturition the plasma levels of estradiol 17 increases sharply in the dam, whereas progesterone levels will suddenly decline. Estrogen, at its maximum, will aid in the expulsion of fetal membranes. On the other hand, glucocorticoids down-regulate collagenases (Youngquist and Threlfall 2007). Hence, either a decrease in estrogen level or the administration of glucocorticoids such as dexamethasone to induce parturition will lead to a failure of the fetal membranes to be expelled. Furthermore, altered hormonal levels also result in the altered release of protease from epithelial cells, which compromises their activity in loosening the fetal membranes.

9.3.3 Nutritional Causes

Cows during the periparturient period (0–20 days postpartum) have a high energy demand for body maintenance and milk production. Inadequate nutrition during this period results in a negative energy balance, which leads to increased concentrations of non-esterified fatty acids (NEFAs) and β-hydroxybutyrate (BHBA) (Reddy et al. 2018). The increased concentrations of NEFA and BHBA result in metabolic diseases like ketosis, milk fever, etc. and reduces the phagocytic capacity of immune cells, which predisposes animals to reproductive disorders like dystocia, RFMs, cystic ovarian degeneration (COD), metritis, etc.

Vitamins deficiencies, viz. vitamin A and vitamin E, reduce epithelialization and antioxidant activity, respectively, at the placental level; this reduced antioxidant activity results in decreased estrogen production, decreased prostaglandin (PG) F2α, and a slow buildup of arachidonic and linoleic acids that further delay the expulsion of fetal membranes. Mineral deficiencies in selenium, calcium, and phosphorus ratios impair the immunity of the animal during the transition period by affecting the local defense mechanism of the uterus at the cellular level and thus predisposes the animal to an RFM.

9.3.4 Immune System

The deviation of normal neutrophil function, i.e. reduced leukocytic infiltration to the site of the signal (placentomes), and the reduced colonization of macrophages due to immunosuppression predisposes the cow to RFMs. Immunosuppression also compromises the protease activity of the leukocytes.

9.4 Physiology of Placental Separation

The placentome is considered the functional unit of the placenta, wherein the fetal cotyledons are attached to the maternal caruncles, which is mediated by villi or microvilli interactions in the cotyledon with the crypts of the caruncle. The placentome is maintained intact from the time of formation until parturition, a series of events during parturition aids the separation of cotyledons from maternal caruncles. Collagen links the interface together at several sites, and the breakdown of this collagen is likely a key factor in placental separation for cattle and buffaloes.

Parturition is initiated by a sequence of events triggered by fetal cortisol, which induces 17α-hydroxylase, aromatase, and several other enzymes that convert progesterone produced by the placenta to estrogen. An increase in the estrogen concentration further upregulates the oxytocin receptor on the myometrium and aids in the secretion of prostaglandins from the endometrium. PGF2α lyses the corpus luteum (CL), initiates myometrial contractions, and decreases the concentration of progesterone. Furthermore, relaxin secretion is aided by decreased progesterone and increased estrogen concentrations that activate the collagenase, which is required for remodeling of the cervix and is a key factor for the separation of maternal and fetal placenta.

The processes that lead to a normal separation and delivery of the placenta are multifactorial and begin before parturition. In addition to the described mechanisms, maturation of the fetal monoamine oxidase enzyme system occurs near parturition, which is important for degradation of serotonin. This results in a reduction of the serotonin concentration, which is vital in maintaining the caruncular attachment with cotyledons. Furthermore, the reduction in the serotonin concentration also activates metallomembrane proteases that aid in placental separation and uterine remodeling leading up to parturition (Beagley et al. 2010).

9.5 Clinical Signs

- Dull and depressed.
- Anorexic.
- Soiled fetal membranes hanging from the vulva, with or without a foul smell (Figure 9.1).
- Foul-smelling discharge from the vagina (long standing cases).

9.6 Treatment

Different treatment modalities have been used for RFMs, ranging from manual removal to collagenase treatment, and are discussed in this section.

9.6.1 Manual Removal

Manual removal (Figures 9.2 and 9.3) is one of the oldest treatments used. However, the manual removal of fetal membranes prolongs the interval from calving to first functioning CL by 20 days (LeBlanc 2008). The removal of placental adhesions damages the endometrium and suppresses uterine leukocyte phagocytosis (Goshen and Shpigel 2006), which leads to bacterial invasion (Fourichon et al. 2000). The combination of endometrial damage, bacterial invasion, and

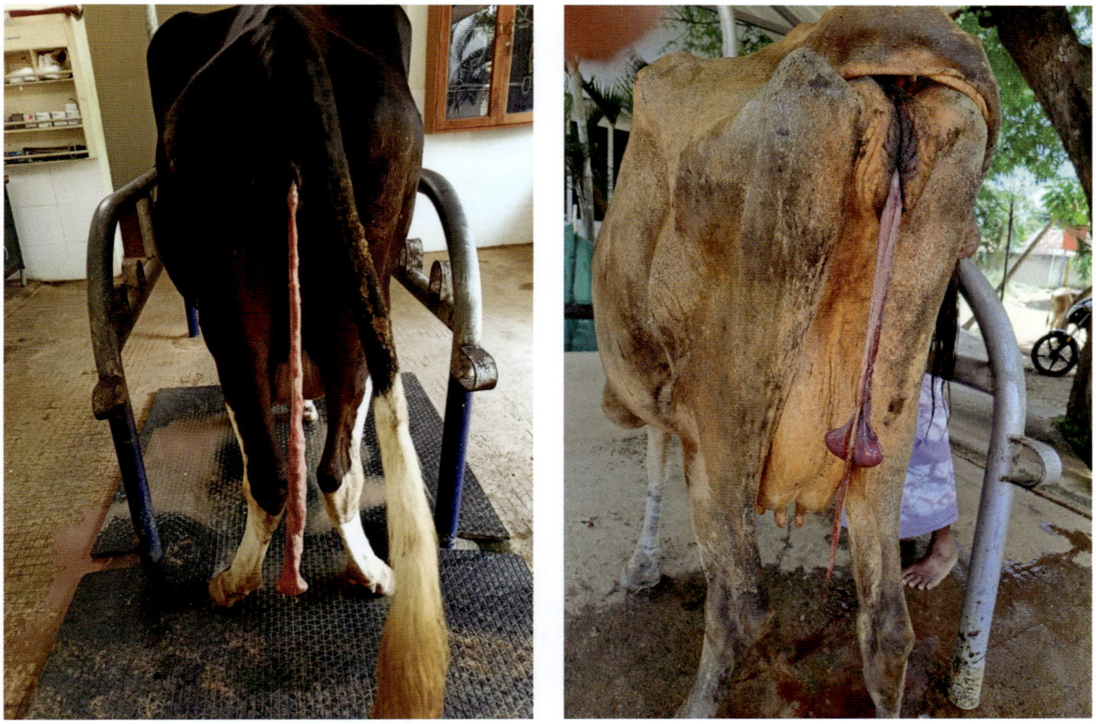

Figure 9.1 A retained fetal membrane hanging from the vulva.

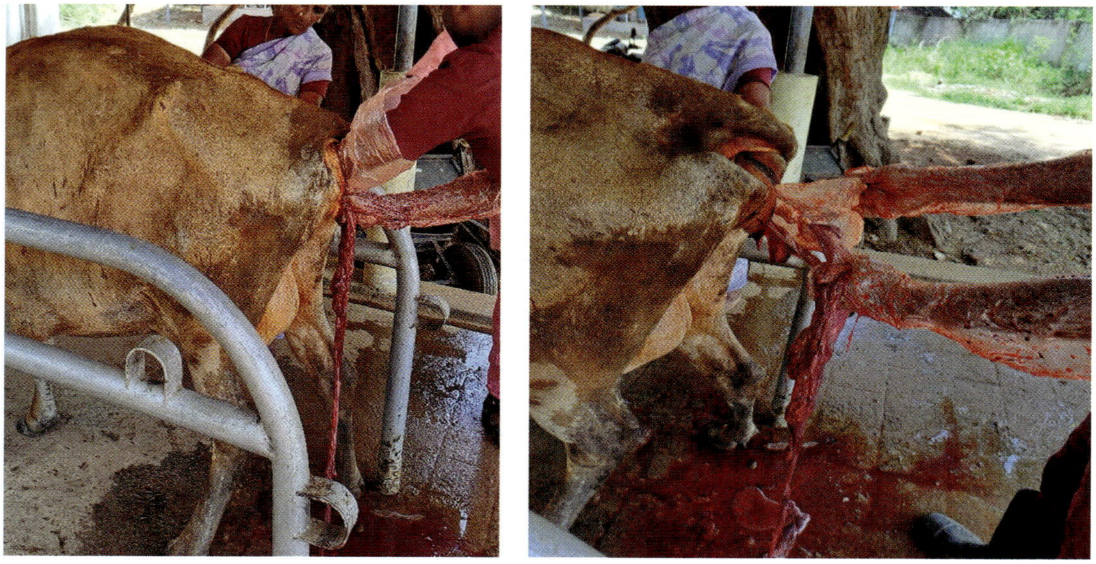

Figure 9.2 Manual separation of the cotyledonary–caruncular complex and removal of the placenta.

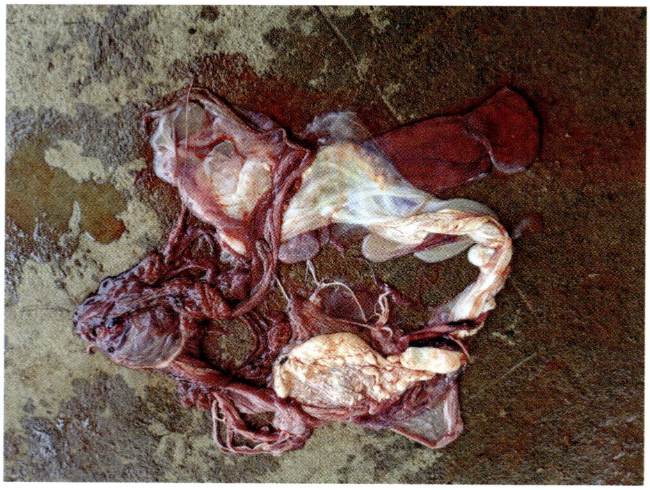

Figure 9.3 Fetal membranes after their removal from a cow affected by a retained fetal membrane.

suppression of phagocytic activity results in an increased likelihood of developing postpartum metritis and subsequent negative effects on fertility. Owing to all these problems, the manual removal of placental membranes is no longer considered an effective treatment for RFMs.

9.6.2 Antimicrobial Therapy

Antimicrobial therapy involves the utilization of various antibiotics for the treatment of RFMs, with conflicting results. Usually, RFMs are comorbid with metritis, with or without systemic involvement. Antibiotics have been tried locally, systemically, and in a combination of both local and systematically. Intrauterine infusions or bolus are the most common forms of intrauterine therapy. Ceftiofur sodium and tetracyclines have been successfully used in treatment as intrauterine infusions. In the recent past, cephalexin, metronidazole, and levofloxacin have been used most often in commercial intrauterine preparations. Although intrauterine preparations have reduced the incidence of metritis in RFM-affected cows by restricting bacterial growth, they interfere with the necrotizing process responsible for the eventual release of RFMs (Roberts 1986). Therefore, systemic antibiotics are believed to be beneficial in RFM cases where a fever is also present (LeBlanc 2008). Systemic antibiotics alone are just as effective as systemic antibiotics in combination with intrauterine treatment (Drillich et al. 2006).

9.6.3 Hormonal Therapy

Hormonal interventions have also been tried in the treatment of RFMs, viz. prostaglandins and oxytocin. These are effective at treating RFMs associated with uterine atony. Oxytocin appears to aid in the expulsion of the placenta only a few hours after parturition due to a reduction of its receptors in later stages. Prostaglandin has not been proven very effective at treating RFMs. However, a few studies have reported the complete expulsion of the placenta within 12 hours when treated with PGF2α after a cesarean section (Stocker and Waelchli 1993).

9.6.4 Collagenase Administration

Collagenase has been considered an important factor in the separation of fetal and maternal placenta; an infusion of collagenase could aid in the destruction of cotyledon–caruncle bonds, which results in placental separation. The injection of 200 000 IU of bacterial collagenase in 1 l of saline into the umbilical arteries of the RFM has been effective at treating RFMs. The administration of collagenase within 24–72 hours after calving aids the expulsion of fetal membranes in 85% (23 of 27) of cows within 36 hours (Eiler and Hopkins 1993). However, the cost incurred when treating with collagenase is high; it may not be considered a viable option for the treatment of RFMs in cattle.

Ozone (O_3) is the most recent method used to treat RFMs. Ozone possesses bactericidal, anti-inflammatory, and immune-stimulating properties that make it a choice for treating RFMs. A recent study has claimed that an intrauterine ozone flush is a potential and cost-effective treatment option for a retained placenta, with positive effects on uterine health and fertility (Zobel and Tkalčić 2013).

The intrauterine ozone flush, therefore, has potential as an efficacious and cost-effective treatment option for retained placentas, with an overall positive effect on puerperal health and fertility in cows.

9.7 Preventing RFMs

The control of RFMs could be achieved by concentrating on predisposing and causative factors like abortions, premature calving, dystocia, and vitamin and mineral deficiencies. Ensuring quality feed during the transition period and preventing a negative energy balance as well as metabolic disorders may be instrumental in preventing RFMs. Furthermore, herds with a higher incidence of RFM can be supplemented with vitamin E and selenium to lower its incidence.

9.8 Conclusion

The expulsion of fetal membranes following parturition is a complex process that involves peripartum endocrine and biochemical changes. Disturbances to any of the normal processes that involve placental separation may result in the retention of fetal membranes. Understanding the pathophysiology of disease helps in understanding the disease and developing different treatment modalities. RFMs are often associated with other complications such as puerperal metritis; treatment of the condition should focus on easing placental separation, preventing bacterial colonization, and not interfering with the uterine cleansing process. Considering the magnitude of the disease, the effective use of available treatment strategies and further exploration of new treatment modalities are warranted.

References

Ahmed, W.M., El-Ekhnawy, K.I., Desouky, H.M. et al. (1999). Investigations on retained fetal membranes in Friesian cows in Egypt. *Egyptian Journal of Comparative Pathology and Clinical Pathology* 12: 160–177.

Beagley, J.C., Whitman, K.J., Baptiste, K.E., and Scherzer, J. (2010). Physiology and treatment of retained fetal membranes in cattle. *Animal Reproduction Science* 24 (2): 261–268.

Drillich, M., Mahlstedt, M., Reichert, U., and Tenhagen, B.A. (2006). Strategies to improve the therapy of retained fetal membranes in dairy cows. *Journal of Dairy Science* 89: 627–635.

Eiler, H. (1997). Retained placenta. In: *Current Therapy in Large Animal Theriogenology* (ed. R.S. Youngquist), 340–348. Philadelphia: WB Saunders.

Eiler, H. and Hopkins, F.M. (1993). Successful treatment of retained placenta with umbilical cord injections of collagenase in cows. *Journal of the American Veterinary Medical Association* 3: 436–443.

Fourichon, C., Seegers, H., and Malher, X. (2000). Effect of disease on reproduction in the dairy cow: a meta-analysis. *Theriogenology* 53: 1729–1759.

Goshen, T. and Shpigel, N.Y. (2006). Evaluation of intrauterine antibiotic treatment of clinical metritis and retained fetal membranes in dairy cows. *Theriogenology* 66: 2210–2218.

LeBlanc, S.J. (2008). Postpartum uterine disease and dairy herd reproductive performance: a review. *Veterinary Journal* 176: 102–114.

Noakes, D.A., Parkinson, T.J., and England, C.C.W. (2003). *Arthur's Veterinary Reproduction and Obstetrics*, 8e. Saunders Co.

Reddy, A.N., Seshiah, C.V., Sudhakar, K. et al. (2018). Effects of shortened dry period on the physical indicators of energy reserves mobilization in high yielding Murrah buffaloes. *Indian Journal of Animal Research* 52: 1656–1660.

Roberts, S.J. (1986). *Veterinary Obstetrics and Genital Diseases*, 373–393. Woodstock, VT: SJ Roberts.

Sheldon, I.M. and Dobson, H. (2004). Postpartum uterine health in cattle. *Animal Reproduction Science* 82–83: 295–306.

Stocker, H. and Waelchli, R.O. (1993). A clinical trial on the effect of prostaglandin F2a on placental expulsion in dairy cattle after caesarean operation. *The Veterinary Record* 132: 507–508.

Youngquist, R.S. and Threlfall, W.R. (2007). *Current therapy in large animal theriogenology*, 2e, 560–572. Saunders Elsevier.

Zobel, R. and Tkalčić, S. (2013). Efficacy of ozone and other treatment modalities for retained placenta in dairy cows. *Reproduction in Domestic Animals* 48 (1): 121–125.

10

Periparturient Immunological Disorders

Amitava Roy[1], *Tanmoy Rana*[2], *and Arkaprabha Shee*[3]

[1] *Livestock Farm Complex, West Bengal University of Animal & Fishery Sciences, Kolkata, West Bengal, India*
[2] *Department of Veterinary Clinical Complex, West Bengal University of Animal & Fishery Sciences, Kolkata, West Bengal, India*
[3] *Dhaanyaganga Krishi Vigyan Kendra, Sargachi, Murshidabad, West Bengal, India*

10.1 Introduction

Health issues that arise during the periparturient period are particularly problematic for dairy cattle because they have a significant impact on the productive efficiency of cows during their subsequent lactation (Pinedo et al. 2010). Dairy cattle are susceptible to increased incidence and severity of disease during this period. In fact, according to LeBlanc et al. (2006), 75% of illness incidence in herds occurs within the first month of lactation, including conditions with economic significance such mastitis, metritis, ketosis, and displaced abomasa. Therefore, to develop more effective management strategies to lower health disorders during periparturient periods, a number of studies have been conducted to better understand the underlying causes of both metabolic and infectious diseases around the time of parturition (Roche et al. 2013). The effectiveness of cows' immune systems affects their capacity to fend off sickness throughout the periparturient phase. The immune system is made up of many biological mechanisms and parts that work together to shield cows against the negative effects of illness. The immune system's main functions are to stop germs from entering the body, get rid of infections that are already present as well as other sources of cellular damage, and return tissues to their normal state of function. Animal immune systems defend against a wide range of pathogenic threats by utilizing a complex network of soluble, cellular, and physical components. In order to preserve a delicate balance between the activation of immunity required to stop the spread of illness and the resolution of activity after the threat of invasion has passed, this integrated system of defense mechanisms is closely regulated. In this chapter, the immune system will be briefly reviewed along with the ways in which inadequate immune responses can lead to disease and the methods currently used to maximize immune responses in food-animal subjects when disease susceptibility is high will be discussed.

10.2 The Immune System in General

Animals with healthy immune systems should be shielded from a range of harmful organisms, such as bacteria, viruses, and parasites. The immune system uses a dynamic and intricate network of defense mechanisms, which are easily divided into two categories (i) innate immunity and (ii) adaptive or acquired immunity (Table 10.1) to carry out this function. Defense systems can be further divided into cell-mediated immunity, soluble or humoral immunity, and physical barriers, within both innate and adaptive immunity.

10.2.1 Adaptive Immunity

When innate immune systems are unable to eradicate a disease, the adaptive immune response is triggered. The production of antigen-specific lymphocytes and memory cells that can identify particular antigenic determinants of a disease are hallmarks of the adaptive immune response. Immunological memory and the clonal growth of antigen-specific effector

Periparturient Diseases of Cattle, First Edition. Edited by Tanmoy Rana.

Table 10.1 Groups within the immune system.

Adaptive immunity	Innate immunity
Immunological memory	No immune memory
Immunization against antibodies	Minutes after exposure, immediately after
Antigen-specific response	Inflammation
Soluble and cellular components	Nonspecific or generic response
Delayed following exposure (days)	Soluble and cellular components
No mechanical or physical obstacles	Physical and mechanical barriers

Table 10.2 Elements of adaptive immunity.

Factor	Main functions
Mastocytes and dendritic cells	Presentation cells for antigens
B lymphocytes	Antigen presentation; develop into plasma cells that produce antibodies
T lymphocytes	$CD4^+$ or T helper cells (Th1, Th2, Th17, Treg); generate the cytokines that control both adaptive and innate immunity; immunoglobulin isotype switching
	$CD8^+$ or T cytotoxic (Tc) cells; assault and destroy virus-infected cells that express foreign antigens
	T cells; prevalent at mucosal surfaces
Immunoglobulin (Ig; antibodies)	The largest and initially generated antibody, IgM, has a function in complement activation and agglutination
	Serum has a high IgG concentration, which is crucial for opsonization
	IgA has an antiviral effect and is present on mucosal surfaces
	Allergies and parasite illnesses are linked to IgE
	Regulation molecule IgD is not secreted
Significant histocompatibility	Identifies self from nonself

cells result in an increased state of immune responsiveness when host cells and tissues are re-exposed to the same antigen. Compared to a primary immune response, a memory immune response would be far quicker, stronger, more durable, and frequently more successful when eliminating an invasive pathogen. As opposed to the innate immune response, the clonal growth of B and T cells that are unique to the invasive pathogen causes adaptive immunity to evolve over several days. A remarkable characteristic of the immune system is the host's capacity to identify and react to billions of distinct antigens that it may come into contact with. It is also critical that the host's own antigens do not trigger an improperly targeted immune response. Because of this, the immune system can differentiate between self and nonself and respond to foreign antigens exclusively. Major histocompatibility complex (MHC) molecules are membrane-bound, genetically heterogeneous proteins that aid in identification. Only when antigens are coupled with an MHC molecule on the surface of particular cells – a process known as antigen presentation – will a particular immune response take place (Sordillo and Aitken 2011). Vaccine techniques are based on the distinct characteristics of the adaptive immune response (Table 10.1).

Antigen-presenting cells and lymphocytes are the two types of cells involved in the generation of efficient specific immunity. By means of membrane receptors unique to the invasive pathogen, lymphocytes are able to identify bacterial antigens. These are the cells that mediate the characteristics that distinguish adaptive immunity, including memory, self/nonself-identification, diversity, and specificity. Two unique subsets of lymphocytes with different functions and protein products are the T and B lymphocytes. T cells, which comprise $CD4^+$ (T helper) and $CD8^+$ (T cytotoxic) lymphocytes (Table 10.2). The percentages of these cells might vary greatly, depending on the tissue (Sordillo and Streicher 2002). One of the effector roles of T cells is to produce cytokines, which control the strength and duration of the immune response, thus promoting cell-mediated immunity.

When T helper lymphocytes (Th1, Th2, Th17, and Treg) recognize antigen–MHC complexes on antigen-presenting cells (B lymphocytes and macrophages), they release cytokines. T helper cells release a range of immunoregulatory cytokines when they are activated. T helper cells are essential for the activation of B and T lymphocytes, neutrophils, macrophages, and other immune response cells due to their capacity to release specific cytokines. Different immune responses are caused by variations in the pattern of cytokines that activated T helper cells produce. For instance, it is believed that the cytokines interleukin (IL)-2 and interferon (IFN)-α may promote some nonspecific cellular processes such as intracellular death and phagocytosis (Sordillo and Aitken 2011). Antibodies, or immunoglobulin (Ig), that identify and neutralize microbial virulence factors are produced and secreted by B lymphocytes unique to antigens. B lymphocytes stimulated by antigens create immunoglobulins, and these cells then divide and mature into plasma cells that secrete antibodies. IgD, IgG, IgA, and IgM are the four classes of immunoglobulins known to affect host defense against infectious diseases; these classes vary in their physiochemical and biological characteristics. For instance, multiple Ig isotypes, including IgG1, IgG2, and IgM, can function as opsonins to promote neutrophil and macrophage phagocytosis. Apart from its function in opsonization, IgM demonstrates efficiency in complement fixation. IgA participates in bacterial agglutination, which can prevent some infections from spreading across particular tissues, but it does not help with bacterial opsonization. The capacity for IgA to neutralize various bacterial toxins is another crucial function. The amount and isotype makeup of immunoglobulin present in tissues can have a significant impact on the development of new infections.

10.2.2 Inflammation

An essential part of the body's natural defense mechanism, inflammation is the result of intricate biological reactions that involve soluble and cellular components to localized tissue damage or trauma. The aim of the host's inflammatory reactions is to eradicate the cause of tissue damage, re-establish immunological equilibrium, and enable tissues to resume their typical functions. The inflammatory cascade causes an increase in leukocyte and plasma component migration from the circulation into infected tissues, in addition to the local increase in antimicrobial agents. According to Mattmiller et al. (2013), redness, heat, swelling, and discomfort are examples of clinical indicators of inflammation. Different modifications in vascular endothelial responses can account for these clinical manifestations. For instance, higher blood flow that results from an expanded vascular diameter causes redness, heat, and pain. Increased vascular permeability causes fluids and proteins that have collected in tissues to leave the bloodstream. This is caused by the dissociation of the tightly packed endothelial cells that line blood vessels. These occurrences explain the edema or swelling connected to inflammation.

The vascular endothelium not only modifies blood flow but also acts as a "gatekeeper," that controls leukocyte migration from blood arteries into impacted tissues. To start the inflammatory cascade, host cells have pattern molecule receptors triggered by pathogen-associated molecular patterns (PAMPs). These receptors subsequently release a variety of inflammatory mediators, including oxylipids and cytokines. These inflammatory mediators directly affect the vascular endothelium, reducing blood flow while simultaneously causing endothelial cells to express more adhesion molecules. To enable leukocyte migration from the circulation to the site of damage, adhesion molecules on leukocytes bind to vascular adhesion molecules (Hodgkinson et al. 2007). Most cells that go through this extravasation process in the early phases of inflammation are neutrophils. In the vicinity of the infection site, neutrophils cling to the local endothelium after first marginating. Adherent neutrophils are stimulated by cytokines, oxylipids, and other mediator molecules to migrate between endothelial cells and cross the basement membrane into the areas of injured tissue. Chemotactic gradients produced at the localized site of infection by inflammatory mediator molecules help neutrophils migrate throughout the tissues. As soon as 30–60 minutes after injury, neutrophil migration can happen, swiftly building up within the damaged tissues (Summers et al. 2010).

Leukocyte populations that were already there and those that were recruited recently work together to eradicate microbial infections. Tissue-resident macrophages release oxylipids and immune-regulatory cytokines in response to bacterial invasion. The ability to phagocytize and eliminate invasive microorganisms is shared by recruited neutrophils and macrophages. The internalization of bacteria within phagosomes that contain hydrolytic enzymes and bactericidal reactive oxygen species (ROS) is the process of phagocytosis. According to Sordillo and Aitken (2009), respiratory burst activity produces superoxide radicals and hydrogen peroxide by activating NADPH oxidase. This process produces ROS. Myeloperoxides have the ability to further combine chloride and hydrogen peroxide to create hypochlorite, which is connected to bacterial activity. Apart from phagocytosis, neutrophils can eliminate germs via extracellular means. In order to capture and eliminate germs, activated neutrophils can create neutrophil extracellular traps (NETs), a web of fibers made of chromatin and serine proteases. According to research, NETs offer highly concentrated foci of antibacterial compounds that bind and destroy bacteria without requiring the mammary gland's phagocytic absorption (Grinberg et al. 2008). Additionally, NETs may operate as a physical barrier to stop bacteria from spreading throughout the mammary gland.

10.2.3 Innate Immunity

In most organisms, the innate immune system serves as the primary host defense mechanism. The immune system's non-specific components, which can react to pathogenic bacteria in a general way, are referred to as innate immunity. Since innate immunity components are already present at the site of exposure or quickly activate, they serve as the first line of defense against invasive pathogens. Following an invasion, germs may be eradicated in a matter of minutes to hours, contingent upon the effectiveness of inherent defenses. The speed and effectiveness of this first line of defense may prevent any appreciable alterations in the tissues' regular physiological processes as a result of the attempted microbial invasion. However, repeated exposure to the same insult does not enhance innate immune responses due to their generic nature. Phagocytes, different soluble mediators, and mechanical and physical barriers are elements of the innate immune system (Table 10.3). Obstacles, both mechanical and physical, are necessary to keep infections out of the body. Skin, tears, and mucus are a few examples of surface barrier defenses that prevent microbial infiltration. The cellular and soluble elements of the innate immune response, however, must move quickly to stop the effective establishment of disease after pathogens have managed to get past this first line of defense (Aitken et al. 2011).

Innate immunity relies heavily on pattern recognition receptors to identify invasive microorganisms that manage to penetrate defenses against surface invasion. Pattern recognition receptors identify a variety of microbial components linked to infectious diseases and can be expressed intracellularly, on cell surfaces, or in secretions. PAMPs are a broad category of conserved motifs specific to particular types of microorganisms. Examples of PAMPs include the lipopeptides found in gram-positive bacteria and the lipopolysaccharide found in gram-negative bacteria (Kumar et al. 2011). Pattern recognition receptors, such as CD14, nucleotide-binding oligomerization domains (NODs), and the family of Toll-like receptors (TLRs), which includes TLR-2, TLR-4, TLR-5, and TLR-9, are present in both immune and nonimmune cells in animals and are capable of differentiating a variety of PAMPs (Kumar et al. 2011). Pattern recognition receptors can directly promote antimicrobial activity or start intracellular signaling cascades that initiate innate immune responses upon binding to their ligand (Aitken et al. 2011).

When an invading bacterium enters the animal successfully, it can encounter several endogenous soluble defenses of innate immunity. Some of these soluble components are either pre-existing or generated by signaling cascades following the recognition of microbial PAMPs by host-cell pattern recognition receptors, depending on the invasion site. One element of the innate defense system is complement, which is a group of proteins found in serum and other bodily fluids. Hepatocytes are the primary cellular source of complement system proteins, but monocytes and tissue macrophages also contribute. Complement components C3 and C5a, which form pore-forming complexes on the surfaces of bacteria, can directly cause

Table 10.3 The elements of innate immunity.

Factor	Main functions
Neutrophils	Phagocytosis and reactive oxygen species generation
Pattern recognition receptors	Monitoring and innate immune response activation
Complement	Bacteriolytic, facilitates phagocytosis
Physical barriers	Stop and capture of microorganisms (skin, tears, mucus)
Oxylipids (prostaglandins, leukotrienes)	Pro-inflammatory and pro-resolving
Endothelial cells	Controls the movement and activation of leukocytes
Dendritic cells	Links innate and adaptive immunity through phagocytosis
Macrophages	Phagocytosis, synthesis of oxylipids and cytokines
Natural killer cells	Targets and aids in the removal of contaminated host cells
Cytokines	Pro-inflammatory and immune suppressive

bactericidal effects when the complement system is activated (Riollet et al. 2000). Opsonizing bacteria and preparing or activating host immune cells for phagocytosis and intracellular death are two other crucial biological roles of complement that support early microbial killing. In the early phases of infection, complement is also a strong chemoattractant for monocytes and neutrophils (Rainard 2003).

When PAMPs activate pattern recognition receptors, soluble innate defenses are triggered, and cytokines are a prime example of this. For instance, when TLRs are activated, the NF-κB signaling cascade is triggered, and one of the main reactions is increased cytokine expression. The cytokine network is made up of a broad range of proteins that are produced by immune and nonimmune cells in many parts of the body and under various conditions. The cytokine network has a sophisticated potential to modulate both the immune system and physiology. Individual cytokines can interact with other cytokines in a variety of cell targets either additively, antagonistically, or synergistically. Due to significant functional redundancy within the cytokine network, many cytokines can have similar effects on biological processes. Because most cytokines have very short half-lives, their synthesis and activity typically happen in bursts (Sordillo and Streicher 2002). High affinity receptors for each cytokine are found on host cells and allow cytokines to affect cellular processes. As a result, the relative expression of cytokine receptors influences the activity of responder cells, in addition to the amount and kind of cytokines present in the tissue milieu.

When it comes to innate immunity, cytokines have a variety of impacts. They can trigger an inflammatory response or make it easier for leukocytes to migrate from blood into infected tissues when local cell populations have recognized the pathogen. Depending on the kind of pathogen that triggers the immune reaction, different cells will express cytokines in different ways. However, compared to gram-positive bacteria, which typically produce a weaker and delayed cytokine response during the early stages of infection, gram-negative bacteria generally initiate a bigger magnitude of pro-inflammatory cytokine responses (i.e. IL-1, IL-6, IL-8, and tumor necrosis factor [TNF]-α). Oxylipids are a class of lipid mediators that control the beginning, intensity, and length of the inflammatory response, hence promoting innate immunity. According to Schmitz and Ecker (2008), ω-3 eicosapentaenoic (EPA) and docosahexaenoic (DHA) acids or ω-6 linoleic and arachidonic acids – polyunsaturated fatty acid substrates – are found mostly in the cell membrane and are the source of oxylipids. ROS or various enzymatic pathways, such as cyclooxygenases (COXs), lipoxygenases (LOXs), and cytochrome P450 pathways, nonenzymatically oxidize these fatty acid substrates to produce a range of oxylipids, such as prostaglandins (PGs), thromboxanes (TXs), leukotrienes (LTs), and lipoxins (LXs).

Certain oxylipids can either resolve or exacerbate the inflammatory response, depending on when and how much they express themselves. By raising vascular permeability, leukocyte infiltration, localized edema, and fever, oxylipids can intensify inflammatory processes. For instance, COX-2 enzyme activity rises in response to microbial stimuli and triggers the manufacture of oxylipids, such as PGE2, PGF2α, and TXA2, with vasoactive and pro-inflammatory characteristics. Nonsteroidal anti-inflammatory medications (NSAIDs) target COX activity to limit the production of PG and TX, and they are used to treat a range of inflammatory illnesses in food animals. Nevertheless, the available research does not support earlier theories that all COX metabolites are exclusively responsible for triggering the inflammatory response (Serhan et al. 2008). PGE2 synthesis is indicative of enhanced COX-2 expression at the start of inflammation, but the resolution of inflammation is linked to the existence of COX-derived PGD2 and 15d-PGJ2 (Prasad et al. 2008). According to Serhan et al. (2008), more recent research has revealed the existence of anti-inflammatory LXs, which are created when the 5-LOX pathway breaks down hydroperoxy fatty acid intermediates. Additionally, COXs and LOXs can oxidize ω-3 fatty acids to create oxylipids that have stronger anti-inflammatory or resolving qualities (Schmitz and Ecker 2008). For instance, 15-LOX converts DHA to D-series resolvins, protectins, and the macrophage-specific maresin, while 5-LOX metabolizes EPA to create E-series resolvins and modified versions of COX-2 (Serhan and Chiang 2008). Full resolution and restoration of homeostasis in the damaged tissues are impeded during uncontrolled inflammation by a confluence of the increased production of pro-inflammatory oxylipids and decreased production of anti-inflammatory oxylipids. Accordingly, one element that influences the inflammatory phenotype of a cell or the surrounding microenvironment is the ratio of pro-inflammatory–anti-inflammatory oxylipid synthesis (Mattmiller et al. 2013).

10.3 Periodic Immune Dysfunction

The effectiveness of the cow immune system alters drastically during the periparturient phase. Many innate and adaptive immune system alterations have been reported in several studies that may affect the transitioning cow's susceptibility to novel diseases (Aitken et al. 2011). Numerous negative outcomes may arise from a compromised immune system.

The exposure of cows to harmful organisms increases the likelihood of infection and the severity of the condition. For instance, dysfunctional inflammatory responses that manifest locally as well as systemically provide particular challenges due to their direct influence on the etiology of diseases in transitioning cows, such as mastitis and metritis. In the early stages of the disease, dysregulation of the inflammatory response can include a hyporesponsive condition marked by the delayed migration of functionally sufficient neutrophils and other innate immune components. Conversely, an excessively strong or persistent inflammatory response that causes significant tissue damage to the host might arise from an improper balance between the start and end of inflammation. The intensity and protracted nature of mastitis in early lactation cows is a prime illustration of the outcome of a malfunctioning immunological response. Research revealed that, compared to cows in mid-lactation, mammary glands in early lactation were able to react more quickly to an endotoxin from *Escherichia coli* (Grommers et al. 1989). When compared to later periods of lactation, the periparturient period was thought to have more severe coliform mastitis due to the delayed migration of neutrophils and their decreased antibacterial activity (Shuster et al. 1996). Many studies have been conducted on the underlying reasons of dysfunctional inflammation during the transition phase, and the evidence suggests that both endocrine and metabolic variables may be involved (Sordillo and Mavangira 2014). For instance, the altered function of neutrophils is caused, at least in part, by increases in multiple steroid hormones around the time of parturition (Burton et al. 2005). It is well recognized that glucocorticoids have strong immunosuppressive effects, and their plasma concentrations rise around calving time. The down-regulation of L-selectin and CD18 adhesion molecules, which are necessary for efficient activation and migration to tissue injury sites, is one way that glucocorticoids can affect blood neutrophil activity (Burton et al. 1995). Moreover, it has been documented that variations in the levels of progesterone and estradiol just before calving affect the capacities of immune-cell populations both directly and indirectly (Roth et al. 1982). Since changes in these steroid hormones do not coincide with the transition period as a whole, it is evident that inflammatory dysfunction is partly a result of other transition-related variables.

The disruption of adequate inflammatory responses has been linked to the involvement of a negative energy balance (NEB) and modifications in food metabolism throughout the transition phase (Sordillo and Raphael 2013). Kimura et al. (2002), and Nonnecke et al. (2003), for instance, conducted a series of sophisticated studies in which pregnant dairy cows were mastectomized in order to preserve the endocrine changes associated with late pregnancy and parturition while evaluating the effects of milk production and NEB on different immune parameters. When compared to cows with intact mammary glands, the mastectomized cows saw only modest increases in non-esterified fatty acids (NEFAs) over the periparturient interval. While mastectomized cows experienced a temporary reduction in immune function around calving, cows with mammary glands experienced a lengthier decline in lymphocyte and neutrophil functions (Nonnecke et al. 2003). Additionally, Kimura et al. (2002) observed that lactation had a deleterious effect on the composition of peripheral blood leukocyte populations. The main finding of these studies was that parturition itself, along with the corresponding alterations in steroid hormone profiles, does not appear to be the primary immunosuppressive factor in periparturient cows. Rather, the detrimental effect on immune-cell populations was probably caused by the higher metabolic needs of early lactation. In fact, there is a plethora of research that show how specific metabolic factors, such as NEFAs, BHBA, variations in glucose, and micronutrient availability, may impact immune-cell populations throughout the periparturient phase (Sordillo and Mavangira 2014). Modifications in the metabolism of nutrients could serve as a common pathway that connects immune system dysfunction to the higher prevalence of viral and metabolic disorders in periparturient dairy cows.

10.4 Optimizing Immunity: Benefits

When both innate and adaptive immune mechanisms are closely controlled to successfully eradicate harmful shocks and restore tissues to homeostasis, host defenses against infectious pathogens are at their best. Infections that are quickly resolved will stop bystander tissue damage and stop any appreciable alterations to the general health and well-being of food animals. However, some viruses possess inherent characteristics that render the immune system unable to effectively eliminate them, and local defense efforts to gain control frequently result in severe tissue damage and lost productivity. Alternative and adjunct therapeutic strategies that target host immune responses are necessary, even if antibiotic therapy is still the cornerstone for the treatment of many infectious illnesses. The difficulty lies in selectively down-regulating detrimental host responses while maintaining favorable responses that aid in the removal of invasive infections. Unlike antimicrobial medications used to treat illnesses in food animals, host response–based techniques reduce the chance of drug residues and the emergence of drug-resistant bacteria. Understanding the factors that weaken host defenses can help create effective immunomodulatory techniques to regulate the onset of illness.

Numerous studies have demonstrated a strong correlation between the physiological stress experienced by dairy calves during their periparturient phase and the malfunctioning of multiple components of their innate and adaptive immune responses (Sordillo et al. 1997). Some of the detrimental impacts on immunity during the periparturient period can be explained by certain hormones connected to parturition. However, oxidative stress can also impair immune-cell populations, particularly when there is inflammation or an increase in metabolism (Sordillo and Aitken 2009). Energy is needed to activate the immune response, and the immune system must fight for vital resources that would otherwise be used for development, the building of muscle, and the production of milk. Uncontrolled acute or chronic inflammatory reactions to infectious pathogens can repartition resources and inflict collateral damage to host tissues, which can lead to sharp declines in animal production and growth (Aitken et al. 2011). Thus, optimizing immunity in animals can be greatly impacted by modifying animal feed and enhancing management to minimize exposure to infectious pathogens.

The occurrence of infections in animals used for food production may be significantly reduced by the development of novel techniques to strengthen an immune response that is otherwise compromised. Gaining a deeper understanding of the intricate relationships between bacterial pathogenesis, host responses required to eradicate pathogens from host tissues, and strategies to boost the immune potential of these factors prior to disease establishment is the current challenge facing researchers.

10.5 Conclusion

It was discovered that the occurrence of various transition issues is significantly influenced by dysregulated immune function. To clarify the underlying mechanism of peripartum diseases, however, trustworthy contemporary predictive technologies can be utilized to evaluate the immunological and inflammatory status of individual transition dairy cows. Several tools can serve as a supplement to the measurement of traditional biomarkers in biological fluids. Additionally, it will create a new field for studies on managing crucial transition periods. Consequently, it would be expected that the immune system's periparturient responses would be impacted by the metabolic and physical demands of pregnancy, parturition, and lactation, which are linked to altered neuroendocrine profiles. It is already known that some acute stressors slow the pace at which immunoglobulin is transferred to the newborn calf. Thus, the health of the cow and the calf are affected by peripartum immunological dysfunction. More investigation is needed to pinpoint the precise role that neuroendocrine factors and the genes that control them play in immune system homeostasis during the peripartum phase.

References

Aitken, S.L., Corl, C.M., and Sordillo, L.M. (2011). Immunopathology of mastitis: insights into disease recognition and resolution. *Journal of Mammary Gland Biology and Neoplasia* 16 (4): 291–304.

Burton, J.L., Kehrli, M.E. Jr., Kapil, S., and Horst, R.L. (1995). Regulation of L-selectin and CD18 on bovine neutrophils by glucocorticoids: effects of cortisol and dexamethasone. *Journal of Leukocyte Biology* 57 (2): 317–325.

Burton, J.L., Madsen, S.A., Chang, L.C. et al. (2005). Gene expression signatures in neutrophils exposed to glucocorticoids: a new paradigm to help explain "neutrophil dysfunction" in parturient dairy cows. *Veterinary Immunology and Immunopathology* 105 (3–4): 197–219.

Grinberg, N., Elazar, S., Rosenshine, I., and Shpigel, N.Y. (2008). Beta-hydroxybutyrate abrogates formation of bovine neutrophil extracellular traps and bactericidal activity against mammary pathogenic Escherichia coli. *Infection and Immunity* 76 (6): 2802–2807.

Grommers, F.J., Van de Geer, D., Van der Vliet, H. et al. (1989). Polymorphonuclear leucocyte function: relationship between induced migration into the bovine mammary gland and in vitro cell activity. *Veterinary Immunology and Immunopathology* 23 (1–2): 75–83.

Hodgkinson, A.J., Carpenter, E.A., Smith, C.S. et al. (2007). Adhesion molecule expression in the bovine mammary gland. *Veterinary Immunology and Immunopathology* 115 (3–4): 205–215.

Kimura, K., Goff, J.P., Kehrli, M.E. Jr. et al. (2002). Effects of mastectomy on composition of peripheral blood mononuclear cell populations in periparturient dairy cows. *Journal of Dairy Science* 85 (6): 1437–1444.

Kumar, H., Kawai, T., and Akira, S. (2011). Pathogen recognition by the innate immune system. *International Reviews of Immunology* 30 (1): 16–34.

LeBlanc, S.J., Lissemore, K.D., Kelton, D.F. et al. (2006). Major advances in disease prevention in dairy cattle. *Journal of Dairy Science* 89 (4): 1267–1279.

Mattmiller, S.A., Carlson, B.A., and Sordillo, L.M. (2013). Regulation of inflammation by selenium and selenoproteins: impact on eicosanoid biosynthesis. *Journal of Nutritional Science* 2 (e28): 1–13.

Nonnecke, B.J., Kimura, K., Goff, J.P., and Kehrli, M.E. Jr. (2003). Effects of the mammary gland on functional capacities of blood mononuclear leukocyte populations from periparturient cows. *Journal of Dairy Science* 86 (7): 2359–2368.

Pinedo, P.J., De Vries, A., and Webb, D.W. (2010). Dynamics of culling risk with disposal codes reported by dairy herd improvement dairy herds. *Journal of Dairy Science* 93 (5): 2250–2261.

Prasad, R., Giri, S., Singh, A.K., and Singh, I. (2008). 15-deoxy-delta12,14-prostaglandin J2 attenuates endothelial-monocyte interaction: implication for inflammatory diseases. *Journal of Inflammation (London)* 5: 14.

Rainard, P. (2003). The complement in milk and defense of the bovine mammary gland against infections. *Veterinary Research* 34 (5): 647–670.

Riollet, C., Rainard, P., and Poutrel, B. (2000). Differential induction of complement fragment C5a and inflammatory cytokines during intramammary infections with Escherichia coli and Staphylococcus aureus. *Clinical and Diagnostic Laboratory Immunology* 7 (2): 161–167.

Roche, J.R., Bell, A.W., Overton, T.R., and Loor, J.J. (2013). Nutritional management of the transition cow in the 21st century? A paradigm shift in thinking. *Animal Production Science* 53 (9): 1000–1023.

Roth, J.A., Kaeberle, M.L., and Hsu, W.H. (1982). Effect of estradiol and progesterone on lymphocyte and neutrophil functions in steers. *Infection and Immunity* 35 (3): 997–1002.

Schmitz, G. and Ecker, J. (2008). The opposing effects of n-3 and n-6 fatty acids. *Progress in Lipid Research* 47 (2): 147–155.

Serhan, C.N. and Chiang, N. (2008). Endogenous pro-resolving and anti-inflammatory lipid mediators: a new pharmacologic genus. *British Journal of Pharmacology* 153 (Suppl. 1): S200–S215.

Serhan, C.N., Chiang, N., and Van Dyke, T.E. (2008). Resolving inflammation: dual anti-inflammatory and pro-resolution lipid mediators. *Nature Reviews. Immunology* 8 (5): 349–361.

Shuster, D.E., Lee, E.K., and Kehrli, M.E. Jr. (1996). Bacterial growth, inflammatory cytokine production, and neutrophil recruitment during coliform mastitis in cows within ten days after calving, compared with cows at midlactation. *American Journal of Veterinary Research* 57 (11): 1569–1575.

Sordillo, L.M. and Aitken, S.L. (2009). Impact of oxidative stress on the health and immune function of dairy cattle. *Veterinary Immunology and Immunopathology* 128 (1–3): 104–109.

Sordillo, L.M. and Aitken, S.L. (2011). Mammary resistance mechanisms - endogenous. In: *Encyclopedia of Dairy Sciences*, 2e, vol. 3 (ed. J.W. Fuquay), 386–391. Cambridge, Massachusetts: Academic Press.

Sordillo, L.M. and Mavangira, V. (2014). The nexus between nutrient metabolism, oxidative stress and inflammation in transition cows. *Animal Production Sciences* 54: 1204–1214.

Sordillo, L.M. and Raphael, W. (2013). Significance of metabolic stress, lipid mobilization, and inflammation on transition cow disorders. *The Veterinary clinics of North America. Food animal practice* 29 (2): 267–278.

Sordillo, L.M. and Streicher, K.L. (2002). Mammary gland immunity and mastitis susceptibility. *Journal of Mammary Gland Biology and Neoplasia* 7 (2): 135–146.

Sordillo, L.M., Shafer-Weaver, K., and DeRosa, D. (1997). Immunobiology of the mammary gland. *Journal of Dairy Science* 80 (8): 1851–1865.

Summers, C., Rankin, S.M., Condliffe, A.M. et al. (2010). Neutrophil kinetics in health and disease. *Trends in Immunology* 31 (8): 318–324.

11

Mastitis

Satyavrat Singh[1], Jitendra P. Singh[1], Rajesh Kumar[2], and Pramod Kumar[3]

[1] *Department of Veterinary Medicine, College of Veterinary Science and Animal Husbandry, Acharya Narendra Deva University of Agriculture and Technology, Ayodhya, Uttar Pradesh, India*
[2] *Department of Veterinary Gynaecology and Obstetrics, College of Veterinary Science and Animal Husbandry, Acharya Narendra Deva University of Agriculture and Technology, Ayodhya, Uttar Pradesh, India*
[3] *Department of Veterinary Physiology and Biochemistry, College of Veterinary Science and Animal Husbandry, Acharya Narendra Deva University of Agriculture and Technology, Ayodhya, Uttar Pradesh, India*

Mastitis, an inflammatory condition of the glandular tissue of the udder, is a multifactorial disease of lactating animals characterized by an apparent (or inapparent) alteration in the consistency or color of the udder or milk. It generally ensues from an interplay between a diverse array of microbial infections, host factors, and environmental and management factors. The National Mastitis Council (NMC) defines it as "an inflammation of the mammary gland mainly caused by bacterial infection" (NMC National Mastitis Council 2007). Owing to the variety of etiological agents and multiple predisposing factors, the worldwide prevalence graph is almost constant and never dips to zero. This disease is, therefore, a topic of indefinite discussion that can rightly be acknowledged as "one of the most widely discussed diseases of dairy animal, still lacking a concrete therapeutic module." It not only lowers the animal's lifetime production potential but also increases the risk of infecting other animals and impairs animal welfare (Von Keyserlingk et al. 2009). It is widely acknowledged as a major reason for economic losses in the dairy industry and the reason behind the prescription of antibiotics to dairy cattle herds (EMA and EFSA 2017). Jingar et al. (2017) argued that losses due to mastitis are not only economical, but issues like animal health and welfare, the quality of milk, antibiotic usage, and the image of the dairy sector are also important reasons to focus on mastitis control programs. Mastitis has enshrined itself as a challenging disease in high yield dairy animals in India, next only to foot-and-mouth disease (FMD) (Varshney and Mukherjee 2002), and it drains considerable funds from the dairy owner's pocket (Schroeder 2012; Winter and Fehlings 2013; Kvapilík 2014).

11.1 Economic Losses

Mastitis is considered the most serious economic offender of the dairy industry and is a major reason for premature culling (Cobirka et al. 2020), reduction in milk production (Bezman et al. 2015; Sánchez-Macías et al. 2020), losses in milk quality and quantity, and losses due to discarded milk, treatment costs, and labor. It is a cause for the use of approximately 60–70% of all antimicrobials administered on dairy farms (Stevens et al. 2016). The losses incurred are due to a drop in milk production, discarded milk, damage to the udder or its quarter, cost of veterinary services and medicine, additional labor, and culling. The estimated economic losses worldwide have been estimated at $35 billion (Wellenberg et al. 2002). Current annual economic losses due to mastitis in India have been estimated to be ₹7165.51 crore, including ₹4151.16 crore and ₹3014.35 crore due to subclinical and clinical mastitis, respectively (Bansal and Gupta 2009).

Realizing the importance of identifying the aspects related to the health of the mammary gland and milk products of buffaloes, scientists and researchers worldwide have highlighted this disease in the world literature, e.g. in India (Singh et al. 2021; Yadav et al. 2020), Brazil (Medeiros et al. 2011), the United States (NAHMS 2007), Pakistan (Hussain et al. 2013), Nepal (Dhakal et al. 2007), Italy (Fagiolo and Lai 2007), Germany (Braun and Preuss 2007), etc.

Periparturient Diseases of Cattle, First Edition. Edited by Tanmoy Rana.

11.2 Etiology

The cause of mastitis is always microorganisms that gain entry into the mammary gland and ignite inflammatory reactions (Shaheen et al. 2016). An interplay of host, environment, and organisms takes place, and the disease develops when microorganisms gain the upper hand, overpowering the host immunity (Singh and Pachauri 2004). Owing to the location of the udder, it is always exposed to a plethora of organisms in the environment and from other infected animals. The udder is, therefore, always at a risk of becoming infected, and it is the competency of the cow's immune system that decides the fate of invading organisms or the development of disease.

The major causal microorganisms are bacteria (Lakshmi 2016). Mycoplasmas, fungi, and algae have also been reported to cause mastitis. About 137 species and subspecies of possible pathogens have been reported to cause mammary gland infections. Based on the etiological agents involved, mastitis can be broadly classified as environmental mastitis and contagious mastitis (USDA 2007).

The primary source of environmental mastitis pathogens is the habitat of the cow, like organic bedding materials, a manure-covered floor, wet or damp areas, soil, plant material, contaminated water, and potential pathogens, usually in the digestive tract. Pathogens thrive in conditions typical to cattle housing, i.e. high humidity, especially if the sheds or bedding are damp, there is pooling of water or slurry, and unhygienic conditions. A fecal–oral transmission cycle may perpetuate and amplify the presence of such pathogens. Primary environmental pathogens include two types of bacteria: (i) coliform bacteria, chiefly *Escherichia coli*, *Enterobacter aerogenes*, *Klebsiella pneumonia,* and *Serratia marcescens,* and (ii) species of streptococci other than *Streptococcus agalactiae.* Other environmental pathogens include *Pseudomonas*, *Proteus*, *Serratia*, gram-positive bacilli, yeast, and *Prototheca*. Coliform bovine mastitis accounts for about 24–40% of clinical cases (Paape et al. 1996). *E. coli* has the ability to persist after an infection and reappear after several months (Bradley 2002). Lipopolysaccharide (LPS) is the key virulence factor that elicits the clinical symptoms associated with *E. coli* infections (Bannerman et al. 2003).

Contagious mastitis is caused by bacterial pathogens that are well adapted for survival in mammary glands (or on the udder skin and lesions of the teat) and are passed between cows during milking or by dirty hands, equipment, and inadequately cleaned milking cloths. The infected gland is the main source, and the transmission of contagious pathogens to uninfected quarters and cows occurs mainly during milking by the hands of milkers, the milking machine, milk-contaminated fomites, or sponges. The pathogens that cause contagious mastitis are *Staphylococcus aureus*, *Strep. agalactiae*, and *Mycoplasma* species (Radostits 2000).

According to Natzke et al. (1972), around 19–40% of cows were infected with this organism and that infected cows produce less milk compared to noninfected cows. Mastitis caused by *Staph. aureus* predominantly causes subclinical mastitis (SCM), which results in a chronic infection that can persist for the life of the animal (Riollet et al. 2000). In gram-positive bacteria, several important virulence compounds have been identified, including lipoprotein (Hashimoto et al. 2006), peptidoglycans (Girardin et al. 2003), and lipoteichoic acid. In contrast to *E. coli* mastitis, *Staph. aureus* mastitis is characterized by a moderate and delayed somatic cell count (SCC) increase, partially due to a limited cytokine response (Bannerman et al. 2004).

11.3 Pathogenesis

- Organisms remain on the udder surface.
- Microorganisms overcome a three-tiered defense of the udder immune system to initiate an inflammatory process; the first line of defense is physical barriers like the teat sphincter and keratin plug, which close the teat opening.
- Organisms enter the teat canal and disrupt the teat canal barrier.
- Organisms move further and affect the udder immune barrier.
- Organisms establish and multiply in the udder and initiate inflammatory reactions.

The teat end serves as the body's first line of defense against infection. A smooth muscled sphincter surrounds the teat canal and functions to keep the teat canal closed, prevent milk from escaping, and prevent bacteria from entering the teat. The cells that line the teat canal produce keratin, a fibrous protein with lipid components (long chain fatty acids) that have bacteriostatic properties. This keratin forms a barrier against bacteria. Teat skin with abrasions, cracks, or smudged with

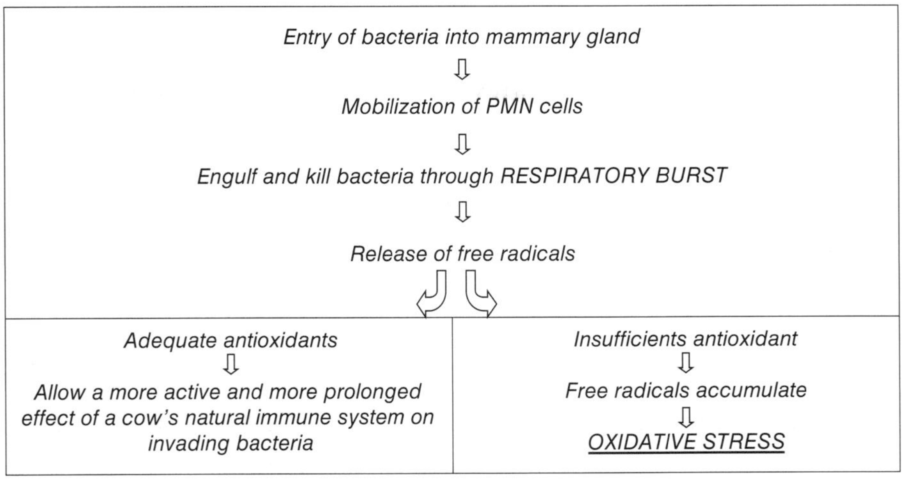

Figure 11.1 Antioxidants and mastitis (PMN = polymorphonuclear).

dirt increases bacterial colonization of the skin, which greatly increases bacterial numbers around the teat sphincter and thus, increases the risk of bacterial penetration through the teat duct. Bacteria may be present near the opening of the teat canal, either through dirty and wet conditions at the teat end, through teat-end lesions or colonization, on contaminated surfaces of milking units (liners or claws), or cow-prep procedures.

An inflammatory response is initiated when bacteria enter the mammary gland, and this is the body's second line of defense. These bacteria multiply and produce toxins, enzymes, and cell-wall components that stimulate the production of nonspecific immune responses including phagocytic cells (i.e. somatic cells), inflammatory response, complement cascade, and lactoferrin. According to Sordillo et al. (1987), the predominant cells found in the mammary tissue and mammary secretions during the early stage of mastitis infection (constituting $>90\%$ of the total leukocytes) are neutrophils. These neutrophils exercise their bactericidal effect through a respiratory burst and produce oxygen and hydroxyl radicals that kill the bacteria. Among the products secreted by neutrophils, nitric oxide (NO), causes an acute or chronic reaction (Lykkesfeldt and Svendsen 2007) with O_2. In an infected mammary gland, the levels of cytokines such as tumor necrosis factor (TNF)-α, interleukin (IL)-1β, IL-6, and IL-8 increase in the cellular system (Notebaert et al. 2008). During phagocytosis, bacteria are also exposed to several oxygen-independent reactants such as peroxidases, lysozymes, hydrolytic enzymes, and lactoferrin. In addition to their phagocytic activities, neutrophils are a source of antibacterial peptides called defensins that kill a variety of mastitis-causing pathogens (Selsted et al. 1993). As a result of mammary invasion by pathogenic species, masses of neutrophils pass between the milk secreting cells into the lumen of the alveoli, which increases the SCC and injures the secretory cells. Somatic cells remain in large concentrations after bacteria are eliminated until the gland heals. *Staph. aureus* can survive within phagocytic cells or become walled off within mammary tissue, thus evading immune detection and preventing its elimination.

The antibacterial activity of neutrophils is diminished by reactive oxygen species (ROS) (Rinaldi et al. 2008). Excessive ROS and diminished amounts of antioxidants lead to oxidative stress (Lykkesfeldt and Svendsen 2007) that leads to both clinical mastitis and SCM (Wakchaure et al. 2015) (Figure 11.1).

11.4 Risk Factors of Mastitis

Mastitis ensues from an altered balance between infectious agents and the local immune system. If the microbes develop an upper hand on innate immunity and succeed at establishing and proliferating in the udder, mastitis occurs, and all those factors that support the growth of, or even help in establishing, infections predispose cows to mastitis. There are several such factors at both the animal and herd levels associated with a higher risk of mastitis.

Busato et al. (2000) summarized and categorized risk factors such as host (breed, high yielder, age, parity, stage of lactation, udder defense, udder confirmation, milking interval, milk SCC, dry period, teat injuries, genetic resistance), pathogen (virulence factor, number of organisms, and blind treatment), management practices (shed and udder hygiene, poor teat condition, poor environmental hygiene, sanitation, large herd size, use of hand washcloth, improper teat dipping, milking technique, and milking machine) and diet (copper, cobalt, zinc, selenium, and vitamin E deficiency). Additional predisposing factors like injury, a defective sphincter, the prevalence of pathogens, and immune status of different quarters also play a role in the development of the disease (Saini et al. 1994).

Animal-related factors such as age, breed, parity, and lactation number, stage of lactation, trauma to udder, teat and teat canal, loose teat sphincters, lesions on teat skin, and the immunological status of each mammary gland are correlated with mastitis prevalence (Joshi and Gokhale 2006; Jingar et al. 2014; Kurjogi and Kaliwal 2014; Oliveira et al. 2015). Other animal-related factors are a previous mastitis record, floor type, the disinfection of fingers, teat dipping, etc. (Karimuribo et al. 2008; Madut et al. 2009). Alemu et al. (2013) insisted that the major sources of pathogens and means of transmission include infected quarters and soiled udder as well as contaminated milking machines, teat cups, milker's hands, washing cloths, flies, and surgical instruments, all of which contribute to the bulk of infections caused by environmental and managemental conditions. The relationship between poor hygiene of the udder and the leg has been correlated with the occurrences of both SCM (Schreiner and Ruegg 2003) and clinical mastitis (Breen et al. 2009). Sant'anna and Paranhos da Costa (2011) found a significant association between the hygiene of the leg, udder, flank, and abdomen and SCC. Ramirez et al. (2014) described udder preparation, milking order, dry period practices, and the use of teat disinfectants as associated factors of mastitis. Other external variables associated with mastitis are season, bedding or floor type, and stall hygiene (Joshi and Gokhale 2006; Kurjogi and Kaliwal 2014; Oliveira et al. 2015). Inadequate sanitation and poor veterinary service have also been suggested as predisposing factors for mastitis.

According to Zeni et al. (2012), absent or incompetent cleaning of milking equipment favors the proliferation of a wide variety of microorganisms that adhere to the inner surface of the equipment and accessories to form biofilms whose removal are quite difficult by normal cleaning methods. Blowey and Edmondson (2010) held the view that mechanical irregularity in the milking system, such as inadequate vacuum pressure, deprived pulse, worn teat cups, or improper removal of the assembly can cause swelling and lesions to the tip of the teats, which facilitates infections such as mastitis, and one of the most common injuries is hyperkeratosis. Joshi and Gokhale (2006) suggested that the genetic makeup of animals plays an important role in determining susceptibility to mastitis and differs from one breed to another. Lakshmi (2016) suggested the selection of animals that are resistant to diseases and the incorporation of this trait in herds as a promising alternative to reduce the problems caused by infectious diseases, including mastitis. The possible association between teat morphometric traits – i.e. teat shape (bottle, conical, cylindrical, and others), teat-end shape (flat, round, and pointed), teat length (TL), teat diameter (TD), and teat end-to-floor distance – and SCM in dairy animals has been established (Yadav et al. 2020).

The most important and ignored risk factor regarding good practices for mastitis is the knowledge and awareness of farmers. Rahman et al. (2018) emphasized collecting such information to better understand the farmers' perspectives regarding mastitis and designing appropriate strategies to help reduce its prevalence and effects; they also concluded that the identification of area- and/or farm-specific risk factors is important for designing mastitis control programs.

Bacterial factors	Host factors	Environmental factors
Ability to survive in the immediate environment of the animal	Genetic predisposition to mastitis: teat shape, sphincter tone, anatomy of the teat canal	Presence of large numbers of potential pathogens in the immediate environment of the animal (poor hygiene)
Ability to colonize the teat duct	Age: older cows, especially after four lactations	Milking machine malfunction or inadequate design
Ability to adhere to mammary epithelium and not be flushed out with the milk flow	Stage of lactation: more susceptible just after calving and for the following 2 months	Milking shed environment, including poor milking techniques and hygiene
Ability to resist phagocytosis and antibacterial resistance to antibiotics	Presence of lesions on the teats	External traumas

11.5 Clinical Findings

The disease is characterized by abnormalities of the udder or its secretion, milk.

Broadly, based on clinical findings, mastitis can be categorized in five forms:

1) **Peracute**: Hot, swollen, and painful quarter; abnormal milk; and a systemic disturbance with fever, depression, anorexia, weakness, and a rapid weak pulse.

2) **Acute:** Severe inflammation but with a less marked systemic reaction.

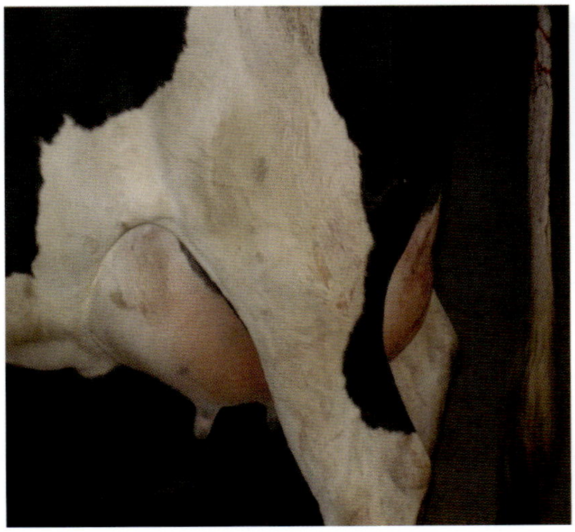

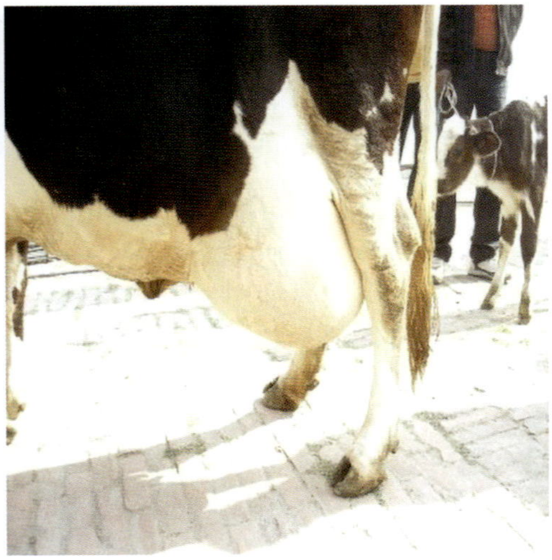

3) **Chronic:** Absence of systemic signs, very few external signs of change in the udder, recurrent episodes of mild inflammation, and a slight change in the milk.

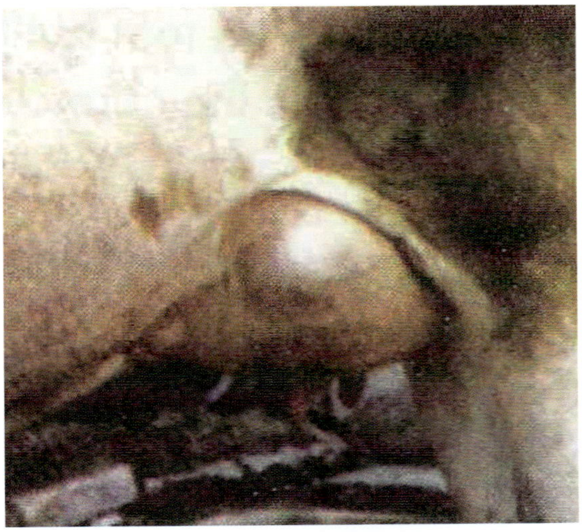

4) **Subclinical:** No visible abnormality in the udder or milk; milk appears normal unless tested in a laboratory.
5) **Gangrenous mastitis:** Characterized by cracked skin on the teats and/or udder that has a reddish to bluish-black discoloration; is hard, cold, and painful with honey-like discharge from fissures; and sloughs off.

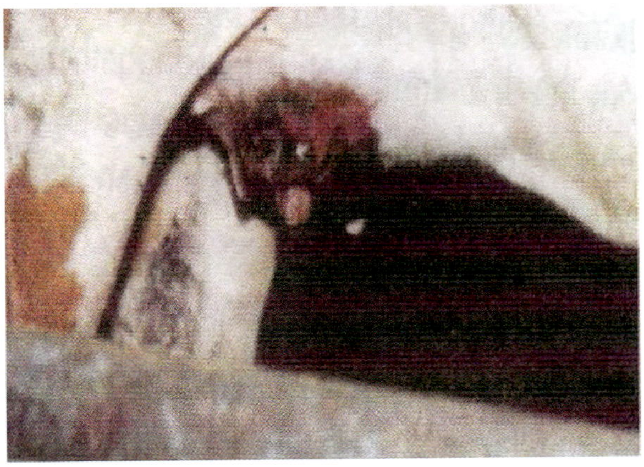

The clinical form of mastitis has multiple visible symptoms, and its severity is commonly scored based on the extent of tissue involvement (Oliveira and Ruegg 2014). Mild clinical mastitis (CM; grade 1) describes an infection limited to clinically abnormal milk; moderate CM (grade 2) also includes an abnormal udder in its clinical presentation; and severe CM (grade 3) corresponds to abnormal milk, an abnormal udder, and systemic signs of disease. In SCM, there is a change in milk composition (SCC, leukocytes and epithelial cells, pH, and ion concentration) with no clinical signs of gross inflammation or milk abnormalities. It cannot be identified without a laboratory or field test and mostly goes unnoticed by farmers; therefore, it is considered a hidden form of mastitis. In a healthy lactating udder, the SCC is usually less than 100 000 cells/ml of milk, but in SCM, the total SCC may be elevated above the normal value of milk. SCM is generally monitored and characterized by an increase in SCC (Schukken et al. 2009).

A meta-analysis of 43 and 22 studies on SCM and CM, respectively, by Krishnamoorthy et al. (2017) revealed:

- The pooled prevalence of
  - SCM: 41% (33–49%), obtained from 25 455 dairy animals.
  - CM: 27% (19–37%), obtained from 6978 dairy animals.
- The pooled prevalence estimates of *Staphylococcus* spp., *Streptococcus* spp. and *E. coli* were 45%, 13%, and 14%, respectively.
- This study showed that the SCM prevalence increased and CM prevalence decreased over a 6-year period (2011–2016).

11.6 Mastitis Diagnostic Approaches

Overview of the steps involved:

- Examination of the udder and individual quarters.
  - Inspection.
  - Palpation.
  - Inspection of the udder secretion.
- Examination of the milk.
  - Detection of alterations in milk due to an inflammatory response.
  - Direct detection of microorganisms in milk by culture.

Inspection

The size and shape of the udder, individual quarters, and the teats should be inspected by viewing it from the front, on each side, and from behind.

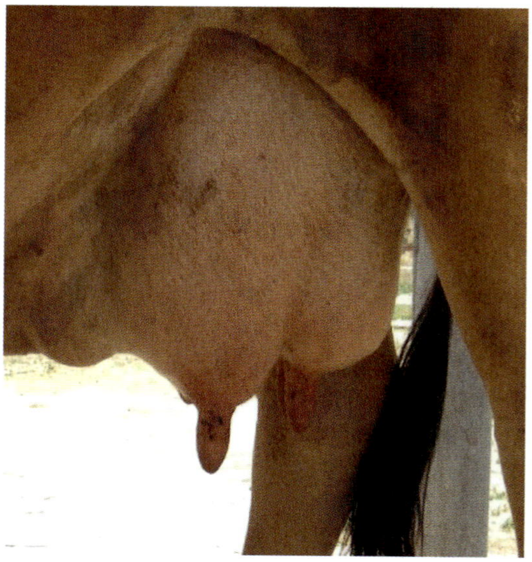

Inspection

Preferably, the udder should be examined from the back with the hindlegs held apart and tail lifted upwards. This position allows a view of the whole udder.

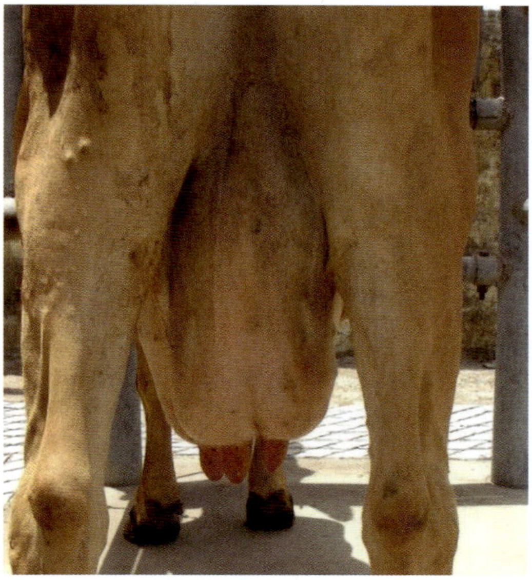

The teat should be palpated with the fingertips.

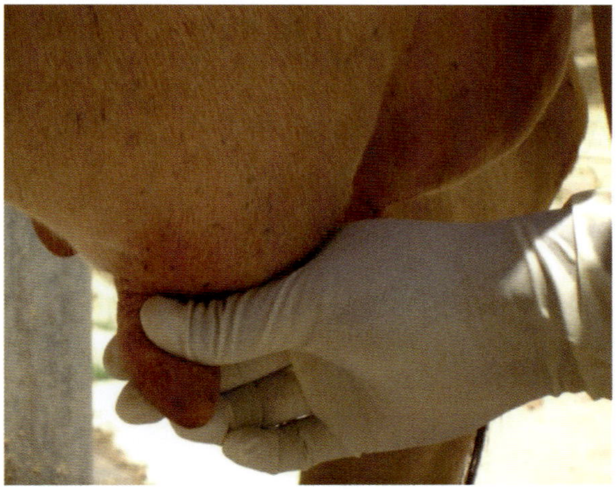

- The quarters should be palpated (preferably after milking) with the flat of the hand, first feeling the surface, then the deeper tissue.
- A convenient procedure is to start at the tip of the teat and proceed upwards.

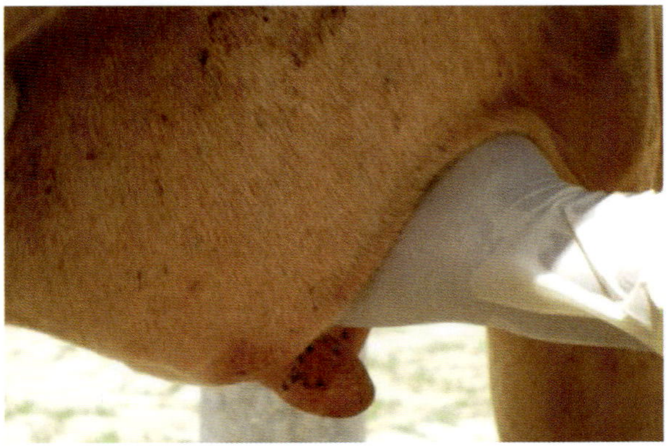

- The teat (streak canal) normally feels firm when rolled between the fingers, and all four teats should feel the same.
- Abnormalities include swelling, injury and neoplasia of the tip and teat canal, abnormal tenderness, and increased warmth.
- Patency of the teat canal is tested by drawing off a few streams of milk (into a stripping cup, not onto the ground).

11.7 Common Tests

11.7.1 Strip Cup Test

- Routine examination of the milk using a filter cup.
- Make first use of the strip cup test for the detection of visible particles of milk.
- Two types of strip cups.
  - Fine-screen type: Filters out the pus, clots, and flakes.
  - Black-background type: Helps to detect a change in color and the presence of particles.

11.7.2 California Mastitis Test (CMT)

The California mastitis test (CMT) is the most sensitive indirect method for the detection of SCM and one of the best methods for detecting it as early as possible at the farm level.

- Add 2–3 ml of milk to an equal amount of CMT reagent.
- Followed by mixing with a gentle circular motion.

  A positive reaction is gel formation and a change of color.

- When the mixture is a distinct deep-purple color the test is positive for alkaline milk.

Reaction	Degree of test
No precipitate or color change	– (Negative)
Slight precipitate	T (Trace)
A distinct precipitate without gel formation and a slight purplish color	1+ (Weak positive)
Viscosity of milk is increased with a moderate gel formation	2+ (Positive)
Immediate thick gel formation, sticking at the bottom	3+ (Strong positive)

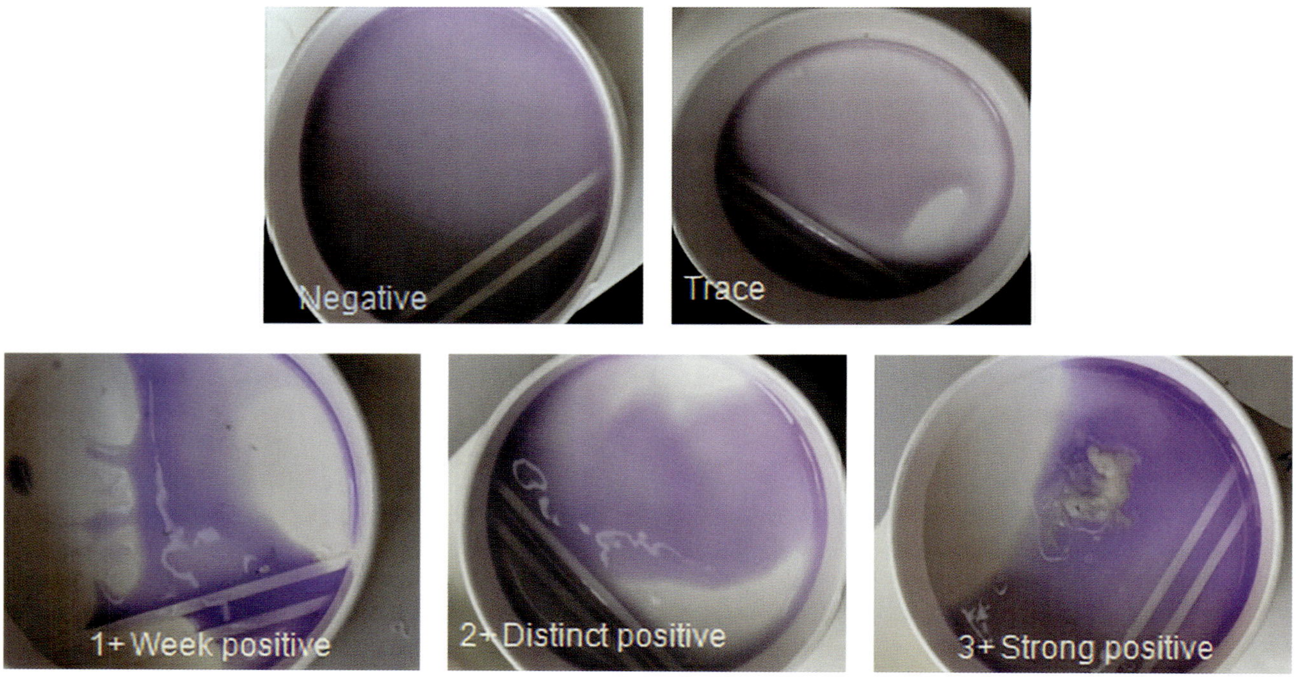

11.7.3 Whiteside Test (WST)

The whiteside test is a commonly applied test based on the reaction between 4% sodium hydroxide and milk.

- Five drops of milk plus two drops of reagent followed by stirring for about 20 s.

Reaction	Degree of test
Mixture remains opaque and free of particles	– (negative)
No apparent reaction during stirring, close inspection reveals finely dispersed particles	±
Thickening during stirring with little or no tendency for the mass to adhere to the stick; upon continued stirring, the mixture separates into milky whey and white particles	1+
Thickening, the coagulum follows the stick and finally separates into a clear whey and white, thread-like whorls	2+
A tenacious mass forms, immediately adhering to the stick; the mass separates into whey and thready, clumped, opaque material	3+
A tenacious coagulum with little or no tendency to break down into whey and particulate material	4+

11.7.4 Somatic Cell Count

In a healthy udder, the majority of an SCC is comprised of macrophages (66–88%), followed by lymphocytes (10–27%), neutrophils (1–11%), and epithelial cells (0–7%). During mastitis, neutrophils (70–80%) become the major cell type present in milk, and the early influx of neutrophils results in an early resolution of infection (Paape et al. 2002). The SCC acts as an indirect indicator of udder health status in dairy cows.

- **Interpretations:**
  - A normal SCC in milk is generally below 200 000/ml.
  - An SCC above 250 000–300 000 is considered abnormal and nearly always indicates a bacterial infection causing inflammation of the udder.

11.7.5 Microbiological Assay

Hillerton (2000) reported that the detection of bacteria in a milk sample was the confirmatory test for the presence of mastitis in cows and argued that the isolation of the microbe was the only test with the highest specificity (100%) for detecting mastitis (Figure 11.2). Sudhan and Sharma (2010) stated that the cultural test was the gold-standard test for detecting an udder infection in dairy cows.

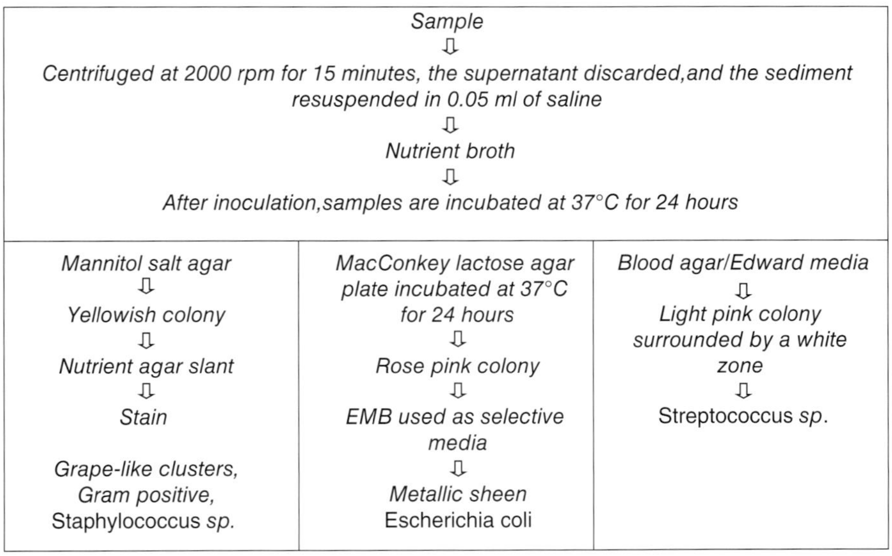

Figure 11.2 Microbiological assay of milk samples (EMB = eosin methylene blue).

11.7.6 Sequencing/Molecular Typing Methods

- Sequencing has become an important mastitis diagnostic tool, not only for the species, subspecies, or strain level identification of microorganisms but also for overcoming resolution problems.
- Polymerase chain reaction (PCR)-based techniques, including multiplex PCR and real-time PCR analyses devices, help identify mastitogens. Moreover, they are being advanced for the identification and quantification of mastitis pathogens in milk. Two-dimensional gel electrophoresis and mass spectroscopy of relevant proteomics techniques are now being used for the identification of several new proteins involved in mastitis that are expressed by invading pathogens. Recent progress in microfluidics and "biochips" have the capability to modernize the early diagnostic procedure for mastitis and to discover and develop specific therapeutic strategies.
- Differentiation of various bacterial strains within a species can be done.
- Various molecular methods can be helpful, such as ribotyping, pulsed-field gel electrophoresis (PFGE), amplified fragment length polymorphism (AFLP), random amplified polymorphic DNA (RAPD), and multilocus sequence typing (MLST).
- DNA is used in these methods, either following digestion of the DNA with restriction enzymes, after employing PCR to amplify the DNA, after analyzing the DNA sequence, or by combining all these approaches.

11.7.7 Infrared Thermography (IRT)

- This could be a very simple future prospect for the diagnosis of SCM in the field.
- Infrared thermography (IRT) is a simple, effective, on-site, and noninvasive diagnostic method based on the heat or thermal difference of the skin or udder surface; hence, it is reflected in the form of images, which are helpful in the diagnosis of udder inflammation.
- For the detection of SCM in cows, the diagnostic sensitivity and specificity of IRT were found to be 95.6% and 93.6%, respectively.

11.7.8 Sensor-based Mastitis Detection Systems

- These diagnostic systems help in sensing mastitis, usually with minimal stress to the animal.
- These diagnostic systems are especially helpful on large farms.
- Appropriate sensing technology includes the in-line monitoring of somatic cell counts (ISCC) and the quarter-based electrical conductivity (EC) of milk for CM cases to be recognized well in time.
- It is expected that such techniques should have a minimum sensitivity of 80%, a specificity of at least 90%, and a detection window of 48 hours.
- Detection of mastitis-specific biomarkers: acute phase proteins (APPs), including haptoglobin (Hp), C-reactive protein (CRP), and mammary-associated serum amyloid α3 (M-SAA3).

11.7.9 Automatic Digital Diagnostics

- Automatic mastitis detection systems are novel diagnostic methods that are field applicable, easy, and rapid (provide instant results).
- These include milk checker, Fossomatic® meter, Dramiński® (Wykrywacz) mastitis detector, DeLaval cell counter, Afimilk® milk meter, UdderCheck® test, and PortaSCC® test and possess a higher accuracy. They are based on either the detection of physical-chemical-biological alterations in the milk or udder or an estimation of biomarkers in body fluids (milk, serum) related to mastitis.

11.8 Treatment

Mastitis is the most common reason for the use of antimicrobials in dairy animals (Mitchell et al. 1998) despite the fact that the bovine mammary gland is a difficult target for antimicrobial treatment. The pharmacokinetic characteristics of a drug, viz. lipid solubility, degree of ionization, extent of binding to serum and udder proteins, and the type of vehicle, decides the penetration of substances into milk when administered parenterally or when infused intramammarily (IMM). Antimicrobials have been used to treat mastitis for several decades, but a consensus about the most efficient, safe, and economical treatment is still lacking. Selected agents should have a low minimum inhibitory concentration (MIC) value for the target pathogen; as for successful antibacterial mastitis therapy, the active medicine must achieve and conserve concentrations above the MIC at the center of infection for long enough to shut down the toxin-producing phase of the causal pathogen. The therapeutic agent should be bactericidal rather than bacteriostatic because phagocytosis is impaired in the mammary gland (Kehrli and Harp 2001). Antibiotic therapy is considered the most effective therapeutic module to treat mastitis, especially CM. The cure rate with antibiotics is variable under field conditions. A longer duration treatment is generally associated with a higher probability of cure (Deluyker et al. 2005) in clinical and SCM. It has been suggested that a 2–3 day treatment is customary for CM (Barkema et al. 2006). The drug may be administered by the intramammary infusion of an ointment or the intramuscular or intravenous injection of antibiotics, such as streptomycin, ampicillin, cloxacillin, penicillin, and tetracycline (Bhosale et al. 2014). A disadvantage of IMM administration is uneven distribution throughout the udder (Ehinger and Kietzmann 2000) and the risk of infecting the quarter when infusing the product via the teat canal, especially if asepsis is not maintained. The best therapeutic response to IMM is observed for mastitis caused by streptococci, coagulase-negative staphylococci, and *Corynebacterium* spp. The only type of mastitis where systemic treatment would be highly effective may be mastitis caused by *Staph. aureus* (Barkema et al. 2006).

Fluroquinolones and cefquinome have shown efficacy in experimental trials (Rantala et al. 2002; Poutrel et al. 2008) and ceftiofur in a clinical field trial (Erskine et al. 2002). Penicillin G or penethamate has been shown to be effective in clinical trials (Pyörälä 2009, Pyorala and Pyorala 1998; McDougall et al. 2016).

The drugs most commonly used for CM cases, as reported by Manimaran et al. (2014), were enrofloxacin (22%), ampicillin with cloxacillin (18.57%), gentamicin (18.29), and ceftriaxone (12.57%). The penicillin group (and their combinations, 29.43%) was found to be the most commonly used group for CM, followed by fluoroquinolones (22%), aminoglycosides (21.43%), and cephalosporins (16.86%). Tetracyclines (9.14%) and chloramphenicol (1.14%) were least often selected, as evidenced by less frequent usage. Marbofloxacin has also been found effective in the treatment of mastitis (Singh et al. 2018).

Reports are pouring in regarding a surge in the resistance of pathogens to the most common antibiotics, which leads to treatment failure (Rossi et al. 2019; Tanzin et al. 2016; Yadav et al. 2020). Antibiotics have been described as a "double-edged sword" (Singh and Pachauri 2001). The time-to-time evaluation of area-specific antibiograms can be a step that promotes the judicious use of antibiotics and improves treatment percentage as well as being a must for the welfare of animals. Recovery can be maximized if the therapy is initiated after assessing the antibiotic sensitivity results.

11.8.1 Alternate Approaches to Treat Mastitis

11.8.1.1 Herbs and Mastitis

Plants are mines of bioactive molecules, most of which probably evolved as chemical defenses against predation or infection (Samie et al. 2010). However, with time and the advent of new generations of antibiotics, the use of herbal drugs took a back seat. Advantages of herbal therapy are:

- They are natural and nontoxic.
- They are cost effective, especially if the potential of locally available plants is exploited.
- The ingredients have antibacterial, anti-inflammatory, analgesic, and immune-stimulatory properties, and thus, they can provide the wide spectrum of activity required in mastitis therapy.
- They are effective against a plethora of organisms, instead of any specific organism.
- The immunopotentiating activity of these drugs enhances the body's defense mechanisms along with udder immunity.
- Singh et al. (2021) studied the in vitro efficacy of different leaves against common mastitis pathogens and found guava leaves, lemongrass, and neem leaves to be effective.
- Plants with the potential to treat mastitis:
  - Fenugreek (*Trigonella graecum foecum*)
  - Fennel (*Foeniculum vulgare*)
  - Asparagus (*Asparagus racemosus*)
  - Ashwagandha (*Withania sonifera*)
  - Giloy (*Tinospora cordifolia*)

- Amla (*Embilica officinalis*)
- Jivanthi (*Leptadenia reticulata*)
- *Aloe vera*
- *Curcuma longa*

11.8.1.2 Essential Oils

Essential oils (EOs) are also now viewed as potent agents to curb mastitis. EOs, unlike antibiotics, are made of many molecules, which prevents bacteria resistance through mutations (Enrico et al. 2004). Curatively and preventively, they are mainly known for their potent antiviral, antimicrobial, antifungal, antiparasitic, expectorant, mucolytic, antipyretic, and anti-inflammatory effects.

The alternative treatment of bovine mastitis with EOs and plant-derived antimicrobials have been assessed in vitro on major bacterial and fungal mastitis pathogens (Baskaran et al. 2009; Ksouri et al. 2017). In fact, EOs are generally regarded as safe, and unlike antibiotics, no resistance has been reported after a prolonged exposure of bacteria to essential oils. Furthermore, synergism between plant metabolites and antibiotics has been described by Hemaiswarya et al. (2008), which suggests the use of EOs as adjuvants.

EOs have antimicrobial and antibiofilm activity against bacteria, parasites (Alexopoulos et al. 2011), fungi (Mari et al. 2003) and viruses (Bishop 1995). More recently, EOs from aromatic and medicinal plants have been tested for their activity against biofilms (Kwiecinski et al. 2009). The EOs target different cellular mechanisms, such as the inhibition of peptidoglycan synthesis (Ogunlana et al. 1987), modification of bacterial membrane hydrophobicity (Cox et al. 2000), and modulation of quorum sensing (Gao et al. 2003).

11.8.1.3 Antioxidant Therapy

Antioxidant supplementation therapy has been proven as an important therapeutic agent and is now being viewed as one of the best alternatives to conventional antibiotic therapy, especially in SCM when an animal's immune system can be potentiated to reverse the infection from subclinical to a normal healthy state (Figure 11.3). The deficiency of many vitamins and micronutrients, particularly vitamin A, vitamin D, vitamin E, selenium, and copper, in the diet leads to the increased incidence of mastitis with infections of longer durations and more severe clinical signs. Antioxidant supplementation could decrease the duration, incidence, and severity of CM (Erskine et al. 1989; Smith et al. 1984) and was associated with a lower prevalence of intramammary infections (IMIs) caused by contagious pathogens (Erskine et al. 1987).

Common antioxidants used in mastitis treatment:

- Vitamin E
- Vitamin A
- Vitamin C
- Selenium
- Zinc

These antioxidants, when combined with other antimicrobial agents, can add to the therapeutic effect of a treatment and thus, are expected to yield better results.

Cells can tolerate mild oxidative stress
⇩
Antioxidants scavenge and minimize the formation of reactive oxygen species; but not 100% effective
⇩
When reactive oxygen species are not effectively removed, oxidative stress impairs health
⇩
Directly: Oxidative damage to important lipids and macromolecules
Indirectly: Changes induced in cell membranes and components
⇩
Tissue injury
Development of disease
"Mastitis"

Figure 11.3 Oxidative stress and disease development.

11.8.1.4 Homeopathy

Homeopathy is useful for treating mastitis, especially chronic cases. Commonly used homeopathic medicines are:

- ***Belladonna* 1m:** For acute postpartum mastitis, when the udder is very hot and red, painful to the touch. The animal is hot, and the pulse is quick and strong. One dose every hour for a total of four doses.
- ***Bryonia alba* 30c:** When the udder is swollen and hard and the pain is less intense when pressed. The animal is often lying down. It is especially good for chronic cases with fibrosis.
  - Acute cases: one dose, every 4 hours, for four doses.
  - Chronic cases: one dose, two times a week, for 1 month.
- ***Phytolacca* 30c:** Clinical cases with sour, coagulated milk. Chronic cases with small clots mid-lactation.
- **Silicea 200c:** When there are a few flakes in thin, yellow milk. Also useful for summer mastitis cases with purulent abscesses. Two doses a week for 4 weeks.
- **Ipecacuanha 30c:** Useful for treating internal bleeding that produces pink or bloody milk. Three doses a day for 3 days (Singh et al. 2004).
- **Calcarea fluorica with silicea:** Chronic mastitis and fibrosis.
- ***Lachesis:*** Udder discoloration, fever, and a putrefied, curd-like appearance of milk.

11.8.1.5 Antimicrobial Peptides

- Antimicrobial peptides (AMPs) are a new generation of antibiotics that destroy invading microorganisms and have a major role in the innate immune mechanism.
- They have broad-spectrum activity against several gram-positive and gram-negative bacteria, including some of the drug-resistant strains.
- AMPs produce synergism when used alongside conventional antibiotics.
- E.g. defensins and cathelicidins.

11.8.1.6 Probiotics

- Lactic acid bacteria can provide protection against mastitis when they are used as feed supplements, a teat dip, and intramammary inoculation due to their potent immunomodulatory activity.
- The lactic acid–producing bacteria colonize the udder and prevent mastitis by forming a protective biofilm, which inhibits the growth of mastitis-causing pathogens.
- Intramammary inoculation of *Lactococcus lactis* subsp. lactis crown-rump length (CRL) 1655 and *L. perolens* CRL 1724 during the dry-off period increased the amount of immunoglobulin (IgG isotypes) in blood and milk. These results suggest that lactic acid–producing bacteria have potent immunomodulatory activity produced by stimulating local and systemic immune responses.

11.9 Prevention Strategies

The prevention of mastitis aims at strengthening the udder immune system through proper management, boosting the host's immune response, and minimizing the number of causative organisms.

11.9.1 Key Points to Minimize Mastitis in Dairy Cows

- **Environment:**
  - Sanitization and udder hygiene.
  - Udder hygiene.
  - Environmental hygiene.
  - Sanitization measures for milker's hands or milking machines.
- **Nutrition:**
  - Balanced rations.
  - Antioxidant therapy.
- **Prompt treatment.**
- **Dry-cow treatment.**
- **Vaccination** (efficacy remains doubtful, however).

Prevention strategies can be designed based on the pathogenesis of mastitis:

- **Invasion stage:**
  - Minimize exposure.
  - Avoid allowing the animals to sit for approximately 10 minutes after calving (prevents the contact of microbes to udder).
  - Teat dipping.
- **Infection stage:**
  - Boost udder immunity by supplementing different antioxidants.
- **Inflammation stage:**
  - Provide immediate medical care.
  - Sick animals should be segregated.

Another way to prevent mastitis is to formulate strategies based on etiology as follows.

- **Contagious mastitis:** Contagious mastitis can be effectively controlled through a rigorous program of teat dipping and dry-cow antibiotic treatment. Teats must be dipped in germicide after each milking (this decreases incidence of the disease). Each quarter must be treated with dry-cow antibiotics at the end of lactation (this decreases prevalence of the disease). Cows with contagious mastitis should be milked last or a separate milking claw should be used for the infected cows. Milking claws should be flushed with hot water or a germicide after milking infected cows (called backflushing). Individual cloth/paper towels should be used to wash/dry teats. Milkers should have clean hands and wear latex gloves. New additions to the herd should be cultured and persistently infected cows should be culled. Teat lesions should be minimized (e.g. from chapping, frostbite, stepped-on teats, lacerations, or machine damage). Heifers can be given dry-cow antibiotic treatment during gestation if *Staph. aureus* is a problem.
- **Environmental mastitis:** Environmental pathogens are more difficult to control than contagious pathogens. Many of these organisms are resistant to the germicides in teat dip and antibiotics in dry-cow therapy. Identification of the source and removal (bedding, ponds, mud) is the key to control. Udders can be clipped to minimize the amount of manure that clings to the glands. Only clean, dry teats should be milked. Teats should be dipped with germicide before milking. Cows should be kept standing after milking (offer them feed). Sterile single-dose infusion products and sterile infusion techniques (alcohol swab) should be used. The milking parlor should be kept clean. The teat dipper should be kept clean; organisms can survive in many germicides.

Must dos:

- Proper and regular disposal of excreta.
- Disinfection of housing premises.
- Sanitization of the cow's udders and milker's hands or milking machines prior to use.
- Pre- and post-milking teat dips with an isopropyl alcohol, chlorhexidine, and 1% sodium hypochlorite solution are effective.
- The rule of thumb rule is to milk primiparous cows first and multiparous cows latter.
- Among these, healthy cows are to be milked first and mastitic cows milked last.
- Hindquarter milking should preferably follow forequarter milking.

11.9.2 General Strategies to Be Adopted

11.9.2.1 Dry-cow Management

Dry-cow management is important in preparing cows for the next lactation and to prevent many disorders, e.g. milk fever, abomasal displacements, retained placentas, uterine infections, and CM. Cows are most susceptible to new mastitis infections during the first 2 weeks of the dry period, the 2 weeks before calving, and the 2 weeks after calving. Dry-cow therapy is 90–93% effective against subclinical *Strep. agalactiae* infections, 70–80% effective against *Staph. aureus*, and 70–90% effective against environmental streptococci.

The Four Goals of Dry-cow Therapy

1) **Cure existing infections at dry off.**
   - Reducing the number of cows that carry infections through the dry period prevents them from flaring up into clinical infections and limits the source of contagious bacteria to other cows in the herd.

2) **Prevent new infections at dry off and throughout the dry period.**
   - Dry period mastitis is difficult to treat, costly, time consuming, and can have long term effects on the cows' production.
   - Prevention is vital, especially when it is difficult to inspect the cows regularly during the dry period.
3) **Protect against mastitis and reduce new infections around the calving period.**
   - Mastitis around calving is common. The cow's immune defenses are lower around the calving period, and there is considerable exposure to environmental bacteria.
4) **Reduce SCC and mastitis going into the subsequent lactation.**
   - Effective dry-cow therapy (DCT) will significantly reduce the SCC.

DCT can be a blanket procedure, i.e. for all cows drying off, or selective, i.e. only to cows who have tested positive for mastitis. While dry treatment is very effective, it must be administered properly, and dry cows must have favorable environmental conditions. If the teat ends are not cleaned properly, there is the possibility of injecting very high numbers of bacteria into the udder that would overwhelm the antibiotic just administered. Unsanitary treatment procedures cause, rather than eliminate, mastitis.

There is no substitute for the proper management of dry cows in mastitis control. If dry cows are exposed to muddy or dirty conditions, the risk of mastitis will increase. This is especially true at calving time; cows are under considerable stress during this period. If an udder is exposed to wet, dirty conditions, the risk of mastitis will increase.

11.9.2.2 Teat Sealant

The use of an internal teat sealant is an important part of a DCT program. The combination of antibiotic DCT and teat sealant provides benefits over antibiotic DCT use alone through the improved prevention of SCM and a reduced ISCC during the first 60 days of lactation.

11.9.2.3 Teat Dips

Pre- and post-milking teat antisepsis is regarded as the single most effective practice for the prevention of mastitis by reducing the new IMI rate in dairy cows and maintaining a low incidence of mastitis.

Teats are the gateway for organisms into the udder, and their health decides the overall health status and productivity of the mammary gland. During milking, milk from the udder flows into individual teats where the milk flows into the teat cistern and then into the teat orifice, in a flow controlled by the teat sphincter muscle. After milking, a drop of milk typically remains on the tip of the teat, which serves as a nidus for the growth of bacteria like *Strep. agalactiae* and *Staph. aureus*. Also, because of their anatomical position, teats are subject to outside influences and are prone to both inflammatory and noninflammatory conditions (Sudhan and Sharma 2010). Teat disinfection pre and post milking is important to reduce the number of bacteria (Dufour et al. 2011), reduce the possibility of mastitis, and the risk of bacterial contamination of milk (Suriyasathaporn and Chupia 2011; Zucali et al. 2011). The primary objective of pre-milking udder preparation and teat sanitization is to achieve an acceptable level of decontamination of the teat skin. This aids in reducing the spread of microorganisms, the incidence of new IMIs, and minimizing the number of bacteria that find their way into the raw milk supply. Post-milking teat dipping is the most effective milking hygiene practice for preventing new infections caused by the two most common contagious mastitis organisms, *Staph. aureus* and *Strep. agalactiae*. Chlorhexidine (0.2%), a commercial iodophor (1% available iodine), a hypochlorite (4% available chlorine), and tap water can be used.

11.9.2.4 Role of Nutrition

Dietary or ancillary supplementation of microelements such as, zinc, copper, cobalt, iron, manganese, chromium, and selenium is essentially required for the optimization of udder immunity. Recommended feeding levels (as per *Nutrient Requirements of Dairy Cattle: Seventh Revised Edition*, 2001, Washington, DC: The National Academies Press):

- **Vitamin E:** 1000 IU/d to dry cows.
- **Selenium:** 3 mg/d for dry cows.
- **Copper:** 10 and 15 ppm of the diet.
- **Vitamin A:** 110 IU/kg body weight (BW).
- **Vitamin D:** 30 IU/kg BW for dry cows.
- **Zinc:** 300 mg/d.

11.9.2.5 Cytokine Therapy

Cytokines are low molecular weight regulatory proteins secreted by white blood cells. Owing to their immunostimulatory properties, they enhance the immune status of the mammary gland. Cytokines regulate the host defense by:

1) Activating B cells, T cells, and macrophages.
2) Inducing clonal expansion of activated B cells, T cells, and macrophages.
3) Initiating secondary secretion of several other cytokines by activated lymphocytes.

Commonly studied cytokines in mastitis are the granulocyte–monocyte-colony-stimulating factor or IL-2, TNF-α, and interferons.

11.9.2.6 Vaccination

Vaccination against mastitis has been attempted but it is seldom used due to the multiple etiological agents involved. Vaccines are available against *Strept. uberis, Strep. agalactiae, Staph. aureus*, and *E. coli*. Vaccines against *Staph. aureus* and *Strep. agalactiae* contain either the whole organism (cellular lysates, inactive, and attenuated vaccines) or subunits (toxins, surface proteins, and polysaccharides). The mutant core antigen J5 is most commonly used to vaccinate against mastitis due to *E. coli*.

11.9.2.7 Prompt Treatment

Cows with SCM should be identified and subjected to short term treatment with effective antibiotics at least for 3–5 days. The clinically affected animals should be provided treatment immediately, and chronic cases should be segregated or culled. This is the only technique to remove the source of the infection. An "extended therapy protocol" or "extended duration of therapy," defined as administering intramammary treatment (mastitis tubes used in the quarter) for 2–8 days consecutively, increases the chance of a complete bacteriological mastitis cure in which all of the bacteria causing the infection are killed. A complete cure often prevents relapses, prevents further damage to the mammary tissue, lowers the SCC, and helps to sustain future milk production.

References

Alemu, A.A., Fikiru, H., Simyalew, A.M., and Yohannes, A. (2013). *Prevalence of Subclinical Mastitis in Lactating Cows in Selected Commercial Dairy Farms of Holeta*, 4. Holeta, Ethiopia: Agricultural Research Center.

Alexopoulos, A., Kimbaris, A.C., Plessas, S. et al. (2011). Antibacterial activities of essential oils from eight Greek aromatic plants against clinical isolates of *Staphylococcus aureus*. *Anaerobe* 17: 399–402.

Bannerman, D.D., Paape, M.J., Hare, W.R., and Sohn, E.J. (2003). Increased levels of LPS-binding protein in bovine blood and milk following bacterial lipopolysaccharide challenge. *Journal of Dairy Science* 86: 3128–3137.

Bannerman, D.D., Paape, M.J., Lee, J.W. et al. (2004). *Escherichia coli* and *Staphylococcus aureus* elicit differential innate immune responses following intramammary infection. *Clinical and Diagnostic Laboratory Immunology* 11: 463–472.

Bansal, B.K. and Gupta, D.K. (2009). Economic analysis of bovine mastitis in India and Punjab-a review. *Indian Journal of Dairy Science* 67: 337–345.

Barkema, H., Schukken, Y.H., and Zadoks, R.N. (2006). Invited review: the role of cow, pathogen, and treatment regimen in the therapeutic success of bovine *Staphylococcus aureus* mastitis. *Journal of Dairy Science* 89: 1877–1895.

Baskaran, S.A., Kazmer, G.W., Hinckley, L. et al. (2009). Antibacterial effect of plant-derived antimicrobials on major bacterial mastitis pathogens *in vitro*. *Journal of Dairy Science* 92 (4): 1423–1429.

Bezman, D., Lembierskiy-Kuzin, L., Katz, G. et al. (2015). Influence of intramammary infection of a single gland in dairy cows on the cow's milk quality. *Journal of Dairy Research* 82: 304–311.

Bhosale, R.R., Osmani, R.A., Ghodake, P.P. et al. (2014). Mastitis: an intensive crisis in veterinary science. *International Journal of Pharma Research and Health Sciences* 2 (2): 96–103.

Bishop, C.D. (1995). Antiviral activity of the essential oil of *Melaleuca alternifolia* (Maiden and Betche) Cheel (tea tree) against tobacco mosaic virus. *Journal of Essential Oil Research* 7: 641–644.

Blowey, R.W. and Edmondson, P. (2010). *Mastitis Control in Dairy Herds*, 2e. London, UK: CAB International.

Bradley, A.J. (2002). Bovine mastitis: an evolving disease. *Veterinary Journal* 164: 116–128.

Braun, P.G. and Preuss, S.E. (2007). Microbial quality of water buffalo milk and milk products in Germany. *Milchwissenschaft* 62: 276–278.

Breen, J.E., Green, M.J., and Bradley, A.J. (2009). Quarter and cow risk factors associated with the occurrence of clinical mastitis in dairy cows in the United Kingdom. *Journal of Dairy Science* 92 (6): 2551–2561.

Busato, A., Trachsel, P., Schallibaum, M., and Blum, J.W. (2000). Udder health and risk factors for subclinical mastitis in organic dairy farms in Switzerland. *Preventive Veterinary Medicine* 44: 205–220.

Cobirka, M., Tancin, V., and Slama, P. (2020). Epidemiology and classification of mastitis. *Animals* 10: 2212.

Cox, S.D., Mann, C.M., Markham, J.L. et al. (2000). The mode of antimicrobial action of the essential oil of *Melaleuca alternifolia* (tea tree oil). *Journal of Applied Microbiology* 88: 170–175.

Deluyker, H.A., Van Oye, S.N., and Boucher, J.F. (2005). Factors affecting cure and somatic cell count after pirlimycin treatment of subclinical mastitis in lactating cows. *Journal of Dairy Science* 88: 604–614.

Dhakal, I.P., Dhakal, P., Koshihara, T., and Nagahata, H. (2007). Epidemiological and bacteriological survey of buffalo mastitis in Nepal. *The Journal of Veterinary Medical Science* 69: 1241–1245.

Dufour, S., Fréchette, A., Barkema, H.W. et al. (2011). Invited review: effect of udder health management practices on herd somatic cell count. *Journal of Dairy Science* 94 (2): 563–579.

Ehinger, A.M. and Kietzmann, M. (2000). Tissue distribution of oxacillin and ampicillin in the isolated perfused bovine udder. *Journal of Veterinary Medicine A* 47: 157–168.

EMA (European Medicines Agency) and EFSA (European Food Safety Authority) (2017). EMA and EFSA joint scientific opinion on measures to reduce the need to use antimicrobial agents in animal husbandry in the European Union, and the resulting impacts on food safety (RONAFA). *EFSA Journal* 15: https://doi.org/10.2903/j.efsa.2017.4666.

Enrico, V., Andrea, P., Francesca, B., and Min, Z.J. (2004). *Experimental Study of Reinforcement of Immunity by Syrup of Father Michel (POE 20)*. Italy: Institute of Naturopathic Sciences.

Erskine, R.J., Eberhart, R.J., Hutchinson, L.J., and Scholz, R.W. (1987). Blood selenium concentrations and glutathione peroxidase activities in dairy herds with high and low somatic cell counts. *Journal of the American Veterinary Medical Association* 190: 1417–1421.

Erskine, R.J., Eberhart, R.J., Grasso, P.J., and Scholz, R.W. (1989). Induction of *Escherichia coli* mastitis in cows fed selenium deficient or selenium supplemented diets. *American Journal of Veterinary Research* 50: 2093–2100.

Erskine, R.J., Barlett, P.C., VanLente, J.L. et al. (2002). Efficacy of systemic ceftiofur for severe clinical mastitis in dairy cattle. *Journal of Dairy Science* 85: 2571–2575.

Fagiolo, A. and Lai, O. (2007). Mastitis in buffalo. *Italian Journal of Animal Science* 6: 200–206.

Gao, M., Teplitski, M., Robinson, J.B., and Bauer, W.D. (2003). Production of substances by *Medicago truncatula* that affect bacterial quorum sensing. *Molecular Plant-Microbe Interactions* 16: 827–834.

Girardin, S.E., Boneca, I.G., Carneiro, L.A. et al. (2003). Nod1 detects a unique muropeptide from gram-negative bacterial peptidoglycan. *Science* 300: 1584–1587.

Hashimoto, M., Tawaratsumida, K., Kariya, H. et al. (2006). Not lipoteichoic acid but lipoproteins appear to be the dominant immunobiologically active compounds in *Staphylococcus aureus*. *Journal of Immunology* 177: 3162–3169.

Hemaiswarya, S., Kruthiventi, A.K., and Doble, M. (2008). Synergism between natural products and antibiotics against infectious diseases. *Phytomedicine* 15: 639–652.

Hillerton, J.E. (2000). Detecting mastitis cow-side. *Proceedings of the 39th Annual Meeting of the National Mastitis Council*, Atlanta, Georgia, USA (13–16 February 2000). Madison, Wisconsin, USA: National Mastitis Council.

Hussain, R., Khan, A., Javed, M.T., and Rizvi, F. (2013). Possible risk factors associated with mastitis in indigenous cattle in Punjab, Pakistan. *Pakistan Veterinary Journal* 32: 605–608.

Jingar, S.C., Mehla, R.K., Singh, M., and Singh, P.K. (2014). Effect of stages and level of milk production on mastitis incidence in cows and murrah buffaloes. *Journal of Bio Innovation* 3 (3): 117–123.

Jingar, S.C., Mahendra, S., and Roy, A.K. (2017). Economic losses due to clinical mastitis in cross-bred cows. *Dairy and Veterinary Sciences Journal* 3 (2): 555.

Joshi, S. and Gokhale, S. (2006). Status of mastitis as an emerging disease in improved and periurban dairy farms in India. *Annals of the New York Academy of Sciences* 1081: 74–83.

Karimuribo, E.D., Fitzpatrick, J.L., Swai, E.S. et al. (2008). Prevalence of subclinical mastitis and associated risk factors in smallholder dairy cows in Tanzania. *Veterinary Record* 163: 16–21.

Kehrli, M. and Harp, J. (2001). Immunity in the mammary gland. *Veterinary Clinics of North America: Food Animal Practice* 17: 495–516.

Krishnamoorthy, P., Suresh, K.P., Saha, S. et al. (2017). Meta-analysis of prevalence of subclinical and clinical mastitis, major mastitis pathogens in dairy cattle in India. *International Journal of Current Microbiology and Applied Sciences* 6 (3): 1214–1234.

Ksouri, S., Djebir, S., Bentorki, A. et al. (2017). Antifungal activity of essential oils extract from *Origanum floribundum Munby*, *Rosmarinus officinalis L.* and *Thymus ciliatus Desf.* against *Candida albicans* isolated from bovine clinical mastitis. *Journal de Mycologie Médicale* 27 (2): 245–249.

Kurjogi, M.M. and Kaliwal, B.B. (2014). Epidemiology of *Bovine mastitis* in cows of Dharwad district. *International Scholarly Research Notices* 1: 1–9.

Kvapilík, J. (2014). Mastitis in dairy cows and production losses. *Veterinářstvi* 64 (7): 550–560.

Kwiecinski, J., Eickb, S., and Wojcika, K. (2009). Effects of tea tree (*Melaleuca alternifolia*) oil on *Staphylococcus aureus* in biofilms and stationary growth phase. *International Journal of Antimicrobial Agents* 33: 343–347.

Lakshmi, R. (2016, 2016). A review on mastitis. *International Journal of Medicine Research* 1 (2): 118–123.

Lykkesfeldt, J. and Svendsen, O. (2007). Oxidants and antioxidants in disease: oxidative stress in farm animals. *Veterinary Journal* 173 (3): 502–511.

Madut, N.A., Gadir, A.E.A., and Jalii, I.M.E. (2009). Host determinants of bovine mastitis in semi-intensive production system of Khartoum state, Sudan. *The International Journal of Biochemistry & Cell Biology* 3: 71–77.

Manimaran, A., Layek, S.S., Kumaresan, A. et al. (2014). Estimation of antimicrobial drug usage for treatment of clinical mastitis cases in organized dairy farm. *Indian Journal of Veterinary and Animal Sciences Research* 43 (2): 140–150.

Mari, M., Bertolini, P., and Pratella, G.C. (2003). Non-conventional methods for the control of post-harvest pear diseases. *Journal of Applied Microbiology* 94: 761–766.

McDougall, S., Abbeloos, E., Piepers, S. et al. (2016). Addition of meloxicam to the treatment of clinical mastitis improves subsequent reproductive performance. *Journal of Dairy Science* 99 (3): 2026–2042.

Medeiros, E.S., Freitas, M.F.L., Saukas, T.N. et al. (2011). Risk factors associated with buffalo mastitis in the Brazilian Northeast. *Pesquisa Veterinaria Brasileira* 31: 499–504.

Mitchell, J.M., Griffiths, M.W., McEwen, S.A. et al. (1998). Antimicrobial drug residues in milk and meat: causes, concerns, prevalence, regulations, tests and test performance. *Journal of Food Protection* 61: 742–756.

USDA (2007). Dairy 2007, Part I: Reference of Dairy Cattle Health and Management in the United States, 2007. Fort Collins, CO: USDA, Animal and Plant Health Inspection Service, Veterinary Services, Center for Epidemiology and Animal Health. *Report No. N480.1007.*

Natzke, R.P., Everett, R.W., Guthrie, R.S. et al. (1972). Mastitis control program: effect on milk production. *Journal of Dairy Science* 55: 1256–1260.

NMC National Mastitis Council (2007). *Guidelines for Evaluating Teat Skin Condition*. USA: Verona.

Notebaert, S., Demon, D., Vanden Berghe, T. et al. (2008). Inflammatory mediators in *E. coli*-induced mastitis in mice. *Comparative Immunology, Microbiology and Infectious Diseases* 31: 551–565.

Ogunlana, E.O., Hoeglund, S., Onawunmi, G., and Skoeld, O. (1987). Effects of lemongrass oil on the morphological characteristics and peptidoglycan synthesis of *Escherichia coli* cells. *Microbios* 50: 43–59.

Oliveira, L. and Ruegg, P.L. (2014). Treatments of clinical mastitis occurring in cows on 51 large dairy herds in Wisconsin. *Journal of Dairy Science* 97: 5426–5436.

Oliveira, C.S., Hogeveen, H., Botelho, A.M. et al. (2015). Cow-specific risk factors for clinical mastitis in Brazilian dairy cattle. *Preventive Veterinary Medicine* 121: 297–305.

Paape, M.J., Lilius, E.M., Wiitanen, P.A. et al. (1996). Intramammary defense against infections induced by *Escherichia coli* in cows. *American Journal of Veterinary Research* 57: 477–482.

Paape, M., Mahrzad, J., Zhaom, X. et al. (2002). Defence of the bovine mammary gland by polymorphonuclear neutrophil leukocytes. *Journal of Mammary Gland Biology and Neoplasia* 7: 109–121.

Poutrel, B., Stegemann, M.R., and Roy, O. (2008). Evaluation of the efficacy of systemic danofloxacin in the treatment of induced acute *Escherichia coli* bovine mastitis. *The Journal of Dairy Research* 75: 310–318.

Pyörälä (2009). Treatment of mastitis during lactation. *Irish Veterinary Journal* 62 (Supplement): 40–44.

Pyorala, S. and Pyorala, E. (1998). Efficacy of parenteral administration of three antimicrobial agents in treatment of clinical mastitis in lactating cows: 487 cases (1989–1995). *Journal of the American Veterinary Medical Association* 212: 407–412.

Radostits, O.M., Gay, C.C., Blood, D.C., and Hinchcliff, K.W. (ed.) (2000). *Veterinary Medicine: A Textbook of the Diseases of Cattle, Sheep, Pigs, Goats, and Horses*, 9e, 563–660. ELBS & Baillier Tindall.

Rahman, M.A., Sarker, Y.A., Parvej, M.M. et al. (2018). Farmers' knowledge, attitude and practices of mastitis in dairy cows at selected areas of Bangladesh. *Bangladesh Journal of Veterinary Medicine* 16 (1): 65–70.

Ramírez, N.F., Keefe, G., Dohoo, I. et al. (2014). Herd- and cow-level risk factors associated with subclinical mastitis in dairy farms from the high plains of the northern Antioquia, Colombia. *Journal of Dairy Science* 97: 4141–4150.

Rantala, M., Kaartinen, L., Valimaki, E. et al. (2002). Efficacy and pharmacokinetics of enrofloxacin and flunixin meglumine for treatment of cows with experimentally induced *Escherichia coli* mastitis. *Journal of Veterinary Pharmacology and Therapeutics* 25: 251–258.

Rinaldi, M., Moroni, P., Paape, M.J., and Bannerman, D.D. (2008). Differential alterations in the ability of bovine neutrophils to generate extracellular and intracellular reactive oxygen species during the periparturient period. *Veterinary Journal* 178 (2): 208–213.

Riollet, C., Rainard, P., and Poutrel, B. (2000). Cells and cytokines in inflammatory secretions of bovine mammary gland. *Advances in Experimental Medicine and Biology* 480: 247–158.

Rossi, R.S., Amarante, A.F., Guerra, S.T. et al. (2019). Efficacy of cefquinome and a combination of cloxacillin and ampicillin for treatment of dairy cows with *Streptococcus agalactiae* subclinical mastitis. *PLoS One* 14 (4): e0216091.

Saini, S.S., Sharma, J.K., and Kwatra, M.S. (1994). Prevalence and etiology of subclinical mastitis among cows and buffaloes in Punjab. *Indian Journal of Dairy Science* 47: 103–106.

Samie, A., Tambani, T., Harshfield, E., and Green, E. (2010). Antifungal activities of selected venda medicinal plants against *Candida albicans*, *Candidi akrusei* and *Cryptococcus neoformans* isolated from South African AIDS patients. *African Journal of Biotechnology* 9: 265–276.

Sánchez-Macías, D., Hernández-Castellano, L.E., Morales-delaNuez, A. et al. (2020). Somatic cells: a potential tool to accelerate low-fat goat cheese ripening. *International Dairy Journal* 102: 104598.

Sant'anna, C. and Paranhos da Costa, M.J. (2011). The relationship between dairy cow hygiene and somatic cell count in milk. *Journal of Dairy Science* 94: 3835–3844.

Schreiner, D.A. and Ruegg, P.L. (2003). Relationship between udder and leg hygiene scores and sub clinical mastitis. *Journal of Dairy Science* 86: 3460–3465.

Schroeder, J.W. (2012). *Bovine Mastitis and Milking Management.* Mastitis Control Programs http://www.ag.ndsu.edu/pubs/ansci/dairy/as1129.pdf.

Schukken, Y.H., Hertl, J., Bar, D. et al. (2009). Effects of repeated gram-positive and gram-negative clinical mastitis episodes on milk yield loss in Holstein dairy cows. *Journal of Dairy Science* 92: 3091–3105.

Selsted, M.E., Tang, Y.Q., Morris, W.L. et al. (1993). Purification, primary structures, and antibacterial activities of the beta defenses, a new family of antibacterial peptides from bovine neutrophils. *The Journal of Biological Chemistry* 268: 6641.

Shaheen, M., Tantary, H.A., and Nabi, S.U. (2016). A treatise on bovine mastitis: disease and disease economics, etiological basis, risk factors, impact on human health, therapeutic management, prevention and control strategy. *Journal of Dairy Research* 4: 1.

Singh, S.V. and Pachauri, S.P. (2001). Antibiotic therapy in bovine mastitis: a double edged sword. *Pashudhan prakash* 16 (8): 1.

Singh, S.V. and Pachauri, S.P. (2004). A note on effect of environmental factors on the occurrence of bovine mastitis. *Indian Journal of Veterinary Medicine* 24 (1): 38–39.

Singh, S.V., Singh, J.P., Jaiswal, S., and Singh, H.N. (2004). Cost efficacy of ipecacuanha in treatment of blood in milk. *Indian Journal of Veterinary Medicine* 24 (2): 100.

Singh, S.V., Singh, N.K., Singh, J.P., and Ramakant (2018). Comparative efficacy of three days injection protocols of morbofloxacin in treatment of mastitis. *Indian Journal of Veterinary Medicine* 38 (1&2): 75–77.

Singh, S., Singh, J.P., Yadav, S.K. et al. (2021). Antibiogram pattern of common plant leaves against *E. coli*, *Staphylococcius aureus* and whole milk culture. *The Indian Journal of Veterinary Sciences and Biotechnology* 17 (1): 63–66.

Smith, K.L., Harrison, J.H., Hancock, D.A. et al. (1984). Effect of vitamin E and selenium supplementation on incidence of clinical mastitis and duration of clinical systems. *Journal of Dairy Science* 67: 1293–1300.

Sordillo, L.M., Nickerson, S.C., Akers, R.M., and Oliver, S.P. (1987). Secretion composition during bovine mammary involution and the relationship with mastitis. *International Journal of Biochemistry* 19: 1165.

Stevens, M., Piepers, S., and De Vliegher, S. (2016). Mastitis prevention and control practices and mastitis treatment strategies associated with the consumption of (critically important) antimicrobials on dairy herds in Flanders, Belgium. *Journal of Dairy Science* 99: 2896–2903.

Sudhan, N.A. and Sharma, N. (2010). *Mastitis: An Important Production Disease of Dairy Animals*, 1e, 72–88. Gurgaon: SSRV Manav Vikas Samiti.

Suriyasathaporn, W. and Chupia, V. (2011). Reduction in numbers of bacteria after pre-milking teat dipping in milking dairy cows. *Chiang Mai University Journal of Natural Sciences* 10: 301–306.

Tanzin, T., Nazir, K.H.M.N.H., Zahan, M.N. et al. (2016). Antibiotic resistance profile of bacteria isolated from raw milk samples of cattle and buffaloes. *Journal of Advanced Veterinary and Animal Research* 3 (1): 62–67.

Varshney, J.P. and Mukherjee, R. (2002). Recent advances in management of bovine mastitis. *Intas Polivet* 3 (1): 62–65.

Von Keyserlingk, M.A.G., Rushen, J., de Passille, A.M., and Weary, D.M. (2009). Invited review: the welfare of dairy cattle–key concepts and the role of science. *Journal of Dairy Science* 92: 4101–4111.

Wakchaure, R., Ganguly, S., Para, P.A. et al. (2015). Mastitis, an economically important disease affecting lactating ruminants: a review. *Chapter 15*. In: *New Dimensions in Microbiology* (ed. M.M.A.A. Khan, J.K. Grandy, E. Dilfuza, et al.), 199–212. Delhi, India: Lenin Media Pvt. Ltd.

Wellenberg, G.J., Van der Poel, W.H.M., and Van Oirschot, J.T. (2002). Viral infections and bovine mastitis: a review. *Veterinary Microbiology* 88: 27–45.

Winter, P. and Fehlings, K. (2013). Aspekte zur therapie von mastitiden in der laktation und zum trockenstellen. *Der Praktische Tierarzt* 94 (6): 21–27.

Yadav, S., Singh, S.V., Ramakant et al. (2020). Status of multi drug resistant *Staphyloccus aureus* in buffaloes of eastern plain zone of Uttar Pradesh having subclinical mastitis. *Buffalo Bulletin* 39 (4): 421–427.

Zeni, O., Sannino, A., and Romeo, S. (2012). Induction of an adaptive response in human blood lymphocytes exposed to radiofrequency fields: influence of the universal mobile telecommunication system (UMTS) signal and the specific absorption rate. *Mutation Research* 747: 29–35.

Zucali, M., Bava, L., Tamburini, A. et al. (2011). Effects of season, milking routine and cow cleanliness on bacterial and somatic cell counts of bulk tank milk. *Journal of Dairy Research* 78 (4): 436–441. https://doi.org/10.1017/S0022029911000598.

12

Downer-cow Syndrome

Samuel U. Felix[1,2], *Chiezey N. Pauline*[1], *Mojetoluwa S. Afolabi*[3], *Bashir M. Darma*[4], *Allam Lushaikyaa*[5], *and Adeniyi Njideka*[3]

[1] *National Animal Production Research Institute, Ahmadu Bello University, Zaria, Nigeria*
[2] *Department of Food and Animal Science, Alabama A&M University, Normal, Alabama, USA*
[3] *Department of Biological Sciences, Alabama A&M University, Normal, Alabama, USA*
[4] *Veterinary Teaching Hospital, Faculty of Veterinary Medicine, Bayero University, Kano, Kano, Nigeria*
[5] *Faculty of Veterinary Medicine, Ahmadu Bello University Zaria, Zaria, Kaduna, Nigeria*

12.1 Introduction

The phrase "downer cow" initially emerged in veterinary literature during the 1950s. It referred to cattle that were too injured, weak, or sick to stand or walk without help (Kumari et al. 2022). In early publications, the definition of this term was vague, describing cattle as "unable to rise" or "unable to stand without assistance," without discussing potential causes, the duration of being unable to stand, or the eventual outcome. More recently, "downer cow" has been used to describe nonambulatory cattle that remain recumbent (lying down) for at least 24 hours without an obvious reason. A further classification of downer cows was proposed, distinguishing between mentally alert nonambulatory cattle that can maintain sternal recumbency ("alert downer cows") and cows with significant mental dullness, abnormal vital signs, and difficulty maintaining sternal recumbency ("nonalert downer cows") (Figure 12.1). Occasionally, the term "creeper cows" is used to describe alert, recumbent cows that cannot bear weight on their hindlimbs but use their forelegs to move short distances (Radostits et al. 2006).

12.2 Causes of Downer-cow Syndrome

Alert downer cows are primarily found lying down due to injuries related to the musculoskeletal or nervous systems. These injuries often involve conditions like sciatic or obturator nerve lesions caused by dystocia (difficult calving), fractures in long bones or the pelvis, hip dislocations, or muscle damage from either direct trauma or extended periods of being recumbent. Nonalert downer cows, on the other hand, include animals with systemic diseases that affect their mental state and overall demeanor. These diseases can encompass conditions like periparturient hypocalcemia (milk fever), septicemia (blood infection), hypovolemia (low blood volume), widespread peritonitis (inflammation of the abdominal lining), severe hepatic lipidosis (fatty liver disease), or neurological disorders that affect the brainstem or cerebral cortex (Simões et al. 2021). In many instances, the syndrome observed in downer cows is a complication of milk fever. Nonambulatory cows often develop myopathies (muscle disorders) and neuropathies (nerve disorders) due to prolonged periods of being unable to stand. These issues frequently involve ischemic myopathy that affects the large muscles in the hindlimbs as well as injuries to the tissues around the hip joint and obturator muscles (Verdon 2023). Such complications become common in cows that fail to fully recover and stand. Injuries to the musculoskeletal system also arise when cows splay their hindlimbs, especially during parturition (giving birth), or when they are made to stand or walk on slippery surfaces shortly

Periparturient Diseases of Cattle, First Edition. Edited by Tanmoy Rana.

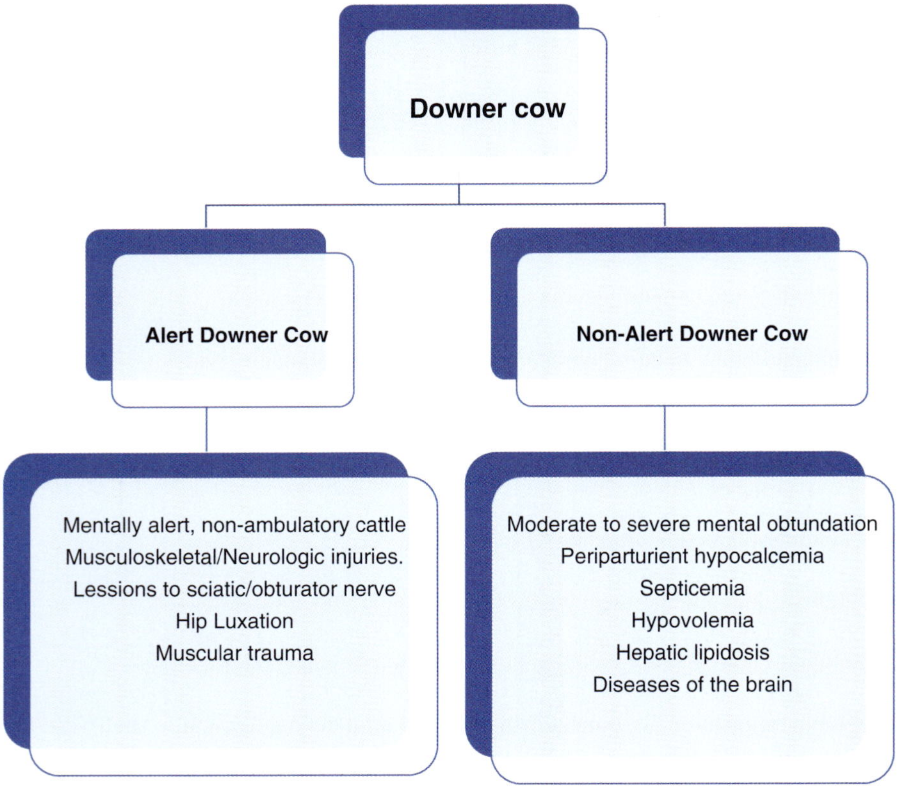

Figure 12.1 Classification of downer-cow syndrome.

before or after calving. A survey of dairy operations in 21 US states revealed that the top three reasons for persistent recumbency among cows were periparturient hypocalcemia (19% of cases), injuries related to calving (22% of cases), and injuries resulting from slipping or falling (15% of cases). Among beef cattle operations, calving paralysis emerged as the most common cause of downer-cow syndrome (Burton et al. 2009).

12.2.1 Disease Surveillance and Occurrence

The disease is most commonly observed in dairy cows and typically arises within the first 2–3 days of giving birth and frequently follows an episode of milk fever. Additional debilitating conditions that affect cows around calving and may lead to prolonged lying down include acute coliform mastitis, septic metritis, and acute rumen acidosis (excessive grain consumption).

In the United States, about 270 000 cattle experienced immobility on farms in 2004. Among these, 57.4% were dairy cows and 31.5% were beef cattle, representing 1.2% of dairy cows and 0.2% of beef cattle that become persistently unable to stand within a year. An earlier survey conducted in 1986 in Minnesota, which involved data from 738 dairy farms and 34 656 cow years at risk, indicated occurrence rates ranging from 0.4% to 2.1% per herd and per year. In this study, the criterium for cases were cows lying on their sides for at least 24 hours without an obvious cause. The overall outcomes revealed that 33% of the recumbent cows recovered, 23% were slaughtered, and 44% died. Owners believed that the downer cows were either high producers (48%) or average producers (46%) with only 6% being low producers. Approximately 58% of cases occurred within the first day of calving, and 37% happened during the initial 100 days of lactation. The highest incidence (39%) was during the coldest months: December to February. Another clinical survey was carried out in New Zealand, which involved 433 recumbent cows around calving. The findings showed a 39% recovery rate, a 30% mortality rate, and 32% of cows needed to be euthanized. This study found that precalving recumbent cows had an 11% higher case-fatality rate than post-calving cows. A survey from 2006 of dairy farms in 21 US states reported that 78.6% of the participating farms had encountered at least one downer cow in 2006. In this study, a downer cow was defined as a cow unable to stand for any duration, including those that eventually regained mobility. Due to the lack of precise clinical definition for this condition and its inclusion of miscellaneous cases that do not fit into other categories, the incidence of downer cows varies based on the veterinarian's assessment and environmental factors in different regions. Regardless, the incidence appears to be on the rise, especially in intensive dairy farming regions, although this perception could stem from an increased emphasis on treating valuable animals (Elena et al. 2021).

12.2.2 Animal Risk Factors

12.2.2.1 Milk Fever

Extended periods of lying down after an occurrence of clinical milk fever, either due to a delay in receiving appropriate treatment or a delayed response to treatment, is recognized as the primary factor contributing to the prevalent condition known as downer-cow syndrome. Reported occurrences of downer-cow syndrome linked to milk fever in literature sources vary from 3.8% to 28.2% among all cases of milk fever. Irrespective of the main cause, prolonged lying down leads to elevated pressure on specific body areas, which restricts blood flow and impairs nerve and muscle function (Adams 2015). A hypocalcemic periparturient cow with an unstable walking stance is at a heightened risk of harm from slipping or falling, which can result in issues like torn muscles, bone fractures, or dislocated hips that ultimately culminate in the development of downer-cow syndrome (Figure 12.2).

Figure 12.2 Downer-cow syndrome.

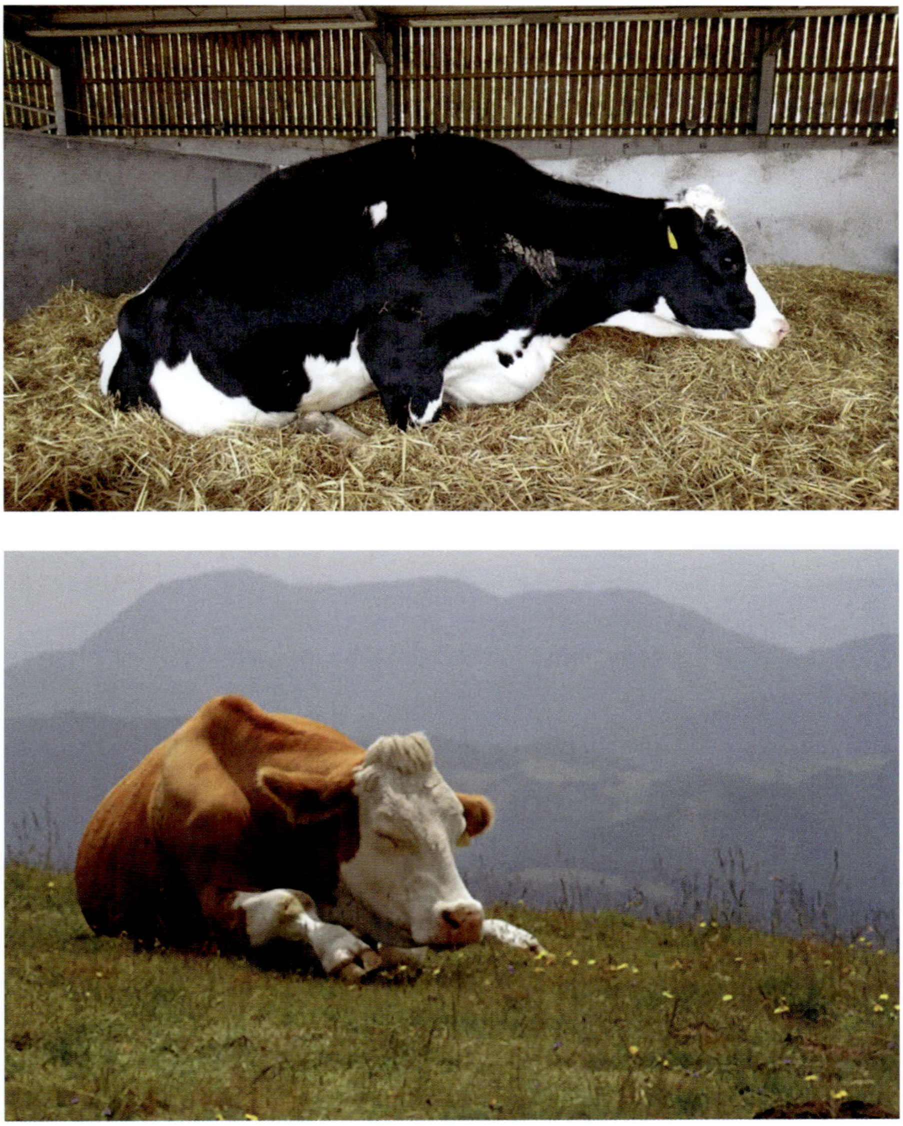

12.2.2.2 Traumatic Injuries to Pelvis

Injuries to the limbs, including bones, muscles, and nerves, can stem directly from the act of giving birth (such as calving paralysis), arise due to weakened muscles and an unsteady walking pattern (seen in cattle with low calcium levels), or result from accidental incidents. Calving paralysis refers to partial or complete loss of motion in one or both hindlimbs due to damage to the obturator nerve and/or the lumbar root of the sciatic nerve during the calving process. These nerves are susceptible to compression between the calf and the bony birth canal during delivery, which leads to nerve impairment. Such nerve damage is most frequently observed after difficult births, the delivery of large calves, or prolonged calving periods. Among beef cattle, calving paralysis is the predominant reason for persistent lying down. Additional nerve injuries in the limbs can emerge as secondary consequences in cows that are immobile due to unrelated causes, which results in pressure-related damage to the superficial nerves (Bradford 2019).

12.2.2.3 Serum Electrolyte Imbalances

In addition to hypocalcemia, other mineral imbalances such as hypophosphatemia, hypokalemia, and hypomagnesemia have been identified as potential factors that might contribute to the occurrence of downer-cow syndrome (Table 12.1). Hypophosphatemia, characterized by low levels of phosphorus, is frequently observed in recumbent periparturient cows and healthy ones. This mineral imbalance is often cited as a risk factor, particularly in "creeper cows," which are alert and mobile but unable to stand. The significance of hypophosphatemia in cows with persistent recumbency has sparked contentious debate, yet an undisputed observation is that recumbent periparturient cows unresponsive to intravenous calcium treatment, especially in the early stages of recumbency, tend to exhibit more frequent or pronounced hypophosphatemia. However, the mechanisms by which phosphorus depletion leads to sustained lying down are not well understood, and the response to treatment that involves the oral or parenteral administration of phosphate salts is inconsistent. Studies of cattle immobile for more extended periods found that lower serum phosphorus levels suggest a positive prognosis, with nonsurvivors typically showing higher serum phosphorus concentrations. This phenomenon could be explained by the fact that cows recumbent for extended periods might have experienced greater muscle damage that lead to the release of intracellular phosphorus into the bloodstream and consequently, elevated serum phosphorus levels.

Long term, mild hypomagnesemia has also been associated with downer-cow syndrome, particularly when it coincides with hypocalcemia. However, this condition usually presents as a tetanic hyperesthetic state, which is not a characteristic of downer-cow syndrome.

In severe cases, hypokalemia (low potassium levels) in cattle results in depression and pronounced skeletal muscle weakness that can lead to recumbency. Instances of significant hypokalemia in individual animals linked to persistent recumbency, with serum potassium concentrations below 2.0 mmol/l, have been documented over the years. These cases are often traced back to the repeated use of isoflupredone, a mineral corticoid with a potent diuretic effect that was commonly employed to treat ketosis in the United States. Mild to moderate hypokalemia is known to occur in early lactating and anorexic cows, but the role of this milder form in the development of downer-cow syndrome requires further investigation. The age and lactation stage of a recumbent cow have been identified as risk factors for nonrecovery. Recovery rates for nonambulatory cows were found to be 10.1% for first-lactation cows, 17.7% for cows in their second to fourth lactation, and 22.2% for fifth-lactation cows. Cows within the first 15 days of lactation had a recovery rate of 28.4%, while cows in later stages of lactation had only a 6.2% chance of making a full recovery. Higher recovery rates in older cows and cows in earlier stages of lactation have been linked to the connection between persistent recumbency and hypocalcemia. Older cows and those in earlier lactation stages are more likely to be recumbent when hypocalcemia is the primary or contributing cause, which generally has a better prognosis than persistent recumbency due to other reasons (Van Saun 2023) (Figure 12.3).

Table 12.1 Serum biochemical and electrolyte composition of cattle.

Serum biochemicals	Reference range (Radostits et al. 2000)
Sodium (mEq/l)	132–152
Potassium (mEq/l)	3.9–5.8
Calcium, total (mg/dl)	9.7–12.4
Calcium, ionized (mg/dl)	4.8–6.2
Phosphorus (mg/dl)	5.6–6.5
Magnesium (mg/dl)	1.8–2.3
Acetoacetate (mg/dl)	0–1.1
Acetone (mg/dl)	0–10.0
β-Hydroxybutyrate (mg/dl)	5.9–13.9
Lactate (mg/dl)	5.0–20.0
Triglyceride (mg/dl)	0–14.0

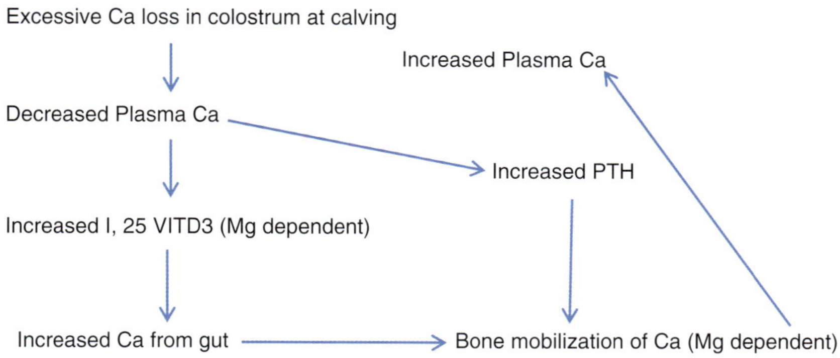

Figure 12.3 Calcium metabolism in the periparturient cow.

12.2.2.4 Fatty Liver Disease (Hepatic Lipidosis)

Hepatic lipidosis, commonly known as fatty liver disease, occurs when excessive fat accumulates in a cow's liver due to an imbalance between the mobilization and metabolism of fat. This issue usually arises when cows have high energy demands, such as during early lactation, which causes their energy requirements for producing milk to surpass the energy they get from their feed. To compensate, the cow's body starts breaking down stored fat to meet the energy deficit. The liver becomes the main site for processing these released fatty acids, especially when the cow's energy demands are very high or feed intake is inadequate. If the liver cannot efficiently process the surplus fatty acids, they accumulate within its cells, which affects normal function.

The liver is crucial for maintaining metabolic balance and supporting various bodily functions. Excessive fat buildup from fatty liver disease compromises the liver's ability to regulate metabolism, detoxify the body, and create essential proteins. This disruption in metabolic processes has ripple effects throughout the cow's body. One result of this disease and its impact on metabolism is the potential effect on muscle function. With the liver's reduced capacity to process and distribute energy, the cow might not have enough energy for proper muscle function. This can lead to muscle weakness and contribute to issues like difficulty standing and walking normally, which ultimately causes downer-cow syndrome (Van Saun 2023).

12.2.2.5 Duration of Recumbency

The duration of recumbency was also identified as a factor linked to the likelihood of complete recovery. Cows that were lying down for less than 24 hours had a recovery rate of 32%, while those that remained recumbent for longer periods had a lower chance of recovery at 8.2%. Furthermore, a high body condition score (BCS) is a recognized risk factor for milk fever and consequently, should be acknowledged as a predisposing factor for downer-cow syndrome. Cows with a BCS exceeding 4.0 out of 5 around the time of calving were determined to be 4.3 times more likely to experience nonambulatory states compared to cows with a leaner body condition. In contrast, cows in poor body condition, with a BCS below 2.5 out of 5, exhibited an 8.1% recovery rate, while 16.6% of cows with a BCS of 2.75 or higher achieved full recovery (Van Saun 2023).

12.2.2.6 Toxic Disorders

Various toxic disorders can lead to bovine recumbency (Radostits et al. 2006). They include:

- **Acute mastitis:** Acute mastitis is the inflammation of the udder tissues due to bacterial infections caused by microorganisms. It is characterized by swelling, hardness, and pain in the cow's udder.
- **Acute puerperal metritis:** Metritis is the inflammation of both the endometrial and muscular layers of the uterus. It is caused by a bacterial infection in postpartum dairy cattle and is characterized by fetid vaginal discharge, fever, and general depression.
- **Peritonitis:** Peritonitis is the inflammation of the serous membrane that lines the peritoneal cavity. It is caused by infectious agents and is characterized by fever, anorexia, pain, and depression.
- **Traumatic reticuloperitonitis:** Traumatic reticuloperitonitis is the inflammation of the reticulum wall due to perforation by a sharp object, e.g. a nail or wire, that may have been ingested by a cow.
- **Abomasal volvulus:** Abomasal volvulus occurs when the abomasum is displaced into the right abdominal cavity.

12.2.2.7 Neurological Disorders

Downer cows, characterized by their inability to stand and walk, often experience muscle weakness as a result of various underlying factors. Among these factors, damage to and functional loss of the sciatic nerve plays a significant role. The sciatic nerve, one of the largest nerves in the body, originates from the lumbar and sacral spinal cord and extends down the hindlimb, providing motor and sensory innervation to several muscles.

Sciatic Nerve Damage The sciatic nerve can be damaged in downer cows through several mechanisms.

- **Direct compression:** When a downer cow lies in a recumbent position for an extended period, the weight of the cow's body and the pressure exerted on the nerves can lead to nerve compression. In particular, the sciatic nerve can be directly compressed against the caudal (rear) femur bone.
- **Muscle swelling:** The muscles surrounding the sciatic nerve can become inflamed and swollen due to the cow's prolonged recumbency. This swelling can further contribute to pressure on the sciatic nerve, which exacerbates the nerve damage.

Muscle Weakness from Sciatic Nerve Damage The sciatic nerve innervates several muscles in the hindlimb, including the hamstrings, gluteal muscles, and muscles of the lower leg. When the sciatic nerve is damaged, the communication between the nerves and the muscles is disrupted, which leads to muscle weakness or paralysis in the affected limb.

12.2.3 Recovery and Factors Affecting Severity

The recovery of a downer cow depends on the extent of damage to the sciatic nerve and the associated muscle weakness. The severity of pressure damage to the muscles and nerve compression is influenced by several factors.

- **Duration of compression:** Prolonged pressure on the sciatic nerve can lead to more severe nerve damage and muscle dysfunction. The longer a cow remains in a recumbent position, the greater the potential for irreversible nerve injury.
- **Regional anatomical factors:** The anatomy of the cow, including size and orientation of the muscles and bones, can influence the specific areas where pressure is exerted on the sciatic nerve. Certain anatomical variations might increase the risk of nerve compression and damage.
- **Surface and environment:** The surface on which the downer cow is lying can also contribute to nerve damage. Hard or uneven surfaces can create localized pressure points that increase the risk of nerve compression. Additionally, the environment's cleanliness and bedding quality can impact the development of muscle swelling and inflammation (Radostits et al. 2006).

12.2.4 Environmental and Management Risk Factors

A slippery ground surface poses a significant risk factor for cattle, particularly during crucial moments such as calving. Cattle are large, heavy animals that rely on sure footing to maintain their balance and mobility. When they are forced to walk across surfaces that are slippery or lack traction, the potential for accidents and injuries increases significantly. During calving, when a cow is giving birth to a calf, both the mother and the newborn calf are in a vulnerable state. The cow's body undergoes significant physiological changes, and her movements might be slower and less coordinated due to the discomfort and physical strain of labor. Similarly, the calf is still adjusting to its new environment and is inherently unsteady on its feet in the initial hours after birth.

If the ground surface is slippery, be it due to mud, ice, water, etc., the risk of accidents and injuries rises dramatically. As the cow tries to navigate across the unstable surface, she may lose her footing and slip. When a cow slips and falls, especially when calving, there are several potential negative consequences.

- **Muscular injuries:** Cattle, like all animals, have powerful muscles in their limbs that help them move and maintain their posture. When a cow slips and falls, she might twist her body unnaturally or land in an awkward position. This can result in strains, sprains, or even tears in the large muscles of her pelvic limbs (hindlegs).
- **Lameness:** If a cow sustains significant muscular injuries from slipping and falling, she may struggle to stand up again. The pelvic limb muscles are crucial for a cow's ability to support her body weight and stand. Injuries to these muscles could render her unable to stand and leave her lying on the ground in distress.

- **Dystocia:** The process of calving is already physically demanding for a cow. An injury caused by slipping and falling could complicate the calving process and lead to delays, difficulties in delivery, or even complications that endanger both the cow and the calf.
- **Stress and pain:** In addition to the physical injuries, slipping and falling can also cause significant stress and pain for the cow. Stress can further hinder the calving process and impact the overall health of the animal (Radostits et al. 2006).

12.3 Pathogenesis

In most instances, downer-cow syndrome arises as a complication stemming from an unrelated, underlying issue that triggers muscle weakness or the continual inability to stand. The primary factors responsible for downer-cow syndrome can be categorized into four main groups: (i) metabolic disorders (such as low calcium or potassium levels), (ii) sudden widespread illnesses (like coliform mastitis or toxic metritis), (iii) problems in the muscles and skeleton (such as fractures or dislocated joints), and (iv) unclear origins. Extended periods of lying down can lead to additional harm due to excessive pressure on limbs caught between the body and the ground or from the animal's efforts to rise. These added injuries can impact muscles, nerves, bones, or joints. Regardless of the original cause, prolonged recumbency will lead to varying degrees of pressure-induced damage that mainly affect the hindlimbs. Research findings suggest that after approximately 6 hours of lying down, tissue damage from excessive weight bearing becomes likely, which emphasizes the urgency of treating any persistently recumbent cow as a medical emergency. Pressure-related damage in downed cattle primarily impacts the significant muscles of the hindlimbs, particularly the semitendinosus muscle, muscles below the knee, and the peripheral sciatic nerve, along with its branches. This localized tissue damage is known as compartment syndrome, while the broader systemic effects caused by this local tissue damage are termed crush syndrome (Radostits et al. 2006).

12.3.1 Compartment Syndrome

A body compartment comprises the muscles and nerves situated within a precisely defined anatomical area enclosed by a rigid layer of muscle fascia. When a cow is lying down, the particularly relevant compartments are mainly the upper section and to a lesser extent, the lower section, of each hindlimb. The initial pressure applied to the hindlimb beneath the cow's body depends on the weight of the body pressing onto the limb and the firmness of the ground beneath the cow. This pressure on the limb immediately results in an escalation of pressure within the specific compartment, which leads to a partial or complete blockage of venous blood flow before the arterial blood flow to the region diminishes. This disparity between the influx and outflow of blood in the compartment adds to the accumulation of pressure within it. The compromised blood supply to the muscles and nerves, accompanied by the resulting deficiency of tissue oxygen, combines with the direct harm caused by mechanical compression (Radostits et al. 2006).

The robust boundaries formed by the muscle fascia that encircle the compartment hinder the expansion of tissues that could alleviate the excessive pressure on the internal structures. Consequently, cellular damage and inflammation occur, which prompts swelling that exacerbates pressure and initiates a sequence of detrimental events. In experimental situations, intentional external compression of the pelvic limb in goats – designed to replicate limb compression in recumbent cows – led to a noteworthy reduction in the conduction velocity of the peroneal nerve. This decrease in nerve conduction velocity correlated with observable impairment in the limb, as evidenced through clinical examination. There are two main types of compartment syndrome:

- **Acute compartment syndrome:** This type of compartment syndrome typically occurs as a result of trauma, such as a broken bone, crush injury, or severe contusion. Swelling and bleeding in response to the injury can cause the pressure within the compartment to rise rapidly. Classic symptoms include severe pain that is out of proportion to the injury, numbness or tingling, swelling, and tenseness of the affected area. Acute compartment syndrome is a medical emergency that requires immediate intervention to relieve the pressure, often through a surgical procedure called a fasciotomy. Failure to treat it promptly can result in permanent damage to muscles, nerves, and blood vessels.
- **Chronic exertional compartment syndrome:** This type of compartment syndrome typically occurs in athletes and individuals who engage in repetitive physical activities. It is caused by increased pressure within the affected muscle compartments during exercise due to muscle swelling and increased blood flow. Symptoms usually occur during or after physical activity and include pain, cramping, and a sensation of tightness in the affected muscles. Rest and conservative

treatments, such as physical therapy and modified activity, are often recommended. In some cases, surgery may be considered if conservative measures are not effective.

12.3.2 Crush Syndrome or Traumatic Rhabdomyolysis

Crush syndrome, also known as crush injury or traumatic rhabdomyolysis, encompasses the collective systemic effects that result from substantial damage to muscle tissue. This condition is attributed to the significant release of breakdown products from muscle tissue into the bloodstream. Notably, there is a substantial elevation in the serum activity of muscle enzymes like aspartate aminotransferase (AST) or creatine kinase (CPK). Concurrently, there are increases in the serum levels of primarily intracellular electrolytes such as potassium and phosphorus. Ultimately, the presence of myoglobin in the urine serves as an indicator of crush syndrome. Myoglobinuria, which involves the presence of myoglobin in the urine, is a potentially life-threatening complication associated with downer-cow syndrome that potentially leads to the development of acute renal failure.

12.3.3 Experimental Sternal Recumbency

Inducing sternal recumbency in experiments, by placing one hindlimb under the body to simulate extended periods of lying down, leads to a swollen and stiff limb within 6–9 hours. After muscle cell injury, the activity of the enzyme CPK in the serum significantly rises around 12 hours after the onset of recumbency. Between 12 and 36 hours after the onset of prolonged recumbency, proteinuria and in severe instances, myoglobinuria occur due to the release of myoglobin from the damaged muscles. In cases where cows attempt to stand but cannot succeed, persistent struggling may cause muscle fiber rupture and bleeding. Approximately 10% of cases involve acute focal myocarditis, which results in a rapid heartbeat, irregular rhythm, and in some cases, an adverse response to intravenous calcium salts. The cause of this heart muscle lesion is unknown, but the excessive administration of calcium salts has been proposed as a potential factor. Prolonged recumbency can lead to additional complications like sudden mastitis (inflammation of the udder), pressure sores, and traumatic injuries to the limbs.

The underlying causes of downer-cow syndrome, particularly when the cow is not alert and responsive, remain unclear. Most such cows have initially experienced milk fever but failed to respond effectively. Within 1–2 days, affected cows display a preference for lying on their sides and exhibit moaning and groaning during exhaling. These nonalert downer cows account for about 2% of all cases of milk fever (Radostits et al. 2006).

12.4 Clinical Findings

Downer-cow syndrome can manifest either independently or follow an apparent recovery after treatment for milk fever, except for the prolonged inability to stand. In a typical scenario, affected cows either exhibit no effort or are incapable of standing following treatment for parturient paresis. Approximately 30% of cows treated for milk fever will remain unable to stand for up to 24 hours after treatment. These affected cows generally maintain their brightness and alertness, with either normal or mildly depressed feed intake, which places them into the category of alert downer cows. Their body temperature is within the normal range, and the heart rate may be normal or elevated, reaching 80–100 beats/minute. Some cows experience tachycardia (rapid heart rate) and arrhythmia (irregular heartbeat), particularly immediately after the administration of intravenous calcium, and sudden death has been observed. The respiratory rate is typically unaffected. While defecation and urination follow the usual pattern, proteinuria (presence of protein in the urine) is frequent and may indicate significant muscle damage if pronounced (Radostits et al. 2006).

In some cases, affected cows might not make any attempt to stand, while others will frequently try to stand but are unable to fully extend their hindlimbs and lift their hindquarters more than 20–30 cm off the ground. On surfaces with grip (bare ground, sand, or deep bedding), certain cows can stand with assistance, provided by lifting their tailheads or using hip slings. Cows that make no effort to stand usually remain unable to do so, even with support from slings, and they typically show stiffness, pain, or numbness in their limbs, which makes them hesitant or unable to bear weight. Hyperflexion of the fetlock joints and damage to the peroneal nerve are usually observed in these cases. Some cows position their hindlimbs extended on either side of their body, which can lead to ischemic myopathy due to the excessive weight placed on the medial thigh muscles.

Complications frequently arise in cases of downer-cow syndrome and can result in death or the need for euthanasia. Coliform mastitis, decubitus ulcers (bedsores) – particularly over the hock and elbow joint prominences – and traumatic injuries related to the use of hip slings are common complications. The course of the disease varies based on the nature and extent of the lesions and the quality of care provided during the initial days. Proper care can help approximately 50% of downer cows stand within 4 days or less. The prognosis is grim for cows that remain recumbent after 7 days, although some cases have shown recovery even after being down for 10–14 days. Death may occur within 48–72 hours after the onset of the syndrome and is often linked to myocarditis (inflammation of the heart muscle) (Radostits et al. 2006).

12.4.1 Clinical Examination of the Downer Cow

A clinical assessment of a downer cow can prove to be quite challenging and is influenced by factors like the environment and the animal's size. Persistent recumbency in cattle can stem from metabolic, musculoskeletal, neurologic, neoplastic, and inflammatory disorders. Therefore, obtaining a thorough history and conducting a comprehensive physical examination are crucial. Vital aspects of the history include the cow's age, lactation stage, duration of recumbency, any prior clinical issues, previous treatments, diet, exposure to new feeds, sudden changes in exercise, and an evaluation of management practices. Observing the surroundings and the ground surface around the downed animal might provide insights into whether the cow slipped, fell, or suffered an injury. A systematic evaluation of all accessible body systems is essential. The cow should be observed from a distance to identify abnormalities in head and neck posture, limb positioning, and any attempts to stand or move. A comprehensive close examination is necessary to assess body temperature, heart rate, pulse, respiratory rate, and the condition of major body systems such as the respiratory, cardiovascular, central nervous, gastrointestinal, mammary, and reproductive systems, any of which might indicate abnormalities linked to shock-induced recumbency.

In recently calved cows, special attention is given to thoroughly examining the udder for mastitis, the uterus for metritis, and the gastrointestinal tract for conditions associated with toxemia, dehydration, and shock (like abomasal volvulus, acute diffuse peritonitis, and carbohydrate engorgement) that can result in recumbency. It is crucial to obtain and test a urine sample for ketones and the presence of myoglobinuria. A systematic musculoskeletal examination involves palpating the muscles, bones, joints, and hooves of each limb, including gently flexing and extending each limb. The coxofemoral joints are inspected for signs of dislocation. The vertebral column is evaluated for potential fractures or dislocations. It is important to examine both sides of the animal, which may require rolling the cow over multiple times for repeated assessments.

A neurologic examination includes evaluating withdrawal reflexes, patellar reflexes, limb sensation, and spinal reflex arcs. Careful scrutiny of the lumbar and sacral areas, including tail sensation and tone, is performed, along with an assessment of the cranial nerves. To further the examination, the downer cow can be lifted using appropriate devices and observed for whether the cow extends its limbs and attempts to bear weight. While assisting the cow to standing, additional examinations of various body parts can be conducted (Radostits et al. 2006).

12.4.2 Clinical Pathology

The serum concentrations of calcium and glucose often fall within the normal range. In contrast, phosphorus and potassium concentrations might be reduced in cows with decreased feed intake or increased in animals with more severe muscle damage and/or dehydration. Initial hematologic exams usually reveal no significant abnormalities during the early stages of recumbency. However, the serum activity of enzymes CPK and AST is typically considerably elevated within 18–24 hours after the onset of recumbency.

A notable elevation of serum CPK activity shortly after recumbency starts, followed by a significant decrease within the subsequent 24–48 hours, points to acute muscle trauma (like muscle rupture) as a potential cause of the recumbency. A moderate increase in serum CPK activity, which tends to rise slightly or remain constant over the following days, suggests continuous and ongoing muscle trauma due to the prolonged compression of muscle tissue. CPK is abundant in muscle tissue, and its plasma half-life in cattle is relatively short, around 8–9 hours. Thus, it serves as a sensitive but transient marker of muscle damage. When assessing the serum CPK activity in a recumbent cow, it is crucial to consider the timing of sample collection in relation to the onset of recumbency.

On the other hand, AST has a significantly longer half-life and remains elevated for several days after the initial trauma. In a study of 262 recumbent dairy cows, serum samples were analyzed for CPK, lactate dehydrogenase (LDH), and AST to predict recovery failure. Optimal cutoff points were determined at 2330 U/l for CPK, 2225 U/l for LDH, and 171 U/l for AST. AST exhibited the best predictive capability for a cow's failure to recover, especially for serum samples taken on the first day of recumbency (Radostits et al. 2006).

In experimental instances of induced recumbency in cows, CPK activity stayed within normal limits for the first 6 hours, but by 12 hours, there was a sharp increase to mean values of 12 000 U/l that climbed to 40 000 U/l by 24 hours. There might also be moderate ketonuria (presence of ketones in urine). Significant proteinuria is typically apparent 18–24 hours after recumbency initiates and can either persist for several days or disappear within a few days. Severe cases might exhibit brown and turbid urine due to severe myoglobinuria.

Elevated serum levels of urea, muscle enzymes, and signs of inflammation are considered the most reliable indicators for an unfavorable recovery prognosis. Cows with a total protein–fibrinogen ratio below 10 : 1, along with evidence of neutropenia (low white blood cell count) and/or a left shift (shift in the distribution of white blood cells), tend to have a lower recovery rate. Cows with serum urea levels that exceed 25 mmol/l and serum creatinine levels above 130 mmol/l have a poor prognosis (Radostits et al. 2006).

12.4.3 Necropsy Findings

Hemorrhages and edema of the skin due to trauma are frequently observed in downer cows. The main pathological alterations involve hemorrhages and deterioration of the medial thigh muscles. Hemorrhages around the hip joint, sometimes accompanied by rupture of the ligamentum teres, are also commonly seen. Localized areas of ischemic necrosis in the muscles (such as the gracilis, pectineus, and adductor muscles) can develop at the front edge of the pelvic symphysis. Eosinophilic infiltration has been noted in the ruptured and necrotic thigh muscles of downer cows. Hemorrhages and edema that affect the nerves of the limbs (like obturator, sciatic, peroneal, and radial nerves) are also frequent and generally linked to severe muscle damage. Upon examination, the heart is dilated and flabby, with a histological analysis that often reveals focal myocarditis. Fatty degeneration is observed in the liver, and the adrenal glands are enlarged. Furthermore, there are degenerative changes in the glomerular and tubular epithelium of the kidneys when analyzed microscopically (Radostits et al. 2006).

12.5 Differential Diagnosis

The diagnosis of downer-cow syndrome is typically made by exclusion of all other known causes of recumbency in a cow persistently recumbent for at least 24 hours while having received two courses of parenteral calcium treatment (Radostits et al. 2006). Differential diagnoses for alert downer cows are:

- **Hypocalcemia:** Also known as milk fever, this condition occurs due to low blood calcium levels, typically after calving. It can lead to muscle weakness and recumbency.
- **Hypokalemia:** Low blood potassium levels can cause muscle weakness and paralysis, leading to downer-cow syndrome.
- **Fractures of the bone or pelvis:** Traumatic injuries like fractures can result in cows being unable to stand.
- **Hip luxation:** Dislocation of the hip joint can lead to paralysis and difficulty standing.
- **Botulism:** Caused by a toxin produced by the bacterium *Clostridium botulinum*, botulism can lead to muscle paralysis and weakness.
- **Calving paralysis:** This refers to paralysis or weakness due to nerve damage after a difficult calving.
- **Spinal lymphosarcoma (bovine leukosis virus [BLV]):** Lymphosarcoma, a cancer that affects lymphoid tissues, can sometimes affect the spinal cord and lead to paralysis.
- **Differential diagnoses for nonalert downer cows include:** Hypocalcemia, hypomagnesemia, coliform mastitis, toxic metritis, hepatic lipidosis/puerperal liver coma, hypovolemic shock, septic shock, generalized peritonitis, acute rumen acidosis, botulism, right-displaced abomasa/abomasal volvulus, hypokalemia, meningoencephalitis, and polio encephalomalacia.

12.6 Treatment

Treating a nonambulatory cow requires addressing both the underlying cause of recumbency and the secondary damage that results from prolonged lying down. If the primary cause of recumbency is known, treatment should primarily target that cause. For specific treatment recommendations based on the identified cause, the relevant chapter of this book is recommended.

However, treating a downer cow also necessitates intensive supportive care to manage secondary damage and prevent further complications. The prognosis of a downer cow is influenced by the initial cause of recumbency and to a significant extent, by the quality of care provided during the period of recumbency. Comprehensive and attentive care during this period can greatly impact the cow's chances of recovery.

12.6.1 Anti-inflammatory Therapy

In recent years, the use of anti-inflammatory therapy as a component of pain management in ruminant production medicine has gained more attention. This is increasingly acknowledged as a crucial aspect of animal welfare by both veterinarians and owners. While there might not be an extensive amount of data supporting the use of steroidal and nonsteroidal anti-inflammatory drugs (NSAIDs) in downer cows, their application appears warranted. Their use helps alleviate pain and discomfort in the sick, nonambulatory cow as well as manage and control the secondary inflammation that arises from recumbency. This inflammation could potentially worsen myopathy (muscle damage) and neuropathy (nerve damage), both of which play a significant role in downer-cow syndrome. NSAIDs may need to be administered repeatedly to adequately manage pain and inflammation, but this increases the risk of adverse gastrointestinal effects, like abomasal ulceration. To mitigate this risk, it is recommended that the owner regularly examines the feces for signs of melena (dark, tarry stools that indicate bleeding).

Some clinicians suggest a single high dose of dexamethasone (0.2–0.3 mg/kg intravenously [IV]) early in the recumbent period. This approach is based on clinical experience and is aimed at controlling and containing inflammatory neuropathy that results from trauma or pressure. However, due to the potential abortive effects of dexamethasone, its use in pregnant cows must be discussed with the animal's owner.

12.6.2 Fluid and Electrolyte Therapy

Fluid and electrolyte therapy is necessary for patients with inadequate water and feed intake. If the cow is drinking normally, multiple electrolytes can be added to the drinking water. While the supplementation of minerals like phosphates, magnesium, or potassium has been suggested, their success has been inconsistent. Oral fluid therapy through drenching is effective for maintaining hydration in alert animals. However, drenching a recumbent cow should only be considered if the cow is alert and possesses a healthy swallowing reflex. Since recumbency increases pressure on visceral organs, the amount of fluid given per treatment should not exceed 40 l to prevent the risk of reflux caused by heightened intraruminal pressure.

12.6.3 Bedding and Clinical Care

The paramount aspect of treatment involves ensuring the most comfortable bedding possible and regularly rolling the cow from side-to-side multiple times a day. This practice aims to minimize the extent of ischemic damage (lack of blood supply) and para analgesia (lack of pain sensation) that results from prolonged recumbency. With dedicated care and the provision of quality bedding, appetizing feed, and ample water, most cows will make attempts to stand, albeit with some difficulty and assistance, within the first 24 hours. Within the next 1–2 days, most cows will regain the ability to stand unassisted and in a normal manner.

For facilitating standing when downer cows make efforts to rise, an ideal ground surface is a sand or dirt pack. If affected cows are left on a slippery surface, their motivation to stand diminishes, and their condition tends to worsen. Additionally, cows should be milked as usual, and extra attention should be given to maintaining udder hygiene. Washing the udder with a germicidal soap before milking and applying post-milking teat dips are recommended practices to ensure udder health.

12.6.4 Assisted Lifting to Aid Standing

When considering whether to lift a recumbent cow that has not attempted to stand shortly after treatment for milk fever, the behavior of the cow should guide the decision. If the cow makes any effort to stand, even with some coaxing, she should be assisted to stand. Creating a good nonslip ground surface, providing deep bedding, and gently lifting on the tailhead when she attempts to stand can aid in this process. Rolling the cow from side-to-side every few hours and encouraging her to stand multiple times a day is also beneficial.

Various cow-lifting devices have been used to assist downer cows in standing. Hip lifters, which fit over the tuber coxae, and body slings designed to wrap around the abdomen and thorax are examples of these devices. They can be helpful if the cow is making some effort to stand. For cows that exhibit this effort, hip lifters or slings can be applied to lift the animal into a standing position. If the cow can bear weight on all four legs, she can be allowed to stand with the aid of the device for 20–30 minutes before being lowered down. This process can be repeated once or twice daily, provided she can support her own weight while standing. In most cases, these downer cows will regain the ability to stand on their own within a few days. Caution is necessary when using hip lifters to prevent traumatic injuries to the tissues around the tuber coxae. Cows lifted with hip lifters should never be left unattended while suspended, as they could weaken and hang in the device, leading to severe trauma. The careful application of these devices is essential to prevent slipping or injuries, which can contribute to persistent recumbency. Body slings that encompass the abdomen and thorax are more suitable for lifting cows that will not readily bear weight after being hoisted. They distribute weight over several areas, unlike hip lifters that focus weight on the tuber coxae. However, these body slings are more cumbersome to apply and require experienced personnel.

More recently, water flotation tanks have been used for managing nonambulatory cows. These systems involve immersing the cow in a watertight container filled with warm water. The cow's head is held above water, and they are allowed to stand in the water for several hours. While labor-intensive, this approach has shown success, particularly when used selectively for suitable cases.

It is important to note that flotation therapy is not appropriate for cows with certain injuries, such as ruptured tendons, fractures, luxated coxofemoral joints, or septic polyarthritis. However, for cases stemming from milk fever, flotation therapy might be effective with a reported success rate of around 37%. Careful case selection can increase this success rate (Radostits et al. 2006).

12.6.5 Handling, Transportation, and Disposition of Nonambulatory Cattle

There has been significant controversy and disagreement among veterinarians and livestock producers regarding the management, transport, and fate of nonambulatory cattle. Economic factors play a substantial role in decision making in such cases. There has been no universal consensus on whether these animals are suitable for transport or slaughter for salvage purposes. When faced with a valuable downer cow and an unclear cause of recumbency, the typical approach is to either provide treatment over several days to monitor progress or consider slaughter for salvage. Valuable breeding animals that experience recumbency due to complications like milk fever, acute carbohydrate engorgement, or peracute mastitis often receive targeted and supportive therapies. For commercially valuable cattle, slaughter for salvage has been a common choice. Producers seek maximum financial return through this option. However, the transportation of compromised animals, particularly due to their size, raises significant animal welfare concerns. Loading an animal weighing 500–800 kg onto a truck, even with forceful measures like lifting, pulling, or dragging, can lead to substantial pain and discomfort for the animal. In the 1990s, global public attention grew around the handling and fate of nonambulatory animals, especially downer cows, regardless of the reason behind their recumbency. As a result, government regulatory agencies responsible for animal health, along with livestock and veterinary associations, started creating regulations related to the care and treatment of nonambulatory animals, including downer cows. The issue of downer-cow syndrome has become an animal welfare matter that prompts veterinarians to take proactive steps.

Society is increasingly concerned about the treatment, handling, and disposition methods for nonambulatory animals. If a downer cow does not show signs of recovery within a few days, the prognosis becomes uncertain. The owner and veterinarian must then decide whether to continue providing clinical care or consider euthanasia for the animal (Radostits et al. 2006).

12.6.6 Euthanasia

The level of care provided to a recumbent cow can quickly raise concerns related to animal welfare, and in such cases, the option of humane euthanasia should always be considered. This is especially true for instances with a poor prognosis or when the attending veterinarian anticipates that sufficient supportive care cannot or will not be given, regardless of the reasons. Proposed "trigger points" for deciding on euthanasia, as suggested in literature, encompass the following criteria:

- Conditions with a grim prognosis.
- Persistent pain and suffering that are not relieved by treatment.

- Prolonged loss of appetite that spans multiple days.
- Nonalert downer cows that are not responsive to treatment within a reasonable timeframe.
- Inability to maintain sternal recumbency (upright resting position).
- An owner unable or unwilling to provide adequate care.
- Development of complications such as pressure sores, mastitis, or other related conditions.
- Worsening condition despite appropriate patient care.
- Absence of response to treatment for a period exceeding 10 days.

These indicators are meant to guide veterinarians and owners in making ethical decisions that prioritize the well-being of the animal and consider their overall quality of life.

12.7 Control

The early identification and management of milk fever can significantly reduce the occurrence and severity of downer-cow syndrome. Ideally, cows should receive treatment during the initial stage of milk fever, before they become recumbent. If a cow does become recumbent, prompt treatment should be administered, without delaying for more than 1 hour. Providing proper bedding, such as ample straw or a soft ground surface, is important for cows with milk fever. For recumbent cows, if feasible, efforts should be made to encourage and assist them in standing after milk fever treatment. If standing is not possible, these cows should be gently rolled from side-to-side every few hours, if circumstances permit. While getting owners to follow this recommendation can be challenging, frequent rolling is crucial for minimizing the occurrence of ischemic necrosis.

In preparation for calving, dairy cows should be placed in comfortable and well-bedded box stalls. They should remain in these stalls for at least 48 hours after giving birth, especially in cases where there is a risk of developing milk fever. This practice helps ensure timely detection and intervention if milk fever does occur (Radostits et al. 2006).

References

Adams, A.E. (2015). Dairy cow management and welfare: practices on dairy operations in the United States that may impact dairy cow welfare, lameness, and beef quality assurance. Doctoral dissertation. Colorado State University.

Bradford, B.J. (2019). Dairy research 2019. *Kansas Agricultural Experiment Station Research Reports* 5 (9): 11.

Burton, A.J., Nydam, D.V., Ollivett, T.L., and Divers, T.J. (2009). Prognostic indicators for nonambulatory cattle treated by use of a flotation tank system in a referral hospital: 51 cases (1997–2008). *Journal of the American Veterinary Medical Association* 234 (9): 1177–1182.

Elena, N., Barbara, C., and Giulio, C. (2021). The welfare of beef cattle in the scientific literature from 1990 to 2019: a text mining approach. *Frontiers in Veterinary Sciences*, Sec. Animal Behavior and Welfare Volume 7 – 2020 https://doi.org/10.3389/fvets.2020.588749.

Kumari, A., Kumar Jain, V., Kumar Nehra, A. et al. (2022). Assessment of haematological and biochemical alterations in recumbent buffaloes. *Biological Rhythm Research* 53 (11): 1670–1691.

Radostits, O.M., Gay, C.C., Blood, D.C., and Hinchcliff, K.W. (2000). *Veterinary Medicine*, 9e, 1819–1822. London: W.B. Saunders.

Radostits, O.M., Gay, C., Hinchcliff, K.W., and Constable, P.D. (ed.) (2006). *Veterinary Medicine E-Book: A Textbook of the Diseases of Cattle, Horses, Sheep, Pigs and Goats*. Elsevier Health Sciences.

Simões, J., Stilwell, G., Simões, J., and Stilwell, G. (2021). Puerperal complications in the dam. In: *Calving Management and Newborn Calf Care: An Interactive Textbook for Cattle Medicine and Obstetrics*, 209–237. Springer, Cham.

Van Saun, R.J. (ed.) (2023). *Ruminant Metabolic Diseases, an Issue of Veterinary Clinics of North America: Food Animal Practice, E-Book*, vol. 39, No. 2. Elsevier Health Sciences.

Verdon, M. (2023). *A Review of Factors Affecting the Welfare of Weaned Replacement Heifers in Pasture-Based Dairy Production Systems*. Animal Production Science.

13

Uterine Infections/Metritis

Sarath Thulasiraman[1], Monica Gunasekar[2], Arunmozhi Narayansamy[3], Kalyaan Udumalpet Sampathkumar[4], Rajesh Kumar[5], and Kabir Alam[5]

[1] *Veterinary College and Research Institute, Salem, Tamil Nadu Veterinary and Animal Sciences University, Attur, Tamil Nadu, India*
[2] *Department of Clinics, Madras Veterinary College, Chennai, Tamil Nadu, India*
[3] *Teaching Veterinary Clinical Complex, Veterinary College and Research Institute, Orathanadu, Tamil Nadu Veterinary and Animal Sciences University, Thanjavur, Tamil Nadu, India*
[4] *Department of Veterinary Gynaecology and Obstetrics, Madras Veterinary College, Tamil Nadu Veterinary and Animal Sciences University, Chennai, Tamil Nadu, India*
[5] *Department of Veterinary Gynaecology and Obstetrics, College of Veterinary Science and Animal Husbandry, Acharya Narendra Deva University of Agriculture and Technology, Ayodhya, Uttar Pradesh, India*

13.1 Introduction

Infection of the uterus is a leading cause of compromised fertility and economic loss in the dairy sector (Butani et al. 2008; Kumar et al. 2008). Bacterial infections of the uterus disrupt the uterine milieu and affect the functions of uterus, the ovaries, and the control centers in the hypothalamus and pituitary gland. The sound diagnosis and treatment of uterine diseases is a key component of all reproductive management programs in dairy animals. After parturition, bacterial contamination of the uterine lumen commonly occurs in cattle, which is primarily due to physical damage to the birth canal during calving and a relaxed cervix 2–3 days after parturition.

Postpartum uterine diseases have two types, viz. clinical and subclinical. Clinical disease is easy to diagnose by vaginal discharge, while subclinical disease is difficult to diagnose due to the absence of vaginal discharge and other signs. Subclinical disease may be diagnosed by rectal or vaginal examination and using diagnostic tools like ultrasounds, etc.

Up to 40% of dairy cows exhibit signs of metritis within a week of parturition. Postpartum metritis will lead to prolonged days open and intercalving periods, which favors more involuntary culling in the herd and results in a higher economic loss (Foldi et al. 2006). Toxic puerperal metritis is also a severe, life-threatening problem. Metritis and endometritis are inflammation of the uterus. Inflammation of the endometrium, the underling glandular tissues, and the muscular layer is termed metritis (Gilbert et al. 2005), whereas endometritis refers only to inflammation of the endometrium and the underlying glandular tissues without any systemic signs. These diseases share common etiological factors, are predisposing factors for each other, and largely, share common treatment (Noakes et al. 2002).

13.2 Incidence

Metritis incidence depends on the definition of the disease, but the maximum for obvious clinical disease is 36–50%, while 18.5–21% of animals have metritis with signs of systemic illness such as pyrexia. About 15–20% of cattle have clinical disease that persists beyond 3 weeks postpartum (endometritis), and about 30% have chronic inflammation of the uterus without clinical signs of uterine disease (subclinical endometritis).

The expression of a clinical uterine infection depends on the balance between factors such as the animal, its immunity, the number and pathogenicity of the microbes, and the uterine environment. Usually, in the first 2 weeks after calving, 25–40% of animals have clinical metritis that persists in up to 20% of animals as clinical endometritis. The clinical type of

Periparturient Diseases of Cattle, First Edition. Edited by Tanmoy Rana.

endometritis can be diagnosed easily based on the type of vaginal discharge, but the subclinical uterine disease is less well characterized and is an emerging condition. In the 40–60 days after calving, around 50% of cows have neutrophils in the uterine lumen or endometrium, concomitant with inflammation of the tissues and subclinical endometritis, which reduces conception rates. Chronic endometrial scarring, obstruction of the uterine fallopian tubes, and adhesion between the ovary and the bursa are other consequences of uterine bacterial infections. The incidence of ovarobursal adhesion in cows is recorded at 2%.

The prevalence of uterine infections is not consistent worldwide, instead variability exists among studies (Lewis 2003). It was reported that the prevalence rate of uterine infection in buffaloes was much higher than in cows, 24.7% in India (LeBlanc et al. 2001). Mansour et al. (2003) found a high prevalence of postpartum infections 38.54% in buffalo cows. Furthermore, Kim and Kang (2003) recorded a 30% prevalence of endometritis among Indian buffaloes. In Pakistan, Usmani et al. (2001) recorded a prevalence of 24% for uterine infections in buffaloes. The higher incidence of uterine infection in buffaloes compared to cows might be due to poor hygiene, vaginal stimulation for milk letdown, and wallowing behavior (Azawi 2006).

13.2.1 Etiology and Risk Factors for Uterine Infection

Uterine disease is commonly associated with *Escherichia coli*, *Trueperella pyogenes* (formerly *Corynebacterium pyogenes, Actinomyces pyogenes,* and *Arcanobacterium pyogenes*), *Fusobacterium necrophorum,* and *Prevotella* species. Except for *E. coli*, the other three organisms act synergistically to enhance the likelihood of uterine disease and increase the risk of clinical endometritis as well as its severity.

Various risk factors have been reported for uterine infections (Correa et al. 1993; Kim and Kang 2003; Sheldon and Dobson 2004; Dubuc et al. 2010; Potter et al. 2010). In general, the risk factors of uterine infection can be classified as follows.

1) Uterine damage associated with dystocia, twins, retained fetal membranes, stillbirth, abortion, uterine prolapse, and delayed uterine involution (Correa et al. 1993; Kaneene and Miller 1995; LeBlanc et al. 2002; Sheldon et al. 2008; Molinari et al. 2023). A delayed uterine involution and cesarean section–associated uterine damage, predispose the cow to uterine infections.
2) Metabolic disorders such as abomasal displacement, hypocalcemia, ketosis, and others (Markusfed 1987; Correa et al. 1993; Whiteford and Sheldon 2005). Postpartum pyrexia can be used as sign of postpartum inflammation, but other signs are needed to confirm uterine infections (Sheldon et al. 2004). Other risk factors are parity (Markusfed 1987), season (Molinari et al. 2022), environmental hygiene, and diet (Sheldon et al. 2008).
3) Balance between pathogenicity and immunity and other miscellaneous causes such as:
   a) <u>Disruption of neutrophil function:</u> Cows that develop metritis or endometritis had decreased neutrophil glycogen stores around the time of calving, thus a disruption of neutrophil function could be a risk factor for uterine disease later in lactation (Galvao et al. 2010).
   b) <u>Dysbiosis of the uterine microbiota:</u> The gravid uterus is not a sterile place, as was previously believed (Perez-Munoz et al. 2017; Appiah et al. 2020; Ault-Seay et al. 2023). A few recent studies have shown that it has its own microbiome (NIH HMP Working Group et al. 2009; Human Microbiome Project Consortium 2012; Moreno and Franasiak 2017; Pelzer et al. 2017; Baker et al. 2018) peculiar to each compartment of the genital tract, i.e. vagina, cervix, and uterus. Furthermore, parturition results in the loss of compartmentalization, which results in the dispersal and mixing of microbiota from different compartments. The delayed differentiation of vaginal and uterine microbiomes (Miranda-CasoLuengo et al. 2019) and dysbiosis may result in the development of a uterine infection (Adnane and Chapwanya 2022). Moreover, Pascottini et al. (2020) observed that the microbiome dynamics of clinical endometriotic cows differed significantly from those of their subclinical or healthy herd mates. They further noted that uterine pathogens are not associated with subclinical endometritis.

13.2.2 Classification of Uterine Infection

Veterinarians use clinical manifestation and attributes of vaginal discharge to diagnose varying degrees of uterine infections in field and farm conditions. Indeed, there are well-established definitions to categorize uterine infections (Sheldon et al. 2006; de Boer et al. 2014; Wagener et al. 2017). The definitions are as follows.

13.2.2.1 Metritis

Metritis is characterized by an enlarged uterus, a purulent uterine discharge that ranges from a watery red-brown fluid to thick off-white pus, and is most frequently encountered within 10 days postpartum (DPP) (Sheldon et al. 2006). However, the incidence of metritis varies by breed, nation, and herd. Metritis can be further graded as follows:

- **Grade 1:** Animals without apparent systemic symptoms of illness but with an unusually enlarged uterus and a purulent vaginal discharge (PVD) of a uterine origin.
- **Grade 2:** Animals that display an unusually enlarged uterus, a PVD of uterine origin, and additional symptoms of systemic illness such as fever, dullness, and a declined milk yield.
- **Grade 3:** Most severe form, often known as toxic or puerperal metritis, characterized by an abnormally enlarged uterus and a PVD of uterine origin accompanied by toxemia symptoms like dullness, depression, inappetence or anorexia, pyrexia (> 39.5 °C), and cold extremities.

13.2.2.2 Clinical Endometritis

Clinical endometritis is characterized by the presence of a purulent or mucopurulent vaginal discharge of uterine origin 21 or more DPP.

13.2.2.3 Subclinical Endometritis

Subclinical endometritis is characterized by inflammation of the endometrium (no deeper than the stratum spongiosum layer) in the absence of clinical signs of endometritis. The importance of subclinical endometritis emerged when cytological evidence of endometritis was associated with reduced fertility (Kasimanickam et al. 2004). The cause of subclinical endometritis is not yet clear and may include resolving bacterial infections, immunopathology, tissue repair, or an abnormal shift in uterine microbiota.

13.3 Pathophysiology of Uterine Infections

In a postpartum cow, the following events must be completed before she is likely to conceive again:

1) Uterine involution,
2) Regeneration of the endometrium,
3) Elimination of bacterial contamination of the uterus, and
4) Return of ovarian cyclical activity.

The expulsion of the fetus, including the fetal membranes and the fluids, is the first step. Uterine involution involves physical shrinkage as well as the necrosis and sloughing of caruncles and the regeneration of the endometrium. After the allantochorion is expelled, the necrosis of uterine caruncles and sloughing will take place within 12 days of parturition. Since the caruncles account for over half of the weight of the uterus, sloughing of the uterine caruncles results in a rapid weight reduction (from 13 kg at parturition to about 1 kg 3 weeks later). The lochial discharge comprises the sloughed caruncles, the remains of fetal fluids, and blood from the ruptured umbilicus. Regeneration of the endometrium takes place initially in the intercaruncular areas, followed by the cells over the caruncle. By 25 days after parturition, the epithelial regeneration is completed, whereas the deeper layers of tissues are not fully restored until 6–8 weeks post calving.

The postpartum uterine environment favors the growth of several aerobic and anaerobic bacteria. Many of these bacteria are contaminants in the uterine lumen and are removed by a range of uterine defense mechanisms (UDMs). The concentrations of steroid hormones decrease to basal values after parturition, and the first postpartum follicular wave emergence is stimulated by an increase in plasma follicle-stimulating hormone (FSH) that occurs within days of calving. Subsequently, around 10–12 days after calving, the first dominant follicle is selected in all postpartum cows irrespective of periparturient disease, environment, or dietary deficiencies. The dominant follicle that emerges from the first postpartum follicular wave has one of the three following fates:

1) Ovulation and formation of the first postpartum corpus luteum (return of ovarian cyclical activity).
2) Atresia with the emergence of one or more follicular waves without ovulation (anestrus).
3) Formation of an ovarian follicular cyst.

Generally, the early return of ovarian cyclicity is considered beneficial for subsequent fertility. However, it is reported that if there is a uterine infection when ovulation occurs during the first postpartum estrus, it may lead to pyometra with the persistence of a corpus luteum. This presence of pus within the uterine lumen will favor the subsequent occurrence of uterine diseases.

13.3.1 Uterine Diseases: Molecular Mechanisms

As the uterus is usually sterile, the presence of microbes or pathogen-associated molecules appears to provoke a substantial immune response. The immune cells within the endometrium and the endometrial stromal and epithelial cells generate a uterine immune response. Indeed, it is the epithelial cells that are the first line of defense against microbes in the uterine lumen. Pathogen-associated molecular patterns (PAMPs) are detected by pattern recognition receptors (PRRs), and the innate immunity of the genital tract is highly dependent on the expression of these PRRs.

These PRRs, such as the family of Toll-like receptors (TLRs), are highly conserved across phyla and detect a range of PAMPs associated with fungi, viruses, and bacteria. The binding of PAMPs to PRRs activates signal transduction pathways for the mitogen-activated protein kinase (MAPK) and NF-κB transcription factors that lead to the secretion of prostaglandins, cytokines, and chemokines. The innate immune receptor for lipopolysaccharide (LPS; endotoxin, a key PAMP of the common uterine pathogen *E. coli*) is TLR-4, which is expressed by epithelial and stromal cells of the uterus. In other species, this concept of endometrial cell expression of PRRs is supported by the expression of other TLRs for bacteria and viruses. However, bovine cell cultures have an advantage over other species as they are free of contamination from professional immune cells (as indicated by zero expression of CD45). The bovine TLR-4 signaling pathways are emerging. Hence, bovines are a useful model for exploring uterine disease and its mechanism in other mammals, including cattle. PAMPs cause inflammation of the uterus and affect endocrine function.

The principal hormones secreted by the endometrium are prostaglandin (PG)F2α and PGE2, and the secretion of these hormones is modulated by *E. coli* or LPS. The prediction from in vitro work is that uterine disease extends the luteal phase, which is observed clinically. Exogenous administration of PGF2α effectively clears uterine infections, and eicosanoids modulate uterine immunity directly.

In vitro, LPS stimulates progesterone secretion from mixed populations of luteal cells (including steroidogenic, endothelial, and immune cell types) to a level similar to that of luteinizing hormone (LH), but at higher concentrations LPS kills the cells.

13.4 Clinical Signs

1) **Septic metritis, puerperal metritis, or toxic metritis:** A fetid, watery, uterine discharge varies in color from brown to amber, gray, or red but is always low in mucous content, purulent, and has an extremely fetid odor with swollen caruncles that occurs within the first 7–10 days after parturition. Signs of illness common in cattle and buffaloes are pyrexia (39.5–41.5 °C), tachycardia, inappetence, decreased production, rumen stasis, depression, dehydration, and diarrhea.
2) **Puerperal metritis:** When a cow has an abnormally enlarged uterus and fetid, watery, red-brown uterine discharge that is associated with signs of systemic illness (decreased milk yield, dullness, or other signs of toxemia) and fever (> 39.5 °C), within 21 days of parturition, it is termed puerperal metritis.
3) **Clinical metritis:** Metritis most commonly occurs within 10–21 days of parturition. An enlarged uterus and a watery, red-brown fluid to a viscous, off-white, purulent, uterine discharge is noticed in metritis, along with a foul odor. Signs of health determine the severity of the disease.
   a) Grade 1 clinical metritis–affected cows will have an abnormally enlarged uterus and a purulent uterine discharge without any systemic signs of ill health.
   b) Grade 2 clinical metritis–affected cows will have additional signs of systemic illness such as decreased milk yield, dullness, and fever.
   c) Animals with signs of toxemia such as inappetence, cold extremities, depression, and/or collapse are classified as having Grade 3 metritis, which has a poor prognosis.
4) **Clinical endometritis:** The presence of purulent (> 50% pus) discharge from the uterus, 21 days or more after parturition or a mucopurulent (50% mucus, 50% pus) discharge from the uterus after 26 days of parturition is observed in

clinical endometritis. Morphological and functional changes in the endometrium that lead to decreased fertility (delayed submission for artificial insemination [AI], repeat breeding) are the major clinical signs exhibited. External uterine discharge may not be observed very often.
   a) Disrupted luteolytic path exposes the uterus to the immune-suppressive action of progesterone.
   b) Decreased milk production.
   c) Ovarian function abnormality observed as a delay in first ovulation and dominant follicular growth impairment in cycling cows.
5) **Subclinical endometritis (SE):** SE in cows is characterized by a clear, mucus discharge with a normal reproductive tract and regular cycle. But the cows will not conceive, even after three or four consecutive inseminations with good quality semen. SE can be diagnosed based on the uterine cytology. Uterine cytology samples collected 21–33 days after calving with greater than 18% neutrophils and samples collected at 34–47 days with greater than 10% neutrophils are indicative of SE.
6) **Pyometra:** The accumulation of purulent material within the uterine lumen with a closed cervix that occurs in the presence of a persistent corpus luteum.

13.4.1 Difference Between Metritis and Endometritis

Metritis is an infection of the endometrium, its lining, and uterine deeper layers. Endometritis is a localized infection of the lining of the uterus, which is inflamed and characterized by mucus mixed with a purulent discharge from the uterus. Since the deeper layers of the uterus are not affected in endometritis, not much thickening of the uterus is observed compared to normal. Clearly, metritis has a higher degree of severity than endometritis and requires a different therapeutic approach for cattle and buffaloes.

Pyometra refers to pus accumulation within the uterine lumen with a closed cervix and the presence of a corpus luteum in the ovary. In endometritis-affected cows, a corpus luteum is often present, but the cervix is patent, often with pus discharging from the uterus into the vagina. Nonetheless, clinical endometritis is common compared to pyometra, which is relatively rare and comprises less than 5% of clinical uterine disease cases.

13.5 Diagnosis

Diagnosis of metritis within the first 10 DPP is relatively easy based on the clinical signs.

1) **Clinical signs:** Metritis-affected cows exhibit clinical signs like the presence of pyrexia, fetid pus within the uterine lumen, and discharge from the vulva accompanied by delayed uterine involution.
2) **Clinical examination:** A clinical examination includes a detailed evaluation of the reproductive tract by rectal examination for the location of the cervix and its texture; location of the uterus and an assessment regarding its contents, texture, and firmness; the presence of discharge from the cervical canal; the condition of the vaginal mucosa; etc.
3) **Vaginoscopic examination:** A vaginoscopic examination aids when assessing the vaginal wall and the nature of vaginal discharge in the anterior vagina as well as the patency of the cervix. Additional information such as the presence of vaginal lacerations will also be acquired.
4) **Laboratory investigations:**
   a) Cytology of the uterine contents yields valuable information and allows for a diagnosis of subclinical infections.
   b) Bacterial culture and sensitivity testing provides important information about the infection and indicates which antibiotic should be used.
   c) Biopsy and histology provide information on the extent of inflammation and the health and functional status of the endometrium. Biopsies are helpful for formulating a prognosis.
5) **Ultrasonography:** A less invasive technique with rapid results such as Doppler ultrasonography (Figure 13.1) can provide satisfactory results regarding the evolution of uterine alterations in uterine disease conditions like endometritis.

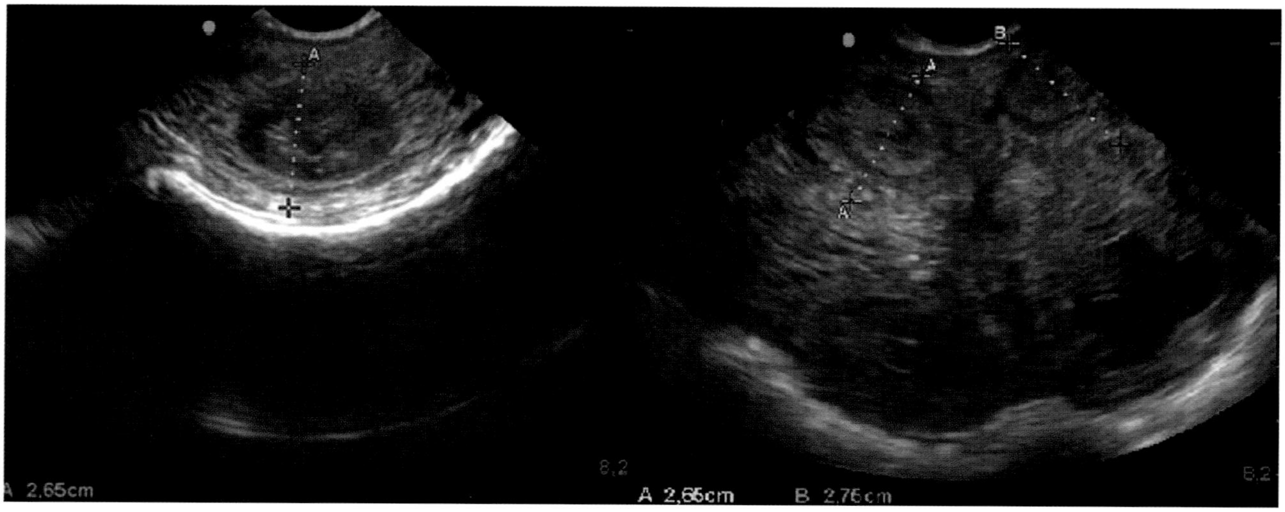

Figure 13.1 Assessment of the bovine uterus with endometritis using Doppler ultrasound. *Source:* Bruno Leonardo Mendonça Ribeiro, Enoch Brandão de Souza Meira Júnior, Mario Augusto Aleman Reyes, Eduardo Carvalho Marques, Alessandra Figueiredo de Castro Nassar, Lilian Gregory October 31, 2019 bioRxiv 826065; https://doi.org/10.1101/826065.

13.6 Therapeutic Approaches

All therapeutic agents available to treat uterine infections are focused in four major areas:

1) **The elimination of bacterial infections or mitigation of bacterial dysbiosis in the genital tract.** Antibiotics used to treat uterine infections must comply with certain criteria including a high activity against the main pathogens whereby injectable formulations must reach high concentrations in the uterine lumen and endometrium. Intrauterine formulations must result in good penetration of the lumen and endometrium, not irritate the endometrium, not have a negative effect on uterine immune cells, and finally, have a short milk withdrawal period.
2) **Improvement of uterine contractility and UDMs.** This results in evacuation of the pathological contents of the uterus.
3) **The elimination of the immunosuppressive influence of progesterone.** There is a role for prostaglandins in the therapy of uterine infections (Lewis 2003).
   a) Luteolysis results in:
      - Improvement of uterine contractility.
      - Elimination of immunosuppressive effect of progesterone.
   b) Direct stimulation of the functions of immune cells in endometrium.
4) **Prevention of recurrent infections during the following luteal phase.** If prostaglandins alone are used to treat endometritis, clinical improvement can be achieved; some bacteria may, however, remain in the endometrial crypts. These bacteria will multiply during the next luteal phase when the immune function of the endometrium is decreased due to the effect of progesterone. This leads to relapses of endometritis.

A combination of proper anti-infective therapy and prostaglandins allows for the elimination of the existing bacterial infection and prevents a recurrence of the condition in the following cycle (Kumar et al. 2009).

13.6.1 Conventional Therapeutic Agents

13.6.1.1 Antiseptics

Many antiseptic agents such as iodine, chlorhexidine, and normal saline have been used widely as intrauterine infusions to treat uterine infections (Zemjanis 1980). Nonetheless, many antiseptics possess irritant properties (Zemjanis 1980) and can compromise UDMs, which leads to irritation and denudation of the endometrium that can lead to transient strain and possibly extend the duration of genital disease. Earlier, an intrauterine infusion of 2–10% Lugol's iodine was advocated for to treat uterine infections (Roberts 1971), but it has been observed that even 0.25% Lugol's iodine may cause significant necrosis and desquamation in the endometrial lining (Kamugisa et al. 1997). Povidone iodine (PVP-I) possesses antibacterial, antifungal, antiprotozoal, and antiviral properties (Schreier et al. 1997) and an intrauterine administration of 0.5–2% PVP-I has been used with varying success to treat repeat breeding syndrome in bovines (Koujan et al. 1996; Butani et al. 2013; Mido et al. 2016). By inducing transient uterine inflammation, it promotes endometrial epithelial cell regeneration and enhances fertility (Yoshida et al. 2020). Unlike antibiotics, it does not require a withdrawal period and does not pass into the milk (Carleton et al. 2008), nor does it pose a problem for acquired resistance or cross-resistance, even after prolonged use (Bigliardi et al. 2017). Chlorhexidine has the potential to enhance uterine tone, blood flow, and defense mechanisms, thereby causing irritation, inflammation, and a reduction of bacterial levels within the uterus that facilitates the evacuation of abnormal uterine fluid; it is the sole nonantibiotic, antimicrobial drug approved for intrauterine treatment in the United States.

13.6.1.2 Antibiotics

Antibiotics as Intrauterine Infusions Antibiotic infusions are commonly used treatments for all types of uterine infections. The objective of local treatment through intrauterine antibiotic infusion is to achieve uniform distribution of an active drug across all uterine layers, minimize systemic absorption, minimize tissue irritation, and maximize antibacterial effectiveness within the uterine environment. Several antimicrobial agents, such as sulphonamides, tetracyclines, penicillins, nitrofurazone, aminoglycosides, and chloramphenicol, can be easily absorbed systemically from the uterus (Gilbert and Schwark 1992). The efficacy of drugs infused into the postpartum uterus is influenced by three main factors: (i) the condition of the uterus after childbirth, (ii) the ability of uterine tissue to absorb the drugs, and (iii) the distribution of the drugs within the body (Masera et al. 1980).

Penicillin is not recommended for local intrauterine therapy in the early postpartum uterus due to the presence of a mixed bacterial population that produces the penicillinase enzyme. This enzyme provides protection to penicillin-sensitive pathogens. An experimental determination of the ratio of penicillin concentration between serum and genital tissue has not been completed. However, it is probable that this level is sufficiently high to effectively combat *Clostridium*, *T. pyogenes*, and gram-negative anaerobes. In the later stages of the postpartum period, when the bacterial population is primarily composed of *T. pyogenes* and gram-negative anaerobes, the administration of penicillin through intrauterine infusion is likely a suitable option.

Sulphonamides exhibit superior absorption in the postpartum uterus compared to other antibiotics. Aminoglycosides are not suitable for treating intrauterine anaerobic infections due to their poor absorption under aerobic conditions (Sheldon et al. 2004).

Cephapirin benzathine is the only antibiotic approved for intrauterine infusion in dairy cows to treat endometritis. However, its approval for this purpose varies across countries. The drug, known as Metricure® and manufactured by Merck Animal Health, is provided in a syringe with a 19-g dose. Each syringe contains 640 mg of cephalexin. The drug has a withdrawal period of 2 days for meat and no withdrawal period for milk. Two randomized clinical trials were conducted on postpartum cows that were 28–42 days into lactation and diagnosed with endometritis. These cows showed an improvement in first-service conception rates of 8–15% compared to cows that were not treated (Denis-Robichaud et al. 2015). In addition, the administration of cephapirin benzathine via intrauterine infusion has been found to enhance reproductive outcomes in cows affected by SE (Kasimanickam et al. 2005), clinical endometritis (LeBlanc et al. 2002) and in cows previously diagnosed with retained fetal membranes, stillbirths, or a vulval discharge after 13 days in milk. The treatment of metritis showed some beneficial effects with intrauterine infusions of procaine penicillin, oxytetracycline (OTC) (Chenault et al. 2004), and chlortetracycline (Goshen and Shpigel 2006). Unfortunately, there is a lack of reported information regarding the length of time that antibiotic residues can be detected in milk and meat after an intrauterine infusion, with the exception of procaine penicillin (up to 3 days in milk) (Manners and Stewart 1982) and OTC (up to 8 days in milk) (Tan et al. 2007). Chloramphenicol is prohibited in food-producing animals in numerous countries due to its potential to cause toxicosis in humans. In addition to its effective anaerobic postpartum activity, OTC also affects a wide variety of microorganisms, which makes it the medicine of choice for treating clinical endometritis through intrauterine infusion (Kaczmarowski et al. 2004). Conversely, Cohen et al. (1995) found that OTC was ineffective at penetrating the uterine wall, failed to eradicate *T. pyogenes* uterine infections, and irritated the endometrial mucosa. For the treatment of clinical endometritis, Makki et al. (2016) found that the reproductive status was better in the OTC group compared to the hyperimmune serum group. Recently, nanoparticle OTC has been reported to be more effective at treating clinical endometritis compared to conventional OTC (Ghallab et al. 2023).

Antibiotics via Systemic Routes Systemic treatment may be more advantageous than intrauterine treatment for all types of postpartum metritis. Systemic treatment improves drug distribution throughout the female genital tract and ovaries (Bretzlaff et al. 1983). It works to prevent contamination of the uterus and injury to the uterine endometrium caused by iatrogenic factors (Paisley et al. 1986). The systemic treatment of postpartum metritis also preserves leukocyte function (Ziv et al. 1983). This may be the best reason to choose systemic antimicrobials over local.

Penicillin is preferred among antibiotics due to its excellent distribution throughout all layers of the uterus, cost effectiveness, and established withholding times for milk and meat when used as directed (Masera et al. 1980). Penicillin given intramuscularly at 22 000 IU/kg for 5 days has been shown to cure metritis in cows (Smith et al. 1998). In addition, penicillin and ceftiofur have been observed to accumulate in uterine tissues after being administered systemically at concentrations that exceed the minimum inhibitory concentration (MIC) necessary to combat uterine disease–causing bacteria (Braun et al. 2009).

OTC exhibits a wide range of antibacterial effects by binding to 30S ribosomes and hampering the process of protein synthesis. Tetracyclines enter bacterial cells through a two-step process. The initial step involves passive diffusion across the outer cell membrane, while the subsequent step involves active transport across the inner cell membrane, which may require the presence of a specific carrier protein. The serum–tissue ratio of OTC in the genital tissue of healthy and diseased cows varies between 1 : 1 and 1.5 : 1. In order to maintain a minimum serum concentration of 5 ug/ml, cattle need to be administered 11 mg of OTC per kg of body weight twice daily. This would lead to a concentration of approximately 5–8 μg/ml of OTC in the uterine tissue (Olson et al. 1984). OTC is also used for the treatment of postpartum metritis. Metritis in cows with mild symptoms is commonly treated with this approach (Gilbert and Schwark 1992). The uterine tissues reach OTC concentrations that are approximately one-third of the desired MIC for common uterine pathogens (Bretzlaff et al. 1983).

Ceftiofur sodium is approved for use in dairy cattle at dose rates of 1 mg/kg in Canada, 2.2 mg/kg in Europe, and 2.2 mg/kg in the United States. It can be administered once daily for 3–5 days either intramuscularly or subcutaneously. Ceftiofur reaches peak concentrations in uterine tissues after the third injection, when administered intramuscularly at a dosage rate of 1 mg/kg once daily (Drillich et al. 2006). Hence, it is advisable to implement a treatment regimen that lasts a minimum of 5 days in order to effectively treat metritis. The absence of a milk or meat withdrawal period is a distinct advantage of the 1 mg/kg dose of ceftiofur sodium. A sterile suspension of ceftiofur hydrochloride salt at 1.1 or 2.2 mg/kg administered daily for 5 days can also be used to treat metritis cases. Studies suggest that the higher dose may result in higher cure rates (Chenault et al. 2004). In cases where the repeated handling and treatment of animals is not feasible, a single injection of ceftiofur crystalline-free acid at a dose of 6.6 mg/kg can be administered in the base of the ear. Typically, a single dose of ceftiofur crystalline-free acid is not sufficient for treating metritis. To enhance the cure rate, a second dose may be given 72 hours after the initial dose, administered in the opposite ear base (McLaughlin et al. 2012). Caution should be used when administering ceftiofur crystalline-free acid, as intra-arterial injection can result in cow fatality. Additionally, ceftiofur and other cephalosporins exhibit the lowest MICs against uterine-specific strains of *E. coli*, *T. pyogenes*, *F. necrophorum*, and *Prevotella melaninogenica*. In contrast, tetracycline demonstrates the highest MIC (Sheldon et al. 2004). Moreover, numerous studies have demonstrated the efficacy of administering ceftiofur at a dosage of 1 mg/kg/day intramuscularly or subcutaneously for a duration of 3–5 days to treat cows diagnosed with toxic puerperal metritis (Zhou et al. 2001).

Sulphonamides are absorbed better by the postpartum uterus than other antibiotics. Under aerobic conditions, aminoglycosides are absorbed well, and therefore, they are poorly suited for the intrauterine treatment of anaerobic infections (Sheldon et al. 2004). Ampicillin is effective against *E. coli* and gram-positive bacteria (de Boer et al. 2015). A study has demonstrated that the administration of ampicillin trihydrate (11 mg/kg intramuscularly for 5 days) resulted in improved cure rates for metritis (Lima et al. 2014).

13.6.1.3 Hormones

Several hormones like estrogen, ergonovine, prostaglandin, and oxytocin have been used by to treat uterine diseases. These drugs either stimulate uterine contractility or augment UDMs (Ahmadi et al. 2019; Verma et al. 2023).

13.6.1.4 Immunomodulators

Parenteral and intrauterine treatments with various antibiotic, antibacterial, and hormonal drugs have inconsistent results. The high cost of treatment, compulsory milk disposal, development of resistance to antibiotics, and inhibition of UDMs have all led to finding alternative therapies to treat uterine infections. In recent years, several immunomodulators like

E. coli LPS (Wakayo et al. 2015), oyster glycogen (Palanisamy et al. 2015), leukotriene B_4 (Krishnan et al. 2015), colostrum (Sahoo and Mohanty 2016), granulocyte–macrophage-colony-stimulating factor (Tizard 1998), bacterial-free filtrate (Deori et al. 2004), levamisole hydrochloride (Singh et al. 2023; Verma et al. 2023), hyperimmune serum (Sarkar et al. 2015), human recombinant interleukin (IL)-8 (Zerbe et al. 2003), polymorphonuclear extracts (Hughes and Couto 1988), mycobacterial cell wall extracts (Rogan et al. 2010), and many herbal drugs like garlic, ashwagandha (Rahi et al. 2013), etc., have been used with varying success to treat uterine infections.

13.6.2 Nonconventional Therapeutic Agents

13.6.2.1 Chitosan

Chitosan, derived from chitin found in specific fungi and yeast, is recognized by the US Food and Drug Administration (FDA). It exhibits a broad range of antimicrobial properties in both neutral and acidic conditions. The pH of the cow's genital tract typically ranges from 6.84 to 7.51. The product claims to enhance the cow's resistance by lowering the presence of bacteria in the uterus. The antimicrobial activity of chitosan microparticles is attributed to their ability to disrupt bacterial cell membranes through interactions with the outer membrane protein A (OmpA), which results in cell death. Cows diagnosed with metritis were treated with 24 g of chitosan particles (diluted in 40 ml of sterile distilled water) in the uterus for 3 days (Jeon et al. 2014).

13.6.2.2 Essential Oils

Essential oils possess antioxidative, anti-inflammatory, and antimicrobial properties, which render them suitable for addressing infectious conditions (Burt 2004). A study was conducted to compare the effects of a compound of certified organic essential oils (Optimum UterFlush®, Van Beek Natural Science, Orange City, Iowa, USA) with intrauterine iodine infusion and a control on toxic puerperal metritis in dairy cows. The compound was infused every other day for a total of three times between 1 and 12 days in milk (DIM). The study included 107 cows in the essential oils group, 113 cows in the iodine group, and 400 healthy cows in the control group, all from organic farms (Pinedo et al. 2015). The conception rates after the first service were 23%, 37%, and 38% in cows treated with iodine, essential oils, and the control group, respectively ($p = 0.05$).

13.6.2.3 Sugar Solutions

The rationale for the use of sugars as an intrauterine remedy for postpartum uterine infections depends on its three properties: (i) sugars interfere with bacterial attachment to tissues; (ii) sugars impair microbial growth; and (iii) sugars, being hypertonic, attract fluid into the uterus and aid in the removal of debris and bacteria during cervical opening. Lectins, which are found on the outer layer of the infectious organism, can attach themselves to specific carbohydrates present on the surface of host tissues (Lefebvre et al. 2021). In order to reduce the incidence or manage metritis and endometritis in cattle and buffaloes, different sugar solutions, viz. mannose and hypertonic dextrose solutions, have been tried as intrauterine infusions to treat uterine infections in bovines with varying success (Bicalho et al. 2012; Brick et al. 2012; Machado et al. 2012; Ahmadi et al. 2019; Verma et al. 2023).

Honey possesses active constituents like glucose, fructose, flavonoids, polyphenols, and organic acids, to which its therapeutic properties are ascribed. Honey products have been found to modulate the immune response by activating lymphocytic function, macrophages, and stimulating cytokine release by monocytes (Sforcin 2007). Moreover, flavonoids in honey can induce apoptosis and inhibit the release of IL-1ß, IL-6, tumor necrosis factor (TNF)-α, inducible nitric oxide synthase (iNOSm), and cyclooxygenase (COX)-2 (Erejuwa et al. 2014). Furthermore, Abdul-Hafeez et al. (2019) reported a 75% conception rate using a 100 ml intrauterine infusion of Egyptian cotton honey (70%) for 3 days in repeat breeder dairy cows with PVD, compared to standard antibiotic therapy.

13.6.2.4 Ozone

Ozone is used in medical treatments and can be found in various products, such as ozonated vegetable oil. These products contain emollient, cicatrizing, antibacterial, and hygienic properties and are available in different forms such as creams, gasses, syringes, paillettes, foam, and boluses (Travagli et al. 2009). Ozone prevents bacterial growth by causing damage to the capsule and cell membrane through peroxidase activity. It can also potentially inhibit bacterial DNA replication. Additionally, ozone is frequently used as a complementary therapy in the treatment of infectious diseases. It suppresses pro-inflammatory cytokines by enhancing the production of immunosuppressive cytokines such as IL-10 and TNF-ß1 in neutrophils, monocytes, and lymphocytes. Ozone has demonstrated positive effects in the prevention and treatment of endometritis and metritis (Escandon et al. 2020).

13.6.2.5 Intravaginal Probiotics: A New Approach to Mitigate Uterine Dysbiosis

According to the Food and Agriculture Organization of the United Nations (FAO), probiotics are live microorganisms that insure health benefits to the subject, when administered in an optimum amount (Fuller 1989). Unlike the vaginal tract of humans, the microbiota of the vaginal tract of dairy cows is not predominated by *Lactobacillus* strains (Miller et al. 2016). Additionally, the vaginal pH of dairy cows and humans differs, with humans having an acidic vaginal pH (3.5–4.5), while cows have a slightly acidic to slightly alkaline pH (pH 6.8–7.35) (Bicalho et al. 2019). As only humans have acidic vaginal pH levels, lactobacilli are known to create lactic acid by hydrolyzing the glycogen found in human vaginal mucosa (Miller et al. 2016). The prevention of bacterial infections is significantly aided by the acidic vaginal pH (Bicalho et al. 2019). In order to make lactic acid, lactobacilli utilize glycogen produced by vaginal epithelial cells. Surprisingly, glycogen has also been found in the uterus of dairy cows (Wrenn et al. 1968). Numerous studies in dairy cows have investigated the possibility of employing intravaginal lactobacilli to prevent vaginal and uterine infections, given that lowering the vaginal pH is a physical barrier to pathogenic bacterial infection globally. The intravaginal administration of a mixture of three strains of lactobacilli (*Lactobacillus sakei*, *Pediococcus acidilactici* FUA 3140, and *Ped. acidilactici* FUA 3138 at 1010–1012 colony-forming units [CFU] of lactobacilli [LAB]/week/cow) in transition dairy cows around calving improved milk yield, lowered plasma haptoglobin (an indicator of uterine infections), and lowered the occurrence of PVDs (Ametaj et al. 2014), but the pregnancy rate did not improve above those of untreated cows. Similarly, a few other researchers have observed promising results using intravaginal probiotics, as evidenced by lower systemic serum amyloid α, elevated vaginal mucus IgA (Deng et al. 2014), lower blood non-esterified fatty acid (NEFA) (Ametaj 2005), and a reduced incidence of uterine infections (Genis et al. 2017) compared to control cows.

Various mechanisms of action for probiotics have been ascribed, like improved function of epithelial barriers (Bermudez-Brito et al. 2012; Hummel et al. 2012), adhesion to the epithelial layer (Juntunen et al. 2001), competition for essential nutrients (Mezzasalma et al. 2017), production of organic acids (Russell and Diez-Gonzalez 1998), production of antimicrobials (Makras et al. 2006), modulation of the immune system (Deng et al. 2014), and modifying vaginal pH (Otero et al. 2006).

13.6.2.6 Prevention and Control of Uterine Infections

During the process of evolution, plants and animals have adopted three tactics to evade infections, i.e. avoidance, tolerance, and resistance (Rausher 2001; Read et al. 2008; Schneider and Ayres 2008). Similarly, Sheldon et al. (2020) opined that the prevention of uterine infections depends upon three premises:

- **Avoidance:** Avoidance mechanisms preserve health by limiting exposure to pathogens and preventing pathogens reaching the uterus (prevent ascending infection) through physical barriers, e.g. the vulva, vagina, and cervical mucus. However, the barrier is breached in certain circumstances, i.e. parturition, dystocia, and poor conformation of vulva and vagina, which allows exposure of the uterus to pathogens. In most animal species, maintaining hygiene is an innate behavior that has developed over thousands of years (Curtis 2007), e.g. animals avoid feces by cleaning themselves and preferring clean and dry bedding. Furthermore, cows groom themselves to keep clean and reduce stress (Newby et al. 2013; Val-Laillet et al. 2009). Moreover, avoidance mechanisms are the least energy expensive compared to tolerance and resistance mechanisms as the animal pays no direct metabolic cost in countering the pathogens.
- **Tolerance:** Tolerance refers to limiting the tissue damage caused by pathogens without affecting pathogenic burden (Read et al. 2008; Schneider and Ayres 2008; Sheldon et al. 2019). Endometrial epithelium and the mucus layer constitute a functional barrier. Moreover, mucus from the reproductive tract contains mucosal glycoproteins, acute phase proteins (haptoglobin, serum amyloid α), and antimicrobial peptides that neutralize bacteria or bacteria-derived toxins (Hein et al. 2002; Adnane et al. 2018). Damage control and tissue repair assist in the tolerance of microbes (Soares et al. 2017; McCarville and Ayres 2018). Furthermore, high yield cows are associated with a declined tolerance to postpartum uterine infections (Sheldon et al. 2019).
- **Resistance:** Resistance limits the pathogens that reach the uterus by killing them. While the study of pathogen avoidance and tolerance is still in its infancy, pathogen resistance mechanisms, notably the functions of innate and adaptive immunity, are well understood. Without requiring prior contact with infections, the innate immune system produces an instantaneous, nonspecific response to pathogens (Medzhitov et al. 2012; Takeuchi and Akira 2010). Because uterine

infections are polymicrobial and fluctuate over the postpartum period, this innate immune response is suitable for treating them. Bacterial DNA, lipopeptides, flagellin, and LPS are only a few examples of PAMPs that are recognized by innate immune cells using PRRs like TLRs. Endometrial stromal and epithelial cells play a part in innate immunity in the uterus by producing inflammatory reactions to bacteria, lipopeptides, and LPS (Turner et al. 2014; Cronin et al. 2012). Antimicrobial peptides, cytokines (including IL-1b and IL-6), chemokines (like IL-8), and PGE2 are frequently released as a result of the immunological response (Takeuchi and Akira 2010; Moresco et al. 2011). By generating vasodilation, luring and activating immune cells, and promoting the creation of acute phase proteins and reactive oxygen species, these inflammatory mediators aid in the tissue's ability to fight off germs (Sheldon et al. 2019; Takeuchi and Akira 2010; Moresco et al. 2011; Healy et al. 2014). The hypothalamic–pituitary–ovary axis is likewise suppressed by inflammatory mediators, which can cause fatigue and a lack of appetite (Wang et al. 2019). An additional nonspecific defense is provided by the complement system, which encourages neutrophils and macrophages to phagocytose pathogens (Wathes et al. 2009).

Acquired immunity takes longer to develop than innate immunity since it is dependent on the prior exposure to particular antigens. With the lymphocytic foci of T cells and B cells, the postpartum endometrium exhibits adaptive immunity (Wagner and Hansel 1969; Bonnett et al. 1991). Additionally, cows with higher levels of circulating antibodies are less likely to develop postpartum uterine illness, and metritis can be prevented by vaccinations made from *E. coli*, *F. necrophorum*, and/or *T. pyogenes* components (Machado et al. 2014). Sadly, domestication and selective breeding have diminished the richness of the major histocompatibility complex antigens, and animals with less variation in these antigens are more likely to have retained fetal membranes (Joosten et al. 1991). The short-lived nature of adaptive immunity in the uterus is another issue. After calving, spontaneous metritis does not offer protection against uterine illness.

Furthermore, a severe negative energy balance (NEB) is a risk factor for persistent endometritis compared to cows with a mild NEB. However, cows with a mild NEB are able to repair their endometrium within 2 weeks postpartum (Wathes et al. 2009). Moreover, a reduced feed intake prepartum (Huzzey et al. 2007) and compromised neutrophil function, secondary to peripartum metabolic changes (Leblanc 2012; Hammon et al. 2006), increase the risk of uterine inflammation. Indeed, glucose or glutamine deficiencies reduce the inflammatory response in the uterine endometrium (Turner et al. 2016; Noleto et al. 2017).

13.7 Conclusion

Uterine bacterial infections and uterine diseases are common after parturition in cattle and cause considerable infertility and economic losses to the dairy industry. Uterine bacterial infections stimulate a robust immune response but also modulate normal reproductive physiology. Increasing knowledge about the interaction between the environment, uterine infections, immunity, and reproduction can lead to improved control and treatment strategies for cattle infertility, thus improving the productivity of cattle and buffaloes.

References

Abdul-Hafeez, M.M., Abdul-Kadder, H.A., Sayed, A.M., and Shehata, S.H. (2019). Intrauterine honey infusion in Holstein Frisian cows with purulent endometritis. *International Journal of Complementary and Alternative Medicine* 12 (1): 53–57.

Adnane, M. and Chapwanya, A. (2022). A review of the diversity of the genital tract microbiome and implications for fertility of cattle. *Animals: An Open Access Journal from MDPI* 12 (4): 460. https://doi.org/10.3390/ani12040460.

Adnane, M., Meade, K.G., and O'Farrelly, C. (2018). Cervico-vaginal mucus (CVM) – an accessible source of immunologically informative biomolecules. *Veterinary Research Communications* 42 (4): 255–263. https://doi.org/10.1007/s11259-018-9734-0.

Ahmadi, M.R., Makki, M., Mirzaei, A., and Gheisari, H.R. (2019). Effects of hypertonic dextrose and paraffin solution as non-antibiotic treatments of clinical endometritis on reproductive performance of high producing dairy cows. *Reproduction in Domestic Animals* 54 (5): 762–771.

Ametaj, B.N. (2005). A new understanding of the causes of fatty liver in dairy cows. *Advanced Dairy Science and Technology* 17: 97–112.

Ametaj, B.N., Iqbal, S., Selami, F. et al. (2014). Intravaginal administration of lactic acid bacteria modulated the incidence of purulent vaginal discharges, plasma haptoglobin concentrations, and milk production in dairy cows. *Research in Veterinary Science* 96 (2): 365–370. https://doi.org/10.1016/j.rvsc.2014.02.007.

Appiah, M.O., Wang, J., and Lu, W. (2020). Microflora in the reproductive tract of cattle: a review (running title: the microflora and bovine reproductive tract), *Agriculture*, 10, (232). *Agriculture 10* (10): 474. http://dx.doi.org/10.3390/agriculture10100474.

Ault-Seay, T.B., Moorey, S.E., Mathew, D.J. et al. (2023). Importance of the female reproductive tract microbiome and its relationship with the uterine environment for health and productivity in cattle: a review. *Frontiers in Animal Science* 4: 1111636. https://doi.org/10.3389/fanim.2023.1111636.

Azawi, O.I. (2006). Clinical, bacteriological and pathological studies of uterine infection in Iraqi buffaloes. Doctoral dissertation. University of Baghdad.

Baker, J.M., Chase, D.M., and Herbst-Kralovetz, M.M. (2018). Uterine microbiota: residents, tourists, or invaders? *Frontiers in Immunology* 9: 208. https://doi.org/10.3389/fimmu.2018.00208.

Bermudez-Brito, M., Plaza-Díaz, J., Muñoz-Quezada, S. et al. (2012). Probiotic mechanisms of action. *Annals of Nutrition & Metabolism* 61 (2): 160–174. https://doi.org/10.1159/000342079.

Bicalho, M.L.S., Machado, V.S., Oikonomou, G. et al. (2012). Association between virulence factors of Escherichia coli, Fusobacterium necrophorum, and Arcanobacterium pyogenes and uterine diseases of dairy cows. *Veterinary Microbiology* 157 (1–2): 125–131.

Bicalho, M.L.S., Zinicola, M., Machado, V.S. et al. (2019). Effects of recombinant bovine interleukin-8 (rbIL-8) treatment on health, metabolism, and lactation performance in Holstein cattle I: production and functional characterization of rbIL-8 in vitro and in vivo. *Journal of Dairy Science* 102 (11): 10304–10315. https://doi.org/10.3168/jds.2019-16334.

Bigliardi, P.L., Alsagoff, S.A.L., El-Kafrawi, H.Y. et al. (2017). Povidone iodine in wound healing: a review of current concepts and practices. *International Journal of Surgery* 44: 260–268.

Bonnett, B.N., Martin, S.W., Gannon, V.P. et al. (1991). Endometrial biopsy in Holstein-Friesian dairy cows. III. Bacteriological analysis and correlations with histological findings. *Canadian Journal of Veterinary Research = Revue canadienne de recherche veterinaire* 55 (2): 168–173.

Braun, M., Zerbe, H., and Kietzmann, M. (2009). Tissue concentration of intrauterine and intravenously administered amoxicillin in the isolated hemoperfused bovine uterus model and in healthy cows. *Berliner und Münchener Tierärztliche Wochenschrift* 122 (1–2): 51–57.

Bretzlaff, K.N., Ott, R.S., Koritz, G.D. et al. (1983). Distribution of oxytetracycline in genital tract tissues of postpartum cows given the drug by intravenous and intrauterine routes. *American Journal of Veterinary Research* 44 (5): 764–769.

Brick, T.A., Schuenemann, G.M., Bas, S. et al. (2012). Effect of intrauterine dextrose or antibiotic therapy on reproductive performance of lactating dairy cows diagnosed with clinical endometritis. *Journal of Dairy Science* 95 (4): 1894–1905.

Burt, S. (2004). Essential oils: their antibacterial properties and potential applications in foods – a review. *International Journal of Food Microbiology* 94 (3): 223–253.

Butani, M.G., Kumar, R., Dhami, A.J. et al. (2008). Incidence of major infertility problems in crossbred cows and buffaloes under field conditions. *Indian Journal of Field Veterinarians* 4 (2): 1–4.

Butani, M.G., Dhami, A.J., Kumar, R. et al. (2013). Therapeutic management of repeat breeding buffaloes under field conditions using hormonal and non-hormonal remedial. *Buffalo Journal* 29 (2): 141–151.

Carleton, C.L., Threlfall, W.R., and Schwarze, R.A. (2008). Iodine in milk and serum following intrauterine infusion of Lugol's solution. *International Journal of Applied Research in Veterinary Medicine* 6: 121–129.

Chenault, J.R., McAllister, J.F., Chester, S.T. et al. (2004). Efficacy of ceftiofur hydrochloride sterile suspension administered parenterally for the treatment of acute postpartum metritis in dairy cows. *Journal of the American Veterinary Medical Association* 224 (10): 1634–1639.

Cohen, R.O., Bernstein, M., and Ziv, G. (1995). Isolation and antimicrobial susceptibility of Actinomyces pyogenes recovered from the uterus of dairy cows with retained fetal membranes and post parturient endometritis. *Theriogenology* 43 (8): 1389–1397.

Correa, M.T., Erb, H., and Scarlett, J. (1993). Path analysis for seven postpartum disorders of Holstein cows. *Journal of Dairy Science* 76 (5): 1305–1312. https://doi.org/10.3168/jds.S0022-0302(93)77461-5.

Cronin, J.G., Turner, M.L., Goetze, L. et al. (2012). Toll-like receptor 4 and MYD88-dependent signaling mechanisms of the innate immune system are essential for the response to lipopolysaccharide by epithelial and stromal cells of the bovine endometrium. *Biology of Reproduction* 86 (2): 51. https://doi.org/10.1095/biolreprod.111.092718.

Curtis, V.A. (2007). A natural history of hygiene. *The Canadian Journal of Infectious Diseases and Medical Microbiology* 18 (1): 11–14. https://doi.org/10.1155/2007/749190.

De Boer, M.W., LeBlanc, S.J., Dubuc, J. et al. (2014). Invited review: systematic review of diagnostic tests for reproductive-tract infection and inflammation in dairy cows. *Journal of Dairy Science* 97 (7): 3983–3999. https://doi.org/10.3168/jds.2013-7450.

De Boer, M., Heuer, C., Hussein, H., and McDougall, S. (2015). Minimum inhibitory concentrations of selected antimicrobials against Escherichia coli and *Trueperella pyogenes* of bovine uterine origin. *Journal of Dairy Science* 98 (7): 4427–4438.

Deng, Q., Odhiambo, J.F., Farooq, U. et al. (2014). Intravaginal lactic acid bacteria modulated local and systemic immune responses and lowered the incidence of uterine infections in periparturient dairy cows. Doctoral dissertation. University of Alberta.

Denis-Robichaud, J. and Dubuc, J. (2015). Randomized clinical trial of intrauterine cephapirin infusion in dairy cows for the treatment of purulent vaginal discharge and cytological endometritis. *Journal of Dairy Science* 98 (10): 6856–6864.

Deori, S., Kumar, H., Yadav, M.C. et al. (2004). Intrauterine administration of bacterial modulins: an alternative therapy for endometritis. *Journal of Applied Animal Research* 26 (2): 117–121.

Drillich, M., Arlt, S., Kersting, S. et al. (2006). Ceftiofur derivatives in serum, uterine tissues, cotyledons, and lochia after fetal membrane retention. *Journal of Dairy Science* 89 (9): 3431–3438.

Dubuc, J., Duffield, T.F., Leslie, K.E. et al. (2010). Risk factors for postpartum uterine diseases in dairy cows. *Journal of Dairy Science* 93 (12): 5764–5771. https://doi.org/10.3168/jds.2010-3429.

Erejuwa, O.O., Sulaiman, S.A., and Wahab, M.S.A. (2014). Effects of honey and its mechanisms of action on the development and progression of cancer. *Molecules* 19 (2): 2497–2522.

Escandón, B.M., Espinoza, J.S., Perea, F.P. et al. (2020). Intrauterine therapy with ozone reduces subclinical endometritis and improves reproductive performance in postpartum dairy cows managed in pasture-based systems. *Tropical Animal Health and Production* 52: 2523–2528.

Foldi, J., Kulcsar, M., Pecsi, A. et al. (2006). Bacterial complications of postpartum uterine involution in cattle. *Animal Reproduction Science* 96 (3–4): 265–281. https://doi.org/10.1016/j.anireprosci.2006.08.006.

Fuller, R. (1989). Probiotics in man and animals. *The Journal of Applied Bacteriology* 66 (5): 365–378.

Galvao, K.N., Flaminio, M.J., Brittin, S.B. et al. (2010). Association between uterine disease and indicators of neutrophil and systemic energy status in lactating Holstein cows. *Journal of Dairy Science* 93 (7): 2926–2937. https://doi.org/10.3168/jds.2009-2551.

Genis, S., Sanchez-Chardi, A., Bach, A. et al. (2017). A combination of lactic acid bacteria regulates Escherichia coli infection and inflammation of the bovine endometrium. *Journal of Dairy Science* 100 (1): 479–492. https://doi.org/10.3168/jds.2016-11671.

Ghallab, R.S., El-Karim, D.R.S.G., Fayed, A.H., and Rashad, A.M.A. (2023). Efficiency of conventional and nanoparticle oxytetracycline in treatment of clinical endometritis in postpartum dairy cows. *Tropical Animal Health and Production* 55 (2): 118. https://doi.org/10.1007/s11250-023-03536-0.

Gilbert, R.O. and Schwark, W.S. (1992). Pharmacologic considerations in the management of peripartum conditions in the cow. *Veterinary Clinics of North America: Food Animal Practice* 8 (1): 29–56.

Gilbert, R.O., Shin, S.T., Guard, C.L. et al. (2005). Prevalence of endometritis and its effects on reproductive performance of dairy cows. *Theriogenology* 64 (9): 1879–1888. https://doi.org/10.1016/j.theriogenology.2005.04.022.

Goshen, T. and Shpigel, N.Y. (2006). Evaluation of intrauterine antibiotic treatment of clinical metritis and retained fetal membranes in dairy cows. *Theriogenology* 66 (9): 2210–2218.

Hammon, D.S., Evjen, I.M., Dhiman, T.R. et al. (2006). Neutrophil function and energy status in Holstein cows with uterine health disorders. *Veterinary Immunology and Immunopathology* 113 (1–2): 21–29. https://doi.org/10.1016/j.vetimm.2006.03.022.

Healy, L.L., Cronin, J.G., and Sheldon, I.M. (2014). Endometrial cells sense and react to tissue damage during infection of the bovine endometrium via interleukin 1. *Scientific Reports* 4: 7060. https://doi.org/10.1038/srep07060.

Hein, M., Valore, E.V., Helmig, R.B. et al. (2002). Antimicrobial factors in the cervical mucus plug. *American Journal of Obstetrics and Gynecology* 187 (1): 137–144. https://doi.org/10.1067/mob.2002.123034.

Hughes, J.P. and Couto, M.A. (1988). Endometritis in the mare. *11th International Congress on Animal Reproduction and Artificial Insemination*, Dublin, Ireland (26–30 June 1988). Dublin, Ireland: University College.

Human Microbiome Project Consortium (2012). Structure, function and diversity of the healthy human microbiome. *Nature* 486 (7402): 207–214. https://doi.org/10.1038/nature11234.

Hummel, S., Veltman, K., Cichon, C. et al. (2012). Differential targeting of the E-Cadherin/β-Catenin complex by gram-positive probiotic lactobacilli improves epithelial barrier function. *Applied and Environmental Microbiology* 78 (4): 1140–1147. https://doi.org/10.1128/AEM.06983-11.

Huzzey, J.M., Veira, D.M., Weary, D.M., and von Keyserlingk, M.A. (2007). Prepartum behavior and dry matter intake identify dairy cows at risk for metritis. *Journal of Dairy Science* 90 (7): 3220–3233. https://doi.org/10.3168/jds.2006-807.

Jeon, S.J., Oh, M., Yeo, W.S. et al. (2014). Underlying mechanism of antimicrobial activity of chitosan microparticles and implications for the treatment of infectious diseases. *PLoS One* 9 (3): e92723.

Joosten, I., Sanders, M.F., and Hensen, E.J. (1991). Involvement of major histocompatibility complex class I compatibility between dam and calf in the aetiology of bovine retained placenta. *Animal Genetics* 22 (6): 455–463. https://doi.org/10.1111/j.1365-2052.1991.tb00717.x.

Juntunen, M., Kirjavainen, P.V., Ouwehand, A.C. et al. (2001). Adherence of probiotic bacteria to human intestinal mucus in healthy infants and during rotavirus infection. *Clinical and Diagnostic Laboratory Immunology* 8 (2): 293–296. https://doi.org/10.1128/CDLI.8.2.293-296.2001.

Kaczmarowski, M., Malinowski, E., and Markiewicz, H. (2004). Influence of various treatment methods on bacteriological findings in cows with puerperal endometritis. *Polish Journal of Veterinary Sciences* 7 (3): 171–174.

Kamugisa, G.M., Patel, D.M., Prajapati, K.S., and Dugwekar, Y.G. (1997). Effect oflugol's iodine and povidone iodine on the histology of the buffalo endometrium. *Buffalo Journal* 3: 397–403.

Kaneene, J.B. and Miller, R. (1995). Risk factors for metritis in Michigan dairy cattle using herd- and cow-based modelling approaches. *Preventive Veterinary Medicine* 23: 183–200.

Kasimanickam, R., Duffield, T.F., Foster, R.A. et al. (2004). Endometrial cytology and ultrasonography for the detection of subclinical endometritis in postpartum dairy cows. *Theriogenology* 62 (1–2): 9–23. https://doi.org/10.1016/j.theriogenology.2003.03.001.

Kasimanickam, R., Duffield, T.F., Foster, R.A. et al. (2005). A comparison of the cytobrush and uterine lavage techniques to evaluate endometrial cytology in clinically normal postpartum dairy cows. *The Canadian Veterinary Journal* 46 (3): 255.

Kim, I.H. and Kang, H.G. (2003). Risk factors for postpartum endometritis and the effect of endometritis on reproductive performance in dairy cows in Korea. *The Journal of Reproduction and Development* 49 (6): 485–491. https://doi.org/10.1262/jrd.49.485.

Koujan, A., Eissa, H.M., Hussein, M.A. et al. (1996). Therapeutic efficacy of povidone-iodine (Betadine) and dichloroxylenol (Septocid) in Holstein cows affected with endometritis and/or cervicitis. *Acta Veterinaria Hungarica* 44 (1): 111–119.

Krishnan, B.B., Kumar, H., Mehrotra, S. et al. (2015). Effect of Leukotriene B_4 and oyster glycogen in resolving subclinical endometritis in repeat breeding crossbred cows. *Indian Journal of Animal Research* 49 (2): 218–222.

Kumar, R., Butani, M.G., Dhami, A.J. et al. (2008). Isolation and antibiogram of genital microflora from repeat breeding cows and buffaloes. *Indian Journal of Field Veterinarians* 4 (2): 5–9.

Kumar, R., Butani, M.G., Dhami, A.J. et al. (2009). Effect of different therapies on fertility and serum progesterone, metabolites and minerals profile in repeat breeding crossbred cows. *Indian Journal of Field Veterinarians* 5 (2): 1–8.

LeBlanc, S.J. (2012). Interactions of metabolism, inflammation, and reproductive tract health in the postpartum period in dairy cattle. *Reproduction in Domestic Animals = Zuchthygiene* 47 (Suppl 5): 18–30. https://doi.org/10.1111/j.1439-0531.2012.02109.x.

LeBlanc, S., Leslie, K., Duffield, T. et al. (2001). The incidence and impact of clinical endometritis in dairy cows. *J. Anim. Sci. Suppl.* 79: 187.

LeBlanc, S.J., Duffield, T.F., Leslie, K.E. et al. (2002). Defining and diagnosing postpartum clinical endometritis and its impact on reproductive performance in dairy cows. *Journal of Dairy Science* 85 (9): 2223–2236.

Lefebvre, R.C., Ali, T., Ali, B., and Stock, A.E. (2021). Alternative treatments of postpartum uterine diseases in dairy cows. *Integrative Journal of Veterinary Biosciences* 5 (3): 1–7.

Lewis, G.S. (2003). Steroidal regulation of uterine resistance to bacterial infection in livestock. *Reproductive Biology and Endocrinology* 1: 117. https://doi.org/10.1186/1477-7827-1-117.

Lima, F.S., Vieira-Neto, A., Vasconcellos, G.S.F.M. et al. (2014). Efficacy of ampicillin trihydrate or ceftiofur hydrochloride for treatment of metritis and subsequent fertility in dairy cows. *Journal of Dairy Science* 97 (9): 5401–5414.

Machado, V.S., Bicalho, M.L.S., Pereira, R.V. et al. (2012). The effect of intrauterine administration of mannose or bacteriophage on uterine health and fertility of dairy cows with special focus on Escherichia coli and Arcanobacterium pyogenes. *Journal of Dairy Science* 95 (6): 3100–3109.

Machado, V.S., Bicalho, M.L., Meira Junior, E.B. et al. (2014). Subcutaneous immunization with inactivated bacterial components and purified protein of Escherichia coli, Fusobacterium necrophorum and Trueperella pyogenes prevents puerperal metritis in Holstein dairy cows. *PLoS One* 9 (3): e91734. https://doi.org/10.1371/journal.pone.0091734.

Makki, M., Gheisari, H., and Ahmadi, M. (2016). Effect of different intrauterine oxytetracycline treatment on reproductive performance of dairy cows with clinical endometritis and determination of oxytetracycline residues in milk. *İstanbul Universitesi Veteriner Fakultesi Dergisi* 42 (1): 80–88.

Makras, L., Triantafyllou, V., Fayol-Messaoudi, D. et al. (2006). Kinetic analysis of the antibacterial activity of probiotic lactobacilli towards Salmonella enterica serovar Typhimurium reveals a role for lactic acid and other inhibitory compounds. *Research in Microbiology* 157 (3): 241–247. https://doi.org/10.1016/j.resmic.2005.09.002.

Manners, J.G. and Stewart, R. (1982). Presence of dihydrostreptomycin and penicillin in cows'milk following intrauterine administration. *Australian Veterinary Journal* 58 (5): 203–204.

Mansour, U.M., Wahba, T.M., Hegazy, M.A., and Essamy, S.A. (2003). Biophysical changes in cervical mucus of buffaloes in response to PGF2 treatment. *Assiut Veterinary Medical Journal* 49: 232–248.

Markusfeld, O. (1987). Periparturient traits in seven high dairy herds. Incidence rates, association with parity, and interrelationships among traits. *Journal of Dairy Science* 70 (1): 158–166. https://doi.org/10.3168/jds.S0022-0302(87)79990-1.

Masera, J., Gustafsson, B.K., and Afiefy, M.M. (1980). Blood plasma and uterine tissue concentrations of sodium penicillin G in cows at intramuscular vs intrauterine administration. *Proceedings of the 9th International Congress on Animal Reproduction and Artificial Insemination*, Madrid, Spain (16–20 June 1980).

McCarville, J.L. and Ayres, J.S. (2018). Disease tolerance: concept and mechanisms. *Current Opinion in Immunology* 50: 88–93. https://doi.org/10.1016/j.coi.2017.12.003.

McLaughlin, C.L., Stanisiewski, E., Lucas, M.J. et al. (2012). Evaluation of two doses of ceftiofur crystalline free acid sterile suspension for treatment of metritis in lactating dairy cows. *Journal of Dairy Science* 95 (8): 4363–4371. https://doi.org/10.3168/jds.2011-5111.

Medzhitov, R., Schneider, D.S., and Soares, M.P. (2012). Disease tolerance as a defense strategy. *Science (New York, N.Y.)* 335 (6071): 936–941. https://doi.org/10.1126/science.1214935.

Mezzasalma, V., Manfrini, E., Ferri, E. et al. (2017). Orally administered multispecies probiotic formulations to prevent urogenital infections: a randomized placebo-controlled pilot study. *Archives of Gynecology and Obstetrics* 295 (1): 163–172. https://doi.org/10.1007/s00404-016-4235-2.

Mido, S., Murata, N., Rawy, M.S. et al. (2016). Effects of intrauterine infusion of povidone-iodine on endometrial cytology and bacteriology in dairy cows with clinical endometritis. *Journal of Veterinary Medical Science* 78 (4): 551–556.

Miller, E.A., Beasley, D.E., Dunn, R.R., and Archie, E.A. (2016). Lactobacilli dominance and vaginal pH: why is the human vaginal microbiome unique? *Frontiers in Microbiology* 7: 1936. https://doi.org/10.3389/fmicb.2016.01936.

Miranda-Caso Luengo, R., Lu, J., Williams, E.J. et al. (2019). Delayed differentiation of vaginal and uterine microbiomes in dairy cows developing postpartum endometritis. *PLoS One* 14 (1): e0200974. https://doi.org/10.1371/journal.pone.0200974.

Molinari, P.C.C., Dahl, G.E., Sheldon, I.M., and Bromfield, J.J. (2022). Effect of calving season on metritis incidence and bacterial content of the vagina in dairy cows. *Theriogenology* 191: 67–76. https://doi.org/10.1016/j.theriogenology.2022.08.001.

Molinari, P.C.C., Davidson, B.D., Laporta, J. et al. (2023). Prepartum heat stress in dairy cows increases postpartum inflammatory responses in blood of lactating dairy cows. *Journal of Dairy Science* 106 (2): 1464–1474. https://doi.org/10.3168/jds.2022-22405.

Moreno, I. and Franasiak, J.M. (2017). Endometrial microbiota-new player in town. *Fertility and Sterility* 108 (1): 32–39. https://doi.org/10.1016/j.fertnstert.2017.05.034.

Moresco, E.M., LaVine, D., and Beutler, B. (2011). Toll-like receptors. *Current Biology: CB* 21 (13): R488–R493. https://doi.org/10.1016/j.cub.2011.05.039.

Newby, N.C., Duffield, T.F., Pearl, D.L. et al. (2013). Short communication: use of a mechanical brush by Holstein dairy cattle around parturition. *Journal of Dairy Science* 96 (4): 2339–2344. https://doi.org/10.3168/jds.2012-6016.

NIH HMP Working Group, Peterson, J., Garges, S. et al. (2009). The NIH human microbiome project. *Genome Research* 19 (12): 2317–2323. https://doi.org/10.1101/gr.096651.109.

Noakes, D.E., Parkinson, T.J., England, G.C.W., and Arthur, G.H. (2002). *Arthur's Veterinary Reproduction and Obstetrics*, 8e, 399–408. Elsevier Sci. Ltd.

Noleto, P.G., Saut, J.P.E., and Sheldon, I.M. (2017). Short communication: glutamine modulates inflammatory responses to lipopolysaccharide in ex vivo bovine endometrium. *Journal of Dairy Science* 100 (3): 2207–2212. https://doi.org/10.3168/jds.2016-12023.

Olson, J.D., Ball, L., and Mortimer, R.G. (1984). Therapy of postpartum uterine infections. *American Association of Bovine Practitioners Conference Proceedings*, 85-88).

Otero, M.C., Morelli, L., and Nader-Macías, M.E. (2006). Probiotic properties of vaginal lactic acid bacteria to prevent metritis in cattle. *Letters in Applied Microbiology* 43 (1): 91–97. https://doi.org/10.1111/j.1472-765X.2006.01914.x.

Paisley, L.G., Mickelsen, W.O.D., and Anderson, P.B. (1986). Mechanisms and therapy for retained fetal membranes and uterine infections of cows: a review. *Theriogenology* 25 (3): 353–381.

Palanisamy, M., Ezakial Napolean, R., Selvaraju, M. et al. (2015). Efficacy of immunomodulators, Lugol's iodine and PGF2α on bacterial load in the endometritis affected cows. *Indian Veterinary Journal* 92 (7): 56–58.

Pascottini, O.B., Van Schyndel, S.J., Spricigo, J.F.W. et al. (2020). Dynamics of uterine microbiota in postpartum dairy cows with clinical or subclinical endometritis. *Scientific Reports* 10 (1): 12353. https://doi.org/10.1038/s41598-020-69317-z.

Pelzer, E., Gomez-Arango, L.F., Barrett, H.L., and Nitert, M.D. (2017). Review: maternal health and the placental microbiome. *Placenta* 54: 30–37. https://doi.org/10.1016/j.placenta.2016.12.003.

Perez-Muñoz, M.E., Arrieta, M.C., Ramer-Tait, A.E., and Walter, J. (2017). A critical assessment of the "sterile womb" and "in utero colonization" hypotheses: implications for research on the pioneer infant microbiome. *Microbiome* 5 (1): 48. https://doi.org/10.1186/s40168-017-0268-4.

Pinedo, P.J., Velez, J.S., Bothe, H. et al. (2015). Effect of intrauterine infusion of an organic-certified product on uterine health, survival, and fertility of dairy cows with toxic puerperal metritis. *Journal of Dairy Science* 98 (5): 3120–3132.

Potter, T., Guitian, J., Fishwick, J. et al. (2010). Risk factors for clinical endometritis in postpartum dairy cattle. *Theriogenology* 74: 127–134.

Rahi, S., Gupta, H.P., Prasad, S., and Bhaithalu, R.K. (2013). Phytotherapy for endometritis and subsequent conception rate in repeat breeding crossbred cows. *Indian Journal of Animal Reproduction* 34 (1): 9–12.

Rausher, M.D. (2001). Co-evolution and plant resistance to natural enemies. *Nature* 411 (6839): 857–864. https://doi.org/10.1038/35081193.

Read, A.F., Graham, A.L., and Råberg, L. (2008). Animal defenses against infectious agents: is damage control more important than pathogen control. *PLoS Biology* 6 (12): e4. https://doi.org/10.1371/journal.pbio.1000004.

Roberts, S.J. (1971). *Veterinary Obestetrics and Genital Diseases Ithaca*, 107–116. New York: Author.

Rogan, D., Fumoso, E., Rodryguez, E. et al. (2010). Use of mycobacterial cell wall extract (MCWE) in susceptible mares to clear experimentally induced endometritis with *Strep. Zooepidemicus*. *Journal of Equine Veterinary Science* 27: 112–117.

Russell, J.B. and Diez-Gonzalez, F. (1998). The effects of fermentation acids on bacterial growth. *Advances in Microbial Physiology* 39: 205–234. https://doi.org/10.1016/s0065-2911(08)60017-x.

Sahoo, S. and Mohanty, D.N. (2016). Effect of uterine immunomodulators on the PMN cell count of uterine fluid in cyclic non breeding cattle in Bhubaneswar area. *Indian Veterinary Journal* 93 (3): 40–42.

Sarkar, P., Kumar, H., and Patra, M.K. (2015). Leukocyte enriched autologous plasma for management of bovine endometritis. *Intas Polivet* 16 (2): 214–217.

Schneider, D.S. and Ayres, J.S. (2008). Two ways to survive infection: what resistance and tolerance can teach us about treating infectious diseases. *Nature Reviews. Immunology* 8 (11): 889–895. https://doi.org/10.1038/nri2432.

Schreier, H., Erdos, G., Reimer, K. et al. (1997). Molecular effects of povidone-iodine on relevant microorganisms: an electron-microscopic and biochemical study. *Dermatology* 195 (Suppl. 2): 111–116.

Sforcin, J.M. (2007). Propolis and the immune system: a review. *Journal of Ethnopharmacology* 113 (1): 1–14.

Sheldon, I.M. and Dobson, H. (2004). Postpartum uterine health in cattle. *Animal Reproduction Science* 82-83: 295–306. https://doi.org/10.1016/j.anireprosci.2004.04.006.

Sheldon, I.M., Rycroft, A.N., and Zhou, C. (2004a). Association between postpartum pyrexia and uterine bacterial infection in dairy cattle. *The Veterinary Record* 154 (10): 289–293. https://doi.org/10.1136/vr.154.10.289.

Sheldon, I.M., Lewis, G.S., LeBlanc, S., and Gilbert, R.O. (2006). Defining postpartum uterine disease in cattle. *Theriogenology* 65 (8): 1516–1530. https://doi.org/10.1016/j.theriogenology.2005.08.021.

Sheldon, I.M., Williams, E.J., Miller, A.N. et al. (2008). Uterine diseases in cattle after parturition. *Veterinary Journal* 176 (1): 115–121. https://doi.org/10.1016/j.tvjl.2007.12.031.

Sheldon, I.M., Cronin, J.G., and Bromfield, J.J. (2019). Tolerance and innate immunity shape the development of postpartum uterine disease and the impact of endometritis in dairy cattle. *Annual Review of Animal Biosciences* 7: 361–384. https://doi.org/10.1146/annurev-animal-020518-115227.

Sheldon, I.M., Molinari, P.C.C., Ormsby, T.J.R., and Bromfield, J.J. (2020). Preventing postpartum uterine disease in dairy cattle depends on avoiding, tolerating and resisting pathogenic bacteria. *Theriogenology* 150: 158–165. https://doi.org/10.1016/j.theriogenology.2020.01.017.

Singh, N., Singh, B., and Kumar, R. (2023). Effect of uterine lavage, levamisole, PGF2α and its combinations on haematological indices and bacterial load in Estrual mucus of Endometritic buffaloes. *The Indian Journal of Veterinary Science and Biotechnology* 19 (2): 28–33.

Smith, B.I., Donovan, G.A., Risco, C. et al. (1998). Comparison of various antibiotic treatments for cows diagnosed with toxic puerperal metritis. *Journal of Dairy Science* 81 (6): 1555–1562.

Soares, M.P., Teixeira, L., and Moita, L.F. (2017). Disease tolerance and immunity in host protection against infection. *Nature Reviews. Immunology* 17 (2): 83–96. https://doi.org/10.1038/nri.2016.136.

Takeuchi, O. and Akira, S. (2010). Pattern recognition receptors and inflammation. *Cell* 140 (6): 805–820. https://doi.org/10.1016/j.cell.2010.01.022.

Tan, X., Huang, Y.J., Jiang, Y.W., and Hu, S.H. (2007). Persistence of oxytetracycline residues in milk after the intrauterine treatment of lactating cows for endometritis. *Veterinary Record* 161 (17): 585–587.

Tizard, I.R. (1998). *Veterinary Immunology an Introduction*, 5e, 531. Singapore: Harcourt Brace and Company.

Travagli, V., Zanardi, I., and Bocci, V. (2009). Topical applications of ozone and ozonated oils as anti-infective agents: an insight into the patent claims. *Recent Patents on Anti-Infective Drug Discovery* 4 (2): 130–142.

Turner, M.L., Cronin, J.G., Healey, G.D., and Sheldon, I.M. (2014). Epithelial and stromal cells of bovine endometrium have roles in innate immunity and initiate inflammatory responses to bacterial lipopeptides in vitro via toll-like receptors TLR2, TLR1, and TLR6. *Endocrinology* 155 (4): 1453–1465. https://doi.org/10.1210/en.2013-1822.

Turner, M.L., Cronin, J.G., Noleto, P.G., and Sheldon, I.M. (2016). Glucose availability and AMP-activated protein kinase link energy metabolism and innate immunity in the bovine endometrium. *PLoS One* 11 (3): e0151416. https://doi.org/10.1371/journal.pone.0151416.

Usmani, R.H., Ahmad, N., Shafiq, P., and Mirza, M.A. (2001). Effect of subclinical uterine infection on cervical and uterine involution, estrous activity and fertility in postpartum buffaloes. *Theriogenology* 55 (2): 563–571. https://doi.org/10.1016/s0093-691x(01)00426-5.

Val-Laillet, D., Guesdon, V., Keyserlingk, M.A. et al. (2009). Allogrooming in cattle: relationships between social preferences, feeding displacements and social dominance. *Applied Animal Behaviour Science* 116: 141–149.

Verma, S.K., Kumar, R., Singh, B. et al. (2023). Impact of different therapies on haematological parameters and therapeutic outcomes in subclinical endometritis. *The Indian Journal of Veterinary Science and Biotechnology* 19 (5): 60–64. https://doi.org/10.48165/ijvsbt.19.5.12.

Wagener, K., Gabler, C., and Drillich, M. (2017). A review of the ongoing discussion about definition, diagnosis and pathomechanism of subclinical endometritis in dairy cows. *Theriogenology* 94: 21–30. https://doi.org/10.1016/j.theriogenology.2017.02.005.

Wagner, W.C. and Hansel, W. (1969). Reproductive physiology of the post partum cow. I. Clinical and histological findings. *Journal of Reproduction and Fertility* 18 (3): 493–500. https://doi.org/10.1530/jrf.0.0180493.

Wakayo, B.U., Brar, P.S., Prabhakar, S., and Arora, A.K. (2015). Evaluation of prophylactic cloprostenol and *E. coli* LPS treatment against endometritis in dairy cows and buffaloes. *Journal of Reproduction and Infertility* 6 (1): 17–21.

Wang, A., Luan, H.H., and Medzhitov, R. (2019). An evolutionary perspective on immunometabolism. *Science (New York, N.Y.)* 363 (6423): eaar3932. https://doi.org/10.1126/science.aar3932.

Wathes, D.C., Cheng, Z., Chowdhury, W. et al. (2009). Negative energy balance alters global gene expression and immune responses in the uterus of postpartum dairy cows. *Physiological Genomics* 39 (1): 1–13. https://doi.org/10.1152/physiolgenomics.00064.2009.

Whiteford, L.C. and Sheldon, I.M. (2005). Association between clinical hypocalcaemia and postpartum endometritis. *The Veterinary Record* 157 (7): 202–203. https://doi.org/10.1136/vr.157.7.202.

Wrenn, T.R., Wood, J.R., Bitman, J., and Brinsfield, T.H. (1968). Vaginal glycogen assay for oestrogen: specificity and application to blood and urine. *Journal of Reproduction and Fertility* 16 (2): 301–304. https://doi.org/10.1530/jrf.0.0160301.

Yoshida, R., Kitahara, G., and Osawa, T. (2020). Intrauterine infusion of povidone-iodine: its effect on the endometrium and subsequent fertility in postpartum dairy cows. *Journal of Veterinary Medical Science* 82 (7): 926–934.

Zemjanis, R. (1980). Repeat breeding or conception failure in cattle. *Current Therapy in Theriogenology* 1: 209.

Zerbe, H., Schuberth, H.J., Engelke, F. et al. (2003). Development and comparison of in vivo and in vitro models for endometritis in cattle and mares. *Theriogenology* 60: 209–223.

Zhou, C., Boucher, J.F., Dame, K.J. et al. (2001). Multilocation trial of ceftiofur for treatment of postpartum cows with fever. *Journal of the American Veterinary Medical Association* 219 (6): 805–808.

Ziv, G., Paape, M., and Dulin, A.M. (1983). Influence of antibiotics and intramammary antibiotic products on phagocytosis of Staphylococcus aureus by bovine leukocytes. *American Journal of Veterinary Research* 44 (3): 385–388.

14

Injuries to the Birth Canal

Rajesh Kumar[1], Daund Sushant Sakhahari[1], Deepak Ningwal[2], and Pramod Kumar[3]

[1] Department of Veterinary Gynaecology & Obstetrics, College of Veterinary Science and Animal Husbandry, Acharya Narendra Deva University of Agriculture and Technology, Ayodhya, Uttar Pradesh, India
[2] Department of Veterinary Gynaecology & Obstetrics, College of Veterinary Science and A.H., Rewa, Madhya Pradesh, India
[3] Department of Veterinary Physiology & Biochemistry, College of Veterinary Science and Animal Husbandry, Acharya Narendra Deva University of Agriculture and Technology, Ayodhya, Uttar Pradesh, India

14.1 Introduction

The birth canal, also known as the reproductive tract or birth passage, plays a crucial role in the process of parturition or birth of young ones. However, this essential anatomical structure is susceptible to injuries for various reasons that may occur before, during, and after the calving process. Understanding these injuries is vital for veterinarians, livestock owners, and animal breeders to ensure the health and well-being of both the dam and the offspring as well as the dam's future fertility.

14.2 Injuries Before Parturition

14.2.1 Vaginal/Cervical Prolapse

During the last stage of pregnancy, crossbred cows are most likely to have eversion and prolapse of the vagina, with or without the involvement of the cervix (Figure 14.1). Many factors are responsible for the condition, viz. hereditary (more often in beef cows than in dairy cows) (Woodward and Quesenberry 1956); bigger breeds like Charolais, Limousin (Coulthard 1991), and Shorthorns; high levels of estrogen in the blood (Miesner and Anderson 2008); and mineral deficiencies. Elevated estrogen levels in advanced pregnancy result in relaxation of the pelvic diaphragm and vagina. Moreover, severe straining during defecation, increased intra-abdominal pressure in advanced pregnancy, and an enlarged rumen make the ligaments around the perineum fragile. Extremely cold weather, too much fat around the vaginal opening, past damage to the vaginal tissues, eating a lot of hard-to-digest roughage, having abnormal vaginal anatomy, and the walls of the Müllerian tubes staying in place all make the animal more likely to suffer from vaginal prolapse. Furthermore, incompetence of the constrictor vestibule and constrictor vulvae muscles may have a role in etiology (Hudson 1986).

The prolapse begins as an intussusception-like folding of the vaginal floor just cranial to the vestibule–vaginal junction. The discomfort caused by this eversion, along with irritation and swelling of the mucosa, makes the animal strain and causes the prolapse to get worse due to a vicious cycle of continuous straining. At some point, the cervix may be visible at the most caudal part of the prolapsed tissue, which means that the whole vagina may have slipped out of place. There may be a bladder or loops of bowel inside a prolapsed vagina. When the bladder moves into the prolapsed vagina, it can block the urethra. The bladder then fills up and gets bigger, making it hard to fix the prolapse unless the bladder is cleared first.

Periparturient Diseases of Cattle, First Edition. Edited by Tanmoy Rana.

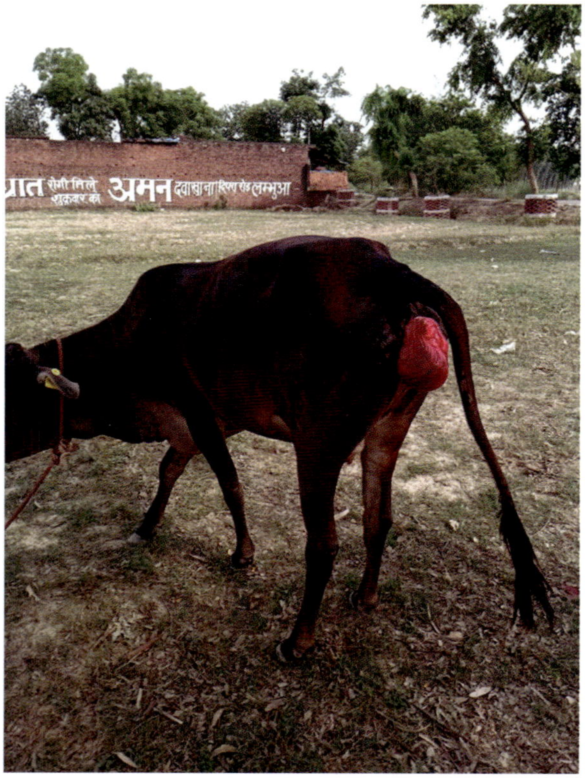

Figure 14.1 Vaginal prolapse in cattle.
Source: Rajesh Kumar.

The bladder could even burst, which is potentially fatal. Based on the severity of eversion, extent of injury, and exposure of the cervix, vaginal eversions are classified as Grades 1, 2, 3, and 4.

- **Grade 1 eversion:** Grade 1 eversions are characterized by a small intermittent protrusion of vaginal mucosa through the vulval lips and are noticed when the animal lies down. They can be readily repaired with a retention suture, however, if they remain untreated, the frequently exposed tissues get dehydrated, traumatized, and progress into Grade 2.
- **Grade 2 eversion:** Grade 2 eversions are characterized by the continuous protrusion of vaginal mucosa through the vulval lips, with the possibility that the bladder becomes trapped in the everted organ. If left untreated, a Grade 2 quickly progresses to a Grade 3 eversion.
- **Grade 3 eversion:** The entire vaginal mucosa and cervix protrude continuously through the vulval lips with a trapped bladder and an exposed cervical mucus plug. The cervical seal may liquefy, allowing bacterial contamination of the uterus that leads to placentitis and fetal death. Often these fetuses become emphysematous and cervical dilation is insufficient for a vaginal delivery. This condition is often erroneously referred to as a cervical eversion but is more correctly referred to as a cervicovaginal eversion. This distinguishes it from the eversion of the cervix alone, as sometimes is observed in *Bos indicus* breeds. In the latter case, only the cervix everts as a pedunculated mass through the vulva.
- **Grade 4 eversion:** The entire vaginal mucosa appears necrotic and fibrosed. Infection is so extensive that the bladder may become involved and peritonitis is a possible result.

14.2.2 Management and Treatment of Vaginal Prolapse

The goal of treatment for pregnant animals is to replace and retain the vagina and cervix in the pelvic canal as well as successfully deliver and care for live offspring. There are many ways to treat vaginal and cervical eversions. These can be put into two main groups: (i) those that aim for permanent reduction and (ii) those that only help for a short time. It is important to remember that one method might not work for all grades. The treatment choice will depend on how bad the eversion is, how long until the fetus is due, the veterinarian's preference, and whether the owner is willing or able to care for the animal after treatment. After seeing how the animal responds to the first treatment plan, it may need to be changed. This is especially important if tenesmus is a problem. If the animal is close to giving birth, an induction is recommended to stop the problem from reoccurring before calving.

As a caudal epidural block, 5–10 ml of 2% lignocaine hydrochloride can be used to avoid straining and desensitize the perineum for suturing. The mass is cleaned with plain water or a gentle antiseptic that does not irritate. It is then gently put back into place with the palm, taking care not to cause trauma to the inflamed and sometimes fragile tissue. After repositioning the everted mass, the retention can be performed using either of the following techniques:

- **Caslick's suture:** This procedure is best suited for Grade 1 vaginal eversions associated with estrus. On some occasions, it can be useful for pregnant animals near parturition that exhibit no signs of discomfort and tenesmus, whereas in many instances this suture method is inadequate as increasing intra-abdominal pressure initiates the sensation of tenesmus, which leads to removal of the suture or protrusion of the vagina beyond the suture line. Moreover, the vulval softening and stretching that occurs near parturition contributes significantly to this phenomenon.
- **Buhner stitch:** This therapeutic modality demonstrates efficacy for conditions characterized by advanced stages and persistence. To achieve a favorable outcome, it is necessary to make a stab incision that penetrates deeply, positioning the retention line as close to the cranial aspect of the vulval lips as is feasible. One drawback of this procedure is that it

requires assistance throughout the calving process to avoid trauma to the vulva, as it hampers normal delivery of the calf that can lead to intrauterine fetal death. After administering epidural anesthesia, the vulva is thoroughly cleansed using soap and water. Subsequently, a stab incision of 1 cm is performed along the midline, positioned below the vulva, and extending as far forward as is feasible. A second surgical cut is performed at a location equidistant between the anus and the dorsal commissure of the vulva. Next, a Buhner needle is inserted deeply, originating from the ventral incision and traversing down one side of the vulva until it emerges through the dorsal incision. The Buhner tape, specifically the nonwicking variant, is threaded through the eye of the needle. The needle is then withdrawn via the ventral incision, simultaneously pulling the tape along. The aforementioned process is repeated on the contralateral vulval lip, and the two extremities are secured, resulting in an approximate two-finger aperture in the ventral vulva to facilitate urination. The preferred method involves tying a bow knot followed by securing the two loops of the bow using a single square knot. This technique enables the manipulation of the knot to achieve a relaxed state while ensuring that the suture remains intact. Consequently, if the animal attempts to evert again, the suture may be repositioned, and the knot can be securely tightened again. This practice can also be conducted during evening hours in cases when continuous animal monitoring for calving is not feasible during nighttime hours. When executed correctly, the tape should not be detectable along the incision on the back, which lowers the risk of fecal matter following the trajectory of the needles (Buhner 1958).

- **Bootlace technique:** This technique is not widely accepted due to the inverted nature of the vulval lips and the labor-intensive process of suturing. Still, it exhibits more strength compared to a Caslick's suture. After the administration of epidural anesthesia and the disinfection of the vulva and its surrounding region, a series of four to five small openings are created using either umbilical tape or hog nose rings. These openings are formed on both sides of the vulva following a dorsal to ventral line, specifically at the point where the hair meets the hairless area on the vulval lips. Following the insertion of eyelets, the vulva is secured with umbilical or Buhner tape, which is employed as if lacing up a boot. As the pattern becomes tighter, the vulvar lips undergo inversion. To prevent significant vaginal trauma during calving, it is imperative to release the bootlace sutures prior to calving (Johansen 1968).
- **Horizontal mattress (Halstead) technique:** This procedure involves the insertion of a needle through the right vulval lip, commencing at a deep point where the labia meet the skin of the rump. The needle is extended along the vulval opening and inserted into the left vulval lip at an equivalent depth as the right. The needle is subsequently reinserted in a left-to-right direction that aligns with the initial trajectory but begins around 2–3 cm ventral to the initial insertion point. This operation may be performed utilizing either a Buhner or a big cutting needle. To achieve appropriate urinary function, it is recommended to employ an adequate number of sutures to narrow the vulva to a width of around two fingers. One drawback of employing this approach is that the occurrence of vulval edema is common and can be fairly severe, even when sutures are not excessively tightened. The reduction of tension in sutures can be achieved through the use of "stents." Polyvinyl chloride tubing with a 1.3-cm diameter can be appropriately sized to match the length of the vulva. Holes can then be drilled at intervals of 2–3 cm. Alternatively, wooden dowels or latex tubing can also be employed. A stent is positioned bilaterally, adjacent to the vulva, and afterward, a horizontal mattress suture is threaded through the perforations and secured (Lamp and Lamp 1981).
- **Deep vertical mattress technique:** This is similar to the horizontal mattress pattern described above. The difference is that a vertical mattress suture pattern is used, and stents are recommended to disperse tension on the vulval lips. This replacement method can also have serious consequences if assistance is not available at the onset of parturition. Moreover, other techniques that allow parturition without jeopardising fixation are available. These include any of the numerous varieties of the Minchev procedure, including those that employ specialist pins, or the Winkler technique (cervicopexy) or Minchev (vaginopexy). By using one of the versions of the Minchev procedure, vaginopexy satisfies the requirement for temporary or "semi-permanent" retention while allowing parturition followed by culling at a more financially favourable time (Sidelinger et al., 2018).

14.2.3 Rupture of the Prepubic Tendon and Ventral Hernia

Most ventral abdominal hernias and tears in the prepubic muscle happen in the last month of pregnancy; the weight of a gravid uterus and peripartum swelling of the ventrum are two main contributing factors for this to occur. Cattle with twins or multiple pregnancies and those with hydrops are also more likely to be affected. Even though it happens more often in multiparous cattle with a sagging belly, this condition can also be encountered in primiparous cattle. Injuries from immediate trauma, such as fighting with other animals, being stuck on inanimate objects, or falling on a slippery surface could cause or contribute to the condition. In cattle, the factors responsible for uterine enlargement are supposed to be major factors like advanced pregnancy (from 7 months onward, twins, etc.) (Roberts 1986).

When the prepubic tendons tear, the fore udder loses all of its shape on both sides and then points in the same direction as the abdominal wall, which is sagging in the same direction. The cow stands like a sawhorse because of severe abdominal pain and the animal does not want to lie down. When the cow is lying down, she tries to do so in a way that does not put pressure on the ventrum to minimize pain. Before a tendon breaks, the owner usually sees an obvious or unusually large amount of abdominal distention. In cows, like mares, the rupture may be preceded by both a large amount of abdominal distention and a large plaque of ventral edema. These signs have been called "impending rupture of the prepubic tendon" and are extremely concerning.

Cattle with ventral hernias have the same risk factors as those with ruptured prepubic tendons but may also exhibit unilateral abdominal sagging and an unusual relationship between the suffering side of the abdomen and the fore udder. They can occur on either side of the body, but the right side is most commonly involved. Both of these conditions are responsible for severe acute pain that might lead to herniation. Typical findings include tachycardia, tachypnea, an apprehensive expression, reluctance to move or lie down, and a sawhorse stance. Prepubic tendon rupture typically causes more obvious pain than a ventral hernia, but this is not always the case; a rectal examination may aid in distinguishing the conditions. When a true rupture of the prepubic tendon has occurred, the cranial rim of the pelvis may be slightly tilted upward, and the hand may be cupped beneath the rim. In ventral hernias, the hernia may or may not be palpable, but the prepubic tendon at its attachment to the pelvic apex can be palpated in the caudal abdomen. Assistance is needed during calving to deliver the live offspring as both these conditions cause severe pain and a lack of the abdominal pressure needed for delivery. In addition, the presence of twins or hydrops increases the likelihood of dystocia. Cows with a ruptured prepubic tendon must be euthanized or saved because of the suffering during this condition. Cows with ventral hernias who do not appear to be in severe discomfort may continue lactating, but they should not be bred again. To prevent herniation or rupture of the prepubic tendon, cows suspected of exhibiting signs of "impending rupture" or suspected of suffering from hydrops should be induced to calve promptly or undergo an elective cesarean section. Cattle that are recumbent and unable to rise or have already developed secondary musculoskeletal complications must be euthanized. When labor is induced in these situations, it must always be monitored. The insertion of a nasotracheal or orotracheal catheter prevents abdominal pressure from exacerbating the abdominal wall rupture, while traction may still be used to deliver the calf. Rupture of the prepubic tendon and ventral hernias are diagnosed based on clinical signs alone; however, they must be differentially diagnosed with large hematomas or abscesses cranial or dorsal to the udder, severe preparturient ventral edema, and inflammatory ventral edema or edema secondary to thrombosis of the mammary vein. Typically, the anatomical relationship between the udder and the ventral abdomen is sufficient to distinguish between these conditions. The use of an ultrasound will aid in reaching a more definitive diagnosis. Anemia is present if there are significant udder hematomas, and a fever could be present if there are abscesses. When a diagnosis is uncertain, ultrasonography could be very useful. Despite surgical measures, Dhillon et al. (2006) opined that oral administration of *Argyreia speciosa* seeds is an economical and effective therapy for vaginal prolapse in cattle and buffaloes, the seeds can circumvent the need for manual manipulation of the genital organs.

14.3 Injuries During Parturition

14.3.1 Perineal Lacerations

Perineal lacerations occur as a result of forced extraction or the expulsive forces generated during labor in the presence of feto-maternal disproportion or fetal malposition (Arthur et al. 1996). Perineal lacerations that commonly affect primiparous females are associated with obstetrical trauma, particularly during assisted deliveries (Rizk and Mosbah 2016). These are usually less frequent in cattle compared to mares (Kazemi et al. 2010).

Perineal lacerations are classified into first, second, and third-degree lacerations, according to the location and degree of tissue damage. First-degree lacerations are superficial wounds of the mucosa of the vulva and vagina, and they often go unnoticed without a close examination after parturition. Meanwhile, second-degree perineal lacerations extend into the submucosa and muscularis layer of the vulva and vagina, the anal sphincter, and the perineal body, which compromises the ability of muscles to constrict the vestibule and causes the perineum to sink cranioventrally (which can predispose the animal to pneumovagina and urine pooling). Lastly, third-degree perineal lacerations will include the rectovaginal septum, the muscles of the vagina and rectum, and the perineal body. They usually create a common rectal and vestibular vault that permits direct fecal contamination and results in bacterial infection of the vagina, cervix, and uterus (Noakes 2009).

Furthermore, fistulae may also form between the rectum and vagina (such as the rectovestibular fistulae and rectovaginal fistulae) as a result of obstetrical trauma, improper repair of third perineal lacerations, trauma during breeding, perineal or perivaginal abscesses, and congenital abnormalities. Perineal lacerations and rectovaginal fistulas create a connection between the rectum and the vaginal vestibule that results in fecal contamination of the vagina. During estrus, the cervix undergoes relaxation, and therefore, endometritis develops with a subsequent decrease in future fertility (Dreyfuss et al. 1990).

Since the reconstruction of third-degree perineal lacerations and rectovaginal fistulas appear necessary to quickly bring cows back to breeding soundness, this retrospective report was performed to shed new light on the occurrence of perineal lacerations and rectovaginal fistulas as well as the evaluation of a one-stage technique for their repair in dairy cows. The anesthesia adopted for such procedures is epidural infiltration anesthesia (Abdullah et al. 2014). Extensive lacerations require careful suturing, whereas minor lacerations heal spontaneously with little care. Moreover, Marien et al. (2023) noted that calving-related injuries of the vestibulum vaginae and the vagina had no statistically significant effect on the reproductive performance of heifers.

14.3.1.1 Surgical Techniques

Numerous surgical techniques and modifications have been reported for the repair of perineal lacerations in cattle (Rizk and Mosbah 2016). Third-degree perineal lacerations are most commonly repaired using the Goetz one-stage surgical technique (Dreyfuss et al. 1990), the Aanes two-stage technique (Aanes 1964), or a modification of these techniques (Woodie 2006; Sato et al. 2019). The goal of any surgical repair is to establish a functional partition between the rectum and the vaginal vestibule and to restore a functional perineal body. This will prevent further contamination and permit the treatment of vaginitis, cervicitis, and metritis, all of which lead to infertility.

14.3.1.2 First-degree Perineal Laceration

First-degree perineal lacerations usually require no medical treatment. However, in deep and severe injuries, perivaginal adipose tissue from the site of injury may protrude into the vagina. As a result, necrosis and infection may occur, which leads to an ascending infection that may affect the reproductive and urinary tracts. Therefore, local or systemic administration of antimicrobial agents may become necessary in first-degree perineal lacerations (Sato et al. 2019).

14.3.1.3 Second-degree Perineal Laceration

For second-degree perineal lacerations, an incision is made along the scar tissue line at the junction between the vaginal vestibule and rectum. Dissection of the rectovestibular shelf starts cranially on a frontal plane and laterally into the submucosal tissues as well as caudally to the level of the perineal skin. Lateral dissection continues until two flaps are created and brought to the midline without any tension. The closure suture is made according to the modified one-stage repair by the Goetz technique (six-bite vertical mattress suture pattern) (Awad and Esam 2016).

14.3.1.4 Third-degree Perineal Lacerations

The tail of the animal is bandaged and tied to one side and aseptic preparation of the perineal region performed. For third-degree perineal lacerations, a modified one-stage surgical repair technique is used for suture and closure of the lacerations (Adams and Fessler 2000). Briefly, the operative area is exposed by holding the skin with Allis tissue forceps near the mucocutaneous margin on each side of the disrupted dorsal commissure of the vulva. An incision is performed through the scar tissue line at the junction between the vestibule/vagina and the rectum to separate the vestibular and rectal mucous membranes horizontally, from the skin caudally, and to the intact perineal body cranially. The incision is deepened about 4–5 cm in normal tissue. All the suture lines are started in the rostral aspect of the laceration and continued caudally using size-1 polydioxanone. First, a continuous horizontal mattress pattern is used to suture the vestibular flap. Second, the perineal body is sutured using a simple interrupted suture. Shelf reconstruction is accomplished by suturing the rectal mucosa as a third line that uses a continuous horizontal mattress suture with the mucosa everted in the rectal lumen. The rest of the perineal tissues, together with the skin, are sutured by interrupted vertical mattress sutures using size-0 Prolene® (Ethicon, LLC, San Lorenzo, Puerto Rico, USA) (Awad and Esam 2016).

14.3.1.5 Post-operative Care

The animal should be given a small amount of feed during the post-operative period, and the careful manual emptying of the rectum is advised, if needed. Skin sutures should be removed 10–14 days after surgery or after complete healing. A gentle digital examination of the surgical site from the vaginal side is recommended 2 weeks after surgery to assess healing. Rectal examinations are not performed for a minimum of 30 days after surgery. Uterine evaluations and treatment of metritis, if present, is recommended before any breeding attempts (Awad and Esam 2016).

The perineum is the tissue that forms the body wall at the pelvic outlet and surrounds the rectum, anus, and urogenital tracts. This region is bounded dorsally by the base of the tail, laterally by the ischial tubers and semimembranosus muscles, and ventrally by the ventral commissure of the vulva. This region is subject to much surgical affection that might affect the fertility of the animals. The affections like rectovaginal and perineum injuries, including rectovaginal fistula, perineal laceration, pneumovagina, and urovagina, cause serious economic loss in dairy bovines. Perineal lacerations occur mostly in primiparous dairy cows with assisted difficult deliveries, and the described techniques to treat perineal lacerations in cows substantially improve the perineal conformation with subsequent improvement of their fertility. The high rectovaginal fistula in cows can be corrected through a vaginal approach, while the low one can be repaired with a single-stage surgical technique. Lastly, breeding after the surgical treatment of perineal lacerations and rectovaginal fistulas in dairy cows is usually advisable.

14.3.2 Uterine Rupture

In cattle, spontaneous uterine rupture has been reported (Azawi et al. 2012; Pascoe 1968). It is usually an unfortunate consequence of dystocia observed occasionally in late pregnancy or during parturition (Pearson and Denny 1975), and it is rare during the prepartum period (Phillips et al. 2015). Although the condition is rarely observed following an unassisted delivery, most cases occur following forced traction, uterine torsions, fetotomy, or the delivery of an emphysematous fetus. Iatrogenic ruptures can also occur as a result of exasperated interventions by a veterinarian who has become fatigued from protracted efforts to relieve dystocia. Prolonged dystocia, emphysematous fetuses, and a failure to adequately lubricate during delivery can increase the resistance and "drag" between the fetus and the maternal reproductive tract, which predisposes the uterus to rupture. The abdominal pressure of the uterus against the pelvic brim may also be responsible for uterine rupture.

In the event of dystocia, it is recommended that a veterinarian be present to do a physical inspection of the cervix and uterus via the vaginal canal after the birth of the calf. Typically, the diagnosis of a full-thickness uterine tear may be made when the tear is in the veterinarian's examination range. In cases when the problem remains initially undiscovered or if veterinary intervention is absent during dystocia, observable symptoms often manifest 1–5 days after parturition. The main signs and symptoms are depression, loss of appetite, elevated body temperature, rapid heart rate, impaired rumen motility, and abdominal tenderness, which are indicative of peritonitis. Certain bovines exhibit the rapid development of septic shock due to extensive contamination of the peritoneal cavity. This condition is particularly prevalent in cases when there is prolonged dystocia, retained fetal membranes, or the presence of a deceased or emphysematous fetus, since these conditions provide an opportunity for bacterial introduction into the uterus that can rapidly disseminate throughout the abdominal cavity. Severe and possibly deadly peritonitis may occur when fetal membranes traverse the uterine rupture and enter the abdominal cavity. Cattle with large uterine tears and tenesmus may have a prolapse of the intestine via the reproductive system, which results in the appearance of these organs at the vulva. Occasionally, an unattended dystocia may lead to a spontaneous rupture that results in the calf or fetus becoming located outside the uterus, inside the abdominal cavity. The prognosis gets considerably worse with the presence of overt peritonitis since the rapid dissemination of fibrinous adhesions throughout the abdominal cavity diminishes the likelihood of successful uterine repair. When there is suspicion of the condition, a manual vaginal examination is recommended, after adequately preparing the perineum and vulva. In cows that have just given birth, the manual entry of a hand into the uterus is easily performed within 48 hours. However, in cows that beyond the 48-hour postpartum period, the passage of the hand through the cervix may become difficult. The use of a speculum may be advantageous; nevertheless, the most reliable method for definitively diagnosing the tear is by manual palpation. Most ruptures are located dorsally and positioned immediately cranial to the cervix. In cases when the uterine tear is minor and located dorsally, conservative therapy (use of broad-spectrum systemic antibiotics and oxytocin) may be considered as a potential approach. The efficacy of conservative treatment is often suboptimal due to the inherent challenges of dystocia, which allows significant bacterial colonization of both the uterus and abdomen. Cattle that encounter minor dorsal uterine tears after the manipulation or birth of a viable calf without contamination of the abdominal cavity by fetal membranes have the most favorable prognosis.

The treatment regimen for this condition includes surgical intervention to rectify the laceration, the administration of potent antibiotics to manage peritonitis, and supportive care. Several authors have reported the repair of uterine rupture either per vaginum, by everting the uterus, or by laparotomy (Pascoe 1968; Pearson and Denny 1975). Surgical repair procedures have been performed through the birth canal; nevertheless, this approach has challenges since it is commonly conducted without direct visualization and has a high rate of failure. The use of an epidural anesthetic and specialized long surgical equipment enhances the feasibility of this approach, but the challenges remain the same. This procedure can only be executed when (i) the issue is promptly identified and (ii) the cervix is sufficiently dilated to permit the use of both hands for manipulation. Surgical intervention after laparotomy is a more favorable option, however, it presents intrinsic challenges due to the tear's location, which is often dorsal and in proximity to the cervix. Consequently, accessing and efficiently suturing the rupture from a flank approach becomes difficult after uterine involution has begun. To enhance visibility and assist in the closure of the rupture, it is necessary to create incisions in the paralumbar fossa positioned as caudally as feasible. The use of assistance to guide the reproductive tract toward the operator by inserting an arm through the birth canal might perhaps assist and facilitate the procedure. In some exceptional instances, the performance of a flank laparotomy becomes imperative when the fetus or fetal membranes are found inside the abdominal cavity. When repairing a uterine tear by a flank approach, a peritoneal lavage using either physiological saline solution and antibiotics or a very diluted solution of Betadine® (Atlantis Consumer Healthcare Inc., Bridgewater, New Jersy, USA) is recommended. Additional supportive treatment, such as intravenous fluids, nonsteroidal anti-inflammatory drugs (NSAIDs), or short-acting corticosteroids, may be necessary for bovines exhibiting the first signs of shock. The prognosis for cattle experiencing uterine rupture is generally considered poor to guarded.

14.3.3 Calving Paralysis

The term "calving paralysis" was used to describe a condition known as post-calving paraplegia. This condition is often believed to result from injury to the nerve roots inside the pelvic region, which may occur when an oversized calf passes through the pelvic canal during calving. The condition mostly affects first-calf heifers; however, it can occur in pluriparous cows. The severity of the condition varies, including symptoms such as weakness and significant abduction of the hindlimbs in animals capable of standing, to the point where they are unable to stand unassisted (Radostitis 2010). Although calving paralysis is well recognized as a prevalent condition in dairy cattle, there is a limited understanding of the various types and extent of nerve injury associated with it. According to Galabinov (1966) and Vermunt et al. (2010), calving paralysis is characterized by sciatic involvement. Additionally, Divers (2004) and Hartnack (2017) suggest that the sciatic nerve is frequently affected in cases of calving paralysis. However, Vermunt et al. (2010) state that obturator paralysis is the most prevalent among the various types of paralysis associated with calving. Throughout the years, the term "obturator paralysis" has often been used simultaneously with "calving paralysis"; nevertheless, it fails to include the fetlock flexion frequently seen in cases of calving paralysis. The occurrence of clinical symptoms associated with calving paralysis can have significant variation, depending upon the degree of nerve damage inside the pelvic canal (Cox 1988).

Cows with calving paralysis may exhibit symptoms of muscular weakening or full immobility after the process of calving. Nerve injury often affects the posterior extremities, which results in a diminished or complete loss of responsiveness and paralysis. Consequently, the bovine may exhibit hindleg dragging during walking, which results in an atypical gait. In some instances, the hindlimbs may exhibit a state of reduced muscle tone, which results in the cow experiencing difficulty sustaining her body weight. Furthermore, there might be impairment in coordination and equilibrium, which makes it difficult for the affected bovine to maintain an upright position or engage in efficient locomotion. The lifting of the affected animal will often show that there is no normal control of the hindlimbs. The fact that the affected leg often does not respond when stimulated confirms the condition, but it needs to be differentiated from other neurological conditions such as hip dislocation and pregnancy toxemia. Immediate identification and thorough evaluation by veterinary professionals are necessary to determine the magnitude of neural impairment and provide suitable treatment and supervision. While some instances of calving paralysis that result from nerve injury may improve with time and a combination of supporting measures, alternative circumstances may need extensive therapy and interventions to facilitate the cow's recovery.

Medicinal treatment along with supportive care can be given to the affected animal, depending on the severity. To reduce the pressure on the affected limb, a soft bedding material can be provided along with regular repositioning of the animal to avoid pressure on the soles and muscle stiffness. Nerve injury in cows may result in considerable pain and discomfort, which makes pain management crucial for reducing suffering and enhancing the cow's movement and ability to stand. To promote healing and regaining muscle function, physical therapy and rehabilitation play a vital role. The cow may be assisted with exercises and gentle movements to maintain joint flexibility and muscle strength. Nutritional supplements, along with medications such as anti-inflammatory drugs, can be given to improve overall health and reduce the swelling around damaged nerves. Mechanical devices can also be used to lift the animal for mobility of the affected leg and massage.

Preventive measures can be taken to avoid such conditions where only adequately grown heifers are bred along with proper nutritional support. The bulls used to breed the heifers must be of suitable breed to ensure appropriately sized calves during calving.

14.4 Injuries After Parturition

14.4.1 Uterine Prolapse

The occurrence of uterine prolapse has been recorded in all species but is frequently seen in cows during the third stage of labor (Roberts 1986) and should always be considered an emergency (Miesner and Anderson 2008). In ruminant species, a prolapse often involves a full eversion of the gravid horn (Arthur et al. 1996).

The occurrence of uterine prolapse is a well-recognized condition among veterinary professionals that specialize in bovine medicine. In the context of dairy cattle, it is widely believed that the problem is not hereditary and seldom reoccurs in successive parturitions. However, it may be difficult to identify the exact etiology; there are many risk factors like dystocia, tenesmus, hypocalcemia, and others that might contribute to the condition. Primiparous cows may have an impact, although pluriparous cows are likely to face a higher susceptibility. The occurrence of uterine prolapse in cattle may be attributed to factors such as confinement, limited physical activity, and the gravitational forces that result from cows calving in a position where their hindquarters are lower than their forequarters. Uterine atony is a prevalent initiating factor and is often linked to hypocalcemia in dairy calves who have given birth several times. Prolapse often manifests shortly after parturition, typically within a few hours, and almost always within 24-hours of calving. Many practitioners have also reported unusual occurrences of uterine prolapse several days after calving (Risco et al. 1984; Potter 2008).

The clinical signs are distinct and provide sufficient evidence for a conclusive diagnosis. At times, those who are new to handling or have not previously encountered the issue may mistakenly conflate uterine prolapse with vaginal prolapse. However, the visual observation of a completely prolapsed uterus is distinct and unlikely to be mistaken for other conditions. The presence of prominent placentomes on the visible endometrium enables the differentiation of the prolapsed uterus from other organs. The cow's overall health may seem unaffected; this is often seen in primiparous cattle. Nonetheless, pluriparous cows suffering from uterine prolapse often exhibit varying degrees of hypocalcemic symptoms such as weakness, depression, subnormal temperature, anxiety, difficulty getting up, or prostration and coma. Tenesmus is a prevalent symptom seen in most cases. It is important to distinguish between signs of shock and hypocalcemia to effectively manage patients with prolapse. This is because a minority of these individuals may have hypovolemic shock due to factors such as blood loss (either internally or externally), injury to the prolapsed organ, or intestine entrapment inside the prolapsed organ. Severe paleness, an elevated heart rate, and extreme physical weakness are significant indicators of a critical condition in bovine animals. The occurrence of cow mortality is infrequent, particularly in cases when calving has taken place without any direct observation. The prolapsed uterus often exhibits significant contamination, including the presence of bedding material, fecal matter, soil, and placental tissue. Bleeding is often seen in cases of placentome or endometrial injuries that result from exposure. If the affected cow can stand and walk, the massive organ hangs near the hocks and can be stretched, traumatized, or lacerated as it flops against the rear quarters.

Uterine prolapse is considered a critical condition in bovines, a timely identification and prompt intervention significantly improves the overall prognosis. When notified of the condition, it is recommended that the veterinarian provide instructions to the owner about maintaining a calm environment for the cow as well as the cleansing and moistening of the exposed organ. A solution of warm water with a 1% concentration of iodine together with a clean towel or sheet will serve the purpose. If feasible, it may be advisable to encourage the owner to raise the organ to the level of ischium or higher to alleviate vascular compromise and consequent edema as well as reduce the risk of damage. The administration of calcium, the choice between repositioning the mass in a recumbent or standing position, the timing of medication administration, and the provision of aftercare are all aspects of specific therapy that exhibit significant individual variation.

The occurrence of edema, tissue damage, and inflammatory changes occur rapidly in a protruded uterine mass, so the early replacement of the prolapsed mass is essential to avoid further complications. An epidural anesthetic (5–7 ml of 2% lignocaine) is administered to relieve tenesmus and avoid resistance by the cow during replacement. The reduction of edema may be achieved with ice packs or hypertonic salt or alum solutions before replacement. The infusion of oxytocin directly into the uterine musculature during pregnancy has been proposed as a potential method for reducing uterine size (Kumar et al. 2013), but it will become difficult to replace the uterus due to its increased tonicity. Fluid therapy and corticosteroids can be given to animals if the overall condition of the animal is suboptimal for stabilization. To relieve the bladder, it is recommended to elevate the uterus, which alleviates pressure on the external urinary meatus (Gnanasubramanian et al. 2000). The insertion of a urinary catheter is recommended in cases when there is impaired urinary flow (Arun et al. 2018). It is essential to ensure that the uterus is placed on a clean sheet of plastic or a sterile cloth. The prolapsed mass should be properly wrapped with a clean cloth to maintain moisture and prevent any unwanted harm to the tissue.

The everted uterine mass is washed with fresh water containing potassium permanganate at a ratio of 1 : 1000 to remove all the dirt and tissue debris present. The lacerations, if any, need to be sutured using chromic catgut. To reduce post-replacement straining, it is recommended to use soft emollient lotions topically and locally apply 4% lignocaine,. To prevent any damage to the uterine wall or delicate cotyledons, it is essential to perform the replacement of the uterus with extreme caution and gentleness. In most situations, the manual repositioning of the uterus may be achieved by inverting the organ from its base and progressing toward its apex. The repositioning of the uterus becomes easier when the animal is in an upright position (Ishi et al. 2010). If the animal is not able to stand, then elevating the hindquarters makes it easier to correct the condition by reducing abdominal pressure (Ishi et al. 2010). The administration of 2–5 l of warm saline into the uterus aids in the repositioning of the organ to its original position as a result of gravitational forces (Miesner and Anderson 2008). It is necessary to remove the surplus fluid by siphoning.

The persistent straining and necrosis of the uterus may be seen if the mass is not properly reduced, which leads to the recurrence of the condition (Miesner and Anderson 2008). This can be prevented using various types of vulvar sutures or a rope truss for retention. The post-operative care of animals after uterine prolapse replacement is dependent upon the animal's health and the duration between the occurrence of the prolapse and its subsequent repositioning. The advised treatment includes the administration of antibiotics, fluid replacements, antihistamines, and uterine motility stimulants such as 20 IU of oxytocin intramuscularly. The administration of intravenous infusions of calcium borogluconate is recommended due to the prevalence of hypocalcemia in animals. Furthermore, the administration of calcium infusions has been shown to enhance myometrial motility, which increases the likelihood of the uterus recovering its normal size and shape. In cases of prolonged uterine prolapse characterized by severe necrosis, circumferential lacerations, and closure of the cervix when repositioning is not feasible, amputating the prolapsed uterus should be considered (Ghuman et al. 2010).

The prognosis for an uncomplicated uterine prolapse in cows is generally favorable, with a high likelihood of successful breeding with the regular monitoring and treatment of metritis. Moreover, there is no evidence to suggest that dairy cows that have had prolapses are more likely to encounter the same issue during subsequent calving. A significant proportion, namely 75% or more, of cows that experience uterine prolapse are expected to have positive outcomes. Among cows that exhibit poor health, a small proportion will experience a recurrence of their condition within a span of 1–3 days. In addition, some cows are unable to be replaced, while others succumb to complications such as intestinal incarceration within the prolapse or fatal bleeding. Furthermore, some cows develop severe peritonitis or perimetritis due to uterine tears, and some cause permanent harm to the prolapsed organ. It is important to inform the owner of the potential fatality of the cow, which may occur either during or after the replacement process, particularly when signs of shock are evident. A repeated prolapse is indicative of a very unfavorable condition, and cows who have recurrent prolapse after the initial repair often exhibit poor outcomes. It is advisable to perform follow-up examinations on all patients with prolapse 3 days after correction to evaluate their general systemic condition and provide targeted advice about metritis or uterine damage. Furthermore, cows with uterine prolapse have a favorable prognosis and chances of conception, if treated early in the correct manner (Carluccio et al. 2020; Ishii et al. 2010).

14.4.2 Vaginal Cystocele

Vaginal cystocele refers to a condition when the bladder is positioned into the vagina or vulva in parturient mares and cows. The condition is encountered in two forms, the first type, which is more common in mares due to the high degree of urethral dilatability and the force used during straining, is bladder protrusion through the urethra. In the second type, the bladder is located inside the vagina, which entails the bladder protruding through a tear in the vaginal floor (Figure 14.2). Here, the serous coat will be the bladder's outermost layer, which is different from the first. The difference between the bladder and the uterus must be understood. This phenomenon is more commonly seen in equine species and is

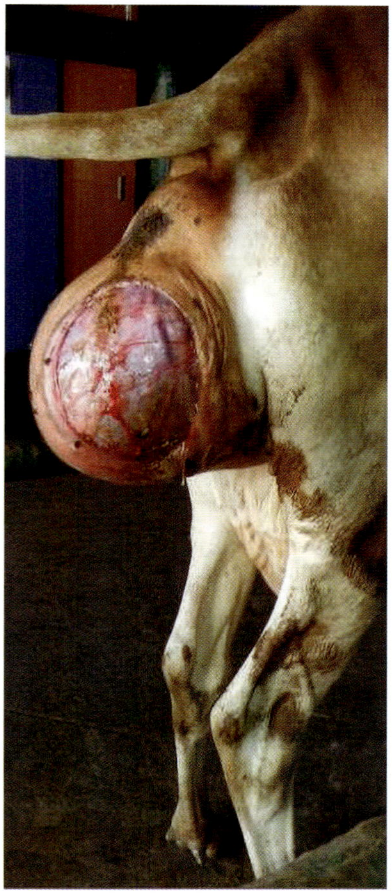

Figure 14.2 Vaginal cystocele in nondescript cattle. *Source:* Rajesh Kumar.

less common in bovine species, whereby the occurrence of a prolapsed bladder and the velvety (villous) texture of the allantochorion exhibit striking similarities sometimes referred to as a "red bag" presentation. In both conditions, the primary objective is to alleviate tension, which is most effectively achieved with the administration of an epidural anesthetic, with or without the concurrent use of sedation (Kumar et al. 2018).

Animals suffering from vaginal cystocele may exhibit symptoms such as urinary difficulties, increased frequency of urination, and exertion during the act of urination since the cystocele hinders the regular passage of urine. Cows that have been impacted may also exhibit indications of distress, such as experiencing abdominal pain or observable swelling in nearby areas of the udder. In instances of significant severity, the presence of a cystocele may result in urinary tract infections or urinary retention in cows, which pose a life-threatening situation if not properly attended to. The diagnosis of vaginal cystocele in cattle frequently involves a comprehensive approach that incorporates clinical examination and diagnostic imaging techniques. During the process of observation, the veterinarian may detect visible signs, such as the protrusion of the bladder into the vaginal canal, distension of the abdomen, or indicators of pain, during the examination. A thorough history, with any associated reproductive or urinary concerns, might provide significant information. To confirm the diagnosis, the veterinarian may perform further examinations, such as a vaginoscopy, to directly see the cystocele and evaluate its extent. The use of ultrasonography or radiography may provide further assistance in assessing the magnitude of the condition and ruling out possible causes for the observed symptoms. Once a diagnosis of vaginal cystocele has been reliably made, relevant treatment options may be explored to effectively manage the condition and enhance the overall welfare of the animal.

It is essential to promptly provide treatment to the animal to mitigate any problems and save its life. An epidural anesthetic, namely lignocaine hydrochloride 2% at 5 ml, may be administered to alleviate excessive straining and promote the efficient retraction of the protruded organ. Following the casting of the animal in a recumbent position, a big towel is used to cover the bladder to minimize the risk of further contamination. A preliminary administration of calcium borogluconate at 450 ml is administered through the intramuscular and subcutaneous routes to alleviate ruminal tympany. The prolapsed mass undergoes a cleansing process using a potassium permanganate solution at a ratio of 1 : 1000 (Khurma et al. 2016), while simultaneously ensuring the removal of any accompanying debris. The bladder surface is cleansed, and then pierced using 16-gauge needles to facilitate urine drainage. Following this, an antibiotic powder is applied to the bladder, and it is carefully repositioned via the vaginal rupture. The ruptured vaginal floor is surgically repaired using chromic catgut no. 2 under the guidance of a vaginal speculum. Approximately 1 hour later, the epidural anesthesia is administered again using a mixture of 2% lignocaine hydrochloride and 0.1 ml xylazine to prolong its effects and prevent the recurrence of prolapse. Additionally, vulvar sutures are applied to further support the repair. Parenteral and oral therapy is provided, including antibiotics, antihistamines, and vitamin supplementation as well as antispasmodics. The vulvar suture can be removed after 7 days or complete healing.

14.4.3 Postpartum Hemorrhage

Postpartum hemorrhage can arise as a result of various factors, such as trauma, lacerations, or tissue ripping. Hemorrhage can occur as a result of the vigorous manipulation of a retained placenta or intrauterine interventions (Markandeya 2011). Postpartum hemorrhage is typical to some extent, but when there is a significant discharge of fresh blood within 24–36 hours of calving, it can be potentially fatal. This is typically caused by the rupture of maternal cotyledon, blood vessels, or trauma to the birth canal following difficulties during labor. The timely identification and management of this condition is essential to prevent the development of shock in the animal and subsequent mortality. It is recommended to perform an examination of the birth canal utilizing a vaginoscope or vaginal speculum to identify the traumatic lesion and if feasible, secure the bleeding spots with ligation. In cases of significant blood loss during calving, it is recommended to consider the use of ice or the infusion of cold normal saline in conjunction with epinephrine. The administration of oxytocin at a dosage of 20 IU through the intramuscular or intravenous route, along with an intravenous infusion of 250–500 ml of calcium borogluconate, is generally beneficial. Severe hemorrhage promptly leads to shock characterized by a weak pulse, cyanotic mucous membranes, cooled extremities, elevated respiratory rate, and reduced urine output, as observed in clinical settings (Markandeya 2011). The use of fluid replacements, hemostats, corticosteroids, and antibiotics is recommended. The utilization of iron–dextran (Salem and Soliman 1979) and iron–sorbitol–citric acid complex (Sarma et al. 2008) has been proposed as an alternative therapy for hemorrhagic problems. Cervical bleeding can occur in cases of cervical dilatation failure as the application of excessive force during traction can lead to the rupture of major blood arteries within the birth canal. The prevention of cervical bleeding can be achieved with local pressure, cold fomentation, and ligation techniques. The retraction of the cervix is recommended as a method for ligating major blood arteries.

14.4.4 Hematoma/Edema

The occurrence of hematomas in the birth canal or vulva in animals is unusual. Typically, these conditions are left untreated, with a general approach that involves the use of anti-inflammatory and analgesic medications. Such local injuries often resolve within 5–10 days. However, in cases when the size and severity are increased, it may be necessary to perform an incision to remove the clots, and then suture the affected area. Vulvar edema can occur as a result of dystocia, improper handling during calving, or as a consequence of using a truss to avoid vaginal prolapse. Typically, edema tends to resolve independently. However, in cases when the edema is widespread, it is recommended to use cold fomentation, diuretics, and anti-inflammatory medications for 3–5 days. The occurrence of vulvar abscesses in animals can happen a few days following parturition, and treatment options include the administration of antibiotics or surgical excision.

References

Aanes, W.A. (1964). Surgical repair of third degree perineal laceration and rectovaginal fistula in the mare. *Journal of the American Veterinary Medical Association* 144: 485–491.

Abdullah, F.F.J., Adamu, L., and Hashim, N.H.B. (2014). Surgical management of a second degree perineal laceration in a buffalo sequel to dystocia. *International Journal of Livestock Research* 4: 146–150.

Adams, S.B. and Fessler, J.F. (ed.) (2000). Third-degree perineal laceration repair. In: *Atlas of Equine Surgery*, 1e, 241–244. Philadelphia, London, Toronto, Sydney: W.B. Saunders Co.

Arthur, G.H., Noakes, D.E., and Pearson, H. (1996). Perineal injuries at parturition. In: *Veterinary Reproduction and Obstetrics*, 7e (ed. G.H. Arthur, D.E. Noakes, H. Pearson, and T.J. Parkinson), 279–284. London: Bailliere Tindall.

Arun, R., Amarna, K., Kumar, D.V., and Bharathi, S. (2018). Management of total uterine prolapse in Jaffarabadi she buffalo: a case report. *Theriogenology Insight* 8: 37–38.

Awad, R. and Esam, M. (2016). Occurrence and surgical reconstruction of perineal lacerations and rectovaginal fistulae in dairy cows. *Journal of Advanced Veterinary Research* 6 (4): 123–129.

Azawi, O.I., Ali, A.J., and Naoman, U.T. (2012). Uterine rupture with alive twins in a Holstein Frisian cow: a case report. *Iraqi Journal of Veterinary Sciences* 26 (1): 27–28.

Buhner, F. (1958). Simple surgical treatment of uterine and vaginal prolapse [translated from German]. *Tierdraztl umsch* 13: 183–188.

Carluccio, A., De Amicis, I., Probo, M. et al. (2020). Prevalence, survival and subsequent fertility of dairy and beef cows with uterine prolapse. *Acta Veterinaria Hungarica* 68 (1): 91–94. https://doi.org/10.1556/004.2020.00017.

Coulthard, H. (1991). Treatment of bovine vaginal prolapse. *Veterinary Record* 129: 151.

Cox, V.S. (1988). Nonsystemic causes of the downer cow syndrome. *The Veterinary Clinics of North America. Food Animal Practice* 4 (2): 413–433. https://doi.org/10.1016/s0749-0720(15)31057-4.

Dhillon, K.S., Singh, B.B., Kumar, H. et al. (2006). Treatment of vaginal prolapse in cows and buffaloes. *The Veterinary Record* 158 (9): 312. https://doi.org/10.1136/vr.158.9.312-b.

Divers, T.J. (2004). Acquired spinal cord and peripheral nerve disease. *Veterinary Clinics Food Animal Practice* 20: 231–242.

Dreyfuss, D.J., Tulleners, E.P., Donawick, W.J., and Ducharme, N.G. (1990). Third-degree perineal lacerations and rectovestibular fistulae in cattle: 20 cases (1981–1988). *Journal of the American Veterinary Medical Association* 196 (5): 768–770.

Galabinov, G. (1966). Zur Atiologie, Pathogenese und Klinik des Festliegens nach der Geburt bei Kühen [On the etiology, pathogenesis and clinical aspects of post-partum lying of cows]. *Monatshefte für Veterinärmedizin* 21 (16): 601–606.

Ghuman, S.P.S., Singh, J., and Honparkhe, M. (2010). Protrusion of an ovary through vaginal tear subsequent to replacement of a postpartum uterine prolapse in a buffalo. *Buffalo Bulletin* 29: 308–310.

Gnanasubramanian, T., Balasubramanian, S., Joseph, C., and Kathiresan, D. (2000). Vagino-cervical prolapse with partial uterine prolapse in a she buffalo. *Indian Journal Animal Reproduction* 21 (2): 161.

Hartnack, A.K. (2017). Spinal cord and peripheral nerve abnormalities of the ruminant. *Veterinary Clinics of North America: Food Animal Practice* 33: 101–110.

Hudson, R. (1986). Genital surgery of the cow. In: *Current Therapy in Theriogenology*, 2e (ed. D.A. Morrow), 346–350. Philadelphia: WB Saunders.

Ishii, M., Aoki, T., Yamakawa, K. et al. (2010). Uterine prolapse in cows: effect of raising the rear end on the clinical outcomes and reproductive performance. *Veterinární Medicína* 55 (3): 113–118.

Johansen, R.D. (1968). Repair of prolapsed vagina in the cow. *Veterinary Medicine, Small Animal Clinician* 63 (3): 252–256.

Kazemi, M.H., Sardari, K., and Emami, M.R. (2010). Surgical repair of third degree perineal laceration by Goetz technique in the mare: 7 cases (2000–2005). *Iranian Journal of Veterinary Research* 11 (2): 184–188.

Khurma, J., Chaudhary, C.R., Sharma, V. et al. (2016). Surgical management of rectal prolapsed in buffalo calf. *International Journal of Science, Environment and Technology* 5 (5): 3409–3414.

Kumar, S., Bhatt, P., and Dhama, K. (2013). Post-partum complete uterine prolapse in buffalo – a case report. *Veterinary Practitioner* 14: 70.

Lamp, J.H. and Lamp, T.M. (1981). A method for correcting vaginal prolapse in a cow. *Veterinary Medicine, Small Animal Clinician* 76 (3): 395–396.

Marien, H., Gundling, N., Hasseler, W. et al. (2023). Do calving-related injuries of the vestibulum vaginae and the vagina affect the reproductive performance in primiparous dairy cows? *Veterinary Sciences* 10 (1): 43.

Markandeya, N.M. (2011). Reproductive emergencies in farm animals. *Intas Polivet* 12: 142–152.

Miesner, M.D. and Anderson, D.E. (2008). Management of uterine and vaginal prolapse in the bovine. *The Veterinary Clinics of North America. Food Animal Practice* 24 (2): 409–419. https://doi.org/10.1016/j.cvfa.2008.02.008.

Noakes, D.E. (2009). Injuries and diseases incidental to parturition. In: *Veterinary Reproduction and Obstetrics*, 9e (ed. D.E. Noakes, T.J. Parkinson, and C.W. Gary), 308–312. London: Elsevier.

Pascoe, R.R. (1968). Rupture of the bovine uterus at parturition. *Australian Veterinary Journal* 44 (7): 329–330. https://doi.org/10.1111/j.1751-0813.1968.tb09116.x.

Pearson, H. and Denny, H.R. (1975). Spontaneous uterine rupture in cattle; a review of 26 cases. *The Veterinary Record* 97 (13): 240–244. https://doi.org/10.1136/vr.97.13.240.

Phillips, P.E., Plummer, P.J., Krull, A.C. et al. (2015). Diagnosis and clinical management of a spontaneous pre-partum uterine rupture in an Angus heifer carrying twins. *Clinical Theriogenology* 7 (2): 109–114.

Potter, T. (2008). Prolapse of the uterus in the cow. *UK Vet Journal* 13: 1–3.

Radostitis, O.M. (2010, 2010). Diseases of the nervous system. In: *Veterinary Medicine: A Textbook of Diseases of Cattle, Horses, Sheep, Pigs, and Goats* (ed. O.M. Radostits, C.C. Gay, K.W. Hinchcliff, and P.D. Constable), 618. Philadelphia, PA, USA: Saunders Elsevier.

Risco, C.A., Reynolds, J.P., and Hird, D. (1984). Uterine prolapse and hypocalcemia in dairy cows. *Journal of the American Veterinary Medical Association* 185 (12): 1517–1519.

Rizk, A. and Mosbah, E. (2016). Occurrence and surgical reconstruction of perineal lacerations and rectovaginal fistulae in dairy cows. *Journal of Advanced Veterinary Research* 6 (4): 123–129.

Roberts, S.J. (1986). *Veterinary obstetrics and genital diseases (theriogenology)*, 3. North Pomfret, VT: S.J. Roberts.

Salem, I.A. and Soliman, F.A. (1979). Intra muscular injection of iron-dextran in Egyptian buffaloes and its effect on milk production and some hematological properties. *Assiut Veterinary Medical Journal* 6: 313–322.

Sarma, G.V.K., Reddy, S.U.M., Subramanyam, P. et al. (2008). Clinical efficacy of iron sorbitol citric acid complex + folic acid + hydroxycobalamin acetate injection in the treatment of hemoprotozoan diseases and post parturient hemorrhagic complications. *Intas Polivet* 9: 64–66.

Sato, R., Kamimura, N., and Kaneko, K. (2019). Surgical repair of third-degree perineal lacerations with rectovestibular fistulae in dairy cattle: a series of four cases (2010–2018). *The Journal of Veterinary Medical Science* 81 (5): 703–706. https://doi.org/10.1292/jvms.19-0004.

Sidelinger, D., Walters, K., Hopper, R., and King, H. (2018). Vaginopexy: a new look at an old technique. *Clinical Theriogenology* 10: 463–467.

Vermunt, J.J., Malmo, J., and Parkinson, T.J. (2010). Lameness: causes and management. In: *Diseases of Cattle in Australasia* (ed. T.J. Parkinson, J.J. Vermunt, and J. Malmo), 710–713. Wellington, New Zealand: Vet Learn.

Woodie, B. (2006). The vulva, vestibule, vagina and cervix. In: *Equine Surgery*, 3e (ed. J.A. Auer and J.A. Stick), 845–852. W.B. Saunders Co: Philadelphia, PA.

Woodward, R. and Quesenberry, J. (1956). A study of vaginal and uterine prolapse in Hereford cattle. *Journal of Animal Science* 15: 119–124.

Kumar, R., Jaisawal, S., Srivastava, S. et al. (2018). Surgical correction of vaginal cystocele in non-descript cow: A case report. *Bulletin of Environment, Pharmacology and Life Sciences.* 7 (2): 43–45.

15

Dystocia in Bovines

Annadurai Thangamani, Abdul Reshma, Sakthivel Manokaran, Ramasamy Rajkumar, Sarath Thulasiraman, and Ayyasamy Elango

Department of Veterinary Gynaecology and Obstetrics, Veterinary College and Research Institute, Tamil Nadu Veterinary and Animal Sciences University, Salem, Tamil Nadu, India

15.1 Introduction

Generally, the causes of dystocia can be classified into maternal and fetal causes of dystocia. Buffaloes are met with a greater incidence of maternally caused dystocia, whereas cattle are met with fetal dystocia (Purohit et al. 2011; Purohit and Gaur 2014).

Anatomical structure	Cow	Buffalo
1) Vulval labia	Tightly apposed	Elongated, wide apart
2) Vagina	Larger and tight	Smaller and less tight
3) Cervix	Conspicuous	Less conspicuous
4) Clitoris	Less developed	More developed
5) Cervical ring	3–5 in number	4–5 in number
6) Uterine horn	Less coiled	More coiled
7) Caruncles	High comparatively	Less, but comparatively larger in size
8) Ovary	Larger than buffaloes	Smaller
9) Pelvis	Less capacious pelvis when compared to buffaloes	More capacious pelvis, larger area of shaft of ilium, free and easily separable fifth sacral vertebrae
10) Pregnancy and parturition		
a) Gestation period (d)	280	River buffaloes: 305–320 Swamp buffaloes: 320–340
b) Time of labor	First stage: 2–6 h Second stage: 0.5–1 h	First stage: 70 min Second stage: 20 min

15.2 Maternal Dystocia

Maternal dystocia in veterinary practice includes either the failure of expulsive forces or constriction of the birth canal (Sloss and Dufty 1980; Noakes et al. 2001).

Periparturient Diseases of Cattle, First Edition. Edited by Tanmoy Rana.

I) **Failure of expulsive forces:**
   a) Uterine inertia (UI; primary and secondary).
   b) Uterine rupture.
   c) Failure of abdominal expulsive forces.

II) **Constriction of the birth canal:**
   a) Abnormalities of the pelvis.
   b) Stenosis of vulvar or vaginal passages.
   c) Neoplasm of the vagina, vulva, uterus, and urinary bladder.
   d) Vaginal cystocele.
   e) Incomplete cervical dilation.
   f) Ventral displacement of the uterus.
   g) Uterine torsion.

15.2.1 Failure of Expulsive Forces

Conditions	Etiology/predisposing factors	Treatment/management
a) Uterine inertia (UI): Sleeping/failure of the uterine contraction that leads to the failure of delivering a fetus	i) Primary UI: Milk fever, hypocalcemia, dropsy of fetus and fetal membranes, weakness of uterine musculature, age, uterine myometrial degeneration, hysteria (nervousness) ii) Secondary UI: Exhaustion due to fetal obstruction in the birth canal (over size, malposition)	• Oxytocin 15–25 IU: intramuscular (IM) or intravenous (IV) • Calcium borogluconate: 350–400 ml, slow IV • Correction of malposition and oversized fetal parts and forced extraction
b) Uterine rupture	Traumatic injuries at late gestation, presence of weak points, complication of uterine torsion	• Vaginal delivery of the fetus in this condition again can aggravate the problems • Laparotomy should be suggested
c) Failure of abdominal expulsive forces	Painful condition of the abdominal cavity that culminates to prevent straining; the condition includes, traumatic pericarditis, weak abdominal muscles, a tear in the muscle, senility, and diaphragmatic hernia	• Fetus can be delivered by casting the dams on the lateral recumbency or by standing cesarean section, a left flank incision is suggested

15.2.2 Constriction of the Birth Canal

Conditions	Etiology/predisposing factors	Treatment/management
a) Abnormalities of the pelvis	Small size of pelvis, exostosis of pelvis after fracture, disease of the bone (osteomalacia), hypoplastic vagina and vulva lips, narrow pelvis	• Traction of fetus after applying copious amount of lubrication like sodium carboxymethyl cellulose (SCMC) • Fetotomy (Figures 15.1–15.3) • Cesarean section indicated • Future breeding should be restricted
b) Stenosis of vulvar or vaginal passage	Congenital stenosis of vagina, fibrous band, perivaginal cyst, failure of relaxation of the vulva, rarely encountered in buffaloes	• Gel that contains prostaglandins like PGE2 applied over the vaginal wall for relaxation • Episiotomy of the lateral wall of the vulva indicated
c) Neoplasm of the vagina, vulva, uterus, and urinary bladder	Vulval tumor: papilloma, fibroma, squamous cell carcinoma (SQCC) Vaginal tumor: leiomyomas, SQCC, vaginal granuloma Cervical tumor: adenoma, SQCC Uterine tumor: lipoma, fibroma Bladder tumor: carcinoma	• Mostly tumors of the reproductive tract, seldom causes dystocia • Resection or cryosurgery indicated

Conditions	Etiology/predisposing factors	Treatment/management
d) Vaginal cystocele	Rupture in the ventral floor of vaginal wall, culminates in prolapse of the urinary bladder through the vaginal wall	Repositioning the bladder into its anatomical position and closure, followed by traction of fetus with ample quantity of lubrication
e) Incomplete cervical dilation	Failure in hormonal cascade mechanism, hypocalcemia, enzyme insufficiency	• Manual massage of cervix with SCMC • Estradiol valerate: 20–30 mg, intramuscular (IM) • Oxytocin 20–40 IU • Epidosin 15–20 ml • Tocolytic drugs – Isoxsuprine at 200–300 mg, intravenously (IV) – Clenbuterol at 0.3 mg, IV • Tried with partial cervicectomy on the lateral wall or dorsal surface of the cervix • Cesarean section is the last resort to solve the condition (Figure 15.4)
f) Ventral displacement of the uterus	Rarely reported in buffaloes, may be due to prepubic tendon rupture	• Fetus may be present beyond reach in a standing animal; if herniation at or around calving, it is better to cast the animal in dorsal or lateral recumbency to assist the delivery of the fetus vaginally • An alternative is to raise the abdominal floor using a wooden plank lifted by two assistants • Cesarean section must be performed if per vaginum attempt fails
g) Uterine torsion	Most common cause of maternal dystocia recorded in buffaloes at referral centers, predisposed to by both maternal and fetal factors, usually due to fetal-associated factors	Simple rotation of dam, Schaffer's method, Sharma-modified Schaffer's method (SMS), vaginal rotation of fetus, cesarean section, termination of pregnancy

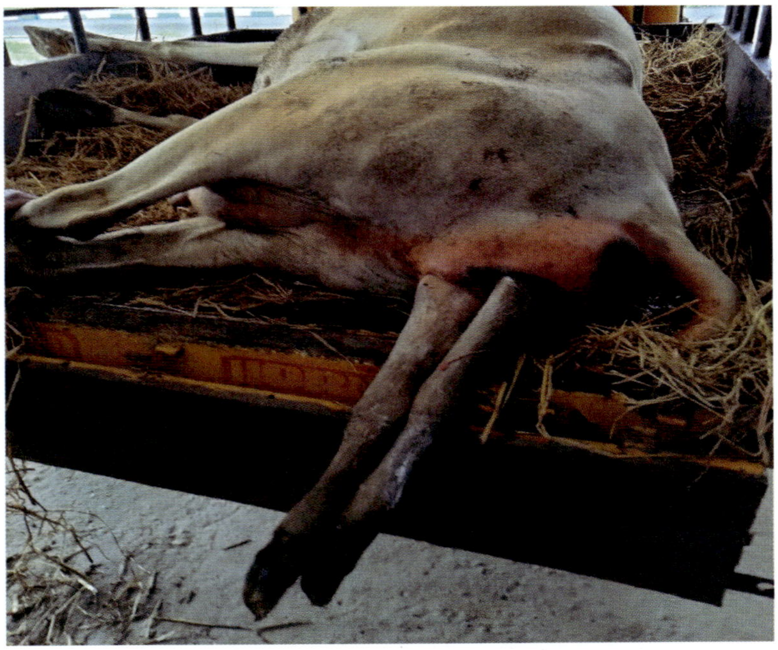

Figure 15.1 Extension of both forelimb outside the vulval lips.

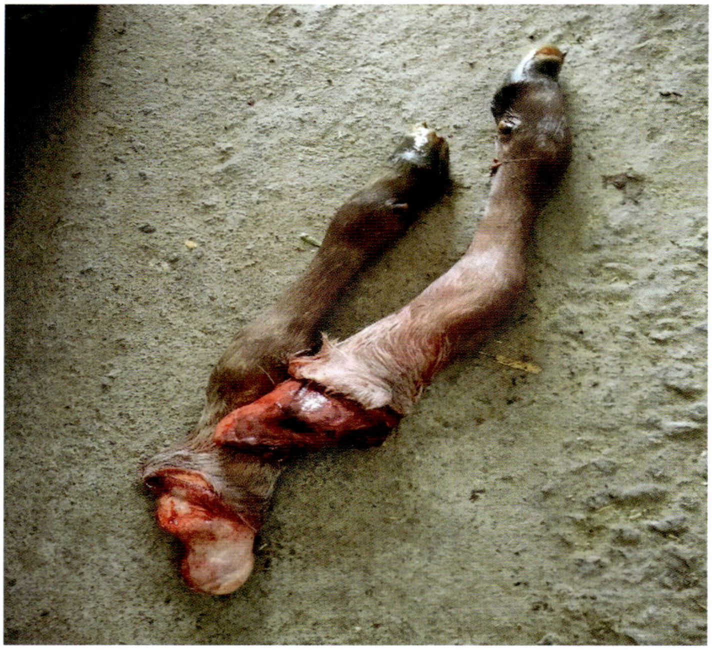

Figure 15.2 Amputated limbs.

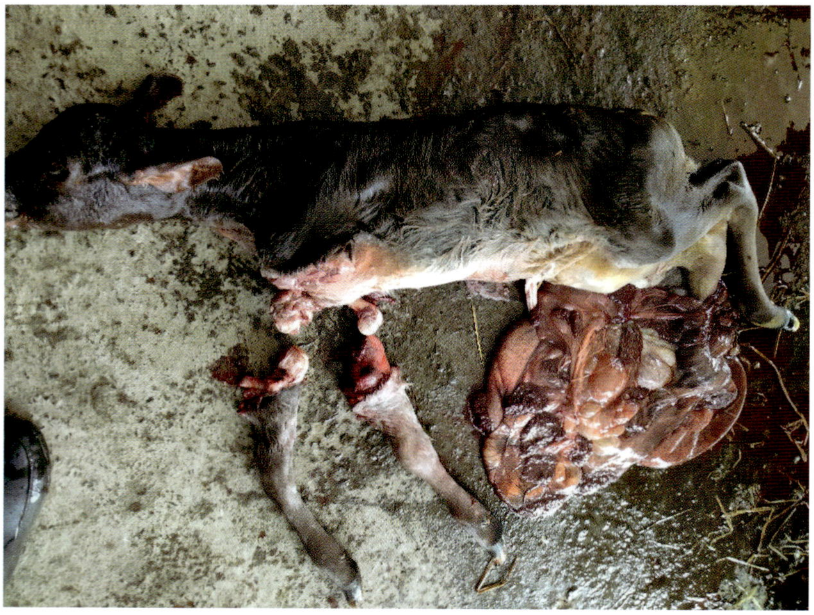

Figure 15.3 A fetus removed by fetotomy.

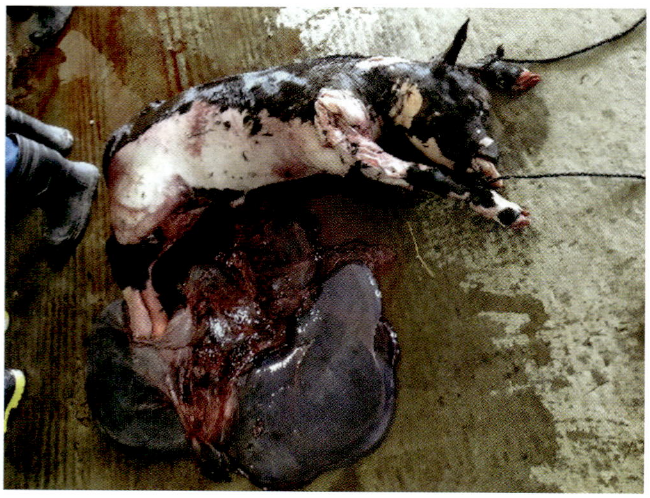

Figure 15.4 A dead emphysematous fetus relieved by cesarean section.

15.3 Uterine Torsion

Uterine torsion in bovines is the single largest cause of maternal dystocia recorded in teaching veterinary clinical complexes, veterinary poly clinics, and veterinary mobile clinics. Diagnostic evaluation of the uterine torsion is by transrectal palpation of the broad ligaments, which deviate from their normal anatomical positions. The success of managing uterine torsion depends on the correct diagnosis and timely presentation of cases followed by medical and obstetrical management. Torsion of the uterus occurs in a gravid uterine horn and is defined as the rotation or twisting of the gravid uterus on its longitudinal axis. The most common cause of dystocia in bovines concerns uterine torsion cases, which are up to 67–83% of the dystocia that presents at referral clinical units.

15.3.1 Predisposing Factors

Predisposing factors for uterine torsion include maternal- and fetus-associated factors.

1) **Maternally associated factors:**
   a) Attachment and musculature of the broad ligament.
   b) Enlargement of the pregnant uterine horn.
   c) Location of the pregnant uterine horn.
   d) Collapsed rumen condition.
   e) Body frame of the dam.
   f) Type of housing.
   g) Sudden movement of the dam.
   h) An unsteady walk.
   i) Age of the dam.
   j) Hormonal profile.
2) **Fetus-associated factors:**
   a) Calf birth weight.
   b) Fetal presentation.
   c) A reduced amount of amniotic fluid.
   d) Fetal movement.
   e) Uterine tone.

Fetus-associated factors are the most probable cause for uterine torsion; moreover, weaker broad ligaments also contribute to torsion of the uterus.

15.3.2 Diagnosis of Uterine Torsion

1) **Post-cervical uterine torsion:** The pregnant uterus rotates about its long axis, with the point of torsion being the anterior vagina, just caudal to the cervix. The cervix is not palpable with the abrupt closing of the vagina.
   - <u>At less than 90°:</u> Hand could be passed to palpate the external os of the cervix with some resistance.
   - <u>At 90–180°:</u> One or two fingers can be passed.
   - <u>At more than 360°:</u> Abrupt stenosis due to the point of torsion being the anterior vagina, just caudal to the cervix.
2) **Pre-cervical uterine torsion:** Less commonly, the point of torsion is cranial to the cervix. The cervix is palpable, and the fetus is not palpable. If less than 90° pre-cervical torsion, the fetus is easily palpable.
3) **Post- and pre-cervical uterine torsion:** Rarely it is noticed that there is partially post-cervical and pre-cervical uterine torsion (personal observation).

a) <u>Per rectum examination:</u>
   - In clockwise or right-side torsion, the ligament and middle uterine artery on the right side are stretched and pulled vertically downward under the uterus, whereas the ligament on the left side is stretched and pulled tightly across the top of the uterine body.
   - In counter-clockwise or left-side torsion, it is contrary to right-side torsion.

b) <u>Per vaginum examination:</u> Abrupt stenosis of the vagina with the vaginal wall spirally twisted, and the external Os of the cervix is not palpable, depending on the degree of torsion (45°, 90°,180°, 270°, 360°, and rarely more than 360°).

15.3.3 Pathophysiological Alterations Following Uterine Torsion

1) **Pathophysiological alterations:**
   a) Altered uterine blood flow.
   b) Loss of viscoelastic (ripening) properties of the cervix.
2) **Altered hemato-biochemical parameters:**
   a) Increased or decreased levels of red blood cells, hemoglobin, packed cell volume, and total leukocyte count.
   b) Increased levels of enzymes like aspartate aminotransferase, alanine transaminase, glutamate dehydrogenase, creatine phosphokinase, and γ-glutamyl transferase.
   c) Decreased levels of serum total protein and albumin.
   d) Increased serum glucose levels.
   e) Decreased levels of antioxidant enzymes like superoxide dismutase, glutathione peroxidase, glutathione reductase, glutathione S-transferase, and glutathione.

15.3.4 Treatment Approach

1) **Simple rotation of the dam:** Principally includes rapidly rotating the body of the animal to overtake the more slowly rotating, inert, gravid uterus.
2) **Schaffer's method (modified rolling technique):** Place a plank (9–12 feet long and 8–12 inches wide) on the animal's abdomen with the lower end of the plank on the ground. An assistant stands on the plank and the animal is slowly rolled in the same direction as the torsion by pulling on ropes around the front- and hindfeet.
3) **Sharma-modified Schaffer's method (SMS):** Modifications were made to the ordinary Schaffer's method (modified rolling technique), and the method is termed Sharma-modified Schaffer's method. The modifications made were:
   a) Alteration in the dimensions of the plank (length: 11.9 feet, width: 9 inches, and thickness: 2 inches) to suit the animals.
   b) While rolling, the plank is anchored by one to two medium weight assistants who stand still upon the lower end of plank while another assistant moves on the plank.
   c) An additional assistant modulates the pressure on the plank by pressing the upper end of the plank.
   d) The animal is rolled quickly.
4) **Per vaginum rotation of fetus:** This technique practiced when there is less than 90° torsion with easy holding of the fetus per vaginum.
5) **Termination of pregnancy:** Medical termination of the pregnancy may be attempted; it will mimic the first stage of labor with prostaglandins, and spontaneous correction due to uterine contractions and fetal movements is expected. Not validated in all cases. Moreover, it may aggravate the degree of torsion in some cases.
6) **Cesarean section:** Irreducible uterine torsion cases directly call for cesarean section.

15.3.5 Post-detorsion Therapy

- **Massive fluid therapy:** Dextrose and sodium chloride, Ringer's lactate, multiple electrolytes, and colloids (hetastarch).
- **Broad spectrum antibiotics:** Strepto–penicillin at 5.0 g, continued for 4 days.
- **Spasmolytic/analgesics:** Flunixin meglumine at 1.1 mg/kg body weight for 3 days.
- **Calcium supplements:** Mifex® (Elanco India Private Ltd, Thane, Maharashtra, India) at 350–400 ml slow IV on the day of detorsion. Ostovet® Forte (Virbac Animal Health India Pvt Ltd, Mumbai, Maharashtra, India) at 100 ml by mouth, daily for 10 days.
- **Liver tonics and iron tonics:** Liv.52® (Himalaya Wellness Company, Makali, Bengaluru, India) and Sharkoferrol® (Alembic Pharmaceuticals Ltd., Vadodara, Gujarat, India).
- **Antioxidant therapy:** Ascorbic acid, selenium, and vitamin E at 10 ml, twice weekly for 3 weeks.

15.3.6 Poor Prognosis Indicators

- Increased levels of blood urea nitrogen, creatinine, and cortisol.
- Decreased levels of magnesium.

- Uterine necrosis, as indicated by increased levels of blood lactate.
- Extent of damage to the tissues and organs, as indicated by decreased levels of antioxidant enzymes.

15.3.7 Conclusion

Cervical dilation failure gives additional challenges after detorsion of the uterus. That can be managed by cervical massage with sodium carboxymethyl cellulose and the administration of 10–15 ml of valethamate bromide (Epidosin®, TTK Limited, Chennai, Tamil Nadu, India) followed by prostaglandin derivatives (PGE2 and PGF2α).

15.4 Fetal Dystocia

Studies on dystocia have revealed that cattle are prone to fetus-caused dystocia, especially fetal maldisposition and abnormal fetal presentations at birth, which contribute to 1–5% of total dystocia cases (Roberts, 2004). In contrast, fetal causes of dystocia are less frequently reported in buffalo.

There are three fetal origins of dystocia in bovines

1) **Over size:**
   a) Absolute (e.g. breed, prolonged gestation).
   b) Developmental defects (e.g., duplication, monsters).
   c) Fetal diseases (e.g., hydrocephalus, ascites, anasarca).
   d) Feto-maternal disproportion (F-MD), an excessive fetal size relative to the maternal pelvis.
2) **Faulty dispositions:**
   a) Presentation (transverse, vertical, or posterior).
   b) Position (ventral or lateral).
   c) Posture, which includes:
      - Anterior limb flexions (like carpal, elbow, shoulder).
      - Posterior limb flexions (like hip flexion, hock flexion).
      - Head flexion (downward, lateral, or upward).
3) **Fetal death:** Includes emphysema, mummification, and maceration.

15.4.1 Maldisposition in Uniparous Animals

It is essential for the sake of accuracy to describe the various presentations, positions, and postures a fetus may assume when it enters the birth canal or pelvis.

1) **Presentation (P_1):** The relationship of the spinal axis of the fetus to that of the dam. Presentations are either (i) longitudinal, (ii) transverse, or rarely, (iii) vertical and refers to the portion of the fetus that is approaching or entering the pelvic cavity or birth canal. The portion of the fetus is anterior or posterior in the longitudinal presentation. The portion of the fetus is dorsal or ventral in the transverse presentation.
2) **Position (P_2):** The relation of the dorsum of the fetus in a longitudinal presentation or the head in a transverse presentation to the quadrants of the maternal pelvis (the sacrum, the right ilium, the left ilium, the pubis).
3) **Posture (P_3):** The relation of the extremities – the head, neck, and limbs – to the body of the fetus.

Presentations	Positions
Anterior longitudinal presentation (ALP)	Dorso-sacral position, right dorso-ilial position
Posterior longitudinal presentation (PLP)	Left dorso-ilial position, dorso-pubic position
Transverse ventral presentation	Right dorso-ilial
Transverse dorsal presentation	Left dorso-ilial

The normal presentation in the uniparous animal is:

P_1: Anterior longitudinal presentation (ALP).
P_2: Dorso-sacral position (DSP).
P_3: Head resting on the metacarpal bones and knees of the extended forelegs.

The normal posterior presentation in the uniparous animal is:

P_1: Posterior longitudinal presentation (PLP).
P_2: Dorso-sacral position (DSP).
P_3: Both hindlegs are extended into the birth canal without any flexion.

4) **Malposture (abnormality in P_3):**

Forelimb	Shoulder flexion, elbow flexion, carpal flexion
Hindlimb	Hip flexion, hock flexion
Head deviation	Right lateral deviation of head, left lateral deviation of head, ventral deviation of head (vertex, nape/poll, true head breast posture), dorsal deviation of head

15.4.2 Dystocia Due to Different Maldispositions

15.4.2.1 Fetal Dystocia in the Anterior Presentation

Dystocia due to forelimbs			
Malposture	**Presentation (P_1)**	**Position (P_2)**	**Posture (P_3)**
Foot nape posture	Anterior longitudinal presentation (ALP)	Dorso-sacral position (DSP), right/left dorso-ilial	One or both forelimbs crossing over the neck with the head in the birth canal
Incomplete extension of forelimbs	ALP	DSP, right/left dorso-ilial	Forelimb incompletely extended in the birth canal
Carpal flexion	ALP	DSP, right/left dorso-ilial	One (unilateral) or both (bilateral) of the forelimbs flexed at the carpal joint (knee) with the head presented in the birth canal
Shoulder flexion (Note: complete unilateral shoulder flexion is known as the swimming posture, whereas the complete bilateral shoulder flexion is known as the diving posture)	ALP	DSP, right/left dorso-ilial	One (unilateral) or (bilateral) both forelimbs flexed at the shoulder joint with the head presented in the birth canal
Crossing over of forelimbs	ALP	DSP, right/left dorso-ilial	One limb crossing over the other with the head in the birth canal
Shoulder lock	ALP	DSP	Shoulder part of the fetus is locked into the maternal pelvis with extended forelimbs and the head in the birth canal

Dystocia due to head deviation			
Lateral deviation of the head (right or left)	ALP	DSP	Head deviated to either the right or left of the fetal body
Downward deviation of the head	ALP	DSP	Vertex presentation: the bridge of the nose rests on the anterior border of the pubis and the forehead is directed into the pelvic inlet Nape/poll presentation: poll region of the head is palpable at the pelvic brim True head breast posture: a ventrally flexed neck lies between the two forelimbs at the pelvic brim, and the head isadjacent to the sternum of the fetus
Upward/backward deviation of head	ALP	DSP	Upward or backward deviation of the head with both forelimbs in the birth canal

Dystocia due to hindlimbs in anterior presentation			
Wedging of hips at the pelvic inlet (hip lock posture)	ALP	DSP	Hips or stifles wedged at the pelvic inlet with the anterior part of the fetus hanging outside or extended in the birth canal
Dog sitting posture (or oblique ventro-vertical presentation; both hindlimbs are extended beneath the body of the fetus in an ALP)	ALP	DSP	All five extremities (four limbs and head) presented in the birth canal

15.4.2.2 Fetal Dystocia in Posterior Presentation

Dystocia due to hindlimbs			
Malposture	**Presentation (P_1)**	**Position (P_2)**	**Posture (P_3)**
Hock flexion	Posterior longitudinal presentation (PLP)	Dorso-sacral position (DSP), right/left dorso-ilial	One (unilateral) or both hindlimbs (bilateral) are flexed at the hock joint
Hip flexion (known as breech or croup presentation)	PLP	DSP	One or both hindlimbs are flexed at the hip joint
Incomplete extension of hindlimbs	PLP	DSP	Hindlimbs are incompletely extended in the birth canal
Hip lock	PLP	DSP	Hips wedged at the pelvic inlet with extended limbs in the birth canal
Shoulder lock	PLP	DSP	Fetus shoulder is wedged at the pelvic inlet with the extended posterior part of the fetus in the birth canal

15.4.2.3 Fetal Dystocia in Transverse Presentation

Fetus lies across the uterus			
Maldisposition	**Presentation (P_1)**	**Position (P_2)**	**Posture (P_3)**
Ventral transverse presentation (sterno-abdominal position or stomach position)	Ventral transverse presentation (VTP)	Right or left cephalo-ilial	All four legs are presented in the birth canal
Dorsal transverse presentation	Dorso-transverse presentation	Right or left cephalo-ilial	Vertebral column of the fetus is palpable at the pelvic inlet and at a right angle to the long axis of the dam

References

Noakes, D.E., Parkinson, D.J., and England, G.C.W. (2001). Maternal dystocias. In: *Arthurs Veterinary Reproduction and Obstetrics* (ed. D.E. Noakes). India: Saunders Harcourt.

Purohit, G.N. and Gaur, M. (2014). Uterine torsion in buffaloes: a critical analysis. *Buffalo Bulletin* 33 (4): 363–378.

Purohit, G.N., Barolia, Y., Shekher, C., and Kumar, P. (2011). Diagnosis and correction of uterine torsion in cattle and buffaloes. *Raksha Technologies Reviews* 2: 11–17.

Roberts, S.J. (2004). Diagnosis and treatment of the various types of dystocia. In: *Veterinary Obstetrics and Genital Diseases (Theriogenology)*, 213–217, 230–333, 337–343, 357–359. Woodstock: Edwards Brothers Inc.

Sloss, V. and Dufty, J.H. (1980). Obstetrical physiology. Obstetrical pathology. Obstetrical procedures. In: *Handbook of Bovine Obstetrics* (ed. V. Sloss and J.H. Dufiy), 39, 105, 108–111, 180–183. Baltimore: Williams and Wilkins.

16

Abomasal Displacements in Cattle

Yogeshpriya Somu[1], *Sowmiya Lakshmanan*[2], *and Shanmugasundaram Murugesan*[3]

[1] *Department of Veterinary Medicine, Veterinary College and Research Institute, Orathanadu, Thanjavur, Tamil Nadu, India*
[2] *Department of Veterinary Public Health and Epidemiology, Veterinary College and Research Institute, Orathanadu, Thanjavur, Tamil Nadu, India*
[3] *Department of Veterinary Clinical Medicine, Veterinary College and Research Institute, Veterinary and Animal Sciences University, Namakkal, Tamil Nadu, India*

16.1 Introduction

Abomasal displacement is a metabolic disorder that primarily affects dairy cattle that were mostly fed a high energy or grain diet with less fiber diet during the pre- and postpartum period. This may be precipitated by conditions like ketosis, metritis, and hypocalcemia that lead to clinical manifestations from inappetence to complete anorexia, a drop in milk production, and a loss of body weight.

The predictive value of clinical and laboratory factors in the diagnosis of displaced abomasa and abomasal volvulus (AV) has been investigated by several authors. The behavior of cows with acute left-displaced abomasa (LDA) is frequently only minimally aberrant, and the rectal temperature, heart rate, and respiration rate are all within or close to the reference ranges. Cows become anorexic, however, and the milk supply plummets as the LDA duration grows (Kuiper 1991). Due to interposition of the abomasum between the rumen and the left abdominal wall, rumen motility is sometimes diminished or absent, and rumen noises become muted. Over the cranial abdominal wall, there may be audible spontaneous abomasal sounds. When air is pumped into the rumen through a stomach tube, auscultation may help distinguish between the rumen and the displaced abomasum.

The abomasum is seen between the abdominal wall and rumen when cows with LDA are examined using ultrasound technology from the left side. On the ventral surface, hypoechogenic to echogenic ingesta can be detected, frequently accompanied with crescent-shaped echogenic abomasal folds. Reverberation artifacts, which appear as a sequence of evenly spaced lines that run parallel to the transducer, are what define the abomasal gas cap dorsally (Constable et al. 2013). The ultrasonographic results in cows with right-displaced abomasa (RDA) and AV acquired from the right side are remarkably similar to those in cows with LDA; the displaced abomasum is located between the right abdominal wall and the liver in the last intercostal gaps. Ultrasounds are unreliable at distinguishing between RDA and AV.

A proper diagnostic procedure is thereby necessary to identify the condition and proceed with treatment. This condition not only affects the production of the animal but also the economy of farmer in terms of treatment cost and animal culling, thereby reducing the national gross domestic product. In this chapter, we discuss abomasal disorders and their clinical symptoms, risk factors, diagnostic approaches, treatment protocols, and preventive methods.

16.2 Abomasal Disorders

Some of the common conditions that affect the abomasum in ruminants are:

- Left-displaced abomasum
- Right-displaced abomasum
- Abomasal ulcer

Periparturient Diseases of Cattle, First Edition. Edited by Tanmoy Rana.

- Abomasal volvulus
- Abomasal impaction

These conditions are commonly noticed in dairy cattle selected for a high milk yield due to their management, feeding of high grain diets to meet that high yield, and their close confinement to save energy.

16.3 Location of the Abomasum

The abomasum is the true stomach and the first glandular part of the digestive system of ruminants. It is located ventral to the omasum near the abdominal floor, fundus near the xiphoid, and predominantly on the right half of the animal, extending beyond the thirteenth rib (Credile and Fubini 2022). The fundus is close to the xiphoid, the body is between the ventral compartments of the rumen, and the pyloric section is inclined to the right to connect the duodenum at the pylorus. The abomasum is largely located on the abdomen floor as an enlarged hollow. The abomasum often occupies the whole right cranioventral abdomen and extends caudally to the right of midline to a point beyond the thirteenth rib. The fundus and body of the abomasum are located in the larger of the two divisions, and the pyloric section is located in the smaller division. In mature cattle, the cranial-most extent of the fundus and body combine to form a pear-shaped sac, which starts 15 cm (5.9 inches) caudal to the xiphoid process and crosses the midline to the left (Brenton and Susan 2022). In nonpregnant animals, the abomasum is wider in size than its length. During gestation, the gravid uterus pushes the rumen forward, which pushes the abomasum forward and results in making it still wider.

The reticulum and ventral ruminal sac, structures to which the abomasum is attached by muscle bundles, are where this section of the abomasum contacts the body wall. The abomasum's fundic region is wider and less uniform, then it passes transversely toward the right body wall, and ascends dorsally to the pyloric zone. The pylorus is the area immediately caudal to the omasum. The fill of various sections of the forestomach, intrinsic abomasal activity, and contractions of the rumen and reticulum all affect the placement and relationship of the abomasum to other abdominal structures. The location of the abomasum is also influenced by age and pregnancy.

As the fetus develops more rapidly inside the uterus during the final 3 months of pregnancy, the abomasal length shortens and the abomasal width widens. During this same time, the abomasum also shifts to a position that is more on the left side of the belly. The uterus returns to its more caudal and right sagittal (nongravid) position within the first 14 days of calving, which allows the abomasum to assume its regular position.

This change is more prominent during the last 3 months of gestation due to the rapid growth of the fetus. About 14 days post parturition, the abomasum regains its normal shape. During this regaining stage, within 6 weeks of parturition, the occurrence of LDA is common (Credile and Fubini 2022).

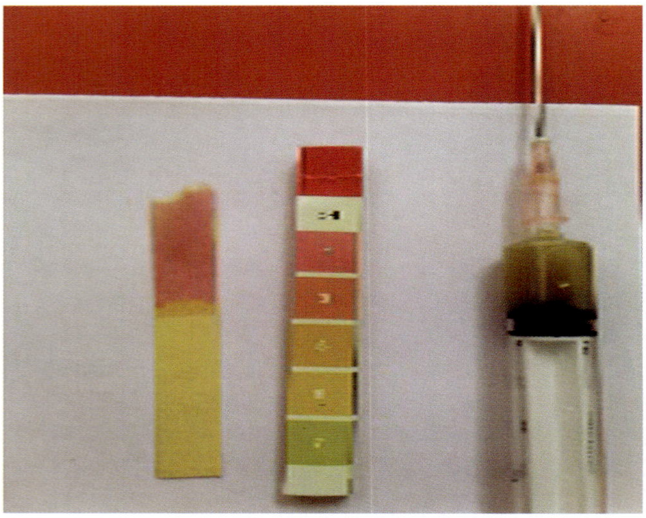

Analysis of pH of abomasal fluid

16.4 Special Diagnostic Techniques

16.4.1 Abomasocentesis

Diagnostic accuracy could be further improved using a combination of abomasocentesis and rumenocentesis with a pH measurement of the aspirated fluid (Gouda et al. 2020).

The sample should be collected 20 cm caudal to the xiphoid process and 5–10 cm lateral to the midline on the right side. Upon evaluation of the pH of the abomasal fluid, it should be acidic with a range of 1.4–4.5.

16.4.2 Ultrasonography

Upon an ultrasound examination on either the left or right side of the midline, the abomasum can be visualized as heterogeneous because of its contents and differentiated from adjacent structures. The abomasum is found between the abdominal wall and rumen, according to an ultrasonographic examination of cows with LDA from the left side (Braun 2009). On the ventral surface, hypoechogenic to echogenic ingesta can be detected that are frequently accompanied by crescent-shaped echogenic abomasal folds. Reverberation artifacts, which appear as a sequence of evenly spaced lines that run parallel to the transducer, are what define the abomasal gas cap dorsally. The ultrasonographic findings in cows with RDA and AV acquired from the right side resemble those in cows with LDA almost exactly; in the last intercostal gaps, the displaced abomasum is located between the right abdominal wall and the liver (Braun and Feller 2008). An ultrasound is unreliable for distinguishing between RDA and AV.

16.5 Left Displacement of the Abomasum

16.5.1 Etiology

- Feeding a high grain diet increases the production of volatile fatty acids, which inhibit the motility of the abomasum to cause gas accumulation and displacement of the abomasum (Constable et al. 2017).
- A reduced rumen volume.
- Diseases like ketosis, retained placentas, metritis, still births, and parturient paresis lead to inappetence, reduced feed intake, and a decreased rumen volume, which predispose the animal to abomasal displacement.
- A decreased plasma calcium concentration around parturition leads to hypomotility of the abomasum, which may result in its displacement.

16.5.2 Risk Factors

Feeding a high concentrate and low roughage diet during the pre- and postpartum periods causes distension and hypomotility of the abomasum (Coppock 1974; Caixeta et al. 2018). The 3–6 weeks following parturition is the critical period in which LDA occurs.

16.5.3 Clinical Signs

- Inappetence.
- Complete anorexia.
- Gradual drop in milk production.
- Signs of ketosis (when treated, relapse occurs).
- Reduced fecal output and pasty dung (Parish 2022).
- Complete refusal of concentrate and a minimum intake of roughage (Parish 2022).

16.5.4 Diagnosis

16.5.4.1 Clinical Examination

- A high-pitched, fluid splashing sound is noticed upon simultaneous auscultation on the upper third of the nineth to twelfth ribs and ballottement of the left lower abdomen just below the paralumbar fossa.
- Simultaneous auscultation and percussion with a plexor or a sharp thump with one's finger between the nineth and thirteenth rib on its upper half reveals a high-pitched ping (tympanitis) sound; this is the characteristic feature of LDA (Parish 2022).
- Simultaneous auscultation on the upper third of the nineth to twelfth ribs and palpation of the left paralumbar fossa for the movement of the dorsal sac of the rumen (Constable et al. 2017).
- A slab-sided abdomen is noticed on the left side because of the smaller rumen size, which is displaced medially by the abomasum (Parish 2022).
- Hypermotility or irregular frequency of abomasal sounds.
- A high-pitched tinkling sound noticed in an area marked by an imaginary line that connects the center of the left paralumbar fossa to just behind the left elbow.

- A normal abomasum is located between the left abdominal wall and rumen and visualized by ultrasonography. Between 1998 and 2022, there were no differences in the diagnostic capability of 3.5 and 5.0 MHz linear and convex transducers. The size and location of the abomasum can be determined with great accuracy by ultrasonography. According to one study, pyloric canal visualization is crucial for the diagnosis of LDA (Dirksen 2002). Combining abomasocentesis, rumenocentesis, and pH testing of the aspirated fluid should further increase the diagnostic accuracy. Obesity-related poor image quality and the buildup of fluid, gas, or fibrin in the belly were two causes of equivocal ultrasonographic findings (Li et al. 2018).
- Rectal examination notices emptiness between the rumen and abdominal wall (Mueller 2011).
- Abomasocentesis (Liptak test) is an analysis of fluid collected by centesis through the tenth or eleventh intercostal space in the middle third of the left abdominal wall that reveals the presence of fluid without protozoa and has an acidic pH (about 2–4). In contrast, rumen fluid will have protozoa and a pH of 6–7 (Mueller 2011).

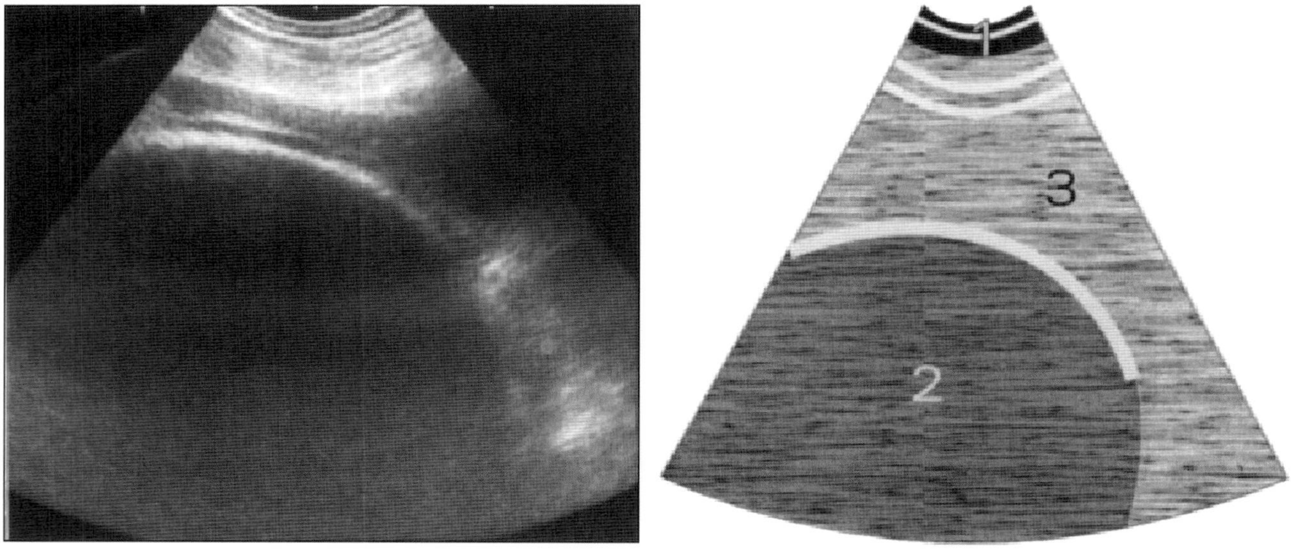

Ultrasonogram and schematic representation of left displacement of abomasum imaged at the twelfth intercostal space. 1 = abdominal wall; 2 = abomasum with hypoechogenic ingesta; 3 = rumen.

16.5.4.2 Serum Biochemistry

- Increased levels of ketone bodies (ketonemia and ketonuria), β-hydroxybutyrate acid (BHBA; 1–1.6 mmol/l), and aspartate aminotransferase (AST; 100–180 U/l) prior to parturition helps predict the occurrence of LDA.
- An elevation of non-esterified fatty acids (NEFAs) during the last week prepartum and BHBA during the first week postpartum are predictive indicators of abomasal displacement (LeBlanc et al. 2005).
- Mild metabolic alkalosis with hypochloremia and hypokalemia (Zachary 2017).
- Gastrointestinal motility hormones like ghrelin, motilin, and gastrin are increased in cattle with LDA.

16.5.4.3 Necropsy Findings

A fatty liver is noticed in cows that have died of LDA. The displaced abomasum was located between the rumen and ventral floor of the abdomen with fluid and gas.

16.5.5 Treatment

1) **Casting and rolling.**
2) **Open surgical techniques:**
   - The most commonly used technique is right-flank omentopexy, wherein the omentum is sutured to the abdominal wall by two U-sutures, 10 cm caudal to the pylorus, by a right-flank approach.
   - Left flank abomasopexy.

- Right paramedian abomasopexy, wherein an animal is restrained in dorsal recumbency to make a ventral incision; after decompression, the abomasum is returned to its normal position and fixed to the abdominal wall.
- Two-step laparoscopic abomasopexy (Janowitz technique), which fixes the abomasum to the ventral abdominal wall using a toggle suture.
- One-step laparoscopic abomasopexy.

3) **Administration of prokinetics and others:**
   - Use of prokinetics post operatively to restore gastrointestinal motility, especially erythromycin at a dose rate of 8.8–10 mg/kg intramuscularly (Constable et al. 2017).
   - Rumen cud transplantation following surgery to improve feed intake.
   - Administration of calcium and potassium in animals with marked hypocalcemia and hypokalemia, respectively (Mueller 2011).

16.5.6 Complications

Perforating abomasal ulcerations and acute local peritonitis with fibrous adhesions occur in some cases of LDA. Abdominal pain and pneumoperitoneum occur.

16.5.7 Prevention

Avoid a negative energy balance and fattening animals during the prepartum period. Treat metabolic and concurrent diseases as early as possible to restore normal feed intake. Promote the maximum intake of roughage during the postpartum period.

16.6 Right Displacement of Abomasum

16.6.1 Etiology

Abomasal atony and gaseous distension due to high grain feed causes dilatation and displacement (Caixeta et al. 2018).

16.6.2 Risk Factor

A high grain diet fed to high yielders during early lactation.

16.6.3 Pathogenesis

A distended abomasum located in the cranial quadrant of the abdomen without displacement of the liver (Constable et al. 2017).

- Dilatation phase
- Displacement phase
- Volvulus phase

RDA progresses to AV when not intervened with as soon as possible.

16.6.4 Clinical Signs

Inappetence, anorexia, dehydration, a history of recent calving, and soft scanty feces (Parish 2022).

16.6.5 Diagnosis

- Upon auscultation and percussion on the lower third of the nineth to thirteenth rib, extending to the right paralumbar fossa, a ping sound is audible (Parish 2022). A pinging sound at the eighth rib indicates displacement of the liver (AV).

- The caudal end of the abomasum reaches to the thirteenth rib or may reach the paralumbar fossa and create a half-moon–shaped distention that can be viewed from behind (Fubini and Ducharme 2017).
- Upon auscultation and ballottement of the right lower to middle third of the abdomen, fluid splashing is audible. These are the characteristic features of RDA.

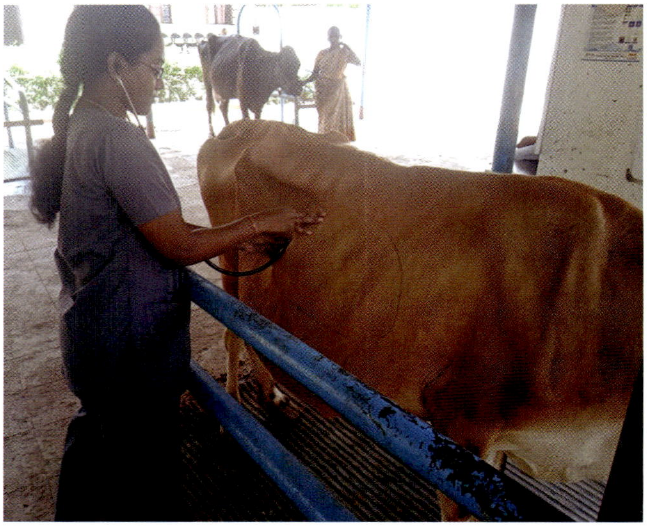

Auscultation and percussion of the right side for a right-displaced abomasum.

16.6.6 Serum Biochemistry

Right displacement of the abomasum reveals hemoconcentration, metabolic alkalosis, hypochloremia, and hypokalemia (Braun et al. 2022).

16.6.7 Treatment

- Right-flank laparotomy.
- Post-operative administration of a prokinetic, like erythromycin, but the use of an antibiotic to increase gastrointestinal motility poses a risk of antimicrobial resistance.
- Intravenous administration of 450 ml of 23% calcium borogluconate to improve motility.
- Administration of fluids with balanced electrolytes like sodium, chloride, potassium, calcium, and a source of glucose.
- Oral administration of sodium chloride and potassium chloride: 50–100 g each.
- Provide good quality hay post operatively.

16.7 Differentiation of LDA and RDA

LDA occurs immediately after parturition, whereas RDA occurs after several weeks of parturition. The dilated abomasum moves caudally and dorsally in the right abdomen because of the high volume of the rumen.

16.8 Abomasal Impaction

There is the presence of abomasal content with less moisture and more volume than normal.

16.8.1 Etiology

Impaction can be either primary or secondary. The primary cause may be the feeding of an abnormal diet, poor quality roughage, or of roughages with soil or sand particles; all of these are factors that predispose an animal to impaction (Constable et al. 2017).

16.8.2 Pathogenesis

Impaction of the abomasum results in obstruction of the upper alimentary tract, so hydrochloric acid produced in the abomasum is unable to reach the duodenum. As a result, hypochloremia and hypokalemia occur.

In any forestomach disorder, it is common to have hypochloremia and hypokalemia.

16.8.3 Clinical Signs

- Anorexia, scanty feces, weight loss, distension of the right lower flank, and the abomasum can be palpated through abdominal wall.
- Heart rate varies from normal to 120 beats/minute in an animal with hypochloremia, alkalosis, and dehydration.
- Increased respiratory rate and expiratory grunt noticed in recumbent cows.

16.8.4 Treatment

- Aggressive intravenous fluid therapy at 100–150 ml/kg body weight.
- Intraruminal administration of 120–180 ml of 25% dioctyl sodium sulfosuccinate with warm water and mineral oil daily for 3–5 days (Constable et al. 2017).
- Right-flank laparotomy for surgical correction of the pyloric antrum and a direct infusion of 100 ml of dioctyl sodium sulfosuccinate.

16.8.5 Prevention

Provide good quality roughage with a balanced amount of grain in the diets of cattle. When low quality roughage is given, analyze its quantity of crude protein and digestible energy. Provide an adequate quantity of fresh drinking water ad libitum.

16.9 Conclusion

Overall, we can conclude that the occurrence of abomasal disorders can be prevented by providing roughage and concentrate in a balanced ratio. The excess feeding of grain results in abomasal displacement, and an excess of low quality roughage results in abomasal impaction. The treatment outcome lies behind the proper diagnosis of each condition and an early intervention. Whatever the condition affecting animals, it results in production loss by affecting milk production, treatment cost, and/or culling (Doll et al. 2009). Therefore, proper care and management should be followed to reduce the economic stress of livestock owners.

References

Braun, U. (2009). Ultrasonography of the gastrointestinal tract in cattle. *The Veterinary Clinics of North America. Food Animal Practice* 2009 (25): 567–590. https://doi.org/10.1016/j.cvfa.2009.07.004.

Braun, U. and Feller, B. (2008). Ultrasonographic findings in cows with right displacement of the abomasum and abomasal volvulus. *The Veterinary Record* 2008 (162): 311–315.

Braun, U., Nuss, K., Reif, S. et al. (2022). Left and right displaced abomasum and abomasal volvulus: comparison of clinical, laboratory and ultrasonographic findings in 1982 dairy cows. *Acta Veterinaria Scandinavica* 64 (40): 1–18.

Brenton, C.C. and Susan, F. (2022). Left displacement of the abomasum. In: *In the Test Book of: Comparative Veterinary Anatomy* (ed. J.A. Orsini, N.S. Grenager, and A. de Lahunta), 1063–1068. Academic Press. ISBN: 9780323910156 https://doi.org/10.1016/B978-0-323-91015-6.00094-7.

Caixeta, L.S., Herman, J.A., Johnson, G.W., and McArt, J.A.A. (2018). Herd-level monitoring and prevention of displaced abomasum in dairy cattle. *Veterinary Clinics of North America: Food Animal Practice* 34 (1): 83–99.

Constable, P.D., Grünberg, W., Staufenbiel, R., and Stämpfli, H.R. (2013). Clinicopathologic variables associated with hypokalemia in lactating dairy cows with abomasal displacement or volvulus. *Journal of the American Veterinary Medical Association* 242: 826–835.

Constable, P.D., Hinchcliff, K.W., Done, S.H., and Grunberg, W. (2017). *In Diseases of Abomasum. Veterinary Medicine: A Textbook of the Diseases of Cattle, Horses, Sheep, Pigs and Goats*, 11e, 500–523. Saunders Elsevier.

Coppock, C.E. (1974). Displaced abomasum in dairy cattle: etiological factors. *Journal of Dairy Science* 57 (8): 926–933.

Credile, B.C. and Fubini, S. (2022). Case 19.2 - Left displacement of the abomasum. In: *Comparative Veterinary Anatomy: A Clinical Approach* (ed. J.A. Orsini, N.S. Grenager, and A. de Lahunta), 1063–1068. Academic Press, Cambridge, Massachusetts.

Delano, M.L., Mischler, S.A., and Underwood, W.J. (2002). Chapter 14 - Biology and Diseases of Ruminants: Sheep, Goats, and Cattle. In: *American College of Laboratory Animal Medicine, Laboratory Animal Medicine*, 2e (ed. J.G. Fox, L.C. Anderson, F.M. Loew, and F.W. Quimby), 519–614. Cambridge, Massachusetts: Academic Press.

Dirksen, G. (2002). Krankheiten des Labmagens. In: *Innere Medizin und Chirurgie des Rindes* (ed. G. Dirksen, H.D. Gründer, and M. Stöber), 473–514. Berlin: Parey Buchverlag.

Doll, K., Sickinger, M., and Seeger, T. (2009). New aspects in the pathogenesis of abomasal displacement. *The Veterinary Journal* 181 (2): 90–96.

Fubini, S.L. and Ducharme, N.G. (2017). *Examination of Surgical Patient: Farm Animal Surgery*, 2e, 1–22. St. Louis, Missouri: Saunders.

Gouda, S.M., Abdelaal, A.M., Gomaa, M. et al. (2020). Diagnostic performance of ultrasonography in clinical management of dairy cattle identified with left-sided ping sounds. *Journal of Advanced Veterinary and Animal Research* 7: 308–313. http://dx.doi.org/10.5455/javar.2020.g422.

Kuiper, R. (1991). Abomasal diseases. *Bovine Practitioner* 26: 111–117.

LeBlanc, S.J., Leslie, K.E., and Duffield, T.F. (2005). Metabolic predictors of displaced abomasum in dairy cattle. *Journal of Dairy Science* 88 (1): 159–170.

Li, X.W., Xu, Q.S., Zhang, R.H. et al. (2018). Ultrasonographic findings in cows with left displacement of abomasum, before and after reposition surgery. *BMC Veterinary Research* 14: 44.

Mueller, K. (2011). Diagnosis, treatment and control of left displaced abomasum in cattle. *In Practice* 33 (9): 470–481.

Parish, S.M. (2022). Non-infectious diseases: displaced abomasum. In: *Encyclopedia of Dairy Sciences*, 3e (ed. P.L.H. McSweeney and J.P. McNamara), 386–390. Cambridge Massachusetts: Academic Press.

Zachary, J.F. (ed.) (2017). Alimentary System and the Peritoneum, Omentum, Mesentery, and Peritoneal Cavity. In: *Pathologic basis of veterinary disease*, 6e. St. Louis, Missouri: Elsevier.

17

Hypomagnesemia

Shivangi Udainiya[1]*, Amita Tiwari*[2]*, Manoj Kumar Ahirwar*[3]*, and Apoorva Mishra*[4]

[1] *Veterinary Polytechnic Bhopal, Nanaji Deshmukh Veterinary Science University, Bhopal, Madhya Pradesh, India*
[2] *Department of Veterinary Medicine, College of Veterinary Science and Animal Husbandry, Jabalpur, Nanaji Deshmukh Veterinary Science University, Jabalpur, Madhya Pradesh, India*
[3] *Department of Veterinary Surgery and Radiology, College of Veterinary Science and Animal Husbandry, Jabalpur, Nanaji Deshmukh Veterinary Science University, Jabalpur, Madhya Pradesh, India*
[4] *Department of Veterinary Surgery and Radiology, College of Veterinary Science and Animal Husbandry, Jabalpur, Nanaji Deshmukh Veterinary Science University, Jabalpur, Madhya Pradesh, India*

17.1 Introduction

Hypomagnesemia is a disorder of ruminants biochemically characterized by low serum magnesium (Mg) (Grunes et al. 1970; Crawford et al. 1998). It most commonly affects grazing cattle, who may be asymptomatic, develop clinical signs, or die abruptly; it sometimes leads to high mortality rates (Grunes et al. 1970; Meyer 1977; Smith and Edwards 1988; Constable et al. 2017; Zelal 2017). Clinical hypomagnesemia may occur when cows are grazing in the pasture under certain conditions (Robinson et al. 1989), but it may also occur at other times. The disease is known by several names, such as grass tetany, grass staggers, and winter tetany, depending upon the circumstances in which it occurs (Fontenot et al. 1989). The condition is associated with tetany and if severe, eventually death, which is caused by a decrease of magnesium levels in the cerebrospinal fluid (CSF) (McCoy et al. 2001) due to decreased levels of magnesium in the plasma. Hypomagnesemia tetany also occurs in younger calves fed for several months on whole milk or milk-replacement diets that provide inadequate magnesium for their maintenance and growth requirements. Hypomagnesemia commonly occurs because of impaired magnesium absorption and may be exacerbated if the animal is stressed, e.g. due to weather conditions or transportation. Magnesium transport between the extracellular and intracellular compartment is affected by stress (Ali et al. 2006), and it has been shown that the hormones related to stress, e.g. adrenaline, decrease plasma magnesium levels. Increases in insulin levels in the plasma are also associated with decreases in the concentration of plasma magnesium, and the rapid change in plasma magnesium levels has been suggested to be caused by movements of magnesium ions from the plasma to the cells (Miller et al. 1980). Clinical hypomagnesemia, in contrast to milk fever, also occurs in beef cows, and as it is associated with dietary factors and sometimes external stressors, it may affect several cows in a herd at the same time (Odette 2005).

Mg is distributed mainly in the bone (60–70%) (Rayssiguier and Larvor 1978), approximately 30% is intracellular and only 1% is in the extracellular space, including the blood (Storry and Rook 1962; Goff 1999). Blood levels of Mg depend on a balance between absorption and excretion rates that is easily altered in cows because Mg in bones is not readily available (Storry and Rook 1962), and only 30% can be mobilized from this site (Alfrey and Miller 1973). In the presence of mineral disorders, it is important to evaluate Mg and calcium (Ca) levels, because both minerals are generally low in the blood (Reinhardt et al. 2011). In cases of Mg deficiency, low Ca values are attributed to hypomagnesemia (Van Mosel et al. 1991).

Periparturient Diseases of Cattle, First Edition. Edited by Tanmoy Rana.

17.2 Etiology

Grass tetany occurs in ruminants grazing early spring grasses, while winter tetany occurs in ruminants consuming cereal forages such as wheat (*Triticum aestivum* Linnaeus), barley (*Hordeum vulgare* Linnaeus), oats (*Avena sativa* Linnaeus), and rye (*Secale cereale* Linnaeus). A concern when livestock are allowed to graze in pastures is grass tetany. It is hypothesized that grass tetany (also called hypomagnesemia tetany, lactation tetany, grass staggers, winter tetany, or wheat pasture poisoning) is caused by a deficiency of Mg in the blood; however, not all animals with hypomagnesemia will develop grass tetany (Harris and Shearer 2003). Grass tetany is typically found in ruminant animals, with lactating cows being the most susceptible (Allison 2003). Grass tetany generally becomes a problem when the diets of cattle are changed from winter stockpiles (silages) to rapidly growing, lush, spring grasses (Caley 1991). Testing may indicate high levels of potassium (K) and nitrogen (N) as well as low levels of Mg, Ca, and sodium (Na) in the soil (Elliot 2009a). Incidences of grass tetany are seasonal and more common when the weather is cool and rainy. Pastures prone to cause grass tetany include but are not limited to a wide variety of warm season grasses, such as orchard grass, perennial rye grass, tall fescue, timothy, and brome grass (Figure 17.1). When grazed, small grains such as wheat, barley, oats, and rye can also cause grass tetany. Lastly, grass tetany can occur in livestock that are wintered on low Mg grass hay or corn stovers (Allison 2003). Throughout the world, there are several types of hypomagnesemia tetany syndromes that can be diagnosed according to the age of cows affected and the etiologic factors that induce the fatal nervous disorder. In beef herds, cows that are older than 6 years, over fat at

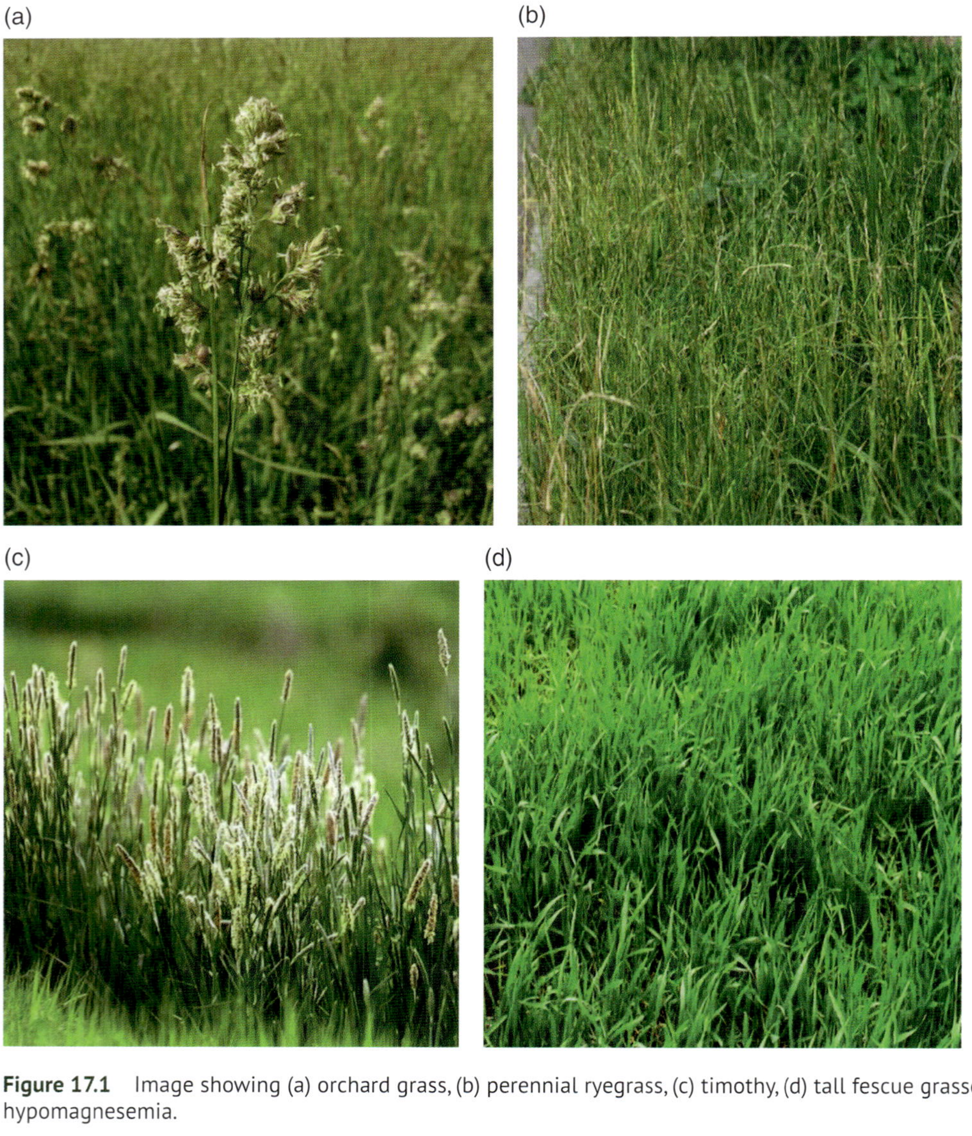

Figure 17.1 Image showing (a) orchard grass, (b) perennial ryegrass, (c) timothy, (d) tall fescue grasses that predispose cattle to hypomagnesemia.

calving (body condition score 4–5 on a 1–5 scale), and lose live weight (up to 1 kg/day) during lactation are more commonly affected by grass tetany than younger cows. Younger cows, 2–3 years old, may also be affected in herds with more complex types of grass tetany syndromes that are associated with low magnesium and high potassium intakes as well as low sodium and phosphorus nutrition (Kronqvist 2011).

17.3 Predisposing Factors

Due to the inability to mobilize Mg from their bones to meet the need for homeostasis in the body fluids, mature animals are far more susceptible to grass tetany than younger ones. The prolonged administration of potassium chloride, however, will lower both plasma Ca and Mg, even in the young animal (Martin et al. 1983). The slow depletion of plasma Mg and Ca probably precludes the occurrence of tetany in younger animals. During spring or rainy season, occurrences of tetany are mostly seen because there is availability of immature and rapidly growing grass or cereal grains. Cool, rainy weather generally accelerates the occurrence of this malady. Tetany seldom occurs when legumes or legume grass mixtures are a major portion of an animal's diet. Legumes may contain twice or more the concentration of Mg that grasses grown on the same soil does. Animals near parturition and until approximately 2 months postpartum are found to be more prone to tetany. Young animals and steers rarely get tetany. Tetany occurs most frequently in beef cows grazing in pastures. Pastures heavily fertilized with high levels of nitrogen or pastures with high soil potassium are more likely to produce tetany-prone pastures, but tetany will occur under other conditions also. Some other predisposing factors are a low energy intake, fasting or sudden changes in feed, transport stress, low phosphorus and salt intake, etc.

17.4 Economic Importance

Hypomagnesemia kills more adult beef cows than any other disease in south-eastern Australia (Champness 2007), and grass tetany is considered the fourth most significant disease that affects southern beef production, after bloat, internal parasites, and pinkeye. They estimated the annual cost to be about $16 million, with two-thirds of that due to increased expenses (Sackett et al. 2006).

While grass tetany deaths also occur in dairy cattle, subclinical hypomagnesemia in dairy cows is associated with reduced milk production and increased susceptibility to milk fever. They also note that chronic hypomagnesemia in dairy cows is associated with wasting, anemia, poor performance, and chronic udder edema ("leather bag"). Economic losses from the death or reduced performance of livestock can be considerable (Mayland and Sleper 1993). Attempts to reduce or eliminate the incidence of grass tetany have focused on increasing the intake of Mg by livestock through pasture fertilization or dietary supplementation. Both methods have limitations. The application of dolomitic lime or other fertilizer sources of Mg has not generally increased forage Mg content (Reinbott and Blevins 1994).

17.5 Pathogenesis

Magnesium is an essential mineral for life and was, for the first time, described in animals by Leroy (1926). It is the second most prevalent intracellular cation after potassium and the fourth most abundant cation in the body. It has various physiological functions, and among them the best function is enzyme activation (Romani and Scarpa 2000). It is also an essential cofactor in numerous enzymatic processes of main metabolic pathways (Martín-Tereso and Martens 2014), an important intracellular second messenger (Li et al. 2011), and participates in osteogenic differentiation (Zheng et al. 2016), neurotransmission (Möykkynen et al. 2001), and muscle function (Goff 1999). Plasma magnesium, just like calcium, is also found in an ionized form, protein-bound, and in complexes, with the ionized magnesium being the most active form. Mg is a constituent of bones (approximately 60–70% of the total body magnesium is present in the skeleton), 30–40% is distributed in the soft tissues, and only about 1% can be found in the extracellular space. Most evidence points to hypomagnesemia as the cause of the tetanic signs observed, but concurrent hypocalcemia may have a contributory effect and even be the dominant factor in many instances. Most clinical cases of the disease have serum magnesium concentrations below 1 mg/dl (0.4 mmol/l), compared to the reference range of 1.7–3.0 mg/dl (0.7–1.2 mmol/l) in cattle, and there is a striking relationship between the incidence of the clinical disease and the occurrence of a seasonal hypomagnesemia. The reduction in serum concentration of magnesium is concurrent with a marked fall in the excretion of magnesium in the urine. In affected herds and flocks, many clinically normal cows and sheep have low serum magnesium concentrations. In some of these circumstances, concurrent hypocalcemia may be the precipitating cause. Magnesium has many influences on impulse transmission in the neuromuscular system, including effects on the release of acetylcholine, on the sensitivity of the motor end plate, on the threshold of the muscle membrane, and on activation of the cholinesterase system. These offer an attractive hypothesis for the muscular irritability seen with the disease. However, it has also been established that magnesium concentrations in the CSF are more predictive of clinical disease than those in serum, which would indicate that alterations in central nervous system (CNS) function are more important than alterations in peripheral nerve function. It is also evident that CSF concentrations of magnesium in hypomagnesemic animals rise significantly after treatment with a magnesium salt. The need for this explains the recovery delay of about 30 minutes after an IV injection because the CSF volume turns over at approximately 1% per minute (Constable et al. 2017).

17.6 Clinical Signs

In cattle, the incidence of hypomagnesemia can be characterized as having acute, subacute, and chronic forms.

17.6.1 Acute Form

Sudden death usually occurs in acute cases, however, if the animal survives then the following symptoms may be seen: an increase in body temperature, increase in heart rate, excitability, muscle twitching, ear flicking, aggressiveness, abnormal gait, vocalization, clonic convulsions, and a frothy discharge from the mouth and nose. During convulsive episodes, the following characteristics are common: opisthotonos, nystagmus, champing of the jaws, frothing at the mouth, pricking of the ears, retraction of the eyelids, etc. (Figure 17.2). Between episodes, the animal lies quietly, but a sudden noise or touch may precipitate another attack. Death of the animal generally occurs within 1 hour of symptom onset (Manju 2021; Constable et al. 2017). Animals generally survive acute cases if treated early.

17.6.2 Subacute Form

In subacute cases, animals remain standing, and signs develop over a period of a few days that include wildness of the facial expression, abnormal gait, excessive blinking, decreased feed intake, weight loss, and decreased milk production. Spasmodic urination and frequent defecation are characteristic. Muscle tremors and mild tetany of the hindlegs and tail with an unsteady, straddling gait may be accompanied by retraction of the head and trismus. Sudden movement or noise, the application of restraint, or the insertion of a needle may precipitate a violent convulsion. The subacute form, if not treated, can also result in death.

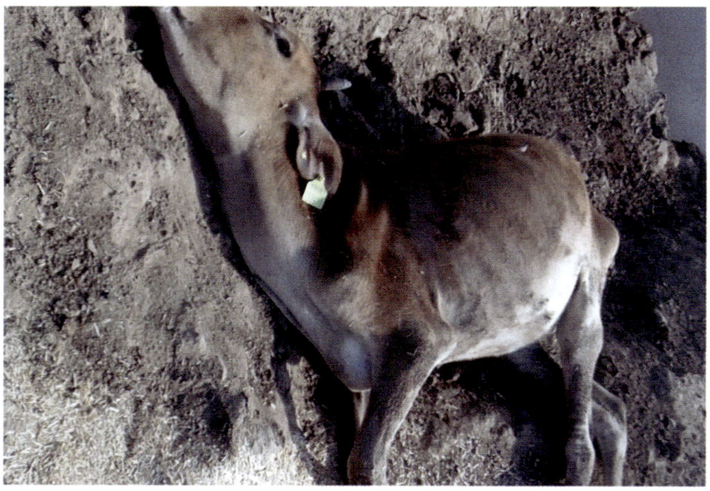

Figure 17.2 A cow affected with acute hypomagnesemia.

17.6.3 Chronic Form

In the chronic form of hypomagnesemia, animals may exhibit the following signs: unthriftiness, weight loss, and decreased milk production. There may be sudden death. Also, in lactating animals, the development of paresis and a milk fever–like syndrome that responds poorly to calcium treatment can be seen. The chronic type may also occur in animals that recover from the subacute form of the disease.

Symptoms of milk fever in lactating cows are quite similar to hypomagnesemia, except animals become paralyzed rather than show violent muscular response. Serum calcium is low in animals with milk fever, which it may or may not be with grass tetany. Calcium deficiency may cause sluggishness in animals, instead of the nervousness they have with magnesium deficiency (Allison 2003).

17.7 Morbidity and Mortality

In all forms of the disease, the morbidity rate is highly variable, reaching as high as 12% in individual herds and up to 2% in particular areas. The incidence varies from year to year, depending largely on climatic conditions and management practices, and the disease is often limited in its occurrence to particular farms and even to individual fields. Although an effective treatment is available, the case-fatality rate is high because of its short course. Because animals die before they are observed to be ill, there are not accurate figures on case fatality, but it is probably about 30% in dairy cattle and considerably higher in beef cattle. There have been few epidemiologic studies that specifically address the importance of the syndrome. In Finland, a lactational incidence that varies between 0.1% and 0.3% has been recorded, with an increase in parity to at least six for lactation tetany that occurs in pastures but not for indoor tetany. No association was found with other diseases, aside for milk fever. In Northern Ireland, approximately 10% of dairy cows and 30% of beef cows have subnormal or deficient blood magnesium concentrations during the grazing season, and hypomagnesemia is considered to be the cause of 20% of all sudden-death mortality in beef cattle. Surveys of beef cattle owners for the relative importance of different diseases invariably rate hypomagnesemia as high in importance (Constable et al. 2017).

17.8 Diagnosis

The diagnosis is made based on history, clinical signs, and a low magnesium concentration in the blood or CSF. Blood is not always an accurate sample in which to measure Mg because muscle damage may cause the leakage of Mg from cells into the bloodstream, causing an artificially high result. Where an animal is dead and hypomagnesemia is suspected, a presumptive diagnosis can be made from samples taken from other at-risk animals in the group or from the vitreous humor of the dead animal. Postmortem samples of CSF that test below 1 mg/dl of magnesium or vitreous humor (fluid within the eye) below 1.34 mg/dl are reliable indicators of hypomagnesemia for approximately 24–48 hours after death. Serum or urinary magnesium concentrations can be used for clinical cases.

17.8.1 Magnesium Concentrations in Serum

In the case of cattle, normal serum magnesium concentrations are 1.7–3.0 mg/dl (0.70–1.23 mmol/l). In seasonal subclinical hypomagnesemia, the serum magnesium concentration may lie between 1 and 2 mg/dl (0.41 and 0.82 mmol/l), but the risk for tetany is not present until the level falls below 1.2 mg/dl (0.49 mmol/l). For clinical signs to develop, the average concentration should be approximately 0.5 mg/dl (0.21 mmol/l). Total serum calcium concentrations are often reduced to 5–8 mg/dl (1.25–2.00 mmol/l), and this may have an important bearing on the development of clinical signs. Serum inorganic phosphate concentrations may or may not be low (Constable et al. 2017).

17.8.2 Magnesium Concentrations in the Vitreous Humor

In the case of a dead animal, the magnesium concentrations in the vitreous humor can be measured because vitreous humor magnesium concentrations remain stable for a longer period of time than magnesium concentrations in serum or CSF. In general, vitreous humor magnesium concentrations less than 0.55 mmol/l up to 48 hours after death indicate the presence of hypomagnesemia in cattle, particularly at ambient temperatures of 4 or 20 °C (Constable et al. 2017).

17.8.3 Magnesium Concentrations in Urine

The occurrence of low urine magnesium levels is good presumptive evidence of hypomagnesemia; however, it is not the most sensitive test. The normalization of urine magnesium to simultaneously determine the urine creatinine concentration will adjust the urine magnesium concentration for animal-to-animal variability in urine concentrations. Further adjustment, by calculating the fraction clearance of magnesium (which requires the simultaneous determination of plasma/serum magnesium and creatinine concentrations), has not been shown to provide additional information beyond that provided by the concentration of urinary magnesium–creatinine alone. Urine magnesium concentrations below 1.0 mg/dl (0.4 mmol/l) indicate a danger for tetany (Constable et al. 2017).

17.8.4 Magnesium Concentrations in Cerebrospinal Fluid

CSF collected up to 12 hours after death can be used diagnostically. In normal animals, CSF concentrations are the same as in plasma, 2.0 mg/dl (0.82 mmol/l) and higher. Magnesium concentrations in CSF of 1.25 mg/dl (0.51 mmol/l) were found in tetanic cows with hypomagnesemia (serum magnesium concentrations of 0.54 ± 0.41 mg/dl; 0.22 ± 0.17 mmol/l). In clinically normal cows with hypomagnesemia, comparable concentrations in CSF were 1.84 mg/dl (0.74 mmol/l) and 0.4 mg/dl (0.16 mmol/l) in serum. The magnesium content of ventricular CSF may be quite different from that of lumbar CSF. Ventricular CSF is also more responsive to changes in serum magnesium concentrations and is preferred for diagnosis at necropsy (Constable et al. 2017).

17.9 Gross, Histologic, and Subcellular Changes

Gross, histologic, and subcellular pathology of the various forms of grass tetany were reviewed (Littledike and Cox 1979). Four principal types of lesions were described: (i) hemorrhagic, (ii) vascular, (iii) deposition of Ca salts, and (iv) degeneration of parenchymatous organs. Widespread vascular lesions, hemorrhagic edema, and calcification in cows with grass tetany may alter the transport of Mg into the CNS as well as other functions, and it may also explain some of the clinical signs and pathogenesis of grass tetany. The extent and reversibility of these lesions at the time of treatment may influence the effectiveness of treatment and final outcome of the disease. Degroot (1960) described alterations in the electrocardiograms (ECGs) of adult cattle that were still present up to 6 months after a hypomagnesemic episode. He ascribed these long changes to calcification in the heart.

17.10 Differential Diagnosis

Hypomagnesemia is sometimes mistaken for other metabolic disorders in cattle. Because of its symptoms, hypomagnesemia can be misdiagnosed as ketosis or milk fever; however, animals that are deficient in Ca will generally appear sluggish, whereas Mg deficient animals will exhibit excitability (Chamblis and Kunkle 2003). Serum Mg concentrations can become extremely low without any physical signs of a deficiency and then any acute excitement may trigger nervous tissue dysfunction to bring about the onset of titanic contractions. Cows can appear apparently normal and then be seriously ill or dead within a few hours (Whitaker 1983). In some outbreaks of hypomagnesemia tetany, there is also hypocalcemia, and although it is less severe than in parturient paresis, there is increasing evidence that the actual onset of clinical tetany may be associated with a rapid fall in serum calcium levels superimposed upon pre-existing hypomagnesemia. This is particularly true for wheat pasture poisoning but can also apply to outbreaks with different predisposing factors. Chronic hypomagnesemia can have a profound effect on calcium homeostasis. Hypomagnesemia reduces production (Constable et al. 2017).

17.11 Treatment

Depending on the clinical stage of the animal at the time of treatment, results may vary from excellent to poor. The quick recovery of an animal can be seen if the treatment is started within 1–2 hours after clinical signs develop. Many animals afflicted with hypomagnesemia die before symptoms are seen. Commonly, 30% or more of treated animals die (Littledike and Cox 1979). The interval between the first signs of hypomagnesemia and death can be as short as 4–8 hours. If the animal is in a comatose condition, then the recovery is quite difficult.

Generally, treating hypomagnesemia involves removal from the pasture and increasing blood serum levels of Mg. The normal treatment is the intravenous injection of a commercial preparation of magnesium and calcium in a dextrose base. A treatment method that has been suggested by the US Department of Agriculture is a dose of 200 ml 50% magnesium sulfate, injected subcutaneously. The most frequently recommended treatment at this time is the intravenous injection of calcium–magnesium–gluconate (200–500 ml). However, it is recommended that an injection of chloral hydrate or magnesium sulfate be given intravenously prior to treatment to calm the animal. There are several commercial preparations available on the market. Mifex® (Elanco India Private Ltd, Thane, Maharashtra, India; 450 ml) is the most popular trade preparation that contains Ca, Mg, and P in the most ideal proportions to meet the normal requirements of a lactating cow. It contains organic phosphate, calcium borogluconate, magnesium, and dextrose (Zelal 2017). Care must be taken while administrating these preparations to avoid any toxic reaction in the animal. Also, approximately 30 g of magnesium sulfate should be given daily (Manju 2021), or 60 g of magnesium oxide (MgO; Causmag®, Causmag International, Young, New South Wales, Australia) should be fed daily after recovery to ensure that the cow's magnesium requirements are met (Elliott 2009b).

An Mg enema is one suggested emergency treatment for affected cattle (Bell et al. 1978). Dissolve 60 g of magnesium chloride in 200 ml of water, place it in a collapsible plastic bottle, and attach it to a plastic tube (an artificial insemination tube works well) for administration. Plasma Mg has increased from 0.65 to 2.22 mg/dl in 20 minutes using this procedure. In addition, it is less expensive, safer to use, and does not require the aseptic techniques that intravenous injections do. Many days are required for plasma Ca and Mg to stabilize within normal ranges after treatment (Littledike et al. 1983). The delay in restoring normal Ca and Mg homeostasis may be the continued poor responsiveness of target tissues or perhaps blood constituents such as Ca and Mg reflect only slow changes in the forage being consumed. A combination of these two processes is most likely. Care must be taken while handling the animal during early stage of hypomagnesemia to avoid creating additional stress. If grass tetany has occurred within a herd, an effort should be made to immediately increase the magnesium intake of other herd members to prevent further losses (Arnold and Lehmkuhle 2014).

17.12 Prevention and Control

The prevention of hypomagnesemia should have two major goals: (i) continuous provision of adequate levels of magnesium in the diet and (ii) maximizing the absorption of this essential mineral. A high rumen magnesium level is achieved by increasing the amount of magnesium in the diet (for example, with a high magnesium mineral mix), and this will allow magnesium to passively flow into the bloodstream of the cow. Determining the factors likely to be important for reducing magnesium absorption in dairy at a specific location enables the recommendation of cost-effective management strategies to prevent hypomagnesemia. Various strategies have been chosen in the prevention and control of hypomagnesemia in cattle (Figure 17.3).

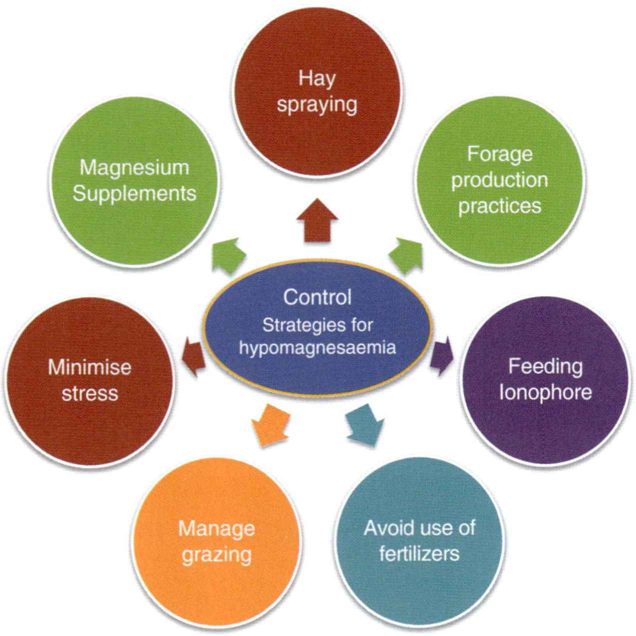
Hay spraying
Magnesium Supplements
Forage production practices
Control Strategies for hypomagnesaemia
Minimise stress
Feeding Ionophore
Manage grazing
Avoid use of fertilizers

Figure 17.3 Various control strategies for hypomagnesemia in cattle.

1) **Supplementation of magnesium:** For the prevention of grass tetany, a general recommendation is to provide a high magnesium mineral supplement during high risk periods and up to 30 days prior to calving (Block 2010). Cows require approximately 17–20 g of magnesium daily or 4 ounces/day of a 15% magnesium mineral mix during the late winter and early spring. Cows depend on a frequent supply of magnesium from the feed since the mobilization of magnesium from the bone is not very efficient. The Ca–P ratio (2:1 is optimum) and energy intake (maintenance or above is desired) of the animal should be adequate.
2) **Ionophores:** Feeding ionophores to the animal has been shown to improve magnesium absorption efficiency. Commonly used ionophores are monensin, lasalocid, etc.

3) **Avoid the use of fertilizers:** If possible, avoid excessive application of nitrogenous, potassium, and phosphatic fertilizers in pastures during the spring (Powell et al. 2013). Fertilizers that are high in nitrogen and potassium should not be given to animals because after consuming high nitrogen-containing forage the animal will produce a large amount of ammonia in the rumen that leads to the conversion of dietary Mg to the unfavorable, insoluble hydroxide form. This lowers the availability of Mg in the blood and tissues (Manju 2021).
4) **Manage grazing:** Manage grazing so that animals are grazing forages greater than 6 inches in height. This technique is referred to as, "holding off pasture until 6 inches tall," because Mg becomes more available in mature, compared to younger, plants (Blasi 1998).
5) **Minimize stress:** Any stress on the cow at the critical time may be enough to trigger grass tetany, such as the first estrus after calving, unnecessary handling and movement, and high fat and protein in the diet, which can depress magnesium uptake (Blasi 1998).
6) **Forage production practices:** In regard to forage grass production for dairy cattle, basic forage production practices can help minimize the risk of low plant Mg or *trans*-aconitate accumulation in forage grasses. These practices include routine soil testing, application of lime to retain a soil pH near optimum levels, avoiding excessive soil K levels, and avoiding the addition of excessive amounts of high K manure to grass forages. Soil tests can be conducted and the danger evaluated prior to crops or grasses being grazed. The soil tests are usually in milliequivalents per 100 g, which need no complex conversions (conyers. M-pers. com. 2002). Simply, the soil tests in milliequivalents can be put straight into the K/(Mg + Ca) ratio and compared to the range K/(Mg + Ca) soil risk (> 0.09 dangerous, 0.08–0.09 hazardous, 0.07–0.08 critical, 0.06–0.07 marginal, and < 0.08 safe) (Elliot 2008). If your soil test contains low Mg levels, use a dolomitic limestone to supply both Ca and Mg to the soil (Hoffman and Peters 2011). Fertilizers that may be applied to raise Mg levels of the soil include dolomitic or high Mg limestone, which contain 12–13% Mg (Reinbott and Blevins 1994). New advances in plant development have led to the production of a variety of tall fescue grasses that are high in Mg (HiMag). These plants are also free of entophytes, which can decrease weight gain and cause reproductive problems in cattle. It was found that the HiMag variety contained 22% more Mg than normal endophyte-free varieties of tall fescue (Au Triumph, Kentucky-31, Martin, and Mozark) as well as 18.5% more Ca and 9% more P. When calculating the risk of this forage causing grass tetany, the tetany ratio was 1.34 (> 2.2 is considered high risk for developing grass tetany). The other varieties averaged 1.65, which was still below the threshold for causing grass tetany (Sleper et al. 1989).
7) **Mg feed supplements:** The feeding of magnesium supplements to cows during the danger period is commonly practiced. The feeding of magnesite (containing not less than 87% magnesium oxide) or other sources of magnesium oxide prevents the seasonal fall in serum magnesium levels (Menzies et al. 1995). Salt–mineral mixes and molasses licks or blocks are the most commonly successful methods. Molasses used in California often contains a large percentage of beet molasses, which is relatively high in Mg. Some molasses supplements are excellent sources of Mg and aid in the prevention of grass tetany. Some molasses supplements contain urea, which breaks down to the ammonium cation ($[NH_4]^+$) in the rumen and increases the risk of grass tetany. Make certain the molasses supplement will help your situation, not make it worse (Maas 2012).
8) **Spray method:** This method of attempting to ensure an adequate intake of magnesium is to spray it on hay and to feed this hay as a supplement during periods of grass tetany risk. The common practice is to mix magnesium with molasses, dilute the mixture with water, spray the mixture on to hay in the windrows when it is being made, inject the mixture into the bales before feeding, or spray it on to the hay at feeding. The level of application is determined by the amount of hay intended to be fed daily and the oral administration of magnesium oxide or magnesium chloride to lactating dairy cows (to provide 10 g magnesium per cow) or administered with a drenching gun just before the cows leave the milking. Stress in any form is to be minimized, as is the provision of shelter during inclement winter weather. Agronomic practices to increase forage magnesium content can be explored. Pasture samples should be periodically monitored to assess the balance between potassium, magnesium, and nitrogen (Radostits et al. 2006).

17.13 Hypomagnesemic Tetany in Calves

Hypomagnesemic tetany most often occurs in 2–4 month-old calves being fed milk with poor quality or no roughage. The efficiency of magnesium absorption falls from 87% at 1 month to 32% at 2 months (Constable et al. 2017). Clinically, it is marked by hyperesthesia, convulsions, and muscular spasms. Clinical signs appear when serum magnesium levels fall below 0.8 mg/dl (Khan 2010).

17.13.1 Etiology

Hypomagnesemic tetany has been observed in calves from 3 months of age and upward when fed an exclusive milk diet (Udall 1992). Magnesium is absorbed in the intestines in calves, but the rumen is the site of absorption in adult cattle. Concurrent coliform- and salmonella-mediated enteritis will hamper intestinal absorption due to reduced transit time. When the amount of magnesium in the diet is inadequate for the requirements of the calf and the efficiency of magnesium absorption from the intestine decreases markedly up to 3 months of age, the maximum susceptibility to the disease occurs, especially for those fed milk replacer or whole milk concentrates or hay and for calves running at pasture with their dams (Constable et al. 2017). Smith (1996) reported that milk tetany occurred in calves that were raised indoors entirely on milk low in magnesium, but since the absorption of magnesium is excellent in neonates, signs of hypomagnesemia do not occur until 2–4 months of age when its absorption has decreased.

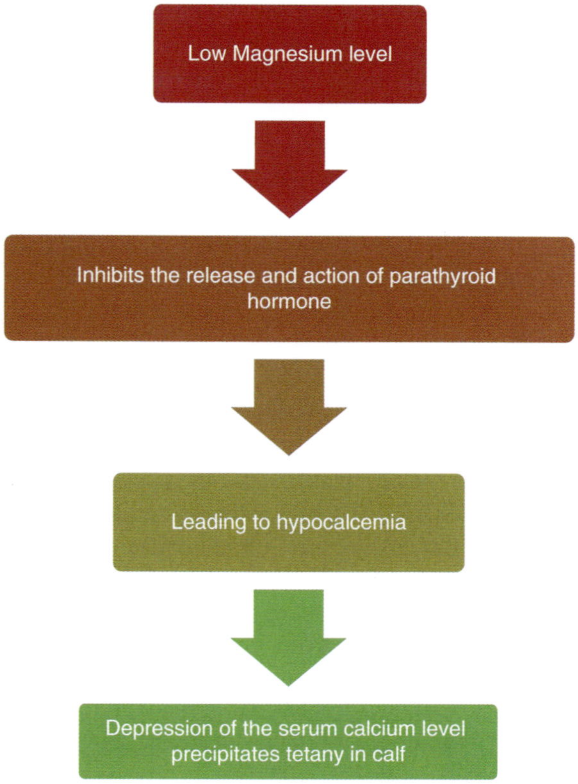

Figure 17.4 The pathogenesis of hypomagnesemic tetany in calf.

17.13.2 Epidemiology

Hypomagnesemic tetany is not common. Cases of this disease usually occur sporadically, or several deaths may occur on one farm within a short period of time (Constable et al. 2017).

17.13.3 Pathogenesis

Magnesium deficiency inhibits the release and action of parathyroid hormone (PTH), which is thought to be the genesis of concurrent hypocalcemia. It is probable that depression of the serum calcium level precipitates tetany in animals rendered tetany prone by low serum magnesium levels (Figure 17.4). Tetanic convulsions can occur in hypocalcemic calves in the absence of hypomagnesemia (Constable et al. 2017).

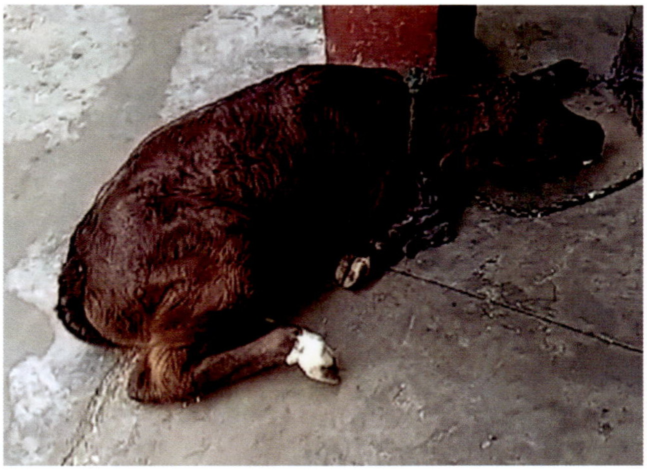

Figure 17.5 A female calf affected with hypomagnesemic tetany.

17.13.4 Clinical Signs

In calves, the clinical signs of hypomagnesemic tetany include stiff walking, nervousness, a great susceptibility to muscular twitching and fright, spasmodic muscular contractions of the limbs and neck muscles, and a partly opened mouth. In the terminal stage, ataxia, hyperesthesia, opisthotonos, and convulsions may be seen (Figure 17.5). Hypomagnesemic tetany in calves is often complicated in field cases by the coexistence of other diseases, especially enzootic muscular dystrophy (Udall 1992; Smith 1996; Constable et al. 2017).

17.13.5 Diagnosis

In hypomagnesemic tetany-affected calves, the blood serum magnesium level is usually less than 1 mg/dl and associated with hypocalcemia, with the blood serum calcium level below normal (5–8 mg/dl), serum phosphorous may be lowered, and there was marked increase in serum aspartate aminotransferase (Udall 1992; Smith 1996; Constable et al. 2017).

Magnesium deficiency inhibits the action and release of PTH, and this is said to be the reason for concurrent hypocalcemia (Schneider et al. 1985). The bone calcium–magnesium ratio is another indicator; normal calves have a ratio of 70 : 1, whereas affected calves have a greater than 90 : 1 ratio. Some affected animals may have concurrent hypocalcemia.

In field cases, there is often calcification of the spleen and diaphragm, and calcified plaques are present in the aorta and endocardium along with hyaline degeneration and musculature. In other cases, necropsy lesions similar to those in enzootic muscular dystrophy occur. In experimentally produced cases, these lesions are not evident, but there is extensive congestion in all organs, and hemorrhages are present in unsupported organs including the gallbladder, ventricular epicardium, pericardial fat, aorta, mesentery wall, and intestinal wall. The lesions are obviously terminal and are associated with a terminal venous necrosis (Constable et al. 2017).

17.13.6 Prevention and Control

The best treatment for hypomagnesemic tetany in calves is a combination of magnesium, phosphorous, and calcium salts (Attia 1999; Constable et al. 2017). To reduce the incidence of hypomagnesemic tetany, preventive measures should be taken by including the supplementary feeding of magnesium with magnesium oxide or magnesium sulfate in the drinking water and vitamin D (70 000 IU/day) (Attia 1999; Constable et al. 2017). The incorporation of hay or silage at 2 months of age will prevent the occurrence of disease.

17.14 Conclusion

Hypomagnesemic tetany is a metabolic disorder of ruminant animals that results from a deficiency of available Mg in the diet or when the serum Mg level is lower than normal. Low blood magnesium can be due to low levels of magnesium in lush spring grass. It mainly affects older, high lactating cows and young calves. Cattle in the first 2 months of lactation and 4–7 years of age are most susceptible, which probably reflects an increased risk due to a higher loss of magnesium in milk. It occurs most frequently in the spring during cool, cloudy, moist conditions when lush, immature grasses start growing rapidly. Morbidity and mortality reach high levels in individual herds. Incidences of grass tetany can be characterized as acute, subacute, or chronic. The diagnosis of clinical tetany is generally made from a combination of history, clinical signs, and response to treatment. A preventive measure is the feeding of magnesium supplements to cows during the danger period. Therefore, based on the above conclusions, the following recommendations are made: Animals at high risk should be moved to low risk pastures during the grass tetany season. Magnesium fertilizer and dolomitic limestone should be applied to the soil to increase the magnesium concentration in plants. In areas where winter pasturing is practiced, the observation that serum magnesium levels fall during the winter and in association with inclement weather suggests that cattle should be provided with shelter at such times.

References

Alfrey, A.C. and Miller, N.L. (1973). Bone magnesium pools in uremia. *The Journal of Clinical Investigation* 52 (12): 3019–3027.

Ali, B.H., Al-Quarawi, A.A., and Mousa, H.M. (2006). Stress associated with road transportation in desert sheep and goats, and the effect of pretreatment with xylazine or sodium betaine. *Research in Veterinary Science* 80: 343–348.

Allison, C. (2003). Controlling grass tetany in livestock. Las Cruces, New Mexico, USA: New Mexico State University, College of Agriculture, Consumer and Environmental Science, Cooperative Extension Service. *Guide B-809*. https://pubs.nmsu.edu/_b/B809/index.html (accessed 29 December 2023).

Arnold, M. and Lehmkuhle, J. (2014). Forage-related cattle disorders: Hypomagnesemic tetany or "grass tetany". Lexington, Kentucky, USA: University of Kentucky College of Agriculture, Food and Environment, Cooperative Extension Service. *ID-226*. https://www2.ca.uky.edu/agcomm/pubs/ID/ID226/ID226.pdf (accessed 29 December 2023).

Attia, M.T.A. (1999). Some studies on hypomagnesaemia in calves under natural and experimental conditions. Master thesis. Zagazig University.

Bell, M.C., Oluokun, J.A., Ramsey, N., and Beckman, G.E. (1978). Magnesium treatment of cows for grass tetany. *Feedstuffs* 50 (6): 24–25.

Blasi, D. (1998). Forage facts: Grass tetany. Manhattan, Kansas, USA: Kansas State University, Agricultural Experiment Station, Cooperative Extension Service. *S-115*. https://bookstore.ksre.ksu.edu/pubs/s115.pdf (accessed 29 December 2023).

Block, E. (2010). Transition cow research – what makes sense today? *2010 Proceedings of the High Plains Dairy Conference*, Amarillo, Texas, USA (11–12 March 2010). Amarillo, Texas, USA: High Plains Dairy Conference.

Caley, H. (1991). Grass tetany. Manhattan, Kansas, USA: Kansas State University, Agricultural Experimental Station, Cooperative Extension Service. *MF-976*. https://www.ksre.k-state.edu/historicpublications/pubs/MF976.pdf (accessed 29 December 2023).

Chamblis, C.G. and Kunkle, W.E. (2003). Grass tetany in cattle. Gainesville, Florida, USA: University of Florida. Institute of Food and Agricultural Sciences Extension. *SS-AGR-64*. https://edis.ifas.ufl.edu/publication/ds137 (accessed 29 December 2023).

Champness, D. (2007). Grass tetany (hypomagnesaemia) in beef cattle. Melbourne, Victoria, Australia: Victoria Department of Primary Industries. *Agriculture Notes AG0579*.

Constable, P.D., Hinchcliff, K.W., Done, S.H., and Grünberg, W. (2017). *Veterinary Medicine*, 11e, 1662–1706. St Louis, Missouri: Saunders Elsevier.

Crawford, R.J., Masie, M.D., Sleper, D.A., and Mayland, H.F. (1998). Use of an experimental high-magnesium tall fescue to reduce grass tetany in cattle. *Journal of Production Agriculture* 11 (4): 491–496.

DeGroot, T. (1960). The influence of the magnesium content of the blood serum on the electrocardiogram in milk cows. *British Veterinary Journal* 116: 225.

Elliot, M. (2008). Grass tetany in cattle – Predicting its likelihood. Sydney, New South Wales, Australia: State of New South Wales Department of Primary Industries. *Primefact 785*. https://www.dpi.nsw.gov.au/__data/assets/pdf_file/0006/226743/Grass-tetany-in-cattle-predicting-its-likelihood.pdf (accessed 29 December 2023).

Elliot, M. (2009a). Grass tetany in cattle. Sydney, New South Wales, Australia: State of New South Wales Department of Primary Industries. *Primefact 420*. https://www.dpi.nsw.gov.au/__data/assets/pdf_file/0013/111334/Grass-tetany-in-cattle.pdf (accessed 29 December 2023).

Elliott, M. (2009b). Grass tetany in cattle –Treatment and prevention. Sydney, New South Wales, Australia: State of New South Wales Department of Primary Industries. *Primefact 421*. https://www.dpi.nsw.gov.au/__data/assets/pdf_file/0008/110888/Grass-tetany-in-cattle-treatment-and-prevention.pdf (accessed 29 December 2023).

Fontenot, J.P., Allen, V.G., Bunce, G.E., and Goff, J.P. (1989). Factors influencing magnesium absorption and metabolism in ruminants. *Journal of Animal Science* 67: 3445–3455.

Goff, J.P. (1999). Treatment of calcium, phosphorus, and magnesium balance disorders. *Veterinary Clinics of North America. Food Animal Practice* 15 (3): 619–639.

Grunes, D.L., Stout, P.R., and Brownell, J.R. (1970). Grass tetany of ruminants. *Advances in Agronomy* 22: 331–374.

Harris, B. and Shearer, J. (2003). Nitrate, prussic acid (HCN) and grass tetany problems in cattle feeding. Gainesville, Florida, USA: University of Florida. Institute of Food and Agricultural Sciences Extension. *DS-6*. https://ufdcimages.uflib.ufl.edu/IR/00/00/47/76/00001/DS16200.pdf (accessed 29 December 2023).

Hoffman, P. and Peters, J. (2011). Grass forages and magnesium status of dairy cattle. *Focus on Forage* 13 (3): 1–3. https://fyi.extension.wisc.edu/forage/files/2014/01/GrassMg-FOF.pdf.

Khan, C.M. (2010). *The Merck Veterinary Manual*, 10e, 505–510. Whitehouse Station, NJ, USA: Merck & CO., INC.

Kronqvist, C. (2011). Minerals to dairy cows with focus on calcium and magnesium balance. Doctoral dissertation. Swedish University of Agricultural Sciences.

Leroy, J. (1926). Requires magnesium for mouse growth. *Sessions of the Society of Biology* 94: 432–433.

Li, F.Y., Chaigne-Delalande, B., Kanellopoulou, C. et al. (2011). Second messenger role for Mg2+ revealed by human T-cell immunodeficiency. *Nature* 475 (7357): 471–476.

Littledike, E.T. and Cox, P.S. (1979). Clinical, mineral and endocrine interrelationships in hypomagnesemic tetany. In: *Grass Tetany: ASA Special Publication Number 35* (ed. V.V. Rendig and V.L. Grunes), 1–50. Madison, Wisconsin, USA: American Society of Agronomy, Crop Science Society of America, and Soil Science Society of America, Inc https://doi.org/10.2134/asaspecpub35.c1.

Littledike, E.T., Stuedeman, J.A., and Wilkinson, S.R. (1983). Grass tetany syndrome. In: *Role of Magnesium in Animal Nutrition* (ed. J.P. Fontenot, G.E. Bunce, K.E. Webb Jr., and V.G. Allen), 173–197. Blacksburg, Virginia, USA: Virginia Polytechnic Institute and State University.

Maas, J. (2012). *Winter Supplementation of Cattle, Part I: Grass Tetany*. UC Davis Veterinary Medicine.

Manju, L. (2021). Hypomagnesemia tetany in cattle. *Just Agriculture* 1 (12): 1–4.

Martin, D.G., Bohman, V.R., Blincoe, C.R., and Hanks, D.R. (1983). Prolonged administration of citric acid and potassium chloride to growing beef heifers. *Proclamation of American Society Animal Science* 34: 320.

Martín-Tereso, J. and Martens, H. (2014). Calcium and magnesium physiology and nutrition in relation to the prevention of milk fever and tetany (dietary management of macrominerals in preventing disease). *Veterinary Clinics of North America. Food Animal Practice* 30 (3): 643–670.

Mayland, H.F. and Sleper, D.A. (1993). Developing a tall fescue for reduced grass tetany risk. *Proceedings of the XVII International Grassland Congress*, Palmerston North, New Zealand (8–21 February 1993). Palmerston North, New Zealand: Dunmore Press.

McCoy, M.A., Hutchingson, T., Davison, G. et al. (2001). Postmortem biochemical markers of experimentally induced hypomagnesaemic tetany in cattle. *The Veterinary Record* 148: 268–273.

Menzies, F.D., Bryson, D.G., McCallion, T.J., and Matthews, D.I. (1995). A study of mortality among suckler and dairy cows in Northern Ireland. *Veterinary Record* 137: 531–536.

Meyer, H. (1977). Pathogenesis of the clinical symptoms of hypomagnesaemia in ruminants. *Veterinary Science Communications* 1 (1): 43–50.

Miller, J.K., Madsen, F.C., Lentz, D.E. et al. (1980). Blood plasma magnesium, potassium, glucose, and immunoreactive insulin changes in cows moved abruptly from barn feeding to early spring pasture. *Journal of Dairy Science* 63: 1073–1079.

Möykkynen, T., Uusi-Oukari, M., Heikkila, J. et al. (2001). Magnesium potentiation of the function of native and recombinant GABA (A) receptors. *Neuroreport* 12 (10): 2175–2179.

Odette, O. (2005). Grass tetany in a herd of beef cows. *The Canadian Veterinary Journal* 46: 732–734.

Powell, J.M., MacLeod, M., Vellinga, T.V. et al. (2013). Feed–milk–manure nitrogen relationships in global dairy production systems. *Livestock Science* 152: 261–272.

Radostits, O.M., Gay, C.C., Hinchcliff, K.W., and Constable, P.D. (2006). *Veterinary Medicine, a Textbook of the Diseases of Cattle, Horses, Sheep, Pigs and Goats*, 10e, 1652–1659. London: Saunders.

Rayssiguier, Y. and Larvor, P. (1978). Mineral bone composition and some elements of calcium metabolism in magnesium-deficient growing rats. *Annales de Biologie Animale, Biochimie, Biophysique* 18 (1): 157–166.

Reinbott, T.M. and Blevins, D.G. (1994). Phosphorus and temperature effects on magnesium, calcium, and potassium in wheat and tall fescue leaves. *Agronomy Journal* 86: 523–529.

Reinhardt, T.A., Lippolis, J.D., McCluskey, B.J. et al. (2011). Prevalence of subclinical hypocalcemia in dairy herds. *Veterinary Journal* 188: 122–124.

Robinson, D.L., Kappel, L.C., and Boling, J.A. (1989). Management practices to overcome the incidence of grass tetany. *Journal of Animal Science* 67: 3470–3484.

Romani, M. and Scarpa, A. (2000). Regulation of cellular magnesium. *Frontiers in Bioscience* 5: d720–d734.

Sackett, D., Holmes, P., Abbott, K., Jephcott, S., and Barber, M. (2006). Assessing the economic cost of endemic disease on the profitability of Australian beef cattle and sheep producers. North Sydney, New South Wales, Australia: Meat Livestock Australia Limited. *AHW.087*. https://www.mla.com.au/contentassets/6359e75d88214978af4273aad56064f0/ahw.087_final_report.pdf (accessed 29 December 2023).

Schneider, K.M., Parkinson, G.B., Houston, J.C., and Leaver, D.D. (1985). 1,25 dihydroxy vitamin D3 increases plasma magnesium and calcium in sheep fed liquid diets low in calcium and magnesium. *Australian Veterinary Journal* 62: 82–85.

Sleper, D.A., Asay, K.H., and Mayland, H.F. (1989). Using plant breeding and genetics to overcome the incidence of grass tetany. *Journal of Animal Science* 67: 56–62.

Smith, B.P. (1996). *Large Animal Internal Medicine*, 2e. USA: Mosby Year Book, Inc.

Smith, R.A. and Edwards, W.C. (1988). Hypomagnesemic tetany of ruminants. *Veterinary Clinics of North America. Food Animal Practice* 4 (2): 365–377.

Storry, J.E. and Rook, J.A.F. (1962). The magnesium nutrition of the dairy cow in relation to the development of hypomagnesaemia in the grazing animal. *Journal of the Science of Food and Agriculture* 13 (12): 621–627.

Udall, R.H. (1992). *The Practice of Veterinary Medicine*. 3rd Indian ed. New Delhi: Oxford and IBH.

Van Mosel, M., Van't Klooster, A.T., and Wouterse, H.S. (1991). Effects of a deficient magnesium supply during the dry period on bone turnover of dairy cows at parturition. *The Veterinary Quarterly* 13 (4): 199–208.

Whitaker, D.A. (1983). Hypomagnesemia in dairy cattle. *Outlook on Agriculture* 12: 77–82.

Zelal, A. (2017). Hypomagnesemia tetany in cattle: review article. *Journal of Advances in Dairy Research* 5 (2): 1–9.

Zheng, J., Mao, X., Ling, J. et al. (2016). Role of magnesium transporter subtype 1 (MagT1) in the osteogenic differentiation of rat bone marrow stem cells. *Biological Trace Element Research* 171 (1): 131–137.

18

Fatty Liver Disease

Subir Singh[1] *and Suman K. Singh*[2]

[1] *Department of Medicine and Public Health, Agriculture and Forestry University, Rampur, Nepal*
[2] *Department of Veterinary Surgery, Medicine, Epidemiology and Public Health, Paklihawa Campus, Institute of Agriculture and Animal Science, Tribhuvan University, Kathmandu, Nepal*

18.1 Introduction

With the rapid demands of producing cattle and a challenge feeding system, dairy cows have been associated with an increase in the incidence of some emerging diseases like "fatty cow syndrome" or "pregnancy toxemia." Fatty liver disease in cattle is a common metabolic disorder of high yielding cattle, who most frequently suffer from it. It is also known as hepatic lipidosis or fatty liver syndrome. This condition significantly impacts both the economic and animal welfare of the livestock industry. It occurs in dairy cattle, most commonly within the first 2 weeks after parturition, and it is associated with periparturient diseases and an increase in the calving–conception interval. In beef cattle, it occurs most commonly in late pregnancy when the nutrient intake is decreased in cattle that were previously well fed and in good body condition (Radostits et al. 2005). Fatty liver can affect cows regardless of their apparent weight at the time of calving. Fatty liver syndrome in cows increases the risk of periparturient metabolic and production complications such as milk fever, ketosis, mastitis, and metritis. They frequently deteriorate and have a poor therapeutic response (Haass and Eness 1984). Overfed cattle during the dry period may develop hepatic lipidosis in just their transition period, due to an increase in the level of blood plasma non-esterified fatty acids (NEFAs) from lipolysis (Gonzalez and Rosendo 2013). Long-chain fatty acids, which make up most of the fat accumulated in liver cells (hepatocytes), are first released from adipose tissue and absorbed by the liver. The condition can be mild, moderate, or severe liver steatosis, depending on the amount of fat in the liver (Kirovski and Sladojevic 2017).

18.1.1 Physiology of the Liver

The liver is a vital internal organ of the body that performs processes vital for life. It is the largest internal organ of the body and has numerous functions, including the production of bile and the regulation of protein, fat, and carbohydrate metabolism (Figure 18.1).

The liver performs a crucial hemopoietic function during fetal development by creating red and white blood cells from tissue located between hepatic cells and artery walls. It detoxifies harmful substances from the bloodstream, such as drugs and toxins.

The liver stores glycogen, vitamins, and minerals, releasing them into the bloodstream when needed. The liver receives a dual blood supply. Oxygenated blood comes from the hepatic artery, while nutrient-rich blood from the digestive system (portal vein) is also directed to the liver for processing. About 70–80% arrives via the hepatic portal vein (nutrient rich) and 20–30% via the hepatic artery (oxygen rich). It has a large blood supply (nearly one-third of cardiac output passes through the liver) (Figure 18.2).

Periparturient Diseases of Cattle, First Edition. Edited by Tanmoy Rana.

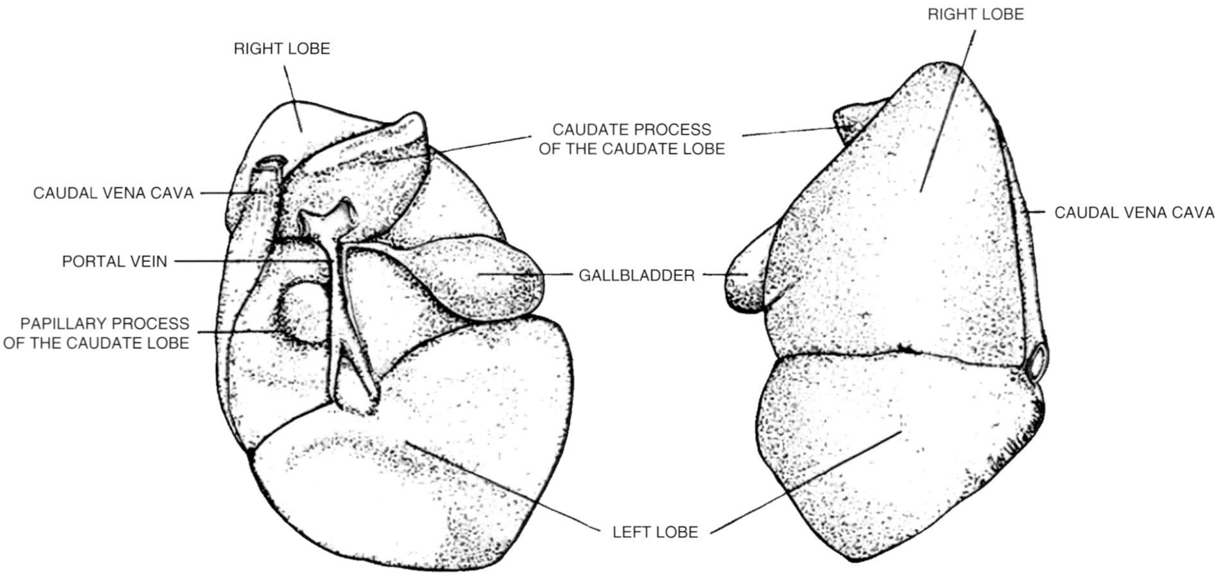

Figure 18.1 Diagram of the ruminant liver. *Source:* Adapted from Sisson et al. (1975).

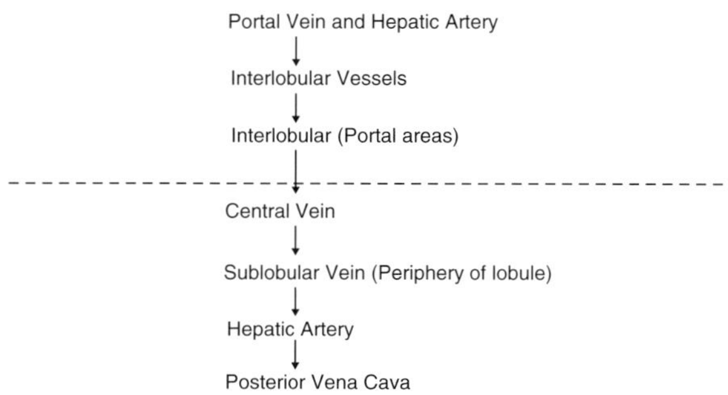

Figure 18.2 Diagram to show that blood flows in and away from the liver. *Source:* Royal Veterinary College.

18.1.2 Metabolism of Nutrients

- **Carbohydrate metabolism:** The liver stores glucose as glycogen and releases it when blood sugar levels drop.
- **Protein metabolism:** It synthesizes and breaks down proteins, converting ammonia to urea for excretion.
- **Lipid metabolism:** The liver is involved in the synthesis and breakdown of fats.
- **Detoxification:** The liver processes and detoxifies various substances, including drugs, chemicals, and metabolic waste products.
- **Regeneration:** The liver has a remarkable ability to regenerate damaged tissue, which is important for recovery from injuries or diseases.
- **Disease and health:** Liver diseases in cattle, such as fatty liver syndrome and infectious diseases, can affect their function and overall health. Proper nutrition and management are crucial for maintaining liver health in cattle. Understanding the physiology of the liver in cattle is vital for managing their health, nutrition, and addressing any potential issues that may arise.

18.2 Etiology of Fatty Liver Disease

Fatty liver is usually a herd problem. It is commonly seen in high producing dairy cows, especially those which are loose housed and fed free choice. According to Morrow (Morrow 1975), at parturition these fat cows appear to be more susceptible to metabolic conditions such as milk fever and ketosis, digestive disorders such as displaced abomasa, infectious diseases such as mastitis and salmonellosis, and reproductive conditions such as retained fetal membranes and metritis. These obese cows are more susceptible to the added stress of disease and frequently die despite treatment. This combination of disease conditions in the obese parturient cows has been termed "fat cow syndrome." It is unusual to see this condition in stanchioned cows that are fed on an individual basis (Bracken 1980).

- **High energy diets:** The over consumption of high energy diets, such as grains or high concentrate diets are at greater risk for dairy cattle. These diets can overwhelm the liver's capacity to process excess energy (De Koster and Opsomer 2012).
- **Negative energy balance:** A low intake of feed during late pregnancy and early lactation causes an excessive amount of body fat to be utilized as an energy source to support production, which may lead to a negative energy balance that causes a drop in blood glucose levels and decreases the production of insulin from the pancreas. Liver enzymes, excess fatty acids, and other energy sources from body stores will rush to the liver, which ultimately fails to convert the fatty acids and others into glucose. Due to the partial metabolism of body lipids, fat accumulates in the liver parenchyma and the surrounding tissues (Wankhade et al. 2017). Compared to other species, the livers of cattle are unable to metabolize triglycerides to very low density lipoprotein (VLDL). Thus, triglycerides accumulate excessively in the liver, which results in impaired hepatic metabolism and leads to fatty cow syndrome (Katoh 2002).
- **Obesity:** Being overweight has serious health issues in both human and animal populations (Daradics et al. 2021). Postpartum hepatic steatosis is an important point in pregnant cows that is influenced by obesity. After parturition, obese cows show a decrease in appetite, which causes a negative energy balance in early lactation that leads to the lipolysis of adipose tissue (Kirovski and Sladojevic 2017). Anorexia in fat cows after calving or any disease and stress condition can lead to excessive fat mobilization and cause a more severe and chronic form of fatty liver. During the transition period, the liver fat blood plasma level significantly increases (Andrew et al. 2008).
- **Disease and stress:** The risk of fat accumulation in the liver following the mobilization of body fat is an anabolic process that triggers an inflammatory response. The amount of body fat mobilization is linked with the inflammatory response, and as the immune system of particular animals becomes suppressed around calving, a high inflammatory response can place the cow at a higher risk of developing other secondary metabolic disorders during the transition period, such as a high somatic cell count or mastitis, metritis, ketosis, and fatty liver disease. Any stress, such as excessive environmental heat and humidity, a lack of shade and comfort, excess mud, overcrowding, and lack of animal welfare, will trigger mechanisms that cause more fat mobilization than normal.

18.3 Pathogenesis

Fatty liver disease is a common metabolic disorder that continuously affects dairy cows in commercial farms across the globe during the dry to early lactation period (Bradford et al. 2015; Shi et al. 2020a,b). Obesity prior to calving, drastic physiological changes, and a reduced appetite are identified risk factors for the development of disease in dairy cows (Bobe et al. 2004). The slow increase in lactose consumption by the body in postpartum dairy animals may lead to an inadequate sugar supply for maintaining energy levels and increased fat mobilization in the liver as alternative energy source. The combination of physiological changes, reduced feed intake, and increased mobilization in the liver leads to immunological stress and a disturbance in metabolism. The metabolism of proteins, fats, and carbohydrates must be balanced for the liver to function as the principal organ for energy and substance metabolism. Furthermore, increased fat mobilization in the liver encourages gluconeogenesis and the liver synthesizes glucose from noncarbohydrate sources. This process can lead to a greatly increased production of NEFAs in the liver (Reid et al. 1983; Shi et al. 2020a,b). NEFAs can be partially re-esterified and form triglycerides (TGs), which form VLDLs; however, especially in dairy cattle, a lack of esterase means that VLDL is not transported out of the liver well. TGs are more likely to build excessively in the liver and result in a fatty liver (Katoh 2002).

The proposed schematic diagrams significant metabolic changes that occur during the pathogenesis of fatty liver disease in dairy cows. During the perinatal period, the metabolism of dairy cattle is in a state of negative energy balance, which promotes the mobilization of fat in the liver. Enhanced fat mobilization promotes a sharp increase in NEFAs in the liver. These NEFAs are more inclined to be involved in re-esterification and therefore, the synthesis of TGs and/or production of ketone bodies instead of β-oxidation because of mitochondrial dysfunction and inflammation that causes certain increased and/or decreased metabolism processes. The excessive accumulation of TGs in the liver leads to fatty liver.

18.3.1 Clinical Pathology

- Neutrophilia with increased band neutrophils is a feature.
- High hemoglobin at 13 g/100 ml. This is due to decreased fluid intake or the impaired ability of the digestive tract to absorb water.
- Hypoglycemia below 40 mg/100 ml.
- Glucocorticoid below 13–20 mg/ml.
- Ketone bodies 80–100 mg/dl (normal is 10 mg/dl).
- Free fatty acids elevated above a normal of 7 mg/dl.
- Aspartate aminotransferase (AST) > 100 units/l is indicative.
- Serum NEFA levels more than 1000 mEq/l in lactating cows and more than 325–400 mEq/l in prepartum cows are abnormal.
- Urea nitrogen above 20 mg/dl.

18.4 Clinical Findings

- The clinical appearance of fatty liver disease can range from mild ketosis to liver failure, depending on the degree of liver TG buildup, with deadly consequences. The fatty liver cow may have initially presented with one of many diseases of periparturient and lactating cows. Conditions such as milk fever, mastitis, metritis, and retained placentas all occur more frequently in fatty liver cows.
- The most common indication is a high incidence of disease around the transitional period (milk fever, ketosis, mastitis, retention of fetal membranes).
- A body condition score greater than 3.5 at calving that quickly drops to less than 2 by 4 weeks post calving.
- Reduced feed intake or complete anorexia.
- Loss of body weight.
- Drop in milk production in high yielding cattle.
- They may appear lethargic and depressed with reduced activity.
- Some cattle may develop jaundice, which is marked by yellowing of the mucous membranes, including the gums and eyes, due to the buildup of bilirubin in the blood.
- Due to the enlarged liver, cattle with fatty liver disease may acquire a swollen or distended abdomen.
- Cattle may show neurological symptoms, including incoordination and head pressing.
- Reduced gut motility causes constipation and decreased manure production.
- Severely affected animals are unable to stand and become recumbent.
- Due to hepatomegaly, pressure against the diaphragm leads to difficulty breathing in some cattle.
- Palpable liver during physical examination.

18.5 Diagnosis

It is difficult to diagnose fatty liver. There are several typical clinical pathological abnormalities. Ketonuria occurs when ketones are produced by the body metabolizing fats for energy instead of carbohydrates. Hypoglycemia occurs because the ability of the liver to regulate glucose is impaired due to excessive fat accumulation. Elevated levels of free fatty acids in the bloodstream are often seen in cows with hepatic lipidosis. This is a result of the breakdown of stored fat in the liver. Liver-derived enzymes like γ-glutamyl transferase (GGT) and AST are usually higher than for a dry cow but are still within normal ranges. Due to decreased functional liver mass, TGs and cholesterol may become low. Serum bile acids are an unreliable indicator of hepatic fatty degeneration (Johnson and Sherding 2006).

18.5.1 Physical Examination

A thorough physical examination by a veterinarian can help identify signs of liver disease, such as an enlarged liver or abdominal discomfort.

18.5.2 Blood Test

Elevated liver enzymes, bilirubin levels, TGs, and ketone bodies (ketosis) as well as low blood glucose levels (hypoglycemia) are typical. A blood sample can be used to measure the concentrations of NEFAs and β-hydroxybutyrate (BHBA), which are often elevated in fatty liver disease.

18.5.3 Liver Biopsy

A biopsy of liver is the most accurate and reliable method for the determination of fatty degeneration severity through the estimation of total lipids and TGs. The most accurate time to biopsy the liver is 8–14 days postpartum. Liver percutaneous biopsies in dairy cows are obtained using a biopsy instrument as described by Samanc and coworkers (Samanc et al. 2010).

18.5.4 Ultrasonography

Ultrasounds can be used to evaluate the size and texture of a liver. The liver may appear enlarged and echogenic (bright) due to the accumulation of excessive fat.

18.5.5 Necropsy (Postmortem Examination)

The excessive infiltration of lipids, especially of TGs, results in microscopic and macroscopic liver changes that become more pronounced as the amount of lipids increases. The liver becomes enlarged and swollen with round edges and a pale-to-yellow appearance (Kapp et al. 1979). Additionally susceptible to excessive TG infiltration are the kidneys, cardiac and skeletal muscles, and adrenal glands (Morrow et al. 1979). Myocarditis; necrosis in the kidneys, ovaries, muscle, and uterine tissues; involution of the pituitary gland; involution of the pancreas and lymphatic system; necrosis; inflammation; and ulceration of the liver are additional gross pathological features in cows with severe fatty livers (Reid 1982).

18.6 Treatment

The treatment of cows with clinically significant fatty liver syndrome is virtually always unsuccessful. Many treatment regimens have been offered, as is the case with most illnesses for which there is no known cure (Bobe et al. 2004). In general, cows that are totally anorexic for 3 days or more will die (Radostits et al. 2005). Cattle that have lost weight but are still eating may be managed with supportive therapy and nutrition (Kahn 2005).

The rationale for treatment is the prevention of fat mobilization that will decrease the fatty acid present in the liver (Morrow 1975) and correction of the pathophysiological effects of ketosis (Radostits et al. 2005).

- Intravenous infusion of 500 ml 50% dextrose solution.
- Protamine zinc insulin can be given after dextrose administration to suppress ketogenesis at 200–300 IU, subcutaneously, twice daily.
- Propylene glycol can be force fed orally to promote gluconeogenesis and minimize the mobilization of fat deposits at 0.5–1 g/kg/day.
- Choline chloride (50%) at 50 g orally, once daily, can be fed. This is essential for the formation of phospholipids that are required for lipoprotein production and the transport of fatty acids (Morrow 1975).
- Anabolic steroids injection.
- Intravenous vitamin B12.
- Rumen juice at 5–10 l to stimulate appetite.
- To decrease the energy output of any cow with pregnancy toxemia, the induction of parturition or removal of the fetus by cesarean section should be considered.
- Affected cattle should be provided with good quality green forage and ample water.
- Fatty cows should be fed good quality feed supplemented with cobalt-iodized salt.
- There are benefits from the forced exercise of dry cows (Blake et al. 1975).

The severity of lipid infiltration and the underlying cause will determine how to treat fatty liver. The flaws that led to the initial lipid invasion must be corrected. The general treatment techniques used to prevent fatty liver are also used to treat mild and moderate fatty liver. By providing fresh premium grass or legume hay, feed consumption should increase. To encourage the oxidation of ketone bodies in muscle, moderate exercise for 1 hour/day is advised. Daily, intramuscular injections of 200 mg prednisolone for 5 days can reduce liver TG concentrations. For 14 days, daily 15-mg subcutaneous doses of glucagon prevent the buildup of liver TGs in older cows. As therapies for fatty liver, glucocorticoids, adrenocorticotropic hormone (ACTH), and glucagon all enhance gluconeogenesis in the liver, which raises plasma glucose levels. These hormones have the drawback of needing frequent injections, which makes them unpractical for usage on farms. It would be ideal to create a subcutaneous implant for the slow release of glucagon and glucocorticoid. The use of glucocorticoids and glucagon raises the possibility that they will boost NEFA release from adipose tissue, which worsens ketosis. Nicotinic acid, dexamethasone-21-iso-nicotinic acid, and glucocorticoids are used in conjunction to suppress the release of NEFAs. The most effective treatment to date involves continuous intravenous infusions of glucagon, glucose, and injections of glucocorticoids, insulin, or both (Haass and Eness 1984).

18.7 Prevention and Control

Several general management techniques can aid in the prevention of fatty liver. The best "cure" is avoiding additional cases once a herd's problematic fat metabolism has been identified. The easiest method to deal with this is to change how and what cows eat (Melendez et al. 2018). On the herd level, it can be prevented by adequate attention to nutrition and health care of cattle in late gestation. The principal method of control is to prevent pregnant cattle from becoming fat during the last trimester of pregnancy, particularly during the dry period in dairy cattle.

It is advised to feed cows a balanced diet that meets their nutritional needs throughout the postpartum period. It is advised to treat infectious and metabolic diseases in cows during the periparturient phase right away and vigorously. To prevent infections, it is crucial to have a clean stall that is well ventilated, sufficient room and exercise, and fresh high quality feed. By providing an additional source of glucose and reducing the mobilization of NEFAs from adipose tissue during the peripartum period, fatty liver can be prevented in dairy cows. For the last 10 days prior to delivery, 1 l/day oral drenches of propylene glycol have been shown to prevent fatty liver and ketosis by raising plasma glucose and insulin levels while lowering plasma BHBA and NEFA levels.

During pregnancy, mature cattle should receive sufficient feed to meet the needs for maintenance and pregnancy, and the total daily nutrient intake must increase throughout the last trimester to meet the needs of the fetus (Radostits et al. 2005).

- Monitor body condition and feed accordingly. For example: 3.0–3.5 during late lactation, 3.5–4.0 at dry off, 3.5–4.0 at calving, and 2.5–3.0 at peak lactation. Animals should be grouped and fed based on body condition scoring.
- Provide high quality forages to fresh cows and bring them onto concentrate feed gradually.
- Supply adequate protein in rations with a proper balance between degradable and undegradable.
- Treat high risk cows with oral propylene glycol prophylactically until they are eating aggressively. For example, high risk cows can be treated with 250 ml of propylene glycol once daily as an oral drench for the first 7–10 days after calving.
- Treat postpartum diseases such as milk fever, mastitis, retained placentas, and ketosis promptly in order to prevent severe fatty infiltration of the liver.
- The use of bovine somatotropin (BST) may help prevent excessive body condition gains in late lactation (Laven and Andrews 1998). This could potentially be a useful tool for cows that have had breeding problems and are putting on excessive amounts of weight in late lactation.

References

Andrews, A., Blowey, R.W., Boyd, H., and Eddy, R.G. (2008). *Bovine Medicine: Diseases and Husbandry of Cattle*, 2e, 781–804. Oxford: Blackwell Science.

Blake, J.T., Olsen, R.C., Lamb, R.C. et al. (1975). Body condition of dairy csattle in confinement. *Journal of Dairy Science* 58: 776.

Bobe, G., Young, J.W., and Beitz, D.C. (2004). Invited review: pathology, etiology, prevention, and treatment of fatty liver in dairy cows. *Journal of Dairy Science* 87 (10): 3105–3124.

Bracken, F.K. (1980). Diseases affecting liver function. In: *Bovine Medicine and Surgery*, 2e, vol. 2 (ed. H.E. Amstutz), 689–691. Santa Barbara, CA: Am. Vet. Pub. Inc.

Bradford, B.J., Yuan, K., Farney, J.K. et al. (2015). Invited review: inflammation during the transition to lactation: new adventures with an old flame. *Journal of Dairy Science* 98 (10): 6631–6650.

Daradics, Z., Crecan, C.M., Rus, M.A. et al. (2021). Obesity – related metabolic dysfunction in dairy cows and horses: comparison to human metabolic syndrome. *Life (Basel)* 11 (12): 1406.

De Koster, J. and Opsomer, G. (2012). Are modern dairy cows suffering from modern diseases? *Vlaams Diergeneeskundig Tijdschrift* 81: 71–80.

Gonzalez, C.I. and Rosendo, O. (2013). Assessment of fatty liver syndrome and its predisposing factors in a dairy herd from Venezuela. *ISRN Veterinary Science* 2013: 191708.

Haass, C.L. and Eness, P.G. (1984). Bovine fatty liver disease. *Iowa State University Veterinarian* 1984 (46): 7.

Johnson, S.E. and Sherding, R.G. (2006). Chapter 71 - Diseases of the Liver and Biliary Tract. In: *Saunders Manual of Small Animal Practice*, 3e (ed. S.J. Birchard and R.G. Sherding), 747–809. Philadelphia, PA: W.B. Saunders.

Kahn, C.M. (ed.) (2005). *The Merck Veterinary Manual*, 9e. USA: Merck & Co., Inc.

Kapp, P., Pethes, G., Zsiros, M., and Schuster, Z. (1979). Contribution to the development of the fatty liver syndrome in high producing dairy cows. *Magyar Allatorvosok Lapja* 34: 458–468.

Katoh, N. (2002). Relevance of apolipoproteins in the development of fatty liver and fatty liver-related peripartum diseases in dairy cows. *The Journal of Veterinary Medical Science* 64: 293–307.

Kirovski, D. and Sladojevic, Z. (2017). Prediction and diagnosis of fatty liver in dairy cows. *SM Journal of Gastroenterology and Hepatology* 3 (1): 1005.

Laven, R.A. and Andrews, A.H. (1998). Control of fatty liver syndrome in a Jersey herd by a change of diet and the use of recombinant bovine somatotrophin. *The Veterinary Record* 142 (2): 36–39. http://veterinaryrecord.bvapublications.com/cgi/content/abstract/.

Melendez, P., Whitney, M., Williams, F. et al. (2018). Technical note: evaluation of fine needle aspiration cytology for the diagnosis of fatty liver in dairy cattle. *Journal of Dairy Science* 101 (5): 4483–4490. https://doi.org/10.3168/jds.2017-13346.

Morrow, D.A. (1975). Fat cow syndrome. *Journal of Dairy Science* 59: 1625–1628. http://www.agromedia.ca/ADM_Articles/content/a1c2h1f1.pdf.

Morrow, D.A., Hillman, D., Dade, A.W., and Kitchen, H. (1979). Clinical investigation of a dairy herd with the fat cow syndrome. *JAVMA* 174: 161–167.

Radostits, O.M., Blood, D.C., Arundel, O.M., and Gay, C.C. (2005). *Veterinary Medicine: A Textbook of the Diseases of Cattle, Sheep, Pigs, Goats and Horses*, 9e. London: Bailliere Tindal. ISBN: 070201592X, 9780702015922.

Reid, J.R. (1982). Fatty liver in dairy cows. *In Practice* 11: 164–169.

Reid, I.M., Rowlands, G.J., Dew, A.M. et al. (1983). The relationship between post-parturient fatty liver and blood composition in dairy cows. *Journal of Agriculture Science (Cambridge)* 101: 473–480.

Samanc, H., Stojic, V., Kirovski, D. et al. (2010). Thyroid hormones concentrations during the mid-dry period: an early indicator of fatty liver in Holstein-Friesian dairy cows. *Journal of Thyroid Research* 2010: 897602,6 p, https://doi.org/10.4061/2010/897602.

Shi, K.R., Li, R.R., Xu, Z.J., and Zhang, Q. (2020a). Identification of crucial genetic factors, such as PPARγ, that regulate the pathogenesis of fatty liver disease in dairy cows is imperative for the sustainable development of dairy industry. *Animals (Basel)* 10 (4): 639.

Shi, K.R., Niu, F.G., Zhang, Q. et al. (2020b). Identification of whole- genome significant single nucleotide polymorphisms in candidate genes associated with serum biochemical traits in Chinese Holstein cattle. *Frontiers in Genetics* 11: 163.

Sisson, S.J.D., Grossman, and Getty, R. (1975). *Sisson and Grossman's the Anatomy of the Domestic Animals*, 5e. Philadelphia: Saunders.

Wankhade, P.R., Manimaran, A., Kumaresan, A. et al. (2017). Metabolic and immunological changes in transition dairy cows: a review. *Veterinary World* 10: 1367–1377.

19

Thelitis

Rajesh Kumar[1], Aakanksha Bhoker[1], Sanjeev Kumar[2], and Anil Kumar[3]

[1] *Department of Veterinary Surgery and Radiology, Bihar Veterinary College, Patna, Bihar, India*
[2] *Department of Veterinary Pathology, Bihar Veterinary College, Patna, Bihar, India*
[3] *Department of Veterinary Medicine, Bihar Veterinary College, Patna, Bihar, India*

19.1 Introduction

Thelitis is the inflammation of teat wall layers, including the skin, canal, and cistern (Hanaa et al. 2011). It is generally characterized by acute inflammation of one or more teats along with ulceration, necrosis, obstruction, and sloughing of the affected teat. Microorganisms can enter the teat canal and ascend toward the mammary parenchyma. In the mammary parenchyma, microorganisms can colonize, multiply, and produce toxins, eventually predisposing the animal to mastitis. Teat health is increasingly important for dairy producers, and any disease condition that involves the teat ultimately affects animal productivity and the farmer's economy. Healthy teat skin is desirable for the welfare, comfort, and health of animals; for aesthetic reasons; to produce wholesome milk; and for the health and comfort of those involved in milking. Teat lesions are quite a common and somewhat neglected problem in bovines. Pure exotic breeds are highly susceptible, followed by crossbred animals, while buffaloes are the least affected. The lower susceptibility of local breeds is primarily due to better immunity levels and low production.

The prevalence of teat lesions varies according to the method of sampling and conditions included in the study. Among teat lesions, mastitis (67.5%), mastitis and thelitis (4.6%), teat obstruction (20.5%), thelitis (2.0%), wounds (0.7%), abscesses (2.0%), psychic agalactia (0.7%), pox (0.7%), teat stricture (0.7%), and ulcers (0.7%) are the most commonly encountered conditions (Thilagar and Dewanmuthumohammed 1992). Obstructive thelitis causes the complete obstruction of milk flow and is associated with hot, painful, and distended teats. Trauma caused during milking is the operating cause. The incidence of obstructive thelitis is noticed most often during the first lactation of cows and buffaloes, predominantly in graded Murrah rather than nondescript animals (Kathirvel and Dharmaceelan 2016). The hindquarters are more commonly affected (left more frequently than right). Cases were usually reported within 10 days of calving during the first lactation. The animals showed no febrile symptoms. The disease either had a peracute or acute onset. Tiwary et al. 2005 reported a 73.33% and 26.66% occurrence of acute and peracute cases, respectively, in buffaloes.

Ulcerative thelitis is an obstacle for the milk-producing capacity of cattle and buffaloes. This condition is characterized by the acute inflammation of one or more teats, ulceration, necrosis, and sloughing of the affected teat with subsequent thickening, narrowing, or closure of the teat canal, which leads to the incomplete drainage of milk. The quality of milk appears to be normal, unlike in clinical mastitis. Conventional treatment with antibiotics and other supportive therapy used to treat mastitis has no curative value in ulcerative thelitis (Lokanadhamu et al. 2005).

Bovine nodular thelitis (BNT) in dairy cows is a chronic and enzootic infection. Four stages, i.e. growth of nodules within the teat wall, rupture and ulceration of the nodules, scarring with deformation of the teats, and secondary infections are reported (Thorel et al. 1990). The disease causes economic loss due to mastitis complications and nonspecific reactions to the intradermal tuberculin test during tuberculosis prevention (Berhomde 1986). It was first reported in France in 1963 and then in Japan and Switzerland (Rüsch et al. 1984; Thorel et al. 1990). This granulomatous dermatitis of the teat was

Periparturient Diseases of Cattle, First Edition. Edited by Tanmoy Rana.

associated with acid-fast bacilli that suggested a mycobacterial origin of infection (Rüsch et al. 1984; Thorel et al. 1990). Tuberculoid nodular thelitis is caused by mycobacterial infection of the teat skin. Clinical presentations of BNT include the occurrence of chronic teat skin lesions and the formation of papules, nodules, and ulcers with differing sizes that undergo spontaneous healing or cicatrization after 6–12 months.

Teat lesions of thelitis are not fatal to animals but can undoubtedly be classified as a disease of great economic importance to the dairy industry. Teat lesions may cause the deterioration of animal health, severe milking problems, prolonged milking time, and the development of mastitis. Teat skin should be kept free from microbial contamination to maintain the health of animals. High stocking density, contaminated floors, wet bedding, poor ventilation, and a hot and humid climate can promote the growth of pathogens and increase cow exposure, which results in a higher occurrence of thelitis.

In goats, skin lesions of the teat or the udder are also very important, particularly in dairy goats, as they represent a potential source of pathogens for both milk and the mammary gland. Viral infections like papillomavirus, bacterial infections like staphylococcal dermatitis, and neoplasia like warts, cutaneous papilloma, or squamous cell carcinoma are among the most prevalent causes of teat and/or udder skin lesions in goats (Smith and Sherman 2009).

19.2 Etiology

Inflammation of the wall of the teat (thelitis) is a nonspecific lesion usually associated with traumatic injury to the lining of the teat cistern. Thelitis or inflammation of the tissues of the teat wall that leads to gangrene is a common complication of gangrenous mastitis and is most commonly associated with peracute *Staphylococcus aureus* mastitis. Photosensitive thelitis occurs due to the photosensitization of the teats. Ulcerative thelitis is caused by a viral agent similar to bovine herpes virus (BHV)-2. Electron microscopic studies of scab tissue and vesicular fluid clearly showed the presence of hexagonal herpes virus–like particles similar to BHV-2, which causes mammillitis in cows. Undescribed species of the genus *Mycobacterium* related to *Mycobacterium leprae* and *M. lepromatosis* are responsible for tuberculoid and lepromatous leprosy as well as a diffuse form of lepromatous leprosy (Han et al. 2008, 2009) and are the causative agent of BNT. *M. leprae* and *M. lepromatosis* are not cultivable on artificial media. *M. uberis* is also isolated from nodular thelitis (Benjak et al. 2018). The pseudogene content of *M. uberis* differs from that of *M. leprae*.

19.3 Epidemiology

Thelitis is most often observed in primiparous animals rather than pluriparous animals (Lokanadhamu et al. 2005). The incidence is high during the first lactation period and is usually noticed within 1–2 weeks (Kathirvel and Dharmaceelan 2016). In buffaloes, the incidence of thelitis is mainly observed in graded Murrah buffaloes rather than in nondescript buffaloes (Rambabu et al. 2011; Kathirvel and Dharmaceelan 2016). Clinical signs in affected animals were found most often in a single teat, especially the right hind teat (Sreedevi et al. 2002). In more than 80% of clinical cases, the condition is limited to a single quarter, and the involvement of two quarters is very rarely seen compared to a single quarter. Various teat lesions have different occurrence rates: thelitis (2.0%), mastitis and thelitis (4.6%), mastitis (67.5%), teat obstruction (20.5%), wounds (0.7%), abscesses (2.0%), psychic agalactia (0.7%), pox (0.7%), teat stricture (0.7%), and ulcers (0.7%) (Thilagar and Dewanmuthumohammed 1992). The cumulative incidence of infectious teat skin lesions in 1 year was 17.3% and 8.5% in cattle and buffaloes, respectively (Sharma et al. 2005). The teat skin is better protected in buffaloes than cattle due to the increased thickness of the teat epithelium. The buffalo teat epidermis also has a comparatively higher amount of melanin than it does in cattle (Kumar 1990). The incidence of obstructive thelitis was noted to be comparatively higher in Murrah buffaloes. The hindquarters are more commonly affected. The cases were mostly reported within 10 days of calving, during the first lactation. The animals showed no febrile symptoms.

BNT is a chronic and enzootic cutaneous disease that was first reported in France in 1963 and then in Japan and Switzerland (Thorel et al. 1990). This granulomatous dermatitis is associated with acid-fast bacilli and is believed to have a mycobacterial origin. Similarly, the first outbreak of caprine nodular thelitis due to *M. uberis* infection was reported in 2012 and published in 2016 (Chartier et al. 2016). After that, several other outbreaks have been identified regularly over the years. Outbreaks of caprine nodular thelitis occur preferably in winter (kidding period and beginning of lactation) and primarily in multiparous goats over 4 years of age. The number of clinical cases increased progressively and after reaching a plateau, decreased slowly. However, the outbreak duration and size are variable, ranging from a couple of months to several years with 1.3–15% of a flock being affected (Brentini et al. 2020). At the individual level, the course of the disease is chronic, lasting from 1 month to more than 6 months.

19.4 Pathogenesis

Teats act as a primary defense barrier against mastitis. This defense function is because of the keratin-lined wall that inhibits bacterial invasion and colonization. Keratin inhibits bacterial growth through its opsonizing property that neutralizes toxins and prevents adherence by lacteal immunoglobulins. Moreover, keratin contains fibrous proteins and fatty acids that electrostatically bind pathogen cell walls and make them more susceptible to osmotic pressure, which thus damages the pathogens. The teat canal also secretes a type of smegma (rich in fatty acids) that inhibits bacterial growth.

But at the same time, the teats are vulnerable to external trauma or injury because of their anatomical location, increased udder and teat size during lactation, faulty methods of milking, repeated trauma to the teat mucosa, injury from calf teeth, being accidentally stepped on, and paralysis that results from metabolic disturbances at parturition.

Teat skin, the teat orifice, and their environment are the main reservoirs for the entry of opportunistic pathogens into the mammary gland. The route of infection appears to be through the teat canal. Wounds that occur via any means will certainly facilitate infection. There is a relationship between teat end callosity (teat skin lesions, hyperkeratosis) and thelitis, which could be caused by mechanical and circulatory impairment of the teat tissue during the milking process. Contaminated milking machine cups, milkers' hands, and farm utensils are other sources of infection.

Many different pathogens have been associated with mammary gland teats; infections may be either viruses, bacteria, parasites, or fungi that occur alone or as a mixed infection. Lesions on teats may be primary diseases that occur mainly on the teat skin, such as bovine herpes mammillitis, pseudocowpox, cowpox, buffalopox, papillomatosis, and udder impetigo, or they may be secondary and incidental symptoms of a generalized disease like foot-and-mouth disease, bovine popular stomatitis, vesicular stomatitis, contagious pustular dermatitis, and lumpy skin disease. Species of *Streptococcus, Staphylococcus, Corynebacterium, Escherichia coli, Pseudomonas, M. tuberculosis, Actinomyces, Actinobacillus,* and *Nocardia* have also been associated with teat inflammation.

Pathogens can invade the teat canal and colonize, multiplying and producing toxin that predispose it to inflammation. The toxic products of these microorganisms and their proteolytic enzymes facilitate entry of the organism from the colonization site into the parenchyma. Four stages were distinguished: (i) the early stage (in which the bacteria enter the teat orifice and can be found in the teat canal and cistern), (ii) the evolutive stage (in which the organisms overcome resistance and multiply), (iii) the ulcerative stage (in which the organisms invade the epithelium and cause pathological lesions like necrosis and hemorrhage), and (iv) the final stage.

Milk is a good medium for the growth of bacteria, hence, lactating cattle, buffaloes, and heifers tend to be more severely affected. The disease is most common in summer and fall or in the calving season in buffaloes. Older cows are more susceptible to infections, probably because of a wider or permanent, partial opening of the teat canal from frequent milking. Furthermore, the mammary epithelium of older cows has increased permeability, mainly because of irreversible damage caused by previous inflammations.

19.5 Clinical Signs

19.5.1 Thelitis

Swelling in the teat increases it to two to three times its normal size and makes it hot, which later becomes hard and painful. Sometimes sloughing of the skin over the teat and the formation of scars on the teat lesion can be seen. The quality of the milk is not generally affected, but the quantity is reduced due to the presence of pain during milking and suckling.

The affected teat skin is cold, edematous, and oozes serum. The subcutaneous aspects are commonly distended with gas. The skin is commonly a dark red to purple-black color. Sloughing of the skin may be evident. The wall of the cistern is thickened, hardened, painful, and in chronic lesions, irregular in its internal lining. The lesion can be felt as a dense, vertical cord in the center of the teat tip. The lesions have historically been intractable to treatment, which usually consists of intramammary antibiotics and refraining from milking. The recent application of teat endoscopy has assisted in identifying cattle most likely to respond to medical or surgical treatment.

19.5.2 Photosensitive Thelitis (Photosensitization of the Teats)

Photosensitive thelitis is a local manifestation of generalized photosensitization. There is a characteristic erythema and hardness of the unpigmented or white parts on the lateral aspect of each teat. The medial aspect is soft and cool. The teats are also painful and apparently irritable in the early stages; affected cows will stand in ponds or waterholes in such a way that the teats are immersed, then rock back and forth. They will also brush the sides of the udder with their hindfeet in a way that could suggest the stamping movements of abdominal pain. In cases where photosensitization is related to the induction of parturition by the administration of corticosteroids, the skin lesions are usually restricted to the teats. In cases due to other causes, there are usually obvious lesions of photosensitive dermatitis on the dorsal aspects of the body that are confined only to the white parts.

19.5.3 Obstructive Thelitis

Obstructive thelitis has either a peracute or acute onset. In the peracute form, the animal is excited during milking, and the teat shows an immediate, balloon-like swelling. In the acute form, the swelling is noticed during the subsequent milking. In both forms, the teats remain painful and cows do not allow the suckling of their calves. The size of the affected teats is increased with a glossy appearance. The hyperemia is followed by soft edema, which later shows induration from the third day onward. Induration is attributed to hyperplastic inflammation and the formation of new connective tissue in abundance (Ramaswamy et al. 2001). These changes lead to the complete obstruction and stoppage of the milk. The milk can be removed by applying pressure on the teats due to decreased elasticity of the tissue. The affected quarter is otherwise normal, except for the thickening of the udder above the base of the teat, which gradually returns to normal in 5–6 days. The case may deteriorate with excoriation of the teat's epithelial layer due to further handling and suckling by the calf. In animals that do not respond to treatment, there might be subsequent yellowish-black discoloration due to necrotic tissue inflammation, which may further slough off and lead to fistula formation. There are no significant changes in vital (rectal temperature, heart rate, and respiration rate), or hematologic parameters (hemoglobin [Hb], total leukocyte count [TLC], differential leukocyte count [DLC]). Milk samples are also within the accepted standards for color, consistency, odor, pH, and somatic cell count (SCC).

19.5.4 Ulcerative Thelitis

The most important clinical signs of ulcerative thelitis include acute inflammation of one or more teats with subsequent thickening, narrowing, and closure of the teat canal. Narrowing of the teat causes the incomplete drainage of milk. Swelling of the teat and subsequent ulcer formation on teat skin is followed by the formation of vesicles and exudation of serous fluid from the dermis upon rupture. This may be followed by necrotic changes in the teat that may eventually lead to either complete or partial sloughing of the affected teat. In some cases, scabs may form over the ulcers, which is followed by healing of the lesions (Turner et al. 1976).

19.5.5 Nodular Thelitis

BNT can be divided into four clinical stages: early, evolutive, ulcerative, and the final stage. The early stage starts with the appearance of a mild localized zone of inflammation (0.5 cm) in the teat wall. Physical examination reveals a painful, pink, well-circumscribed, and indurated area with edema. The cut section appears homogeneous or dotted with orange-yellow foci. The stage is brief in milking cows (8 days) and of an unknown length in heifers. The evolutive stage is associated with the rapid spread of edema and inflammation. The developing papules increase in size to nodules or assume a plague-like appearance. The lesions mature quickly and appear a purplish-pink color. Swelling emerges with a middle point of relative fluctuation, which is hot and painful upon palpation. The lesions may occupy from a quarter to a third of the teat, with marked teat deformation. This stage can last from a few hours to a few days. The ulcerative stage describes the development of a wide but superficial ulcer over the fluctuant areas. A small quantity of reddish, serous drainage develops. The pain generally decreases, but bleeding often occurs after milking. The final stage varies with the degree of any secondary infections, which depends on hygiene conditions on the farm. There can be either a quick healing with scar formation and deformation of the teat or an infection with pyogenic organisms. In infective cases, the teat keeps swelling and the pyogenic process ensues along the lymphatic vessels, which results in the appearance of a string of abscesses that contain a yellowish-creamy pus (a few mm to 1–2 cm in diameter), and the teat becomes nonfunctional. The clinical evolution to further successive stages can be arrested by early detection followed by quick therapy without any delay (authors' unpublished observations). Good results can be obtained in the absence of ulceration when the teat, although deformed, remains functional.

In nodular thelitis in goats, lesions are generally restricted to the lower part of the udder and the upper part of the teat. Initially, the lesions are circular, indurated, and erythematous on the teat skin. The lesions may progress to form dark, raised, hemorrhagic crusts that slough to reveal an underlying ulcerative plaque. In some clinical cases, the supramammary lymph node may become enlarged. Lesions are moderately painful in the early stage and become painless in the latter stage. It is generally associated with a decrease in milk production or secondary mastitis.

Common clinical signs of thelitis in bovines.

- Inflammation of the teat.
- Thickening, narrowing, and closure of the teat canal.
- Erythema and hardness of the unpigmented or white parts on the lateral aspects of the teat in photosensitive thelitis.
- Acute inflammation of one or more teats with subsequent thickening, narrowing, and closure of the teat canal in ulcerative thelitis.
- Nodular lesions in the teat wall and ventral portion of the udder in nodular thelitis.

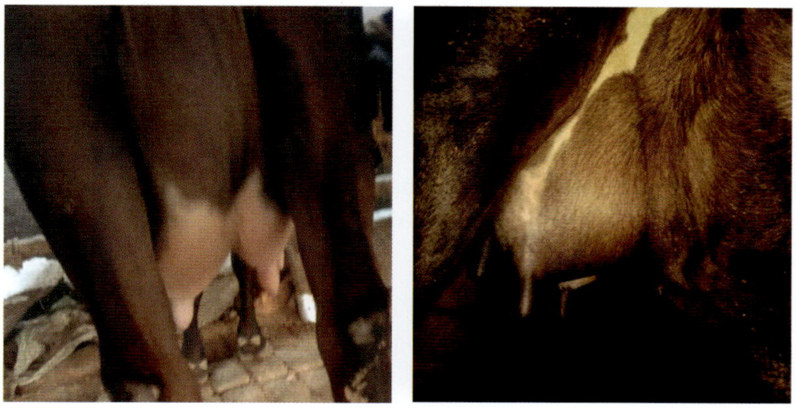

Inflammation of teat

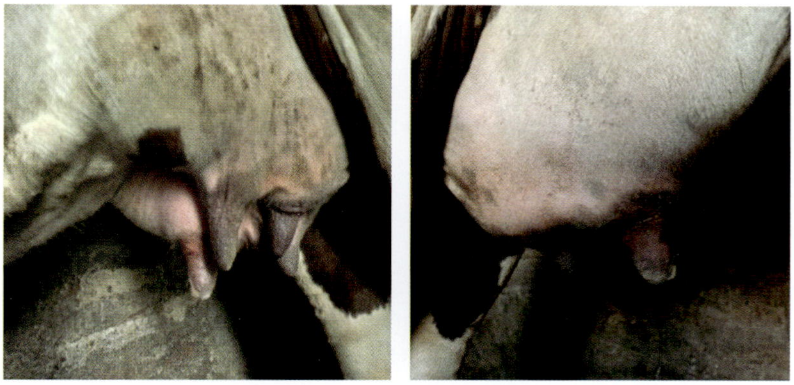

Inflammation of teat with sloughing of teat skin

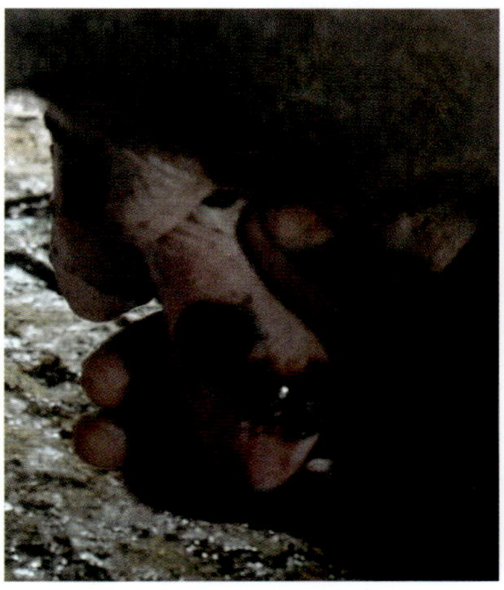

Ulcerative theilitis

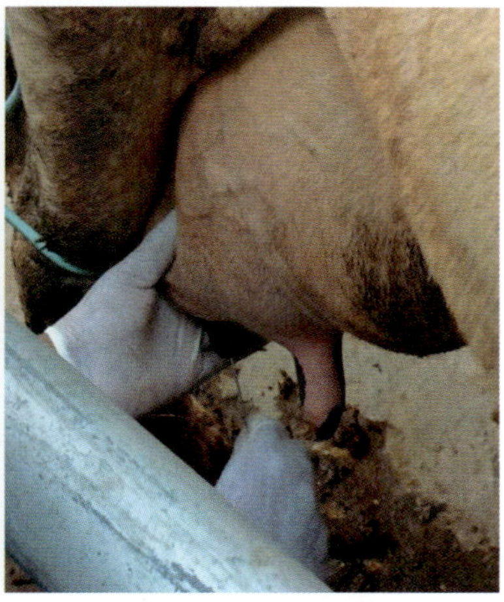

Obstructive theilitis

19.6 Diagnosis

19.6.1 Clinical Signs and Symptoms

Most cattle show no signs of systemic illness. The lesions may be confined to one teat or involve all the teats. The disease is typically sudden in onset with swollen, tender teats. The affected teat initially presents with reddening and swelling. Irregularly shaped vesicles may be seen, but sloughing and ulceration are usually also noted. A severe infection leads to destruction of the affected teat. Complete destruction results from untreated teats.

19.6.2 Milk Sample Examination

Milk samples collected from animals affected by different types of thelitis revealed no changes in color or consistency, as is generally observed in clinical mastitis. Milk samples tested negative with different mastitis diagnostic tests, viz. the California mastitis (CMT), bromothymol blue (BTB), bromocresol purple (BCP), whiteside (WST), and chloride tests. The pH of the milk samples remain within the normal range of 6.5–6.7. The values for electrical conductivity and the SCC remain normal.

19.6.3 Cultural Examination of the Milk Sample

Culture examination indicates that bacteria isolated from the milk of the affected quarter could be the natural inhabitants of the udder and teat or environmental contaminants (Ramaswamy et al. 2001; Rao et al. 2003).

19.6.4 Ultrasonographic Examination

The sonographic examination shows a thick, hyperechoic teat wall lining that replaces the typical central hypoechoic images of the teat canal. The gland cistern and udder parenchyma appear distended with anechoic images due to the obstruction of milk flow.

19.6.5 Intradermal Whey Testing in Rabbits

The bacteria-free filtrate of whey obtained from the milk of affected teats can be used to test the pathogenicity of the etiological agent by the intradermal inoculation of rabbits. The experimental reproduction of lesions in the rabbit gives strong evidence for the etiological agent of thelitis.

19.6.6 Histopathological Examination

Histopathology of the scab tissue in ulcerative thelitis reveals congestion, hyperkeratinization, thinning and fracture of stratum corneum, intraepidermal vesiculation, and the presence of moderate cellular infiltration, mainly lymphocytes, into the epidermis. In some cases, extensive calcification with intracellular edema in the dermis can be observed (Lokanadhamu et al. 2005). In nodular thelitis, histopathological examination of the teat, udder, and body skin lesions show chronic multifocal coalescing and moderate to severe granulomatous dermatitis with variable ulceration that are associated with granulomatous lymphadenitis of varying intensity. This type of lesion is tuberculoid, composed of a central zone with neutrophil granulocytes, surrounded by epithelioid macrophages and some Langhans-type multinucleate giant cells that are, in turn, surrounded by lymphocytes and fibroblasts.

19.6.7 Bacteriological Isolation

The collected specimens should be cultured in the desired culture media for 24 hours at 37 °C. Suspected colonies should be picked and subcultured on selective media for identification by microscopic and biochemical analyses.

19.6.8 Mycological Examination

Sabouraud's dextrose agar containing 0.05 mg/ml chloramphenicol (to inhibit bacterial growth) is the medium of choice, and cultures should be incubated at 25 °C for 7 days.

19.6.9 Serologic Tests

Serologic tests like agar gel precipitation and neutralization tests could also be performed.

19.7 Differential Diagnoses

19.7.1 Ulcerative Mammillitis

- Ulcerative mammillitis is caused by bovine herpes virus-2.
- Highly contagious and characterized by the development of inflammatory and ulcerative lesions on the udder and teats.
- Most clinical cases occur within the first 2 months of lactation.
- The disease often has a seasonal association with cold weather over other seasons.

19.7.2 Foot-and-Mouth Disease

- Teat lesions along with characteristic vesicles, bullae, and ulcerated areas on the muzzle, tongue, and coronary bands that cause profuse salivation and lameness.
- Affected animals are anorexic and pyretic.

19.7.3 Pseudocowpox

- Initially, it appears as small, red, raised sores on the teats and udders.
- Progresses to vesicles, scabs, and nodules.
- May form a "ring" or "horseshoe" of scabs over the course of several weeks.
- In humans, pseudocowpox can cause localized skin lesions, whereas thelitis has no zoonotic potential.
- Inclusion bodies are seen inside the cytoplasm and not in the nucleus (George et al. 2008).

19.7.4 Cowpox

- Initial erythema is followed by firm, raised papules light in color with a zone of hyperemia around the base.
- Vesicles are yellow-colored blisters with a pitted center that are followed by a pustular stage and then the development of thick, red, tenacious scabs 1–1.5 cm in diameter.
- Initially, typical pox lesions are seen primarily on the udder and teats, but later on, the lesions may spread to the base of the horns, inside the thighs, and on the perineal region.
- Udder lesions are primarily proliferative.
- Cowpox has zoonotic potential, unlike thelitis.

19.7.5 Papillomatosis

- Hyperplasia or benign neoplasms on the epidermis (Lancaster and Olson 1982).
- The virus may produce papillomas on cutaneous body parts, viz. the head, neck, shoulders, ventral abdomen (bovine papillomavirus type-2 or 3 [BPV-2,3]), and alimentary tract (BPV-4).
- Teat warts may regress during the dry period and recur in the next lactation. Teat warts usually have an increased frequency with age (Radostits et al. 2007).

19.7.6 Udder Impetigo

- The lesions start with the appearance of numerous small, cream-yellow pustules on the udder with a 2–4 mm diameter.
- The lesions are mostly observed on the lateral sides as well as in the well of the udder; lesions may present on hairless skin at the base of the teats (Francis 1984; Faull et al. 1991).

19.8 Treatment

Enrofloxacin along with antihistamines, a combination of vitamins A, D_3, and E (AD_3E), and supportive treatment are found to be effective along with a mineral mixture that contains probiotics (Babu et al. 2017). Strepto–penicillins, antihistamines, vitamin AD_3E, and candidemia ointment is more effective for thelitis with skin sloughing of the teat (Kathivel and Dharmaceelan 2016). Boric acid and glycerin pastes are effective for horizontal scars, whereas a copper sulfate solution is effective for vertical scars. In obstructive thelitis, treatment with antibiotic (amoxycillin–cloxacillin) and antihistamine (chlorpheniramine maleate) drugs as well as intralesional hyaluronidase and corticosteroid is very effective. Methylprednisolone (0.4 ml, 40 mg/ml) is comparatively more effective (1000%) than prednisolone (2 ml, 10 mg/ml) and dexamethasone (0.75 ml, 4 mg/ml), reducing painful teat conditions and restoring milk flow in 80% of cattle (Tiwary et al. 2005). The swelling generally subsides 2–3 days after the use of intralesional methylprednisolone, whereas it takes 3–5 days with the prednisolone and 4–7 days with dexamethasone.

The treatment of ulcerative thelitis with conventional therapy (enrofloxacin, diclofenac sodium, and pheniramine maleate) is not systemically effective (Lokanadhamu et al. 2005); conventional drugs had only a 12.5% cure rate in 35 days. Conventional drugs along with acyclovir both orally and topically had a cure rate of 62.5% in 12 days. However, the topical application of acyclovir along with conventional drugs had a comparatively lower cure rate (37.5%), within 26 days. Lysine may be applied as a topical paste on the affected teat since lysine reduces the severity of herpes simplex virus infections in humans (Griffith et al. 1987). *M. uberis* is responsible for nodular thelitis and is susceptible to the antileprosy drugs rifampin, dapsone, and ofloxacin. It is also susceptible to clofazimine and clarithromycin, as is *M. haemophilum* (Lindeboom et al. 2011).

19.9 Alternative Treatment

Alternative treatments include homeopathic medicine like *Arnica* and *Bryonia*. Varshney (2006) reported successful results in five teats from three dairy animals (two Holstein crosses and one Murrah buffalo) with *Arnica* 30c at 10 pills orally, thrice daily, on the day of referral; followed by *Bryonia* 30c at 10 pills orally, thrice daily, from the second day onward for 2–3 days; and the topical application of *Bryonia* cream (*Bryonia alba* Q 8% volume per weight) thrice daily from the first day for 3 days. Ruddock (1991) reported that *Bryonia* generally relieves inflammation quickly, and when it is associated with trauma, a few doses of *Arnica* should precede it.

Common drugs used to treat thelitis.

Drug	Dose (mg/kg body weight)
Ceftriaxone	10, intramuscularly (IM)
Amoxicillin–sulbactam	10, IM
Enrofloxacin	5–10, IM
Meloxicam	0.1, IM
Ketoprofen	2, IM
Chlorpheniramine maleate	05–1.0, IM
Acyclovir	1–2, slow intravenous

19.10 Control and Prevention Measures

The control and prevention of diseases in bovines are to prevent the occurrence of diseases in cattle. A series of management steps can be taken when controlling diseases in cattle that include disease prevention, treatment, supervision, quarantine, access restrictions, and awareness. The most effective way to control a disease is prevention. Prevention is carried out by maintaining sanitation practices in the livestock environment, paying attention to feed quality, and maintaining cleanliness. With prevention, farmers can minimize the possibility of spreading disease to cattle and prevent disease outbreaks that can cause large economic losses. Maintaining the sanitation of the livestock environment is also important to prevent the spread of disease. The farmer must ensure that cow pens are clean and dry, livestock waste is properly disposed of, and the cattle have adequate access to clean water. Paying attention to feed quality is also important for preventing disease in cattle. The owner must ensure that the feed given to cattle meets the required nutritional standards. Farmers must pay attention to the cleanliness of cows, including cleaning and caring for cow skin so that they are not easily infected with a disease. In addition, the following points should be considered:

- The milker's hands should be cleaned before each milking.
- Teat dipping after each milking may be effective in preventing pathogen entry into the teat.
- Affected animals should be given earlier treatment to avoid destruction of the teat.
- Udder hygiene and proper milking methods.
- Proper installation, function, and maintenance of milking equipment.
- Dry-cow management and therapy.
- Appropriate therapy.

The environmental conditions and management practices of herds have decisive effects on animal health and welfare. Keeping the herd clean and comfortable can reduce the incidence and severity of mastitis. Quarantine is also important to prevent the spread of disease to healthy cattle populations. In practice, quarantine is maintained for several weeks, depending on the disease suspected or on the health condition of the newly purchased cattle. During the quarantine period, cattle are isolated and intensively observed by farmers or veterinarians to ensure the health of the cattle. During the quarantine period, farmers or veterinarians also carry out health checks. If the cattle are declared free from disease, then the cattle can be returned to other cattle populations. Restricting access can be done by limiting the people or vehicles that enter the farm or cattle shed. In practice, access restrictions are carried out by installing a fence or gate around the farm.

References

Babu, G.S., Divya, T., and Raja, K. (2017). Management of thelitis in graded Murrah buffaloes. *International Journal of Scientific Research* 6 (10): 552–553.

Benjak, A., Avanzi, C., Benito, Y. et al. (2018). Highly reduced genome of the new species Mycobacterium uberis, the causative agent of nodular thelitis and tuberculoid scrotitis in livestock and a close relative of the leprosy bacilli. *mSphere* 3 (5): 10–1128.

Berhomde, N. (1986). Contribution to the epidemiological study of nodular thelitis. National epidemiological survey among veterinary technical groups. Doctoral dissertation. National Veterinary School of Alfort.

Brentini, M., Peroz, C., Dagher, E. et al. (2020). Caprine nodular thelitis due to Mycobacterium uberis: a series of 26 cases in 11 dairy goat farms in Western France. *Preventive Veterinary Medicine* 181: 105060.

Chartier, C., Albaric, O., Cesbron, N. et al. (2016). Tuberculoid nodular thelitis in a dairy goat flock. *The Veterinary Journal* 209: 199–200.

Faull, W.B., Hughes, J.W., and Ward, W.R. (1991). Teat problems. In: *A Mastitis Handbook for the Dairy Practitioner*, 5e. Liverpool: Liverpool Univ. Press.

Francis, P.G. (1984). Teat skin lesions and mastitis. *British Veterinary Journal* 140 (5): 430–436.

George, L.W., Divers, T.J., Ducharme, N., and Welcome, F.L. (2008). Diseases of the teats and udder. In: *Rebhun's Diseases of Dairy Cattle* (ed. T.J. Divers and S.F. Peek), 328–394. St. Louis, Missouri, USA: Saunders Elsevier.

Griffith, R.S., Walsh, D.E., Myrmel, K.H. et al. (1987). Success of L-lysine therapy in frequently recurrent herpes simplex infection. *Dermatology* 175 (4): 183–190.

Han, X.Y., Seo, Y.H., Sizer, K.C. et al. (2008). A new Mycobacterium species causing diffuse lepromatous leprosy. *American Journal of Clinical Pathology* 130 (6): 856–864.

Han, X.Y., Sizer, K.C., Thompson, E.J. et al. (2009). Comparative sequence analysis of Mycobacterium leprae and the new leprosy-causing Mycobacterium lepromatosis. *Journal of Bacteriology* 191 (19): 6067–6074.

Hanaa, A.E.-H., Saad, M.A., and Kadry, R.M. (2011). Histopathological and microbiological studies on the teat affections in she-camel. *Global Veterinaria* 7 (2): 129–137.

Kathirvel, S. and Dharmaceelan, S. (2016). Thelitis in buffaloes-reveiw of 12 clinical cases. *Indian Veterinary Journal* 93 (10): 73–74.

Kumar, S. (1990). Studies on mastitis in buffaloes with emphasis on resistance, chemotherapy and control. Master thesis. Punjab Agricultural University.

Lancaster, W.D. and Olson, C.A.R.L. (1982). Animal papillomaviruses. *Microbiological Reviews* 46 (2): 191–207.

Lindeboom, J.A., Bruijnesteijn van Coppenraet, L.E., van Soolingen, D. et al. (2011). Clinical manifestations, diagnosis, and treatment of Mycobacterium haemophilum infections. *Clinical Microbiology Reviews* 24 (4): 701–717.

Lokanadhamu, M., Sreedevi, B., and Reddy, T.V. (2005). Studies on etiology, symptomatology, diagnosis and therapy in ulcerative thelitis of buffaloes in Andhra Pradesh (India). *Buffalo Bulletin* 24 (3): 56–69.

Radostits, O.M., Gay, C.C., Constable, P.D., and Hinchcliff, K.W. (2007). *Veterinary Medicine*, 9e, 1242–1260. London: WB Saunders Company Ltd.

Ramaswamy, V., Rajendran, N., Chandrasekran, D., Rajeshwar, J. J., and Sukumar, K. (2001). *Studies on the Etiology and Effect of Obstructive Thelitis in Buffaloes: Indian Council of Agricultural Research Ad Hoc Scheme, Final Report (Period from 31.12.1997 to 31.3.2001).* Chennai, India: Tamil Nadu Veterinary and Animal Sciences University.

Rambabu, K., Sreenu, M., Sureshkumar, R.V., and Rao, T.S.C. (2011). Incidence of udder and teat affections in buffaloes. *Tamilnadu Journal of Veterinary Animal Science* 7 (6): 309–311.

Rao, U.M., Sreedevi, B., and Reddy, T.V. (2003). Studies on ulcerative mammillitis of buffaloes in Andhra Pradesh (India). *Buffalo Bulletin* 22 (4): 80.

Ruddack, E.H. (1991). *The Pocket Manual of Homeopathy. Veterinary Medicine*, 3e. New Delhi: B. Jain Publishers (P) Ltd.

Rüsch, P., Corboz, L., Ossent, P. et al. (1984). Enzootic nodular-ulcerative mamillitis in dairy cows caused by unclassified mycobacteria [in German]. *Schweizer Archiv für Tierheilkunde* 126: 467–478.

Sharma, S., Singh, K.B., Bansal, B.K., and Sharma, D.K. (2005). Clinical symptomatology and epidemiological observations on teat skin lesions in buffaloes. *Buffalo Bulletin* 24 (1): 12–16.

Smith, M.C. and Sherman, D.M. (2009). Mammary gland and milk production. In: *Goat Medicine, Second* (ed. M.C. Smith and D.M. Sherman), 647–689. Ames, Iowa, USA: Wiley-Blackwell.

Sreedevi, B., Rao, U.V.N.M., and Reddy, T.V. (2002). In: *Round Table on Mastitis: Proceedings of the Indian Veterinary Congress; VIII Annual Conference of the Indian Association for the Advancement of Veterinary Research, 22-23 February 2001, Ludhiana* (ed. R. Verma), 33–35. Amedabad: Indian Association for the Advancement of Veterinary Research.

Thilagar, S. and Dewanmuthumohammed, M.S. (1992). A clinical survey of bovine teat and udder lesions. *Indian Veterinary Journal* 69 (7): 645–646.

Thorel, M.-F., Morand, M., Fontaine, J.-J., and Gourreau, J.-M. (1990). Bovine nodular thelitis: a clinicopathological study of 20 cases. *Veterinary Dermatology* 1: 165–170. http://dx.doi.org/10.1111/j.1365-3164.1990.tb00095.x.

Tiwary, R., Hoque, M., Maiti, K.S. et al. (2005). Comparative evaluation of therapeutic regimens of obstructive thelitis in buffaloes. *Buffalo Journal* 21 (1): 75.

Turner, A.J., Morgan, I.R., Sykes, W.E., and Nicholls, W.A. (1976). Bovine herpes mammillitis of dairy cattle in Victoria. *Australian Veterinary Journal* 52 (4): 170–173.

Varshney, J.P. (2006). Thelitis in dairy animals. *Homeopathic Links Winte* 19: 218.

20

Acute Hypokalemia

Samuel U. Felix[1], Chiezey N. Pauline[1], Nathaniel Ogunkunle[2], and Allam Lushaikyaa[3]

[1] National Animal Production Research Institute/Faculty of Veterinary Medicine, Ahmadu Bello University Zaria, Zaria, Kaduna State, Nigeria
[2] Department of Food and Animal Science, Alabama A&M University, Normal, Alabama, USA
[3] Faculty of Veterinary Medicine, Ahmadu Bello University Zaria, Zaria, Kaduna State, Nigeria

20.1 Introduction

Potassium is a monovalent cation that is fundamental for cell functions. It is involved in cell homeostasis, osmotic volume regulation, and acid–base regulation. It plays crucial roles in maintaining cell stability, controlling acid–base equilibrium, establishing the resting membrane potential, transmitting nerve signals, and enabling muscle contractions. Its metabolic process is intricate and dynamic. Potassium is acquired through dietary intake, distributed within and outside cells, and primarily expelled through urine. Milk contains roughly 1.4 g of potassium per liter, which makes it a notable contributor to the elimination and loss of potassium from the body, particularly in highly productive dairy cows (Plöntzke et al. 2022).

Disorders in potassium balance maintenance can have life-threatening implications. Hypokalemia and hyperkalemia correspond to extracellular potassium levels that fall below or rise above the normal physiological range of 3.9–5.2 mmol/l, respectively. Hypokalemia is commonly observed in cows brought to veterinary clinics. Clinical records encompass conditions like displaced abomasum, sometimes with volvulus, mastitis, retained placentas, metritis, and hepatic lipidosis. Severe hypokalemia is indicated by a serum potassium concentration below 2.5 mmol/l that results in pronounced weakness or recumbency in most animals. Moderate hypokalemia, indicated by a serum potassium concentration of 2.5–3.5 mmol/l, leads some cattle to become recumbent or display weakness along with reduced gastrointestinal motility (Viera and Wouk 2015).

Potassium equilibrium is predominantly regulated by the interplay between the absorption of potassium from the gastrointestinal (GI) tract and its subsequent removal through the kidneys (in all animals) and saliva (specifically in mature ruminants). Potassium movement within the small intestine is passive, and it becomes active within the colon, driven by the presence of aldosterone. The central influencer of potassium elimination via the kidneys and saliva is aldosterone, a hormone discharged from the glomerulosa zone in the adrenal gland in response to heightened potassium levels and other stimuli. A key function of aldosterone is to amplify the discharge of potassium ions in the distal tubules of the kidneys and collecting ducts (Table 20.1) (Luna et al. 2023).

At least 95% of potassium in the body is intracellular with skeletal muscle containing 60–75% of that intracellular potassium. Marked changes in serum or plasma potassium concentrations alter the resting membrane potential of cells because the potassium gradient generated by the Na^+/K^+-ATPase is primarily responsible for the negative electric potential across cell membranes (Russell and Roussel 2007). Therefore, hypokalemia or hyperkalemia alters the resting membrane potential, which results in clinically important changes to cellular and organ function. Hypokalemia usually indicates the whole-body depletion of potassium, unless identified in animals with hyperinsulinemia due to hyperglycemia, in which case potassium may have translocated intracellularly. Whole-body potassium status during hyperkalemia cannot be inferred because many animals with hyperkalemia have concurrent acidemia and whole-body potassium depletion (Yamada et al. 2023).

Periparturient Diseases of Cattle, First Edition. Edited by Tanmoy Rana.

Table 20.1 Classification of hypo- and hyperkalemia.

Type of condition	Mild (mEq/l)	Moderate (mEq/l)	Severe (mEq/l)
Hypokalemia	3.0–3.5	2.5–2.9	< 2.5
Hyperkalemia	5.5–6.4	6.5–7.5	> 7.5

The depletion of whole-body potassium can lead to muscle weakness and may or may not coincide with reduced plasma potassium levels (hypokalemia). More frequently, animals without potassium depletion may appear hypokalemic on a serum biochemistry profile due to potassium redistribution. The significance of hypokalemia requires the consideration of other electrolytes and the acid–base balance. Additionally, determining whether an intervention is necessary relies on a physical examination and comprehensive history. As it is predominantly intracellular, potassium levels in the bloodstream (serum potassium concentration) offer limited insight into an animal's potassium status. To better gauge potassium depletion, measuring the intracellular potassium concentrations of erythrocytes or muscle cells is more precise, but this is often impractical due to current technological limitations (Sattler and Fecteau 2014).

Plasma potassium concentrations hinge on both external and internal potassium balances. External balance relates to potassium intake and absorption from the GI tract as well as kidney-mediated potassium excretion. The primary potassium source in the normal ruminant diet is forage. An animal with a healthy appetite usually maintains normal serum potassium levels. Almost all ingested potassium is absorbed, particularly for animals with forage-based diets like lactating dairy cows. These cows might consume over 10 times their daily potassium requirement. Consequently, well-developed renal mechanisms in cattle eliminate excess potassium. However, when intake is disrupted, these mechanisms might not respond promptly, which leads to potassium depletion. Partial or complete anorexia in cows often results in moderate hypokalemia, although without evident weakness. Conditions like diarrhea, third-space loss, and alkalosis can exacerbate potassium loss from fluid compartments. Certain corticosteroids with mineralocorticoid effects, such as isoflupredone acetate, elevate potassium excretion, while diuretics like furosemide contribute to renal potassium loss. After relieving urinary obstruction, a diuretic phase may cause substantial potassium depletion. Internal balance concerns the potassium distribution between intracellular fluid (ICF) and extracellular fluid (ECF) compartments. The acid–base equilibrium notably influences this distribution. Acidosis prompts potassium movement from the ICF to the ECF, which leads to hyperkalemia, while alkalosis triggers the opposite and results in hypokalemia. Insulin also aids in shifting potassium from the ECF to the ICF. Thus, administering dextrose or insulin could induce hypokalemia or alleviate existing hyperkalemia (Kim et al. 2023).

20.2 Etiology

Hypokalemia is most common in lactating dairy cattle and is secondary to several conditions (Bairwa et al. 2023).

20.2.1 Anorexia due to Clinical Mastitis and Retained Placentas

Clinical mastitis, an infection that affects the udder, and a retained placenta, when the placenta does not expel after calving, can both result in a reduced appetite (anorexia). This diminished food intake can contribute to hypokalemia.

20.2.2 Obstruction in the Upper Gastrointestinal Tract

Conditions like left-displaced abomasum, right-displaced abomasum, abomasal volvulus, and abomasal impaction can block the upper gastrointestinal tract. Such blockages can hinder nutrient and electrolyte absorption, including that of potassium.

20.2.3 Inevitable Potassium Loss Through Milk

Lactating dairy cows lose potassium through milk production. The passage highlights that approximately 1.4 g of potassium is lost for every liter of milk produced, leading to the development of hypokalemia.

20.2.4 Hyperinsulinemia and Shifting of Potassium Within Cells

Elevated levels of insulin due to high blood glucose can prompt a movement of potassium from the ECF to the ICF, causing a drop in blood potassium levels.

20.2.5 Activation of the Sympathetic Nervous System

Activation of the fight-or-flight response through the sympathetic nervous system can influence blood potassium levels. This can lead to greater potassium absorption by cells, which contributes to hypokalemia.

20.2.6 Aldosterone Release

Aldosterone, a hormone that manages sodium and potassium levels in the body, is discharged in response to factors like low blood volume (hypovolemia) and the necessity for sodium retention. However, its actions can also lead to potassium loss.

20.2.7 Diminished Total Body Potassium Reserves

Dairy cows usually have a lower muscle mass compared to other cattle breeds. This reduced muscle mass equates to lower overall potassium reserves in the body, which can contribute to hypokalemia.

20.2.8 Severity of Hypokalemia

In most conditions of hypokalemia among lactating dairy cows, the deficiency in potassium is not severe enough to induce weakness and recumbency (inability to stand). This suggests that even though hypokalemia might be present, its consequences might not always be substantial enough to trigger muscle-related complications.

20.3 Epidemiology

Hypokalemia is a commonly observed condition in lactating dairy cattle that experience prolonged periods of reduced appetite (more than 2 days), but it is infrequent in adult ruminants with a sufficient dry matter intake as well as in neonatal calves, lambs, and kids. Hypokalemia occurs more frequently in lactating dairy cows compared to beef cows or animals in feedlots. This discrepancy can be attributed to the additional loss of potassium through milk, the lower muscle mass in dairy cows that leads to decreased overall potassium stores, and the utilization of glycogen and skeletal muscle protein for energy during early stages of lactation. Milk typically contains about 36 mmol/l of potassium. Consequently, high yielding dairy cows are at a higher risk of developing hypokalemia, and the occurrence of hypokalemia after giving birth increases as milk production rises (Wallig et al. 2023).

During the early lactation phase, dairy cows experience a significant negative energy balance. The breakdown of intracellular glycogen and protein results in increased potassium excretion through urine, which leads to whole-body potassium depletion due to the binding of potassium to glycogen. The kidneys excrete potassium through distal tubular cell secretion. Substances like aldosterone and other steroids with mineralocorticoid activity enhance this distal tubular secretion by making tubular luminal membranes more permeable to potassium and thus, increase potassium loss through urine. Hypokalemia and whole-body potassium depletion are frequently observed in lactating dairy cattle that receive corticosteroid injections for conditions like ketosis, especially when the corticosteroids possess mineralocorticoid activity, as isoflupredone acetate does. This effect is due to the increased renal and gastrointestinal (saliva and colon) loss of potassium caused by the mineralocorticoid activity of isoflupredone. Hypokalemia typically reaches its lowest point, around 60–70% of the normal value, approximately 72 hours after the first of two 10-mg injections.

The release of exogenous or endogenous insulin that results from hyperglycemia following intravenous (IV) dextrose administration or corticosteroid use can induce hypokalemia through the intracellular movement of potassium alongside glucose. This shift in potassium represents movement within the cell and not whole-body depletion. Generally, higher alkaline pH levels in the blood decrease serum potassium concentrations, whereas more acidic pH levels increase it. Therefore, hypokalemia is often seen in ruminants experiencing metabolic alkalosis.

In experimental cases, the induction of metabolic alkalosis through the oral administration of sodium bicarbonate in Jersey cows led to marked metabolic (strong ion) alkalosis (base excess ranging from 14 to 19 mEq/l), hypokalemia (potassium levels between 2.6 and 3.1 mEq/l), and a rise in muscle potassium concentrations by 6–10%. This suggests an intracellular shift of potassium from the extracellular space to the intracellular space. In healthy dairy cattle, immediately after calving, whole-body potassium depletion might be present, based on potassium balance studies and research that documents decreased skeletal muscle potassium content and urinary potassium concentrations post calving (Mezzetti and Trevisi 2023).

20.3.1 Intracellular and Extracellular Potassium Gradients

The disparity in potassium concentrations between the ICF and ECF compartments has significant influence on cellular membrane potentials and the generation of action potentials. This gradient dictates the baseline membrane potential, which is crucial for maintaining muscle activity and transmitting nerve signals. While the plasma potassium concentration does not solely dictate this gradient, the difference between ICF and ECF potassium concentrations is pivotal. This gradient is fundamental to standard cellular activities, and deviations can lead to muscle weakness and other symptomatic outcomes.

20.3.2 Muscle Damage and Rhabdomyolysis

Hypokalemic myopathy in cattle can manifest with varying degrees of muscle damage that span from subtle effects to severe impacts. The exact causes behind the extent of muscle damage remain uncertain, and the reasons for the varying degrees of severity among individual animals are still ambiguous. Severe cases may involve structural muscle damage, including necrosis, which suggests a potential link between the severity of muscle damage and the occurrence of substantial rhabdomyolysis. Nevertheless, the precise factors that dictate the distribution of cattle into groups with varying severity in muscle damage have not been definitively established.

20.3.3 Cardiac Electrical Irregularities

Hypokalemia can affect the electrical activity of the heart, which leads to dysrhythmias and other arrhythmogenic phenomena. Some possible mechanisms include the hyperpolarization of cardiac cells that results in spontaneous automatic activity, conduction issues due to disparities between resting membrane and threshold potentials, prolonged action potential durations due to slow repolarization, and changes in responses to stimuli. These irregularities can contribute to an increased likelihood of cardiac dysrhythmias in cattle with hypokalemic myopathy. Moreover, the presence of necrotic muscle cells can amplify the risk of cardiac dysrhythmias, which underscores the significance of comprehending the muscle pathology linked to the condition.

20.3.4 Muscle Lesions and Hypokalemic Myopathy

Despite cardiac dysrhythmias and muscle damage being possible outcomes of hypokalemia, consistent evidence of muscle lesions characteristic of hypokalemic myopathy has not been universally documented in cattle cases where the syndrome is reported. This discrepancy raises queries about the direct correlation between hypokalemia and the necrosis of muscle cells in cattle. Further investigation is necessary to unveil the relationship that connects hypokalemia, muscle damage, and clinical indications in cattle.

20.4 Pathogenesis

Potassium equilibriums in mature cattle hinge on the interplay between potassium absorption from the GI tract and its subsequent elimination through the kidneys and salivary glands. Potassium transport is passive in the small intestine and active in the colon, driven by aldosterone. The most influential hormone that impacts renal and salivary potassium excretion is aldosterone, which is released from the zona glomerulosa of the adrenal gland in response to hyperkalemia and other factors. Around 95% of the body's total potassium resides within cells, with skeletal muscles containing between 60%

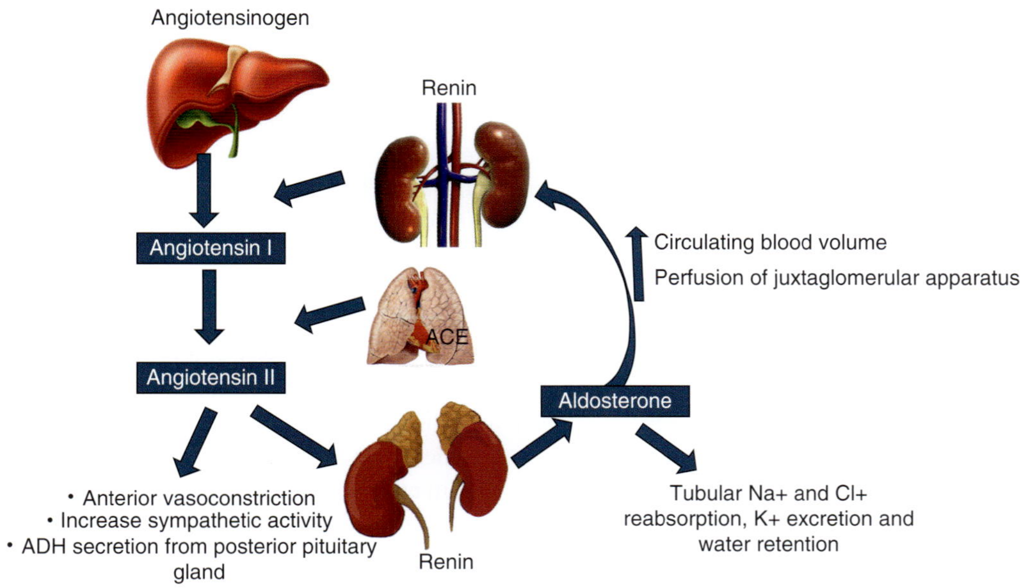

Figure 20.1 Pathogenesis of hypokalemia.

and 75% of this intracellular potassium. Total potassium losses in lactating cattle comprise 75% in urine, 13% in feces (primarily endogenous), and 12% in milk. Notably, these losses are obligatory (Figure 20.1).

Significant fluctuations in serum or plasma potassium levels bring about changes in the resting membrane potential of cells, primarily due to the potassium gradient established by Na^+/K^+–ATPase, which contributes to the negative electric potential across cell membranes. Consequently, hypokalemia disrupts this resting membrane potential, which leads to substantial shifts in cellular and organ functions. Hypokalemia generally signifies a depletion of whole-body potassium, unless it is the result of hyperglycemia and hyperinsulinemia.

The potassium content in cattle is approximately 2.2 g/kg body weight. Lactating dairy cows should consume diets that contain at least 0.7% potassium on a dry-weight basis, although high producing dairy cows require higher dietary potassium concentrations that often range from 1.3% to 1.4%. The absorption efficiency of potassium in a standard lactating dairy cow diet spans from 74% to 88%, with absorption primarily occurring in the small intestine and forestomach, with the former being more predominant. Rumen fluid in cattle usually holds a potassium concentration between 24 and 85 mEq/l, and both rumen fluid potassium concentration and potassium absorption rely heavily on intake. This indicates that augmenting potassium intake, particularly raising rumen potassium concentration, directly leads to heightened potassium absorption.

Hypokalemia development in cattle is influenced by factors such as anorexia and dehydration. A reduction in dietary potassium intake necessitates 24–48 hours for the mammalian kidney to adapt. Dehydration impacts hypokalemia via the activation of aldosterone. There appears to be a sensor in the gut or hepatoportal system that detects potassium intake and prompts the kidney to increase potassium excretion upon heightened potassium ingestion. However, the specific location of this sensor and the molecular pathway for signal transmission remain unknown. Despite this, the activation of this sensor causes increased potassium excretion by the kidneys, even before a noticeable increase in serum potassium concentration follows heightened potassium intake.

Regarding abomasal physiology, reduced potassium concentrations may impact muscle contraction. Decreased potassium concentrations in the tissue bath of cow abomasal corpus circular muscle reduce the amplitude of contraction. In bulls, there is a minor, statistically insignificant, decrease in force developed by abomasal smooth muscle when the in vitro potassium concentration drops from 5.4 to 2.0 to 3.0 mmol/l. Consequently, hypokalemia might lead to a diminished abomasal emptying rate that elevates the risk of conditions like left-displaced abomasum, abomasal volvulus, and potentially, retained placentas and metritis in dairy cattle. While the link between potassium concentrations and skeletal muscle tone in cattle has not been established, studies in humans suggest that marked hypokalemia (<2.0–2.5 mEq/l) is necessary to influence skeletal muscle tone (Walter et al. 2022).

20.5 Clinical Findings

Affected animals have generalized muscle weakness, decreased gastrointestinal motility, and depression. Severely affected animals are unable to stand or lift their heads from the ground. Cows with severe hypokalemia (< 2.0 mEq/l) are usually recumbent and profoundly weak, appear flaccid, and lie in sternal or lateral recumbency. They are unable to support the weight of their heads off the ground and commonly hold their heads on their flanks. Profound weakness of the lateral cervical muscles may occur. Anorexia is common. Cardiac arrhythmias are often detectable upon auscultation, and atrial fibrillation may be present upon electrocardiography. Cardiac arrhythmias are associated with abnormal serum potassium concentrations, both hypokalemia and hyperkalemia. In an unpublished study of 110 adult cattle with atrial fibrillation, hypokalemia was common before the induction of atrial fibrillation (Çinar and İsmail 2022). Although there do not appear to be any large-scale studies that examine the association between hypokalemia and cardiac arrhythmias in adult cattle, hypokalemia, hypocalcemia, and alkalemia are common in lactating dairy cattle with left-displaced abomasum and atrial fibrillation. In a recent study, 2 of 15 lactating dairy cows with experimentally induced hypokalemia and alkalemia developed atrial fibrillation that resolved within 24 hours of administering KCl, which was accompanied by an increase in plasma potassium concentrations and a decrease in blood pH. Atrial fibrillation in other studies was diagnosed in 4 of 10, 2 of 14, and 5 of 17 cows with naturally acquired hypokalemia and in 1of 7 lactating dairy cows with experimentally induced hypokalemia following intramuscular (IM) administration of two 20-mg doses of isoflupredone acetate at a 48-hour interval. Taken together, these findings suggest that hypokalemia plays an important role in the development of atrial fibrillation in adult cattle. Signs of chronic potassium depletion in cattle include anorexia; pica characterized by hair licking, floor licking, and chewing of wooden partitions; rough hair coat; muscular weakness; irritability; paralysis; and tetany (Mann et al. 2019).

20.6 Clinical Pathology

The order of sensitivity and specificity in determining whole-body potassium depletion is as follows: skeletal muscle > serum/plasma > milk > erythrocyte/whole blood > urine > saliva (Mekroud et al. 2023; Yasaswin et al. 2023) (Figure 20.2).

20.6.1 Skeletal Muscle Potassium Content

Measuring the skeletal muscle potassium concentration is considered the most sensitive and specific method for assessing whole-body potassium status and therefore is the gold standard test. Skeletal muscle is considered the best tissue to sample because it contains approximately 75% of whole-body potassium stores. A standardized muscle should be evaluated in cattle because differences in potassium content greater than 15% are present in individual animals, and this muscle-to-muscle variation is greater than that produced by breed.

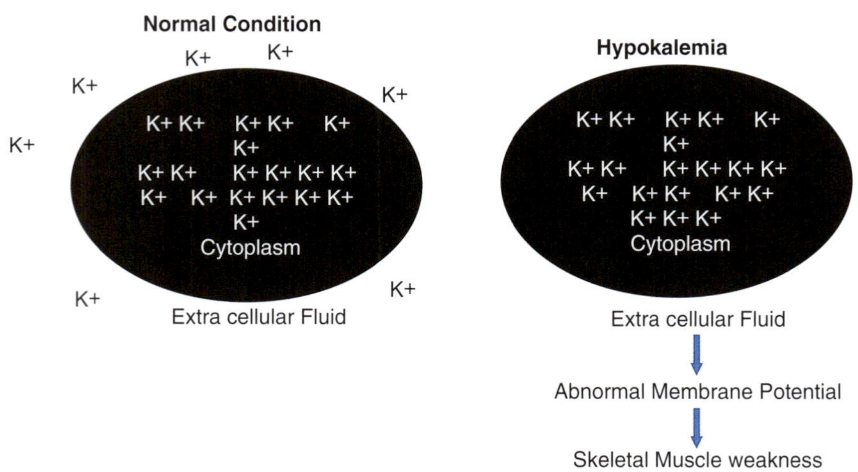

Figure 20.2 Relationship between cytosolic and extracellular potassium levels in hypokalemia.

20.6.2 Plasma Potassium Concentration

The determination of the serum/plasma potassium concentration is required to confirm a suspected diagnosis of hypokalemia. A serum potassium concentration less than 2.5 mEq/l reflects severe hypokalemia, and most animals will be weak or recumbent. A serum potassium concentration of 2.5–3.5 mEq/l reflects moderate hypokalemia, and some cattle will be recumbent or appear weak, with depressed gastrointestinal motility. In addition to the measurement of serum potassium concentration, determining the serum concentrations of sodium, chloride calcium, and phosphorus as well as the serum activities of creatine kinase and aspartate aminotransferase can be very helpful in guiding the treatment of cattle with hypokalemia. Serum potassium concentrations are usually a little higher than plasma potassium concentrations because platelet activation releases potassium. In summary, a serum/plasma potassium concentration below the normal range provides unequivocal evidence of hypokalemia unless there is concurrent hyperinsulinemia or alkalemia. However, because more than 95–98% of whole-body potassium stores are intracellular, it is likely that serum/plasma potassium concentrations are not as sensitive as the skeletal muscle potassium content for indicating whole-body potassium depletion.

20.6.3 Milk Potassium Concentration

Milk potassium concentrations are theoretically more sensitive than serum/plasma potassium concentrations for detecting whole-body potassium depletion in individual cows because milk concentrations of potassium are constant for an individual cow. Potassium depletion in lactating dairy cows causes the milk potassium concentration to decrease from 1.45 to 1.28 g/l; this is a greater percentage decrease than that in the plasma or whole blood of cattle with whole-body potassium depletion. However, there is marked individual variation in the milk concentrations of potassium in healthy cattle, with variations up to 50% between cows. This variability appears to be a result of changes in milk fat, protein, and lactose percentages, with the highest correlation of milk potassium concentrations being with milk lactose concentrations ($R = -0.53$ or -0.74). The relationship between potassium and lactose can be attributed to the fact that these are important contributors to milk osmolality, which is constant and isotonic. Milk potassium concentration also changes during lactation, being 42 mmol/l in early lactation, 40 mmol/l in mid-lactation, and 27 mmol/l in late lactation, with a mean bulk milk potassium concentration of 37 mmol/l. The large cow-to-cow variability in milk potassium concentrations and dependence on milk lactose concentrations make it difficult to produce a suitable cutoff point for identifying whole-body potassium depletion in sick, lactating dairy cows. However, milk potassium concentrations have clinical utility in monitoring potassium homeostasis over time in an individual cow.

20.6.4 Erythrocyte Potassium Concentration

Erythrocyte potassium concentrations are determined by measuring the plasma potassium concentration and hematocrit, adding sufficient distilled water to hemolyze the erythrocytes, and then measuring the potassium concentration of the hemolyzed fluid, which is followed by a mathematical calculation. There is marked cow-to-cow variability in the erythrocyte potassium concentrations (7–70 mmol/l) and sodium concentrations (15–87 mmol/l) of healthy cattle that has a genetic basis with no breed influence. There are two main cellular potassium concentration peaks, one at 20 mmol/l and the second at 50 mmol/l. In lactating dairy cattle with induced whole-body potassium deficiency, whole-blood potassium concentrations changed similarly to plasma potassium concentrations. However, in 180 cows, a relationship between plasma potassium concentrations and erythrocyte potassium concentrations was not found. The measurement of erythrocyte or whole-blood potassium concentrations is not currently recommended for evaluating whole-body potassium status.

20.6.5 Urine Potassium Concentration

The concentration of potassium in urine, referred to as urine potassium concentration, is typically found to be high, with an average value of 454 ± 112 mEq/l. However, this concentration can vary significantly, as indicated by a mean fractional clearance of 82% and a coefficient of variation of 61%. This substantial variability in urine potassium concentration poses challenges in establishing a definitive threshold for identifying cases of whole-body potassium depletion. Despite the challenges in setting a specific cutoff point, analyzing urine potassium concentrations remains useful in certain contexts. For instance, when studying an individual cow that maintains a consistent diet over an extended period, monitoring urine potassium concentrations can provide insights into the cow's potassium balance and overall homeostasis. In addition to urine potassium concentrations, the pH level of urine, known as urine pH, could offer valuable information as a more effective preliminary screening test. If there is a significant drop in the urine potassium concentration, it might lead to the occurrence of aciduria, where the urine becomes more acidic than usual. This acidic urine response could indicate a substantial reduction in urine potassium concentration and alert clinicians to the possibility of underlying potassium-related issues.

20.6.6 Salivary Potassium Concentration

The salivary potassium concentration is influenced by various factors, primarily aldosterone in response to changes in serum sodium concentrations. Comparing salivary potassium concentrations to salivary sodium concentrations (with a one-to-one exchange) as well as considering the ratio of serum sodium–potassium is necessary to derive any clinical value from these measurements. This approach accounts for sodium homeostasis and provides insights into potassium balance. The normal range for salivary potassium concentrations is quite broad, spanning from 4 to 70 mEq/l. This wide range is largely affected by sodium homeostasis, which exerts the most significant influence on these concentrations. However, when interpreting salivary potassium concentrations, it is important to note that it is not just the concentration itself but also its relationship with the salivary sodium concentration and serum sodium–potassium ratio that matters. A study conducted on cattle with conditions like left-displaced abomasum, right-displaced abomasum, or abomasal volvulus found no meaningful correlation between salivary and serum potassium concentrations. This implies that the salivary potassium concentration might not reliably reflect the potassium status of the entire body. Collectively, the evidence suggests that measuring the salivary potassium concentration offers limited insight into the overall potassium status of an individual. The complex interplay between aldosterone, serum sodium concentrations, and the sodium–potassium balance complicates the use of salivary potassium concentrations as a reliable indicator of whole-body potassium levels. Therefore, while salivary potassium concentrations can be measured, their clinical utility in assessing overall potassium status appears to be minimal.

20.7 Necropsy Findings

Autopsies performed on cattle that have experienced hypokalemia-induced recumbency unveil the presence of muscle necrosis in the pelvic limbs. Muscle necrosis refers to the demise of muscle tissue. When blood circulation and oxygen delivery are compromised, as can occur in cases of severe hypokalemia, muscle cells can incur damage and eventually perish. This phenomenon leads to muscle necrosis, where the impacted muscles lose both their functional capacity and structural integrity.

The identification of muscle necrosis in the pelvic limbs suggests that these muscles endured insufficient blood circulation and oxygen provision due to hypokalemia, which lead to tissue harm. The examination of non-weight bearing muscles at a microscopic level reveals the presence of multifocal myonecrosis coupled with infiltration by macrophages and vacuolation of myofibers. These histological findings align with the pattern of hypokalemic myopathy observed in humans and dogs. Importantly, it is worth noting that hypokalemic myopathy can also manifest in muscles not subject to recumbency-associated ischemia (Chen et al. 2022).

20.8 Treatment

Treating hypokalemia in lactating dairy cows should focus on the methods described in this section (Constable et al. 2014; Ferraro et al. 2023).

20.8.1 Surgical Correction of Abomasal Displacement

In cases where hypokalemia is associated with abomasal displacement (a condition where the stomach shifts out of its normal position), surgical correction of the displacement may be necessary. The abomasum is the fourth compartment of the stomach in ruminants, including cows. Abomasal displacement occurs when the abomasum shifts from its normal anatomical position. This displacement can have various causes, including changes in the abdominal cavity's pressure and positioning of other organs. Hypokalemia can be associated with abomasal displacement due to the disruption of normal digestive processes and nutrient absorption that occurs when the abomasum is displaced. This can lead to imbalances in various electrolytes, including potassium. Abomasal displacement, also known as abomasal volvulus or twisted stomach, is a condition that primarily affects ruminant animals such as cattle, sheep, and goats. In this condition, the abomasum becomes displaced from its normal position within the abdominal cavity. Surgical correction of abomasal displacement is a veterinary procedure aimed at repositioning the displaced abomasum back to its original anatomical location and restoring normal digestive function.

20.8.2 Increasing Potassium Intake

Increasing the intake of potassium is an important aspect of treatment. This can be achieved by promoting higher dry matter intake, which includes the consumption of potassium-rich feeds. Potassium is one of the key electrolytes, along with sodium and chloride, that help maintain the balance of fluids and electrolytes in the body. This balance is crucial for maintaining proper hydration, nerve function, and muscle contraction. Ruminants, including cattle, have a unique digestive system that produces volatile fatty acids during the fermentation of ingested feed. These acids can lead to changes in the acid–base balance. Potassium helps regulate the acid–base balance, particularly when metabolic disturbances like metabolic acidosis are present. Potassium is essential for proper muscle function, including the muscles involved in digestion and abomasal movement. Increasing potassium intake can aid in restoring normal gastrointestinal motility, which is particularly important in cases of abomasal displacement. Promoting a higher dry matter intake is an important strategy to increase potassium intake. This is significant because potassium-rich feeds, such as alfalfa, clover, and certain grains, can contribute to higher potassium levels in the diet. These feeds can be selected based on their nutritional content and suitability for the specific animal's needs.

20.8.3 Oral Administration of Potassium Chloride (KCl)

The preferred method for treating hypokalemia is oral potassium supplementation. Oral potassium administration is the method of choice for treating hypokalemia. Inappetent adult cattle should initially be treated with 120 g of potassium chloride (KCl) orally (PO), followed by an additional oral treatment of 120 g KCl 12 hours later, for a total treatment of 240 g KCl (0.4 g/kg body weight [BW]) within 24 hours 0.6 g/kg. Higher oral doses of KCl are not recommended because they can lead to diarrhea, excessive salivation, muscular tremors of the legs, and excitability. Administering KCl orally is effective for raising potassium levels. The treatment plan might involve specific dosages and timing. Hypokalemia is typically diagnosed through blood tests that measure the concentration of potassium in the blood. The severity of the condition is determined by the level of potassium depletion. The underlying cause of hypokalemia should also be identified and addressed, as additional treatments may be needed to target the root cause.

The oral administration of KCl is a safe and effective way to increase potassium levels in the body. KCl is available in various forms, including tablets, powders, and solutions. It is important to choose the appropriate form and dosage based on the animal's size, condition, and dietary requirements. The treatment plan for oral KCl supplementation will involve specific dosages and timing. The dosage is often calculated based on the severity of hypokalemia and the target potassium level. Veterinarians will carefully determine the appropriate dosage to avoid excessive potassium intake, which could lead to hyperkalemia. The dosages may need to be divided into multiple doses throughout the day to ensure a steady and controlled absorption. Regularly monitoring potassium levels in the blood is crucial to assess the effectiveness of the treatment. The animal's response to supplementation will determine whether adjustments to the dosage and timing are necessary.

20.8.4 Intravenous Administration of Potassium Chloride (KCl)

Intravenous administration of potassium is reserved for severe cases of hypokalemia, especially when the animal is recumbent (unable to stand). However, IV administration carries risks and is typically used only in critical situations. Potassium is rarely administered intravenously; the IV route is used only for the initial treatment of recumbent ruminants with severe hypokalemia and rumen atony because it is much more dangerous and expensive than oral treatment. The most aggressive IV treatment protocol is an isotonic solution of KCl (1.15% KCl), which should be administered at less than 3.2 ml/kg per hour, equivalent to a maximal delivery rate of 0.5 mEq of potassium/kg BW per hour. Higher rates of potassium administration run the risk of inducing hemodynamically important arrhythmias, including ventricular premature complexes that can lead to ventricular fibrillation and death. Palatable hay and propylene glycol administered orally are recommended. In a series of 14 cases, treatment consisting of KCl given intravenously and orally for an average total daily dose of 0.42 g/kg BW (26 g orally and 16 g IV) for an average of 5 days, resulted in the recovery of 11 cases after an average of 3 days. During recumbency, affected cattle require special attention to minimize ischemic necrosis of pelvic limb muscles. The IV administration of KCl is considered when oral supplementation is not feasible or when the immediate correction of potassium levels is required due to life-threatening complications associated with severe hypokalemia. This can include cases where the animal is unable to eat, absorb oral medications, or is in a critical condition. The IV administration of KCl is not without risks. A rapid infusion of potassium can cause cardiac arrhythmias, which can be fatal. Therefore, it must be performed with careful monitoring and at an appropriate dilution to reduce the risk of hyperkalemia-induced heart disturbances. The proper equipment and experienced personnel are essential to manage the administration safely. KCl is usually administered intravenously as a diluted solution to minimize the risk of complications. The concentration and rate of infusion are carefully determined by a veterinarian based on the animal's size, potassium level, and overall health. The goal is to gradually raise potassium levels within safe limits.

20.8.5 Potential Complications of High Oral Doses

This passage notes that excessively high oral doses of potassium can lead to adverse effects like diarrhea, salivation, muscular tremors, and excitability.

- **Diarrhea:** High doses of potassium can irritate the gastrointestinal tract, leading to diarrhea. This is because excessive potassium intake can disrupt the normal balance of electrolytes and fluids in the intestines, which causes the muscles in the intestines to contract more frequently and forcefully and results in loose and frequent bowel movements.
- **Salivation:** Excessive potassium intake can stimulate the salivary glands, which leads to increased saliva production. This can result in a sensation of excessive saliva in the mouth that might be uncomfortable for those experiencing it.
- **Muscular tremors:** High doses of potassium can affect the nervous system and lead to muscular tremors or involuntary shaking of muscles. This is likely due to a disrupted balance between potassium and other electrolytes like sodium and calcium that is essential for proper muscle function.
- **Excitability:** Elevated potassium levels can influence nerve cell function and increase nerve excitability. This heightened excitability can result in restlessness, nervousness, and even muscle spasms.

20.8.6 Special Attention During Recumbency

When cattle are unable to stand (recumbent), there is a risk of muscle damage due to reduced blood circulation. Special care is needed to minimize ischemic necrosis (tissue damage from reduced blood flow) of the muscles in the pelvic limbs. When cattle are unable to stand and are lying down (recumbent), it could be due to various factors such as illness, injury, or weakness. Recumbency for extended periods can lead to a range of complications, including reduced blood circulation to certain body parts.

- **Risk of muscle damage:** Reduced blood circulation to the muscles in the pelvic limbs can lead to muscle damage. The lack of proper blood flow can result in decreased oxygen and nutrient supply to the muscles, which ultimately leads to tissue damage.
- **Ischemic necrosis:** Ischemic necrosis refers to tissue damage that occurs as a result of reduced blood flow (ischemia). When blood flow to a specific area is compromised, the tissues in that area can begin to die due to a lack of oxygen and nutrients. In the context of recumbent cattle, ischemic necrosis can occur in the muscles of the pelvic limbs due to reduced blood circulation to those areas.
- **Minimizing damage:** To minimize the risk of ischemic necrosis and muscle damage, special care is needed for recumbent cattle. This care may include regularly changing the animal's position, providing supportive bedding to cushion their body and prevent pressure sores, and ensuring proper hydration and nutrition.

- **Veterinary attention:** It is important to involve a veterinarian in cases of recumbent cattle. They can diagnose the underlying cause of the recumbency and provide appropriate treatment. Additionally, a veterinarian can advise on proper care techniques to prevent complications such as muscle damage and ischemic necrosis.

20.8.7 Use of Glucocorticoids

Glucocorticoids like dexamethasone and isoflupredone acetate are used to treat conditions like ketosis (a metabolic disorder). These medications can affect potassium levels and mineralocorticoid activity.

Glucocorticoids are a class of steroid hormones that have a wide range of effects on the body's metabolism, immune response, and other physiological processes. Dexamethasone and isoflupredone acetate are examples of glucocorticoid medications commonly used in veterinary medicine.

Glucocorticoids can influence electrolyte balances, including potassium levels, in the body. They may cause an increase in urinary potassium excretion that potentially leads to lower potassium levels in the blood (hypokalemia). This effect is due to the impact of glucocorticoids on renal (kidney) function and the regulation of potassium ions. While glucocorticoids primarily affect metabolism and immune responses, they can also have some mineralocorticoid-like effects. Mineralocorticoids are another class of steroid hormones that regulate electrolyte and fluid balances, primarily sodium and potassium. Glucocorticoids can interfere with the balance between glucocorticoid and mineralocorticoid effects, which potentially disrupts electrolyte regulation. When using glucocorticoids to treat conditions like ketosis, it is important to monitor the animal's electrolyte levels, including potassium, to ensure that imbalances are not occurring. Veterinarians will consider the potential effects on potassium levels and other electrolytes and adjust treatment protocols accordingly. Monitoring can involve regular blood tests to assess the animal's overall health and electrolyte status.

20.8.8 Monitoring and Judicious Use

Monitoring the animal's condition, plasma potassium levels, and any signs of weakness or recumbency is crucial, especially when using glucocorticoids that could impact potassium levels. Regular and thorough monitoring of the animal's overall condition is essential during treatment. This involves observing changes in behavior, appetite, mobility, and other relevant indicators. Monitoring plasma (blood) potassium levels is a direct way to assess the effectiveness of treatment and the response to interventions. Regular blood tests can help track potassium levels and guide adjustments in treatment. Hypokalemia can lead to muscle weakness and even recumbency (inability to stand). Monitoring these signs is crucial to catch any decline in the animal's condition promptly. Glucocorticoids, which are used to treat various conditions including ketosis, can affect potassium levels. Certain glucocorticoids may lead to potassium loss or affect the potassium balance. Due to the potential impact on potassium levels, the administration of glucocorticoids should be approached with caution. Veterinarians often carefully evaluate the need for glucocorticoid treatment, the specific glucocorticoid to be used, and the appropriate dosage. Glucocorticoids can provide benefits in terms of addressing specific health issues, but their use should be balanced against potential side effects, including impacts on potassium levels. Monitoring and judicious use allow for personalized treatment plans tailored to the animal's condition and response. This helps optimize treatment effectiveness while minimizing risks.

20.8.9 Effectiveness and Considerations

The effectiveness of treating potassium-related issues with oral KCl can be significant in certain cases. Oral KCl supplementation is commonly used to address potassium deficiencies, particularly when there is an imbalance in the body's potassium levels. However, the response to treatment can vary based on factors that include the underlying cause of the potassium imbalance, individual animal characteristics, and the specific condition being treated. When considering treatment with oral potassium chloride, several important considerations should be taken into account:

- **Underlying cause:** It is crucial to identify and address the underlying cause of the potassium imbalance. Whether the deficiency is due to dietary factors, medical conditions, medications, or other factors, addressing the root cause is essential for effective treatment.
- **Dosage:** Determining the appropriate dosage of oral potassium chloride is important. Dosage requirements can vary depending on the severity of the potassium deficiency and the individual's overall health. Veterinarians will often prescribe specific dosages based on careful assessment.

- **Monitoring:** Regular monitoring of potassium levels during treatment is necessary to ensure that supplementation achieves the desired effect. Blood tests to assess serum potassium levels help healthcare providers adjust the treatment plan as needed.
- **Duration:** The duration of treatment depends on the underlying cause and the individual's response to supplementation. Some conditions might require short-term supplementation, while others may necessitate long term management. Veterinarians will determine the appropriate duration based on the condition.
- **Side effects and safety:** Oral potassium chloride supplementation can sometimes lead to side effects such as gastrointestinal disturbances, including nausea, vomiting, and abdominal discomfort. In severe cases, excessive potassium intake can lead to hyperkalemia, a condition characterized by high potassium levels in the blood, which can be dangerous. Monitoring for adverse effects and regular communication with healthcare providers are important for maintaining safety.
- **Interaction with medications:** It is important to consider potential interactions between oral potassium chloride and other medications the individual might be taking. Some medications can affect potassium levels, either by causing depletion or increasing levels.
- **Individual variation:** Responses to treatment can vary between animals. Factors such as age, underlying health conditions, kidney function, and overall electrolyte balance can influence how an individual responds to oral potassium chloride supplementation.

Treatment with oral potassium chloride may be required in some cases. It is important to note that the response to treatment may vary, and considerations regarding dosage and duration are necessary.

20.9 Control

The basic principle of hypokalemia control is centered on maintaining physiological levels by exploring different methods (Constable et al. 2014).

20.9.1 Oral Administration of Potassium

Providing potassium through oral supplementation is a necessary part of managing fluid and electrolyte balances in lactating dairy cattle, especially those that are not eating adequately for various reasons such as illness or stress. Potassium is an essential mineral that plays a vital role in maintaining proper cellular function, nerve conduction, and muscle contraction.

Potassium is a crucial mineral that has various physiological roles within the body. These roles include maintaining the proper function of cells, facilitating nerve signals (nerve conduction), and enabling muscle contractions. These functions are especially important for the overall health and productivity of dairy cattle.

20.9.2 Fluid and Electrolyte Administration

When dairy cattle are inappetent, they may not be consuming enough feed to meet their nutritional needs. This can lead to imbalances in electrolytes like potassium. Fluid and electrolyte administration, including oral potassium supplementation, helps restore these imbalances and support the overall health of the animals. Electrolytes, including potassium, are involved in maintaining the balance of fluids and ions within the body. A proper electrolyte balance is essential for maintaining normal bodily functions, such as regulating blood pressure, supporting organ function, and ensuring the proper distribution of nutrients and waste products.

20.9.3 Preventing Hypokalemia

One of the specific concerns mentioned is preventing hypokalemia. Hypokalemia can occur when the levels of potassium in the bloodstream drop too low. This can lead to muscle weakness, cardiac irregularities, and other health issues. Preventing hypokalemia is essential for maintaining overall health and normal bodily functions. For dairy cattle, in whom potassium is required for muscle function, nerve transmission, and milk production, avoiding hypokalemia becomes crucial for their well-being and productivity.

20.9.4 Balanced Nutrition

Ensuring an appropriate dietary intake of potassium through proper feeding practices is a primary method to prevent hypokalemia. This can involve providing potassium-rich feeds or supplements, especially in situations where feed intake might be compromised. Incorporating feeds that are naturally rich in potassium can help maintain proper potassium levels. Different feeds have varying potassium content, so formulating diets with appropriate feed sources is crucial.

20.9.5 Dry Matter Intake

This passage highlights that the best method for preventing hypokalemia in lactating dairy cattle is to ensure an adequate dry matter intake. Dry matter intake refers to the amount of feed consumed without accounting for moisture content. Encouraging cattle to eat a sufficient amount of feed helps maintain their potassium levels within a healthy range. Proper feeding practices, such as providing nutritionally balanced diets and monitoring feed consumption, play a significant role in promoting adequate dry matter intake. Dry matter intake directly affects the amount of potassium and other nutrients that cows receive. When cows consume an appropriate amount of feed, they are more likely to absorb sufficient potassium to maintain potassium levels within a healthy range.

References

Bairwa, J.K., Venkatesakumar, E., Sivaraman, S., and Madheswaran, R. (2023). Demographic study of hypokalemic syndrome in dairy cows in and around Namakkal, Tamil Nadu. *The Pharma Innovation Journal* 12 (7S): 1951–1954.

Chen, C., Guo, Z., Shi, X. et al. (2022). H_2O_2-induced oxidative stress improves meat tenderness by accelerating glycolysis via hypoxia-inducible factor-1α signaling pathway in postmortem bovine muscle. *Food Chemistry: X* 16: 100466.

Çinar, Z.T. and İsmail, Ş.E.N. (2022). Determination of potassium levels in dairy cows in the periparturient period. *Manas Journal of Agriculture Veterinary and Life Sciences* 12 (1): 88–92.

Constable, P.D., Hiew, M.W.H., Tinkler, S., and Townsend, J. (2014). Efficacy of oral potassium chloride administration in treating lactating dairy cows with experimentally induced hypokalemia, hypochloremia, and alkalemia. *Journal of Dairy Science* 97 (3): 1413–1426.

Ferraro, S., Rousseau, M., Dufour, S. et al. (2024). Evaluation of potassium monopersulfate footbath solution for controlling digital dermatitis in lactating dairy cattle. A randomized clinical trial. *Research in Veterinary Science* 170: 105180, ISSN 0034-5288, https://doi.org/10.1016/j.rvsc.2024.105180.

Kim, M.J., Valerio, C., and Knobloch, G.K. (2023). Potassium disorders: hypokalemia and hyperkalemia. *American Family Physician* 107 (1): 59–70A.

Luna, M.A.E., Roldan, M.S.T., Reyes, L.A. et al. (2023). Importance of minerals in the diet of cattle in the tropical climate of Mexico. In: *Landraces - Its Productive Conservation in Animals and Plants* (ed. A. González-Reyna and P. Kaushik). London, United Kingdom: IntechOpen https://doi.org/10.5772/intechopen.100873.

Mann, S., McArt, J., and Abuelo, A. (2019). Production-related metabolic disorders of cattle: ketosis, milk fever and grass staggers. *In Practice* 41 (5): 205–219.

Mekroud, M., Khelifi-Touhami, N.A., Titi, A. et al. (2023). Hematological profile in Holstein dairy cows according to the different physiological stage. *Veterinária* 72 (2).

Mezzetti, M. and Trevisi, E. (2023). Methods of evaluating the potential success or failure of transition dairy cows. *Veterinary Clinics: Food Animal Practice* 39 (2): 219–239.

Plöntzke, J., Berg, M., Ehrig, R. et al. (2022). Model-based exploration of hypokalemia in dairy cows. *Scientific Reports* 12 (1): 19781.

Russell, K.E. and Roussel, A.J. (2007). Evaluation of the ruminant serum chemistry profile. *Veterinary Clinics of North America: Food Animal Practice* 23 (3): 403–426.

Sattler, N. and Fecteau, G. (2014). Hypokalemia syndrome in cattle. *Veterinary Clinics: Food Animal Practice* 30 (2): 351–357.

Viera, A.J. and Wouk, N. (2015 Sep 15). Potassium Disorders: Hypokalemia and Hyperkalemia. *American Family Physician* 92 (6): 487–495. PMID: 26371733.

Wallig, M.A., Usborne, A., and Keenan, K.P. (2023). Nutritional toxicologic pathology. In: *Haschek and Rousseaux's Handbook of Toxicologic Pathology, Volume 3* (ed. W.M. Haschek-Hock, C.G. Rousseaux, M.A. Wallig, and B. Bolon), 105–180. Academic Press.

Walter, L.L., Gärtner, T., Gernand, E. et al. (2022). Effects of parity and stage of lactation on trend and variability of metabolic markers in dairy cows. *Animals* 12 (8): 1008.

Yamada, Y., Yoshida, T., Murakami, H. et al. (2023). Body cell mass to fat-free mass ratio and extra-to-intracellular water ratio are related to maximal oxygen uptake. *The Journals of Gerontology: Series A* 78 (10): 1778–1784.

Yasaswini, D., Kumari, K.N., Shobhamani, B. et al. (2023). Risk factors, clinical indicators, and pathological findings of abomasal ulcers in tropical dairy buffaloes. *Veterinary Research Communications* 47 (3): 1139–1154. https://doi.org/10.1007/s11259-023-10070-9.

21

Stillbirth

Suryakant S. Parikh[1], *Rajesh Kumar*[2], *Tapas K. Patbandha*[3], *and Pramod Kumar*[4]

[1] *Cattle Breeding Farm, Kamdhenu University, Junagadh, Gujarat, India*
[2] *Department of Veterinary Gynaecology & Obstetrics, College of Veterinary Science & Animal Husbandry, Acharya Narendra Deva University of Agriculture & Technology, Kumarganj, Ayodhya, Uttar Pradesh, India*
[3] *Polytechnic in Animal Husbandry (Livestock Production & Management), CoVSc & Animal Husbandry, Kamdhenu University, Junagadh, Gujarat, India*
[4] *Department of Veterinary Physiology & Biochemistry, College of Veterinary Science & Animal Husbandry, Acharya Narendra Deva University of Agriculture & Technology, Kumarganj, Ayodhya, Uttar Pradesh, India*

21.1 Introduction

Stillbirths and dystocia are major contributing factors that affect the productive (Bicahlo et al. 2008) and reproductive life of dairy cattle (Maizon et al. 2004; Bicahlo et al. 2007; Uematsu et al. 2013). Stillbirth is an international animal health and welfare issue (Mee 2013a). It is an economically important trait defined as the death of a calf just prior to, during, or within 24–48 hours of calving following a gestation period of at least 260 days, irrespective of the cause of death or the circumstances related to calving (Chassange et al. 1999; Berglund et al. 2003; Mahnani et al. 2018; John et al. 2019). It has multifactorial origins (Berglund et al. 2003; Mellado et al. 2017) and is also termed perinatal weak calf syndrome (characterized by the birth of full-term calves that either failed to breathe or did not breathe for longer than 10 minutes) (Rice et al. 1986; Smyth et al. 1992). The incidence rate of stillbirth is much greater in heifers compared to cows (Szucs et al. 2009). The direct effects of stillbirths on dairy cattle may result in loss of both the calf and dam, reduced fertility and production performance of the dam, delayed genetic progress, and a higher culling rate in the long term (John et al. 2019). It may cause indirect economic losses due to additional veterinary services, labor, and treatment (Szucs et al. 2009). Calf (size) and dam (pelvic diameter) factors are considered to be the most important determinants for stillbirths in dairy cattle (Szucs et al. 2009). Due to rising incidences of stillbirth in dairy cattle (Bicalho et al. 2007; Bicalho et al. 2008; Berglund et al. 2003; Mee et al. 2011; Mee et al. 2014), efforts are needed to support the further investigation of various risk factors, diagnostic approaches, and preventive measures to mimic the stillbirth rate in dairy cattle.

The rising trend in stillbirths is not acceptable, as far as the economic and animal welfare of a dairy farm are concerned. Similarly, the calving process and its postpartum aftermath are very critical times in the cow–calf production cycle, and that is why knowledge and novel scientific findings should be considered (Szucs et al. 2009). The aim of this review is to reduce such significant economic losses, improve the welfare status of animals, and increase the availability of milk and dairy products to end users.

21.2 Role of Infection and Immunity in Stillbirth Syndrome

Stillbirths in dairy cattle may have either infectious or noninfectious causes, although infectious causes are diagnosed less frequently because in utero infections may compromise fetal development without causing death (Jawor et al. 2021). Infectious causes of perinatal mortality involve various underlying mechanisms associated with the relationship between pathogens and the host. This relationship depends on the types of infectious agents, occurrence of coinfection, principles of primary and secondary pathogens, in utero versus postnatal infections, and the concepts of exposure to infections

Periparturient Diseases of Cattle, First Edition. Edited by Tanmoy Rana.

and causality (Mee et al. 2021). Infectious forms of stillbirth syndrome (SBS) may occur either from the direct effects of an in utero infection or the fetal response to such an infection, which leads to fetal inflammatory response syndrome (FIRS). Both of these (in utero infection and FIRS) cause multiorgan damage and compromise the life of the fetus (Figure 21.1).

21.2.1 Development of the Fetal Immune Response Against Infection

The fetal immune response develops throughout the pregnancy; phagocytic cells (granulocytes and monocytes) appear in fetal blood at approximately the one-hundred-thirtieth day of pregnancy. But during the perinatal period, the fetal immune response (bactericidal activity of neutrophils) is reduced due to a rise in cortisol levels (Tizard 2000). Bacterial *Eschericha coli* infections are very common during the early postpartum period. In case of such a gram-negative bacterial infection, fetal death may occur from the response to the bacterial cell wall–component lipopolysaccharide (LPS) (Nguyen et al. 2018). The fetal inflammatory response is very common against infection. Interleukin (IL)-6 is a good biomarker for the inflammatory response in bovine fetuses. Increased fetal plasma IL-6 concentrations were not observed in stillborn calves with infections, although IL-6 was higher in the plasma and abomasal fluid of live calves compared to dead calves, which might be due to the short half-life (minutes to hours in rats) of cytokines (IL-6) or if the infection occurred during early pregnancy (Castell et al. 1988; Jawor et al. 2018). The bovine fetus can produce a humoral response (immunoglobulins like IgM and IgG) by the second trimester (Ellis et al. 1978).

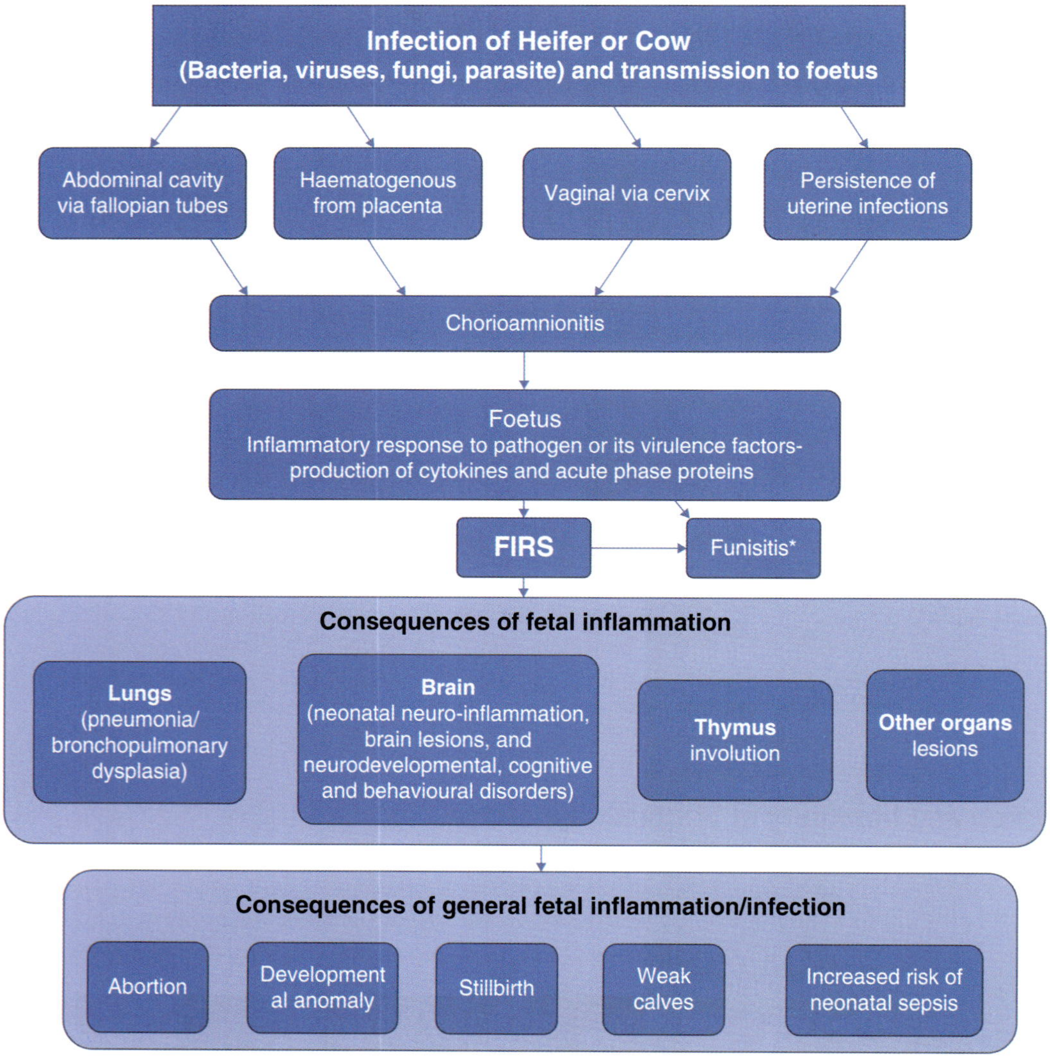

Figure 21.1 Possible sequelae of an intrauterine infection in dairy cattle. *Source:* Jawor et al. (2021).

21.3 Etiological Agents

Dystocia, infections, anoxia/hypoxia, congenital defects, omphalorrhagia, premature placental separation (PPS), and trace element disorders are considered causative agents of stillbirths in dairy cattle (John et al. 2019).

21.3.1 Dystocia

A frequent cause of stillbirths in dairy cattle is dystocia, as reported by previous researchers (Meyer et al. 2001; Berglund et al. 2003; Eriksson et al. 2004; Barrier et al. 2013; John et al. 2019). It is considered to be the cause of half (50%) of stillbirths with a noninfectious etiology (Berglund et al. 2003). The basic causes of dystocia in primiparous and pluriparous cows are relative fetal over size and malposition. Dystotic calves may experience higher physiological stress, acidosis, and hypoxia (Eriksson et al. 2004; Bicalho et al. 2008; Barrier et al. 2013) at the time of calving. A larger percentage of bull calves (40.0%) required calving assistance compared with heifer calves (33.0%) (Lombard et al. 2007). Mee et al. (2013b) also reported various traumatic lesions in stillborn calves associated with dystocia, viz. fractured and dislocated ribs; fractured spine, legs, and mandible; diaphragmatic hernia; hepatic rupture; etc.

21.3.2 Infections

Infections (pathogenic microbes, e.g. bacteria, viruses, parasites, and fungi, and sometimes multiple pathogens) are a minor diagnosed cause (~15%, varying between 5% and 35%) of stillbirths as reported in previous studies (Mee et al. 2021). The variable stillbirth rates in dairy cattle caused by infections might be due to the conflation of data from stillborn calves, geographic differences in infection prevalences and control methods (e.g. vaccination, eradication, etc.), differences in definitions of "infection," and differences in sampling protocols (Mee et al. 2021). Infections rank as the second or third most common cause of SBS. Fetal infections (*Bacillus licheniformis*, *Leptospira*, bovine viral diarrhea virus, and *Neospora caninum* infections) are associated with an increased risk of stillbirths in dairy cattle (Smyth et al. 1999; Graham et al. 2009; Brickell et al. 2010; Mee et al. 2021). The most common pathogens associated with stillborn calves (weak calf syndrome) are *Bacillus* spp. and bovine viral diarrhea virus (BVDV). In the case of fungi, *Aspergillus fumigatus* (primary) as well as *Aspergillus niger* and *Mucor* spp. are sporadically detected in perinatal mortality studies (Mee et al. 2021). The most common diagnostic criterion for infections as a cause of death in cases of perinatal mortality is the presence of an inflammatory lesion indicative of bacterial infection (e.g. bronchopneumonia, encephalitis, and pericarditis). In utero infections are most common, although postnatal infections can also cause stillbirths in cattle (Mee et al. 2021). The transmission of an infection from the dam to the fetus involves migration of the pathogen from the abdominal cavity through the fallopian tubes, hematogenous spread through the placenta, and passage through the cervix from the vagina (Goldenberg et al. 2000).

21.3.3 Anoxia/Hypoxia

Impaired oxygen delivery to cells and decreased tissue perfusion may cause anoxic (absence of oxygen reaching the tissues) or hypoxic (reduced oxygen level) conditions, which may affect cardiac function and cause cardiovascular disorders (Aydogdu et al. 2016; John et al. 2019). Calves with prolonged hypoxia may have more pronounced gross pathological lesions (Mee 2008; Mee 2014; Norquay 2018). The majority (73–75%) of calves without pathological changes during the perinatal period might die due to direct or indirect asphyxia (body is deprived of oxygen) (Greene 1978). Similarly, Schuijt (1990) reported a 58.3% prevalence rate of asphyxia in calves during the perinatal period.

21.3.4 Congenital Defects

Congenital defects may occur as a result of genetic mutation, exposure to infectious agents, pharmaceutical teratogens, and toxins (Whitlock et al. 2008). Various congenital defects, viz. intestinal atresia, arthrogryposis, cerebellar hypoplasia, cleft palate, omphalocoele, ventricular septal defect, schistosomus reflexus, and hydrocephalus, were reported at postmortem examinations of stillborn calves (Mee 2013a).

21.3.5 Omphalorrhagia

Omphalorrhagia is defined as bleeding from one or both umbilical arteries (John et al. 2019). The prevalence of omphalorrhagia as a cause of stillbirths is unknown (Mee 2013b). Affected calves tend to die between 1 and 48 hours after birth, without premonitory clinical signs, due to internally profuse bleeding that leads to anemia and death (Norquay 2018). The most frequent sign of this condition is conjunctival pallor (a sign of anemia). Blood transfusions and surgical ligation are effective with variable success (John et al. 2019).

21.3.6 Premature Placental Separation

PPS is recognized as a minor cause (in utero) of stillbirths, and it has been associated with "premature birth and maldisposition" or "weak calf syndrome" in heifers (Mee 2008; Mee et al. 2014; Aydogdu et al. 2016). Dead calves following PPS may occur due to anoxia or hemorrhage in utero or during calving. For diagnostic purposes, placental tissue should be examined when available (Anderson 2007). In fresh cases, red cotyledons with a clear, translucent, intercotyledonary area are present; when autolysis has occurred, the cotyledons are dull brown and the placental intercotyledonary area is less translucent (Anderson 2007). The measurement of placental functions using various biochemical substances, viz. bovine pregnancy-specific protein B, pregnancy-associated glycoprotein (PAG), and estrone sulfate, are useful to indicate fetal viability in dairy cattle (Kornmatitsuk et al. 2003).

21.3.7 Trace Element Disorders

The deficiency of micronutrients in the dam may directly affect the micronutrient status of the calf (Mee 2013b). The deficiency of various micronutrients such as iodine, selenium, copper, and zinc may result in fetal, neonatal, and postnatal losses of calves (Mee 2008; Mee 2013b; Waldner and Blakley 2014). Iodine and selenium deficiencies in heifers are associated with higher stillbirth rates (Mee 2013b). Perinatal mortality and weakness in beef calves may be considered a cause of congenital selenium deficiency, as reported by previous scientists (Abutarbush and Radostits 2003; Waldner and Blakley 2014; Davis and Myburgh 2016). Thyroid insufficiency is also considered a cause for stillbirths, and the birth of premature or weak calves with low birth weights may occur (Cutler and Jones 2003). In trace element deficiency–induced respiratory distress syndrome (RDS; e.g. selenium, copper, zinc, and iodine), the calves may survive calving, but they have greater difficulty breathing. Even an early diagnosis followed by treatment may not guarantee their survival (Mee 1994; Mee 1999).

21.4 Incidences and Risk Factors for Stillbirth in Dairy Cattle

In Holstein heifers, higher incidences of stillbirth (6.9%, 10.3%, and 10.7%) have been reported by previous researchers (Chassagne et al. 1999; Berglund et al. 2003). Cuttance and Laven (2019) reviewed studies from 1990 to 2019 and reported variable stillbirth (mortality) percentages that ranged from 2.4% to 9.7% in different breeds of dairy cattle. Earlier scientists (Heins et al. 2006; Gulliksen et al. 2009; Olson et al. 2009) have also reported variable stillbirth rates (3.4%, 4.7%, and 5.2%) in different breeds (Norwegian Red, Scandinavian Red, and Jersey crosses, respectively) of cattle. Higher stillbirth rates are observed in beef breeds of cattle compared to dairy breeds (Bleul 2011). The variation in incidence across different studies might be attributed to the definition that the authors followed, reliability of data collected, study design, etc. There are several factors that affect stillbirth. Stillbirth is directly affected by the genetic variation of the calf as well as the genetic variation of the dam (maternal effect). The calf's genetic makeup, particularly its size, describes the calf's ability to survive at birth. The maternal effect on stillbirths describes the ability of a cow to birth a live calf (Al-Samarai 2012).

Both genetic and nongenetic factors cause stillbirths in dairy cows, which include breed (Svensson et al. 2006; Mee et al. 2014), sire (Svensson et al. 2006; Benjaminsson 2007); sire predicated transmitting ability (Mee 2008); parity and age of the dam (Meyer et al. 2000; Svensson et al. 2006; Benjaminsson 2007; Uematsu et al. 2013; Mee et al. 2014); incompatibility between calf size and dam size or pelvic and vulvar conformation (Berglund et al. 2003), age at first calving (Chassagne et al. 1999; Benjaminsson 2007); year and season of calving (Svensson et al. 2006; Mee et al. 2013a; Uematsu et al. 2013); gestation length (Meyer et al. 2000; Hradecka et al. 2006; Svensson et al. 2006; Benjaminsson 2007; Mee 2011; Mellado et al. 2017); insufficient placental development; metabolic disorders of the dam; congenital malformations of the calf

(Berglund et al. 2003); sex, birth weight, multiple birth, twinning, degree of inbreeding status of the pregnancy or breeding method (Johanson and Berger 2003; Steinbock et al. 2003; Svensson et al. 2006; Benjaminsson 2007; Del Rio et al. 2007; Mee et al. 2014; Waldner 2014; Mellado et al. 2017; Szelenyi et al. 2019); level of nutrition during gestation, nutrition deficiencies, and nutritional body energy reserves (Chassagne et al. 1999; Mee 1999; Meyer et al. 2000; Uematsu et al. 2013; Mellado et al. 2017); infections (e.g. BVDV) (Grooms 2006); management factors (e.g. care of the pregnant cow) prepartum and at calving, precalving movement, calving location, calving supervision, calving intervention policy, and calving assistance (Svensson et al. 2006; Mee et al. 2013a; Palombi et al. 2013; Mee et al. 2014; Mahnani et al. 2018); larger herd size (> 20 cows; Mee et al. 2013a); and serum hormones alterations, changes in endocrine profiles in late bovine pregnancy, or other in utero causes (Kindahl et al. 2002; Berglund et al. 2003). Other factors, viz. prepartum body condition, dirtiness scores, biochemical, and hematologic blood parameters measured during the last 2 months of gestation, calving conditions, hour of calving, and moderate or extreme heat stress during the peripartum period (Chassagne et al. 1999; Gustafsson et al. 2007; Szucs et al. 2009; De Rensis et al. 2015; Mellado et al. 2017) may also contribute to the occurrence of stillborn calves. However, at certain times (in 35% of cases), the cause of death or the occurrence of stillborn calves, especially during the perinatal period, cannot be determined (Berglund et al. 2003).

Risk factors can be classified into modifiable (age at first calving, breeding method, sire, calving management, feto-maternal health status, and gestational nutrition), moderately modifiable (calf breed, sex, gestation length), and nonmodifiable (primiparity, history of previous perinatal mortality, fetal plurality, fetal presentation, herd, herd size, calving day of the week, season, and year) factors as reported by previous researchers (Mee et al. 2013b; Mee et al. 2014). Maternal, fetal, environmental, and management factors may influence stillbirth rates in dairy bovine.

21.4.1 Dam Factors

21.4.1.1 Parity of the Dam

Parity is also considered a major risk factor for SBS in dairy bovines (Mellado et al. 2017). Primiparous cows are more prone to stillborns compared to pluriparous cows (Meyer et al. 2000; Meyer et al. 2001; Berry et al. 2007; Bicalho et al. 2008; Mee et al. 2008; Bleul 2011; Al-Samarai 2012; Uematsu et al. 2013). There is a steady increase of stillbirth rates (10–13%), especially in Holstein–Friesian heifers (Harbers et al. 2000; Meyer et al. 2001; Hansen 2004; Murray 2008), although the reasons are not clear. The number of calvings has a significant effect on the stillbirth rate, as it is twice as high in primiparous as pluriparous cows (Hradecka et al. 2004; Benjaminsson 2007).

21.4.1.2 Gestation Length

The most important predictor of stillbirths after dystocia is gestation length (Meyer et al. 2000). Calves born after a short gestation are more susceptible to SBS than those after a long gestation (Bleul 2011). This might be due to organ immaturity (Johanson and Berger 2003; Benjaminsson 2007; Bleul 2011; Briana and Malamitsi-Puchner 2013; Sangild et al. 2013; Caminita et al. 2015). The gestation length (GL; 30% < 278 days), dystocia (29%), and birth weight (19.3% < 35 kg) of calves are major contributing factors for stillborn calves, as reported by Mellado et al. (2017).

21.4.2 Calf Factors

21.4.2.1 Birth Weight of the Calf

Larger calves are more susceptible to dystocia, which may result in anoxia, metabolic, and respiratory acidosis that lead to reduced immunoglobulin absorption and increased disease susceptibility (Norquay 2018). Some scientists support the fact that lighter calves are more susceptible to stillbirths than calves heavier at birth (Tarres et al. 2005; Mellado et al. 2017), whereas Linden et al. (2009) did not observe any effect of birth weight on stillborn calves. Chassagne et al. (1999) suggested that a higher body condition score (BCS; > 4) precalving was a significant risk factor for stillbirth.

21.4.2.2 Sex of the Calf

The sex of the calf had a significant effect on stillbirth percentages (Eriksson et al. 2004; Al-Samarai 2012). Male calves tend to have longer gestations (over 1 day) than female calves, which increases the risk of dystocia and stillbirths; the risk is also considerably higher in multiple births (Maltecca et al. 2006; Benjaminsson 2007; Gulliksen et al. 2009; Mee 2011; Dhakal et al. 2013; Mellado et al. 2017; John et al. 2019). Conversely, Meyer et al. (2001) reported that female calves (12%) had a higher stillborn percentage than male calves (7%) born from primiparous cows. Heifer calves were found to be stillborn similarly to bull calves in different breeds of cattle (Holstein, Jersey, and crossbreeds) as reported by Olson et al. (2009). Calf sex contributes to similar incidences of stillbirth (7.6% in male versus 7.0% in female) in dairy cattle managed in hot environments (Mellado et al. 2017).

21.4.3 Managemental Factors

21.4.3.1 Breeding Method

The breeding method is an important risk factor for SBS in dairy cattle (Mee et al. 2014). Calves produced by embryo/nuclear transfer, timed artificial insemination, natural service (in primipara), or repeat inseminations had higher stillbirth rates than those from artificial insemination at spontaneous estrus (Kruip and den Daas 1997; Ambrose et al. 2006; Hardarson 2012). The relative risk for stillbirths increases linearly quite rapidly as the degree of inbreeding of the calf increases (Benjaminsson 2007). The stillbirth rate was significantly ($p < 0.01$) higher (19.5% versus 5.3%) in twin carriers compared to singleton carriers (Szelenyi et al. 2019).

21.4.3.2 Feeding Management

Concentrate feeding at high levels (ad libitum) during the last month of pregnancy leads to an increased risk of stillbirth (Benjaminsson 2007) due to maternal and fetal over size (Mee et al. 2014). In pregnant primiparous cows, a BCS more than 4 is a risk factor for stillbirths (Chassagne et al. 1999; Vernooy et al. 2007). Prepartum maternal dietary imbalances (energy, protein, or micronutrient deficiency) are also major risk factors for stillborn calves (Murray et al. 2008; Micke et al. 2010; Gao et al. 2012).

21.4.3.3 Precalving Management

Precalving movement of dairy cattle to calving pens can influence the risk of stillbirths, with lower rates (2.5 times less) in cows moved during stage 2 compared to stage 1 of calving (Carrier et al. 2006; Mee et al. 2014). Calving at pasture is associated with a higher risk of stillbirths due to the lack of calving supervision (Vernooy et al. 2007). Similarly, Gulliksen et al. (2009) reported that calving in tie stalls has been associated with a lower stillbirth rate than calving in free stalls. Frequent calving supervision, particularly at night or on holidays, and other parameters like use of a camera surveillance system, farm issues and bonus payments to farm personnel/management, farm personnel training, and obstetrical skills of farmer are associated with reduced stillbirth rates in dairy cattle (Vernooy et al. 2007; Schuenemann et al. 2011; Szenci et al. 2012; Mee et al. 2014).

21.4.3.4 Calving Time

The time of calving is also an important risk factor for stillbirths in Holstein cows in a hot environment (Mellado et al. 2017). They found an upward trend for stillbirth rates when cows calved between 18:00 and 19:00 hours (at sunset), compared with all other hours throughout the day, which might be due to insufficient monitoring around parturition and a high ambient temperature (Gundelach et al. 2009; Mellado et al. 2017).

21.4.4 Environmental Factors

21.4.4.1 Calving Season

The effect of calving season on stillbirth percentages was significant ($p < 0.01$); the highest estimates were for summer calving, which were 14.60% in heifers, 10.71% in cows, and 11.36% in both, but the lowest estimates were for winter calving (Meyer et al. 2001; Al-Samarai 2012). That may result from variation in temperatures, diseases, and nutrition (Al-Samarai 2012). Conversely, Uematsu et al. (2013) reported the highest stillbirth rates in winter season (3.18%) rather than in summer (2.01%) and autumn (2.07%). This might be due to the fact that in the winter season, the average temperatures decreased and there was a subsequent increase in calf birth weights and dystocia cases (Deutscher et al. 1999). During the winter season, hyperthyroidism due to selenium deficiency in pregnant cows is the main cause of stillborn calves (Kohrle and Gartner 2009; Foroughi et al. 2013). The percentage of stillbirths differs significantly each year of calving (Meyer et al. 2001; Hansen et al. 2004; Al-Samarai 2012). That might be due to differences in management between years (Al-Samarai 2012).

21.4.4.2 Heat Stress

Environmental conditions that affect stillbirth rates in beef calves were studied by Azzam et al. (1993) and Meyer et al. (2001). Heat stress definitely causes both productive and reproductive loss in dairy cows (Garcia-Isperto et al. 2006, 2007;

De Rensis et al. 2015). The heat stress (temperature humidity index [THI]) during prepartum and at parturition may lead to stillborn calves with an incidence rate of 5.9–8.6% (Mellado et al. 2017). The offspring of cows heat stressed during the prepartum period have impaired cell-mediated immune function and compromised passive immunity (Tao and Dahl 2013). Mellado et al. (2017) reported that during late gestation, dairy cattle with in utero heat stress and greater incidences of stillbirth might be due to the fact that fetal development increases the dam's respiration rate and core temperature during the last month of gestation, which compromises their structural and physiological functions. Such homeokinetic changes due to heat stress provoke a redistribution of blood flow from the body core to the periphery, which reduces perfusion of the placental blood vessels and compromises placental development through fetal hypoxia, malnutrition, and eventually, fetal growth impedance (Hansen 2009; Tao et al. 2012; Mellado et al. 2016). It also alters blood metabolite profiles and reduces the secretion of prolactin, insulin, and insulin-like growth factor (Guo et al. 2016; Monteiro et al. 2016a), which could be linked to the occurrence of stillbirths (Monteiro et al. 2016b).

21.5 Effect of Stillbirths on Dam Survival, Productivity, and Reproductive Performance in Dairy Cattle

The major loss of a calf (71.0% of the total cost) is not the only cost associated with stillbirths; the costs behind dystocia (7.6%), culling, and replacement expenses (6.3%) are the next most important components of economic loss from stillbirths (Mahnani et al. 2018). The financial consequences are related to various factors, viz. management, hygiene levels, and climatic factors, although multiple researchers have studied financial consequences at the individual cow level in high income countries (Maizon et al. 2004; Bicalho et al. 2007; Mahnani et al. 2018).

Bicalho et al. (2007) reported that losses (the dam's lactation and reproductive performance) from stillbirths are far greater than just the value of the calf. They stated that cows having stillbirths increased the risk of culling or death (higher hazard rate: 40.9%) throughout lactation as well as median days open (calving–conception interval) by 88 (170 versus 258 days) (Bicalho et al. 2007) and 49 days (198 versus 149 days) (El-Tarabany 2015) compared to cows that had live calves. Similarly, cows that gave birth to stillborn calves had significantly ($p < 0.01$) increased days open (14.6 ± 2.6 days) and inseminations per conception (0.22 ± 0.0) compared with cows that gave birth to live calves (Mahnani et al. 2018). They also reported that the hazard ratio for being diagnosed pregnant was 24.1% lower for the cows with a history of still birth compared to cows that had live calves. The sequelae of this condition are metritis, retained placentas, uterine prolapse, displaced abomasa, repeat breeding, and a reduced conception rate (Correa et al. 1993; Emanuelson et al. 1993; Moss et al. 2002; Maizon et al. 2004), which can lead to increased calving intervals and decreased cow survival (Mahnani et al. 2018). Hence, it is clearly indicated that cows with a history of stillbirth had significantly reduced reproductive performance.

Stillbirths significantly ($p < 0.05$) reduced the 305-day milk yield by 5% (582.0 ± 159.5 kg/cow per lactation) in pluriparous cows but had no significant effects on the production performance of primiparous cows (Mahnani et al. 2018). Bicalho et al. (2007) and Atashi et al. (2011) also reported similar findings. In general, there are no significant effects of stillbirths on the productive and reproductive performance of primiparous cows compared to multiparous cows (Mahnani et al. 2018). Moreover, there were no significant effects from a stillbirth on the 305-day fat and protein percentages in either primiparous or multiparous cows (Mahnani et al. 2018). Conversely, Atashi et al. (2011) observed that milkfat and protein percentages were significantly reduced by stillbirths in dairy cattle. Primiparous cows are severely affected by stillbirths; hence, it indicates that this syndrome significantly reduced the milk yield of cows in their first parity (Bicalho et al. 2007). A higher occurrence of placental retention, lower fertility, and a lower 305-day milk yield are common consequences of a stillbirth.

21.6 Clinicopathological and Novel Diagnostic Approaches of SBS

The standard operating procedure for a stillbirth investigation involves three criteria, viz. (i) collect a history, (ii) examine pregnant animals or the dam, and (iii) examine the fetus or placenta (Mee 2020; Mee et al. 2021).

I) **Collect a history:** Collect the history of the dam, the calf, and their herd to assess possible risk factors associated with the loss. From an infection point of view, different aspects regarding most recent vaccinations against fetopathogens, the new arrival of animals at farm, grazing areas, etc. should be considered (Mee et al. 2021).

II) **Examine pregnant animals:** Animals are examined to assess their general health, BCS, and feeding management. The criteria include a proper clinical examination of the dam for signs of infection like pyrexia, diarrhea, and respiratory signs; the collection of fecal/blood/maternal serum samples; and repeat sampling to monitor fluctuations in antibody status (Mee et al. 2021).

III) **Examine the fetus and its placenta:** This involves external and internal examinations and sampling of the carcass (Mee 2016).

a) An external examination involves animal identification, body weight (lower body weight), estimation of gestational age using the crown rump length (CRL), developmental defects, and discharges related to the fetus.

b) An internal examination involves gross evidence of an infection with confirmation by microbial and pathological testing of the different samples (perinatal septicemia, pericarditis, meningitis, etc.) (Jawor et al. 2017a,b).

c) Sampling the carcass involves laboratory investigations of different samples, viz. microbiological samples, abomasal contents (for culture, PCR, and microscopy), serological samples (determination of fetal infection using biomarkers like acute phase proteins [APPs] and nonpathogen-specific immunoglobulins), histopathological samples (brain, lung, liver, thyroid, and heart), and trace elements like selenium, iodine, etc. (Herdt and Hoff 2011; Ibrahim et al. 2016; Mee 2016; Jawor et al. 2018; Mee 2020; Mee et al. 2021) (Figure 21.2).

21.6.1 Novel Diagnostic Approaches of SBS in Dairy Cattle

In response to infections, measuring concentrations of immunoglobulins and APPs (antibodies/elements) may be used to diagnose SBS (Jawor et al. 2021). In utero infections can be detected by the presence of specific inflammatory lesions in internal organs (brain, lung, thymus, liver, heart, etc.) at fetal necropsy. Novel approaches for the diagnosis of a stillbirth include monitoring fetal responses (fetal humoral immune response, acute phase response, and metabolic response) and dam nonspecific responses (Jawor et al. 2021).

21.6.1.1 Monitoring Fetal Responses

- **Fetal humoral immune response:** An estimation of immunoglobulin concentrations (IgG and IgM) in precolostral serum is a novel method to diagnose in utero infections pertaining to stillborn calves (Tierney and Simpson-Morgan 1997) because the antibodies detected in stillborn calves are likely to have originated from the fetal, humoral immune response to the infection (Jawor et al. 2021). The classes of immunoglobulins are detected based on the type and time of infection. A higher concentration of IgM in the precolostral sera indicates a bacterial infection (detected at full term) in stillborn calves (Jawor et al. 2017a,b). Higher concentrations of immunoglobulins (IgG1 and IgG2 but not IgM) were also observed in the blood of stillborn calves with other infections (parasitic, viral, or bacterial) (Jawor et al. 2018). Bovine fetuses

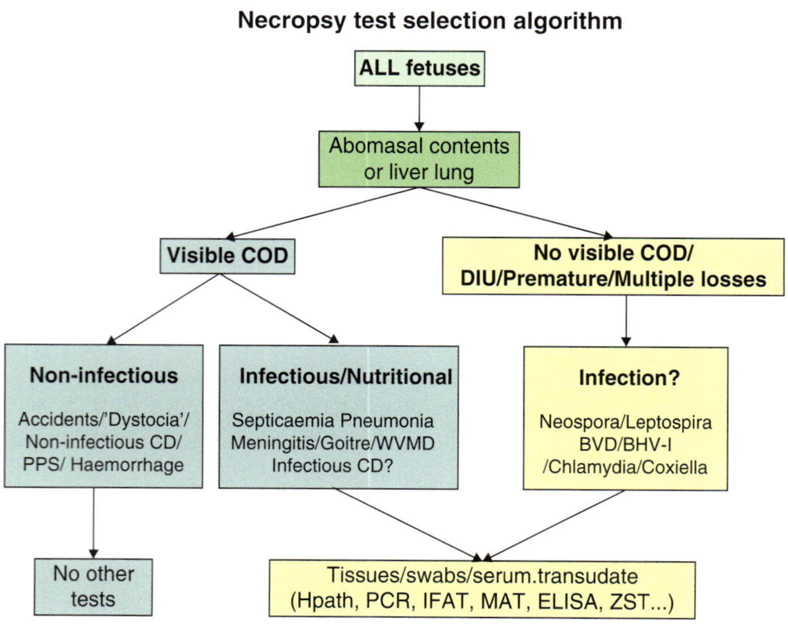

Figure 21.2 Necropsy sample selection decision tree for stillborn fetuses (COD = cause of death; CD = congenital defect; DIU = dead in utero). *Source:* Mee (2020).

infected with the BVDV had precolostral serum with an IgM concentration about 15 times higher and an IgG concentration five times higher than that of healthy calves (Ivanoff 1975). Infected animals also showed a significant upward trend of cytokine messenger (m)RNA levels in the caruncle at the time of death (Regidor-Cerrillo et al. 2014).

- **Fetal acute phase response:** The estimation of APPs like haptoglobin (Hp) and serum amyloid α (SAA) levels may be used as biomarkers for a fetal acute inflammatory response in stillborn calves (Jawor et al. 2021). They are used for the early and precise detection of inflammation, although SAA seems to be a better nonspecific biomarker than Hp for the diagnosis of bacterial infections in stillborn calves. Some other conditions may also influence APP levels in dairy bovine; for example, the concentrations of APPs are also increased in calves that live several hours after birth due to calving phenomena (Jawor et al. 2018).
- **Fetal metabolic response:** The specific metabolic profiles of a calf or its dam are used to detect calves infected in utero. Generally, it is used to detect a specific disease or condition at certain period of time, like stillbirths in dairy cattle (Jawor et al. 2019). Using metabolomics, they suggested metabolic profiles in calves with different times of death, irrespective of the cause. Huang et al. (2020) observed good results with metabolic profiles in the diagnosis and treatment of calves with diarrhea. Similarly, using metabolic profiles, Blakebrough-Hall et al. (2020) identified dairy bovines suffering from respiratory diseases.

21.6.1.2 Monitoring Dam Nonspecific Responses

The other approach to diagnose stillborn calves in dairy cattle is to measure the endocrine profile of the dam (Jawor et al. 2021). Sorge et al. (2008) reported that heifers with stillborn calves had a lower estradiol-17β concentration during the last 2 weeks of pregnancy and on the day of parturition, whereas the prepartum (day 15 to day 11 prepartum) progesterone concentration was greater than in heifers with live calves. As per earlier studies in human medicine (Oh et al. 2019; Lis-Kuberka et al. 2019), changes in fetal fibronectin (FN) concentrations (lower) and the occurrence of FN–fibrin complexes in maternal plasma might be associated with stillborn calves. Similarly, Jawor et al. (2020) reported a higher molecular mass of circulating soluble FN–fibrin complexes in cows (1300–1900 kDa) that delivered stillborn calves compared to control dams (750–1000 kDa) that delivered healthy calves. So, these biomarkers can be used to detect SBS in dairy cattle.

21.7 Protocols for Predicting an Exact Time of Calving (a Tool to Decrease Stillbirth Rates)

Due to the negative effects of SBS on the performance of dairy bovines, it is essential to pay attention to careful surveillance and obstetrical assistance, particularly at calving (Szenci 2017). Some management controlled risk factors, like age at first calving, sire genetic merit for direct stillbirth, predicting the onset of calving, good calving supervision (particularly during stage 2 of calving), and the degree of assistance should be focused on to reduce the prevalence of stillbirths at the dairy farm level (Steinbock et al. 2003; Mee et al. 2008; Gundelach et al. 2009; Szenci 2017). Hence, certain protocols should be considered to predict the exact time of calving and thereby decrease the stillbirth rate in dairy cattle (Szenci 2017).

- Changes in body temperature (Burfeind et al. 2011).
- Controlling the degree of relaxation of the pelvic ligaments, swelling of the vulva, mammary gland expansion, and teat feeling (Streyl et al. 2011).
- Performing ultrasound examinations (Wright et al. 1988).
- Measuring blood estrone sulfate and estradiol-17β or progesterone concentrations (Matsas et al. 1992; Shah et al. 2007; Streyl et al. 2011).
- Determining electrolyte concentrations in mammary gland secretions (Bleul et al. 2006).
- Monitoring the animals by cameras (Cangar et al. 2008).
- Using electronic data loggers attached to legs (Titler et al. 2015).
- Measuring rumination time (Kovacs et al. 2017).
- Measuring heart rate and heart rate variability (Kovacs et al. 2015).
- Using electronic systems (C6 Birth Control by Sisteck, Sassuolo, MO, Italy) with GSM (Global System for Mobile Communication) technology (Paolucci et al. 2010).
- Using intravaginal GSM devices (Palombi et al. 2013).

- Using vaginal thermometers (Paolucci et al. 2010; Szenci 2017).
- Using genetics, the *spp1* gene is considered a good candidate gene for predicting stillbirths in dairy cattle (Chakraborty et al. 2010).

On a large dairy farm, there are no visible clinical signs of the onset of calving, hence it is difficult to recognize. Choukeir et al. (2013) stated that inserting a vaginal thermometer into the vagina may contribute to reducing the rates of stillbirth, delayed calving assistance, and its consequences.

21.8 Conclusions

The incidence rates of SBS from infectious causes are variable between different studies; hence, it is necessary to standardize the diagnostic approaches that pertain to necropsy examination. Various parameters like the loss of a calf, culling, and replacement expenses (financial consequences) should be considered when evaluating possible management options to reduce the incidence of stillbirth. Both fetal and dam immunity are compromised during calving, which can be controlled by proper nutrition, vaccination, and other managemental interventions.

21.9 Future Perspectives

Direct (loss of calf, death of dam, labor, and veterinary assistance) and long term (culling rate, milk yield, fertility) expenses with respect to rising rates of stillbirth must be evaluated and interpreted. The effects of nongenetic factors (dystocia, parity, calving season, gestation length, sex and birth weight of the calf, and faulty management) and their supposed modes of action must be considered. Further research is required to determine the potential roles of immunoglobulins, APPs, different metabolites, endocrine fluctuations, fetal FN concentrations, and the occurrence of FN–fibrin complexes in maternal plasma in diagnosing fetal and dam immune responses for the diagnosis of SBS in dairy cattle.

References

Abutarbush, S.M. and Radostits, O.M. (2003). Congenital nutritional muscular dystrophy in a beef calf. *The Canadian Veterinary Journal* 44 (9): 738–739.

Al-Samarai, F. (2012). The effect of some factors on stillbirth in primiparous and multiparous Holstein cattle in Iraq. *Global Journal of Medical Research* 12 (3): 23–29.

Ambrose, D.J., Govindarajan, T., and Goonewardene, L.A. (2006). Conception rate and pregnancy loss rate in lactating Holstein cows of a single herd following timed insemination or insemination at detected estrus. *Journal of Animal Science* 84: 213–214.

Anderson, M.L. (2007). Infectious causes of bovine abortion during mid-to late-gestation. *Theriogenology* 68 (3): 474–486.

Atashi, H., Zamiri, M.J., and Sayyadnejad, M.B. (2011). Non-genetic factors affecting stillbirth and its effects on longevity, production, and reproductive performance in Holstein cows of Iran. *Iran Agricultural Research* 30: 73–82.

Aydogdu, U., Yildiz, R., Guzelbektes, H. et al. (2016). Cardiac biomarkers in premature calves with respiratory distress syndrome. *Acta Veterinaria Hungarica* 64 (1): 38–46.

Azzam, S.M., Kinder, J.E., Nielsen, M.K. et al. (1993). Environmental effects on neonatal mortality of beef calves. *Journal of Animal Science* 71 (2): 282–290.

Barrier, A.C., Mason, C., Dwyer, C.M. et al. (2013). Stillbirth in dairy calves is influenced independently by dystocia and body shape. *The Veterinary Journal* 197 (2): 220–223.

Benjamínsson, B.H. (2007). Prenatal death in Icelandic cattle. *Acta Veterinaria Scandinavica* 49 (1): 1–3.

Berglund, B., Steinbock, L., and Elvander, M. (2003). Causes of stillbirth and time of death in Swedish Holstein calves examined post mortem. *Acta Veterinaria Scandinavica* 44 (3): 1–10.

Berry, D.P., Lee, J.M., Macdonald, K.A., and Roche, J.R. (2007). Body condition score and body weight effects on dystocia and stillbirths and consequent effects on post-calving performance. *Journal of Dairy Science* 90 (9): 4201–4211.

Bicalho, R.C., Galvao, K.N., Cheong, S.H. et al. (2007). Effect of stillbirths on dam survival and reproduction performance in Holstein dairy cows. *Journal of Dairy Science* 90 (6): 2797–2803.

Bicalho, R.C., Galvao, K.N., Warnick, L.D., and Guard, C.L. (2008). Stillbirth parturition reduces milk production in Holstein cows. *Preventive Veterinary Medicine* 84 (1–2): 112–120.

Blakebrough-Hall, C., Dona, A., D'occhio, M.J. et al. (2020). Diagnosis of bovine respiratory disease in feedlot cattle using blood 1H NMR metabolomics. *Scientific Reports* 10 (1): 115–126.

Bleul, U. (2011). Risk factors and rates of perinatal and postnatal mortality in cattle in Switzerland. *Livestock Science* 135 (2–3): 257–264.

Bleul, U., Spirig, S., Hassig, M., and Kahn, W. (2006). Electrolytes in bovine prepartum mammary secretions and their usefulness for predicting parturition. *Journal of Dairy Science* 89 (8): 3059–3065.

Briana, D.D. and Malamitsi-Puchner, A. (2013). Small for gestational age birth weight: impact on lung structure and function. *Paediatric Respiratory Reviews* 14 (4): 256–262.

Brickell, J.S., McGowan, M.M., and Wathes, D.C. (2010). Association n *Neospora caninum* seropositivity and perinatal mortality in dairy heifers at first calving. *Veterinary Record* 167 (3): 82–85.

Burfeind, O., Suthar, V.S., Voigtsberger, R. et al. (2011). Validity of prepartum changes in vaginal and rectal temperature to predict calving in dairy cows. *Journal of Dairy Science* 94 (10): 5053–5061.

Caminita, F., van der Merwe, M., Hance, B. et al. (2015). A preterm pig model of lung immaturity and spontaneous infant respiratory distress syndrome. *American Journal of Physiology – Lung Cellular and Molecular Physiology* 308 (2): L118–L129.

Cangar, O., Leroy, T., Guarino, M. et al. (2008). Automatic real-time monitoring of locomotion and posture behaviour of pregnant cows prior to calving using online image analysis. *Computers and Electronics in Agriculture* 64 (1): 53–60.

Carrier, J., Godden, S., Fetrow, J., Stewart, S., and Rapnicki, P. (2006). Predictors of stillbirth for cows moved to calving pens when calving is imminent. *Proceedings of the Thirty-Ninth Annual Conference of the American Association of Bovine Practitioners,*Saint Paul, Minnesota, USA (21–23 September 2006). Fort Collins, Colorado, USA: Frontier Printers, Inc.

Castell, J.V., Geiger, T., Gross, V. et al. (1988). Plasma clearance, organ distribution and target cells of interleukin-6/hepatocyte-stimulating factor in the rat. *European Journal of Biochemistry* 177 (2): 357–361.

Chakraborty, D., Sharma, A., Tantia, M.S. et al. (2010). Role of secreted phosphoprotein 1 (SPP1) gene in bovines – a review. *Agricultural Reviews* 31 (3): 184–193.

Chassagne, M., Barnouin, J., and Chacornac, J.P. (1999). Risk factors for stillbirth in Holstein heifers under field conditions in France: a prospective survey. *Theriogenology* 51 (8): 1477–1488.

Choukeir, A., Szelenyi, Z., Bajcsy, A., Kovacs, L., Albert, E., Aubin-Wodala, M., Boldizsar, S., and Szenci, O. (2013). Monitoring the onset of calving by a calving alarm thermometer. *Proceedings of the 23rd International Congress of the Hungarian Association for Buiatrics*, Siofok, Hungary. Budapest, Hungary: Hungarian Association for Buiatrics.

Correa, M.T., Erb, H., and Scarlett, J. (1993). Path analysis for seven postpartum disorders of Holstein cows. *Journal of Dairy Science* 76 (5): 1305–1312.

Cutler, K.L. and Jones, I.G. (2003). The trace element nutrition of beef suckler cattle. *Cattle Practice* 11 (2): 117–120.

Cuttance, E. and Laven, R. (2019). Estimation of perinatal mortality in dairy calves: a review. *The Veterinary Journal* 252: 1–7.

Davis, A.J. and Myburgh, J.G. (2016). Investigation of stillbirths, perinatal mortality and weakness in beef calves with low-selenium whole blood concentrations. *Journal of the South African Veterinary Association* 87 (1): 1–6.

De Rensis, F., Garcia-Ispierto, I., and Lopez-Gatius, F. (2015). Seasonal heat stress: clinical implications and hormone treatments for the fertility of dairy cows. *Theriogenology* 84 (5): 659–666.

Del Rio, N.S., Stewart, S., Rapnicki, P. et al. (2007). An observational analysis of twin births, calf sex ratio, and calf mortality in Holstein dairy cattle. *Journal of Dairy Science* 90 (3): 1255–1264.

Deutscher, G.H., Colburn, D., and Davis, R. (1999). Climate affects calf birth weights and calving difficulty. *Nebraska Beef Cattle Reports Paper* 400: 7–9.

Dhakal, K., Maltecca, C., Cassady, J.P. et al. (2013). Calf birth weight, gestation length, calving ease, and neonatal calf mortality in Holstein, Jersey, and crossbred cows in a pasture system. *Journal of Dairy Science* 96 (1): 690–698.

Ellis, W.A., Logan, E.F., and O'Brien, J.J. (1978). Serum immunoglobulins in aborted and non-aborted bovine foetuses. *Clinical and Experimental Immunology* 33 (1): 136–152.

El-Tarabany, M.S. (2015). Impact of stillbirth and abortion on the subsequent fertility and productivity of Holstein, Brown Swiss and their crosses in subtropics. *Tropical Animal Health and Production* 47 (7): 1351–1356.

Emanuelson, U.L.F., Oltenacu, P.A., and Grohn, Y.T. (1993). Nonlinear mixed model analyses of five production disorders of dairy cattle. *Journal of Dairy Science* 76 (9): 2765–2772.

Eriksson, S., Nasholm, A., Johansson, K., and Philipsson, J. (2004). Genetic parameters for calving difficulty, stillbirth, and birth weight for Herford and Charolais at first and later parities. *Journal of Animal Science* 82: 375–383.

Foroughi, M.A., Dehghani, H., Mahdavi-Shahri, N., and Bassami, M.R. (2013). Sodium selenite increases the transcript levels of iodothyronine deiodinases I and II in ovine and bovine fetal thyrocytes *in vitro*. *Journal of Trace Elements in Medicine and Biology* 27 (3): 213–220.

Gao, F., Liu, Y.C., Zhang, Z.H. et al. (2012). Effect of pre-partum maternal energy density on the growth performance, immunity, and anti-oxidation capability of neonatal calves. *Journal of Dairy Science* 95 (8): 4510–4518.

Garcia-Ispierto, I., Lopez-Gatius, F., Santolaria, P. et al. (2006). Relationship between heat stress during the peri-implantation period and early fetal loss in dairy cattle. *Theriogenology* 65 (4): 799–807.

Garcia-Ispierto, I., Lopez-Gatius, F., Santolaria, P. et al. (2007). Factors affecting the fertility of high producing dairy herds in North-Eastern Spain. *Theriogenology* 67 (3): 632–638.

Goldenberg, R.L., Hauth, J.C., and Andrews, W.W. (2000). Intrauterine infection and preterm delivery. *New England Journal of Medicine* 342 (20): 1500–1507.

Graham, D.A., Beggs, N., Mawhinney, K. et al. (2009). Comparative evaluation of diagnostic techniques for bovine viral diarrhoea virus in aborted and stillborn fetuses. *The Veterinary Record* 164 (2): 56.

Greene, H.J. (1978). Causes of dairy calf mortality. *Irish journal of agricultural research* 17: 295–301.

Grooms, D.L. (2006). Reproductive losses caused by bovine viral diarrhoea virus and leptospirosis. *Theriogenology* 66 (3): 624–628.

Gulliksen, S.M., Lie, K.I., Loken, T., and Osteras, O. (2009). Calf mortality in Norwegian dairy herds. *Journal of Dairy Science* 92 (6): 2782–2795.

Gundelach, Y., Essmeyer, K., Teltscher, M.K., and Hoedemaker, M. (2009). Risk factors for perinatal mortality in dairy cattle: cow and foetal factors, calving process. *Theriogenology* 71 (6): 901–909.

Guo, J.R., Monteiro, A.P.A., Weng, X.S. et al. (2016). Effect of maternal heat stress in late gestation on blood hormones and metabolites of new-born calves. *Journal of Dairy Science* 99 (8): 6804–6807.

Gustafsson, H., Kindahl, H., and Berglund, B. (2007). Stillbirths in Holstein heifers–some results from Swedish research. *Acta Veterinaria Scandinavica* 49 (1): 1–3.

Hansen, M. (2004). Quantitative genetic analysis of mortality in Danish Holstein calves. Doctoral dissertation. Royal Veterinary and Agricultural University.

Hansen, P.J. (2009). Effects of heat stress on mammalian reproduction. *Philosophical Transactions of the Royal Society, B: Biological Sciences* 364 (1534): 3341–3350.

Hansen, M., Misztal, I., Lund, M.S. et al. (2004). Undesired phenotypic and genetic trend for stillbirth in Danish Holsteins. *Journal of Dairy Science* 87 (5): 1477–1486.

Harbers, A., Segeren, L., and de Jong, G. (2000). Genetic parameters for stillbirth in the Netherlands. *Interbull Bulletin* 25: 117–117.

Hardarson, G. (2012). Still born calves in first calving heifers: a farm survey. *Reproduction in Domestic Animals* 47: 62–63.

Heins, B.J., Hansen, L.B., and Seykora, A.J. (2006). Calving difficulty and stillbirths of pure Holsteins versus crossbreds of Holstein with Normande, Montbeliarde, and Scandinavian Red. *Journal of Dairy Science* 89 (7): 2805–2810.

Herdt, T.H. and Hoff, B. (2011). The use of blood analysis to evaluate trace mineral status in ruminant livestock. *Veterinary Clinics: Food Animal Practice* 27 (2): 255–283.

Hradecka, E., Cítek, J., and Rehout, V. (2004). Population genetic evaluation of perinatalmortality in Czech dairy cattle. Abstracts from International Symposium Agroregion. *Journal Central European Agriculture* 5 (3): 235.

Hradecka, E., Cítek, J., and Rehout, J. (2006). The evaluation of stillbirths in Czech Pied cattle. *Acta fytotechnica et zootechnica* 1: 222.

Huang, M.Z., Cui, D.A., Wu, X.H. et al. (2020). Serum metabolomics revealed the differential metabolic pathway in calves with severe clinical diarrhoea symptoms. *Animals* 10 (5): 769–780.

Ibrahim, M., Wagener, K., Drillich, M. et al. (2016). *Trueperella pyogenes* isolated from a cow with clinical endometritis showed a higher growth rate and increased mRNA expression of virulence factors compared with a strain isolated from a healthy cow. *Reproduction in Domestic Animals* 51: 58–58.

Ivanoff, M.R. (1975). Weak calf syndrome: serum immunoglobulin concentrations in precolostral calves. *American Journal of Veterinary Research* 36 (08): 1129–1131.

Jawor, P., Krol, D., Mee, J.F. et al. (2017a). Infection exposure, detection and causes of death in perinatal mortalities in Polish dairy herds. *Theriogenology* 103: 130–136.

Jawor, P., Stefaniak, T., and Mee, J.F. (2017b). Immune and inflammatory biomarkers in cases of bovine perinatal mortality with and without infection in utero. *Journal of Dairy Science* 100 (2): 1408–1416.

Jawor, P., Mee, J.F., and Stefaniak, T. (2018). Perinatal immuno/inflammatory responses in the presence or absence of bovine fetal infection. *BMC Veterinary Research* 14 (1): 1–7.

Jawor, P., Zabek, A., Wojtowicz, W. et al. (2019). Metabolomic studies as a tool for determining the post-mortem interval (PMI) in stillborn calves. *BMC Veterinary Research* 15 (1): 1–10.

Jawor, P., Krzyzanowska-Gołab, D., Bajzert, J. et al. (2020). Changes of plasma fibronectin and fibronectin-fibrin complexes in dams of stillborn dairy calves. *Irish Veterinary Journal* 73: 1–8.

Jawor, P., Mee, J.F., and Stefaniak, T. (2021). Role of infection and immunity in bovine perinatal mortality: part 2. Fetomaternal response to infection and novel diagnostic perspectives. *Animals* 11 (7): 2102.

Johanson, J.M. and Berger, P.J. (2003). Birth weight as a predictor of calving ease and perinatal mortality in Holstein cattle. *Journal of Dairy Science* 86 (11): 3745–3755.

John, M., Ismail, S., Kizi, A.A. et al. (2019). Risk factors for, and causes of, perinatal calf mortality and implications for calf welfare. *Manas Journal of Agriculture Veterinary and Life Sciences* 9 (1): 35–41.

Kindahl, H., Kornmatitsuk, B., Konigsson, K., and Gustafsson, H. (2002). Endocrine changes in late bovine pregnancy with special emphasis on fetal well-being. *Domestic Animal Endocrinology* 23 (1–2): 321–328.

Kohrle, J. and Gartner, R. (2009). Selenium and thyroid. *Best Practice & Research Clinical Endocrinology & Metabolism* 23 (6): 815–827.

Kornmatitsuk, B., Franzen, G., Gustafsson, H., and Kindahl, H. (2003). Endocrine measurements and calving performance of Swedish Red and White and Swedish Holstein dairy cattle with special respect to stillbirth. *Acta Veterinaria Scandinavica* 44 (1): 1–13.

Kovacs, L., Tozser, J., Kezer, F.L. et al. (2015). Heart rate and heart rate variability in multiparous dairy cows with unassisted calvings in the periparturient period. *Physiology and Behavior* 139: 281–289.

Kovacs, L., Kezer, F.L., Albert, E. et al. (2017). Seasonal and maternal effects on acid-base, l-lactate, electrolyte, and hematological status of 205 dairy calves born to eutocic dams. *Journal of Dairy Science* 100 (9): 7534–7543.

Kruip, T.A. and Den Daas, J.H.G. (1997). *In vitro* produced and cloned embryos: effects on pregnancy, parturition and offspring. *Theriogenology* 47 (1): 43–52.

Linden, T.C., Bicalho, R.C., and Nydam, D.V. (2009). Calf birth weight and its association with calf and cow survivability, disease incidence, reproductive performance, and milk production. *Journal of Dairy Science* 92 (6): 2580–2588.

Lis-Kuberka, J., Berghausen-Mazur, M., Kątnik-Prastowska, I., and Orczyk-Pawiłowicz, M. (2019). Delivery-associated presence of supramolecular fibronectin-fibrin complexes in puerperal and cord plasma. *The Journal of Maternal-Fetal and Neonatal Medicine* 32 (21): 3581–3588.

Lombard, J.E., Garry, F.B., Tomlinson, S.M., and Garber, L.P. (2007). Impacts of dystocia on health and survival of dairy calves. *Journal of Dairy Science* 90 (4): 1751–1760.

Mahnani, A., Sadeghi-Sefidmazgi, A., and Keshavarzi, H. (2018). Performance and financial consequences of stillbirth in Holstein dairy cattle. *Animal* 12 (3): 617–623.

Maizon, D.O., Oltenacu, P.A., Grohn, Y.T. et al. (2004). Effects of diseases on reproductive performance in Swedish Red and White dairy cattle. *Preventive Veterinary Medicine* 66 (1–4): 113–126.

Maltecca, C., Khatib, H., Schutzkus, V.R. et al. (2006). Changes in conception rate, calving performance, and calf health and survival from the use of crossbred Jersey × Holstein sires as mates for Holstein dams. *Journal of Dairy Science* 89 (7): 2747–2754.

Matsas, D.J., Nebel, R.L., and Pelzer, K.D. (1992). Evaluation of an on-farm blood progesterone test for predicting the day of parturition in cattle. *Theriogenology* 37 (4): 859–868.

Mee, J.F. (1994). Resuscitation of newborn calves-materials and methods. *Cattle Practice* 2: 197–210.

Mee, J.F. (1999). Stillbirths – what can you do? *Cattle Practice* 7 (3): 277.

Mee, J.F. (2008). Newborn dairy calf management. *Veterinary Clinics of North America: Food Animal Practice* 24 (1): 1–17.

Mee, J. (2011). *Bovine Neonatal Survival: Is Improvement Possible*, vol. 23, 161–174. WCDS Advances in Dairy Technology.

Mee, J.F. (2013a). Why do so many calves die on modern dairy farms and what can we do about calf welfare in the future? *Animals* 3 (4): 1036–1057.

Mee, J.F. (2013b). Impacts of nutrition pre-calving on periparturient dairy cow health and neonatal calf health. *Recent Advances in Animal Nutrition*, 45th University of Nottingham Feed Conference, Loughborough, UK (25–26 June 2013). Nottingham, UK: Context Nottingham Press.

Mee, J.F. (2014). Schmallenberg virus as a cause of perinatal mortality and traumatic dystocia in dairy herds. *Cattle Practice* 22: 290–290.

Mee, J.F. (2016). A practitioner's guide to post-mortem examination of an aborted or stillborn calf. *Livestock* 21 (1): 38–43.

Mee, J.F. (2020). Investigation of bovine abortion and stillbirth/perinatal mortality-similar diagnostic challenges, different approaches. *Irish Veterinary Journal* 73 (1): 20.

Mee, J.F., Berry, D.P., and Cromie, A.R. (2008). Prevalence of, and risk factors associated with, perinatal calf mortality in pasture-based Holstein-Friesian cows. *Animal* 2 (4): 613–620.

Mee, J.F., Berry, D.P., and Cromie, A.R. (2011). Risk factors for calving assistance and dystocia in pasture-based Holstein–Friesian heifers and cows in Ireland. *The Veterinary Journal* 187 (2): 189–194.

Mee, J.F., Sanchez-Miguel, C., and Doherty, M. (2013a). An international Delphi study of the causes of death and the criteria used to assign cause of death in bovine perinatal mortality. *Reproduction in Domestic Animals* 48 (4): 651–659.

Mee, J.F., Grant, J., Sanchez-Miguel, C., and Doherty, M. (2013b). Pre-calving and calving management practices in dairy herds with a history of high or low bovine perinatal mortality. *Animals* 3 (3): 866–881.

Mee, J.F., Sanchez-Miguel, C., and Doherty, M. (2014). Influence of modifiable risk factors on the incidence of stillbirth/perinatal mortality in dairy cattle. *The Veterinary Journal* 199 (1): 19–23.

Mee, J.F., Jawor, P., and Stefaniak, T. (2021). Role of infection and immunity in bovine perinatal mortality: part 1. Causes and current diagnostic approaches. *Animals* 11 (4): 1033.

Mellado, M., Lopez, R., de Santiago, A. et al. (2016). Climatic conditions, twining and frequency of milking as factors affecting the risk of fetal losses in high-yielding Holstein cows in a hot environment. *Tropical Animal Health and Production* 48: 1247–1252.

Mellado, M., Chavez, M.I., Macias-Cruz, U. et al. (2017). Prevalence and risk factors for stillbirths in Holstein cows in a hot environment. *Spanish Journal of Agricultural Research* 15 (2): e0403. (1–8).

Meyer, C.L., Berger, P.J., and Koehler, K.J. (2000). Interactions among factors affecting stillbirths in Holstein cattle in the United States. *Journal of Dairy Science* 83 (11): 2657–2663.

Meyer, C.L., Berger, P.J., Koehler, K.J. et al. (2001). Phenotypic trends in incidence of stillbirth for Holsteins in the United States. *Journal of Dairy Science* 84 (2): 515–523.

Micke, G.C., Sullivan, T.M., Magalhaes, R.S. et al. (2010). Heifer nutrition during early-and mid-pregnancy alters fetal growth trajectory and birth weight. *Animal Reproduction Science* 117 (1–2): 1–10.

Monteiro, A.P.A., Guo, J.R., Weng, X.S. et al. (2016a). Effect of maternal heat stress during the dry period on growth and metabolism of calves. *Journal of Dairy Science* 99 (5): 3896–3907.

Monteiro, A.P.A., Tao, S., Thompson, I.M.T., and Dahl, G.E. (2016b). In utero heat stress decreases calf survival and performance through the first lactation. *Journal of Dairy Science* 99 (10): 8443–8450.

Moss, N., Lean, I.J., Reid, S.W.J., and Hodgson, D.R. (2002). Risk factors for repeat-breeder syndrome in New South Wales dairy cows. *Preventive Veterinary Medicine* 54 (2): 91–103.

Murray, B. (2008). Stillbirths and calf survival. *The Cattle Site*. https://www.thecattlesite.com/articles/1271/stillbirths-and-calf-survival (accessed 3 January 2024).

Murray, R.D., Williams, A.J., and Sheldon, I.M. (2008). Field investigation of perinatal mortality in Friesian cattle associated with myocardial degeneration and necrosis. *Reproduction in Domestic Animals* 43 (3): 339–345.

Nguyen, D.N., Thymann, T., Goericke-Pesch, S.K. et al. (2018). Prenatal intra-amniotic endotoxin induces fetal gut and lung immune responses and postnatal systemic inflammation in preterm pigs. *The American Journal of Pathology* 188 (11): 2629–2643.

Norquay, R. (2018). Perinatal losses in beef herds in Orkney: Assessing incidence and associated pathology from general practice. Doctoral dissertation. University of Glasgow.

Oh, K.J., Romero, R., Park, J.Y. et al. (2019). A high concentration of fetal fibronectin in cervical secretions increases the risk of intra-amniotic infection and inflammation in patients with preterm labor and intact membranes. *Journal of Perinatal Medicine* 47 (3): 288–303.

Olson, K.M., Cassell, B.G., McAllister, A.J., and Washburn, S.P. (2009). Dystocia, stillbirth, gestation length, and birth weight in Holstein, Jersey, and reciprocal crosses from a planned experiment. *Journal of Dairy Science* 92 (12): 6167–6175.

Palombi, C., Paolucci, M., Stradaioli, G. et al. (2013). Evaluation of remote monitoring of parturition in dairy cattle as a new tool for calving management. *BMC Veterinary Research* 9 (1): 1–9.

Paolucci, M., Sylla, L., Di Giambattista, A. et al. (2010). Improving calving management to further enhance reproductive performance in dairy cattle. *Veterinary Research Communications* 34: 37–40.

Regidor-Cerrillo, J., Arranz-Solis, D., Benavides, J. et al. (2014). Neospora caninum infection during early pregnancy in cattle: how the isolate influences infection dynamics, clinical outcome and peripheral and local immune responses. *Veterinary Research* 45 (1): 1–15.

Rice, D.A., McMurray, C.H., Kennedy, S., and Ellis, W.A. (1986). Lack of effect of selenium supplementation on the incidence of weak calves in dairy herds. *The Veterinary Record* 119 (23): 571–573.

Sangild, P.T., Thymann, T., Schmidt, M. et al. (2013). Invited review: the preterm pig as a model in pediatric gastroenterology. *Journal of Animal Science* 91 (10): 4713–4729.

Schuenemann, G.M., Bas, S., Gordon, E., and Workman, J. (2011). Dairy calving management: assessment of a comprehensive program for dairy personnel. *Journal of Dairy Science* 94 (1): 483.

Schuijt, G. (1990). Iatrogenic fractures of ribs and vertebrae during delivery in perinatally dying calves: 235 cases (1978–1988). *Journal of the American Veterinary Medical Association* 197 (9): 1196–1202.

Shah, K.D., Nakao, T., Kubota, H., and Maeda, T. (2007). Peripartum changes in plasma estrone sulfate and estradiol-17β profiles associated with and without the retention of fetal membranes in Holstein-Friesian cattle. *Journal of Reproduction and Development* 53 (2): 279–288.

Smyth, J.A., McNamee, P.T., Kennedy, D.G. et al. (1992). Stillbirth/perinatal weak calf syndrome: preliminary pathological, microbiological and biochemical findings. *The Veterinary Record* 130 (12): 237–240.

Smyth, A., Fitzpatrick, D.A., and Ellis, W.A. (1999). Stillbirth/perinatal weak calf syndrome: a study of calves infected with Leptospira. *Veterinary Record* 145 (19): 539–542.

Sorge, U.S., Kelton, D.F., and Staufenbiel, R. (2008). Prepartal concentration of estradiol-17β in heifers with stillborn calves. *Journal of Dairy Science* 91 (4): 1433–1437.

Steinbock, L., Nasholm, A., Berglund, B. et al. (2003). Genetic effects on stillbirth and calving difficulty in Swedish Holsteins at first and second calving. *Journal of Dairy Science* 86 (6): 2228–2235.

Streyl, D., Sauter-Louis, C., Braunert, A. et al. (2011). Establishment of a standard operating procedure for predicting the time of calving in cattle. *Journal of Veterinary Science* 12 (2): 177–185.

Svensson, C., Linder, A., and Olsson, S.O. (2006). Mortality in Swedish dairy calves and replacement heifers. *Journal of Dairy Science* 89 (12): 4769–4777.

Szelenyi, Z., Gyori, D., Boldizsar, S. et al. (2019). Pregnancy and stillbirth losses in dairy cows with singleton and twin pregnancies. *Acta Veterinaria Hungarica* 67 (1): 115–126.

Szenci, O. (2017). Importance of monitoring calving to decrease stillbirth rate in Holstein-Friesian dairy farms. *Lucrari Stiintifice: Seria Medicina Veterinara* 68: 3–11.

Szenci, O., Nagy, K., Takacs, L. et al. (2012). Farm personnel management as a risk factor for stillbirth in Hungarian Holstein-Friesian dairy farms. *Magyar Allatorvosok Lapja* 134 (7): 387–393.

Szucs, E., Gulyas, L., Cziszter, L.T., and Demirkan, I. (2009). Stillbirth in dairy cattle. *Scientific Papers Animal Science and Biotechnologies* 42 (2): 622–636.

Tao, S. and Dahl, G.E. (2013). Invited review: heat stress effects during late gestation on dry cows and their calves. *Journal of Dairy Science* 96 (7): 4079–4093.

Tao, S., Monteiro, A.P.A., Thompson, I.M. et al. (2012). Effect of late-gestation maternal heat stress on growth and immune function of dairy calves. *Journal of Dairy Science* 95 (12): 7128–7136.

Tarres, J., Casellas, J., and Piedrafita, J. (2005). Genetic and environmental factors influencing mortality up to weaning of Bruna dels Pirineus beef calves in mountain areas. A survival analysis. *Journal of Animal Science* 83 (3): 543–551.

Tierney, T.J. and Simpson-Morgan, M.W. (1997). The immune response of foetal calves. *Veterinary Immunology and Immunopathology* 57 (3–4): 229–238.

Titler, M., Maquivar, M.G., Bas, S. et al. (2015). Prediction of parturition in Holstein dairy cattle using electronic data loggers. *Journal of Dairy Science* 98 (8): 5304–5312.

Tizard, I.R. (2000). Immunity in the fetus and newborn. In: *Veterinary Immunology: An Introduction* (ed. I.R. Tizard), 210–221. Philadelphia, PA, USA: Saunders.

Uematsu, M., Sasaki, Y., Kitahara, G. et al. (2013). Risk factors for stillbirth and dystocia in Japanese Black cattle. *The Veterinary Journal* 198 (1): 212–216.

Vernooy, E., Leslie, K., Kelton, D., Hand, K., Muir, B., and Duffield, T. (2007). Management risk factors associated with stillbirth. *Proceedings of the Fortieth Annual Conference, American Association of Bovine Practitioners*, Vancouver, British Columbia, Canada (20–22 September 2007). Fort Collins, Colorado, USA: Frontier Printers, Inc.

Waldner, C.L. (2014). Cow attributes, herd management and environmental factors associated with the risk of calf death at or within 1 h of birth and the risk of dystocia in cow–calf herds in Western Canada. *Livestock Science* 163: 126–139.

Waldner, C.L. and Blakley, B. (2014). Evaluating micronutrient concentrations in liver samples from abortions, stillbirths, and neonatal and postnatal losses in beef calves. *Journal of Veterinary Diagnostic Investigation* 26 (3): 376–389.

Whitlock, B.E.A., Kaiser, L., and Maxwell, H.S. (2008). Heritable bovine foetal abnormalities. *Theriogenology* 70 (3): 535–549.

Wright, I.A., White, I.R., Russel, A.J. et al. (1988). Prediction of calving date in beef cows by real-time ultrasonic scanning. *The Veterinary Record* 123 (9): 228–229.

22

Digestive Disorders

Gowdaiahnadoddi K. Chetan Kumar, Bagur K. Bhagya, Ashok Ashwini, and Rayal S. Sagar

Department of Veterinary Medicine, Veterinary College, Bangalore, Karnataka, India

The periparturient period encompasses parturition as well as the events that occur in the weeks preceding and following parturition. Dairy cows are more vulnerable to digestive issues during this period due to changes in energy requirements and decreased digestive function. To prevent the occurrence of probable digestive diseases during the periparturient phase, all animals should have free access to good quality feed and water. Simple indigestion, diaphragmatic hernia, vagal indigestion, ruminal impaction, left-side abomasal displacement, traumatic reticulopericarditis, traumatic reticuloperitonitis (TRP), subacute ruminal acidosis (SARA), and ruminal tympany are common digestive disorders that occur around the time of parturition.

22.1 Simple Indigestion

Simple indigestion is common in dairy cattle and stallfed beef cattle due to feed quality inconsistency and excessive feed consumption. Animals are susceptible to secondary simple indigestion during the periparturient period due to metabolic conditions (hypocalcemia), endotoxemic infection (endometritis), and abomasal disease (left-sided abomasal displacement [LDA]). Simple indigestion is characterized by partial or complete anorexia (lack of appetite), ruminal atony, and a modest decrease in milk output. The most prevalent causes of primary simple indigestion are minor dietary anomalies such as indigestible roughages; inadequate protein intake; moldy, overheated, and frosted feeds; the ingestion of relatively excessive grains and concentrates; and an abrupt change in feed. A quick change in grain source, such as from oats to wheat or barley, may produce primary simple indigestion. To overcome a negative energy balance during high production, there will be sudden changes in the diet that will lead to primary simple indigestion in the periparturient period. Changes to the ruminal microbiota result from a lack of potable drinking water, excessive indigestible roughages such as straw, and extended or severe oral antibiotic therapy, all of which cause simple indigestion.

Indigestion causes a shift in the ruminal pH in either the acidic or alkaline direction. Indigestion caused by excessive grain consumption results in acidity. Alkalinity can be increased by feeding a lot of legumes or urea with a lot of protein. The rumen's motility is affected by changes in the pH of its contents. Ruminal atony can also be caused by spoiled feed. Protein putrefaction can also contribute to the development of ruminal atony. Ruminal function may be physically hampered if indigestible feed accumulates. The drop in milk production is most likely due to a significant fall in volatile fatty acid synthesis within a hypotonic reticulorumen.

The most common clinical signs of simple indigestion are partial or complete anorexia, a slight decrease in milk output, and the animal appearing dull and dejected. There will be a reduction in or cessation of ruminative activity. There could be mild tympany. The rumen can be firm and doughy without being distended. There will be no systemic reaction, such as an increase in body temperature, heart rate, or respiration rate. On the first day, feces are reduced in amount and drier than

Periparturient Diseases of Cattle, First Edition. Edited by Tanmoy Rana.

normal; nevertheless, diarrhea may occur 24–48 hours later with copious and malodorous excrement that is softer than normal. In most situations, spontaneous recovery is possible, and with modest treatment, the animal will recover within 48 hours (Constable et al. 2017).

Acetonemia, traumatic reticulopericarditis, lactic acidosis, abomasal displacement, abomasal volvulus, vagal indigestion, phytobezoars, and secondary ruminal atony should be distinguished from simple indigestion. For successful animal recovery, a modest amount of fresh, high quality hay should be fed daily to encourage feeding and increase rumen and reticulum motility. Rumenotorics are recommended to enhance appetite and reticulorumen motility. Rumenotorics that contain nux vomica, and ginger may be utilized because ginger is a prokinetic agent in ruminants (Mamaghani et al. 2013). When there is acidity, alkalizing agents such as magnesium hydroxide are employed; when there is alkalosis, acidifying agents such as acetic acid or vinegar might be utilized to address simple indigestion. If the animal has been anorexic for a long time, cud transplantation is indicated. Rumen fluid is primarily obtained from abattoirs. The rumen fluid should be filtered and delivered orally or through a stomach tube.

22.2 Diaphragmatic Hernia

Diaphragmatic hernia is characterized by chronic ruminal tympany, anorexia, and heart displacement due to reticulum herniation through a perforated diaphragm. Water buffalo have a high incidence of diaphragmatic hernias. Water buffalo may have reticulum herniation accompanied by abomasums. Diaphragmatic hernia occurs as a result of diaphragm weakness caused by traumatic reticulopericarditis lesions. It can happen in some animals due to congenital diaphragm problems or from a foreign body. Increased intra-abdominal pressure during parturition is the primary cause of diaphragmatic hernias during the periparturient period.

As a result of reticulum herniation, there is either achalasia of the reticulo-omasal sphincter due to vagus nerve involvement or impairment of esophageal groove function due to reticulum fixation to the ventral diaphragm. Food can enter the rumen but not the abomasum due to a disruption in the forestomach. Rumen hypermotility may be caused by rumen distension and induce foamy bloat. Respiration is not impaired by diaphragmatic hernias; however, heart displacement and compression are prevalent (Constable et al. 2017).

The animal with a diaphragmatic hernia has persistent, moderate, ruminal tympany and an erratic appetite. Rumen distension, loss of body condition, and grinding of the teeth are common clinical signs. Feces may be pasty or low in volume. Although rumination may be absent, regurgitation may be observed when the stomach tube is passed. Both breathing and temperature are within normal limits. Bradycardia and systolic murmurs are noticed. The intensity of cardiac sounds may indicate heart displacement (Figure 22.1). When viscera other than the reticulum herniate, the severity increases. Because of inanition, affected animals usually die 3–4 weeks following the onset of bloat (Constable et al. 2017).

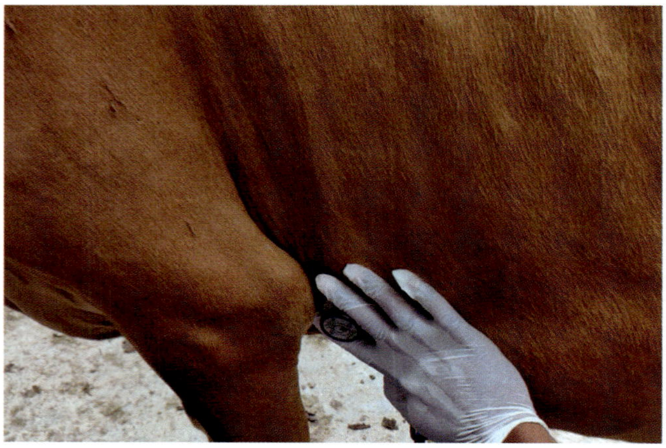

Figure 22.1 Auscultation as a method for detecting the cranial displacement of heart sounds caused by a herniated mass in the thoracic cavity.

During the postmortem examination, if the diaphragmatic hernia is caused by a complication of TRP, a fistulous tract will be discovered in the diaphragmatic rupture. The rumen will be overfilled with foamy material, and the reticulum will be adhered to the surrounding structure. In rare situations, parts of the reticulum, omasum, and abomasum will be herniated. Thoracic radiography and a thorough physical examination are used to make the diagnosis. Thoracic auscultation demonstrates the absence of lung sounds or the presence of gastric sounds. Thoracic radiography may reveal a loss of diaphragmatic contour and abdominal viscera in the thorax. In rare cases, contrast radiography may be required to make the diagnosis. Advanced imaging, such as ultrasonography, computed tomography (CT), or magnetic resonance imaging (MRI), may be indicated in some circumstances if it is accessible. The ideal treatment is surgery to replace the abdominal contents and repair the diaphragm. If the animal is in respiratory distress, it should be stabilized before operation (Kahn 2005).

22.3 Vagal Indigestion/Hoflund Syndrome

Vagal indigestion is a collection of gastrointestinal illnesses that occur in cattle and buffaloes as a result of a mechanical or functional obstruction of the forestomach and/or abomasum outflow (Neal and Edwards 1968; Rebhun et al. 1986). A reduced appetite or anorexia, scarce stools, decreased milk production, gradual abdominal distension leading to a papple-shaped abdomen, dehydration, weight loss, and eventually, weakness and recumbency describe vagal indigestion.

In his 1940 experimental investigation, Hoflund induced chronic indigestion in cattle to simulate functional stomach abnormalities following selective vagotomy. He determined that vagus nerve injury was the primary etiological cause in the development of chronic indigestion and thus developed the name "vagal indigestion." Hoflund syndrome is another name for vagal indigestion.

There are numerous causes of vagus indigestion, but reticular adhesions or vagal nerve injury caused by TRP are currently thought to be the most prevalent. Because of the increased intraabdominal pressure at the time of parturition, the incidence of TRP is high during the periparturient period. Achalasia of the reticulo-omasal orifice is caused by dorsal vagal nerve injury and prevents ingesta from the reticulorumen from passing into the omasum and abomasum, which results in a bloated rumen with aberrant rumen contents. Achalasia of the pylorus is caused by an injury to the pyloric branch of the vagal nerve, which slows the passage of ingesta from the abomasum to result in abomasal impaction. Scattered stools with undigested large feed particles were the result of both anterior and posterior functional stenosis. Vagal tension receptors placed in the medial reticular wall may interfere with forestomach motility and esophageal groove reflexes in the absence of clinical abnormalities. The most common cause of vagal indigestion is reticular adhesion. Reticular adhesions impair reticular motility and produce esophageal groove dysfunction. A perireticular abscess near the reticulo-omasal orifice in cattle can cause vagal indigestion. Late pregnancy indigestion is also regarded as a kind of vagal indigestion in which the rumen and abomasum are excessively distended, but the actual etiology is uncertain.

Anorexia, dehydration, scanty feces, depression, muscular weakness, apathy and indifference to normal stimuli, sunken eye balls, a dry mouth, cold extremities, and gradual abdominal distension are the most common clinical manifestations of vagal indigestion (Pope and Bennett 1961; Hussain et al. 2014).

Progressive abdominal distension is the most important clinical symptom. The main cause of the distension is an accumulation of gas and fluid in the rumenoreticulum. When viewed from behind, abdominal distension usually encompasses the entire left side of the abdomen and the right ventral quadrant of the belly, giving the left side an "apple-shaped" look and the right side a "pear-shaped" appearance. When both shapes are combined, they form a "papple shape" (Iggo and Leek 1967; Braun et al. 2009). Although a papple-shaped abdomen is regarded a common characteristic in cattle, it has only been seen in a few cases in buffaloes (Hussain et al. 2014). Fecal flow decreases progressively as the number of undigested particles increases and feces may sometimes stop completely. Feces are typically pasty in consistency. Melena can appear in rare circumstances as a result of abomasum ulceration. Weight loss occurs in all circumstances but may go unreported by the owner because belly swelling conceals the animal's reduction in muscle mass. Milk production in dairy animals decreases gradually.

Rectal temperature is typically normal; however, subnormal temperatures have been documented. In most cases, respiration is unchanged, but it may be enhanced due to significant abdominal distension. Bradycardia is a characteristic symptom of vagus indigestion in cattle, but it is not always present. An increased pulse rate may arise as a result of pyloric blockage.

Hematologic alterations are inconsistent, and they typically depend on how persistent the condition is and how dehydrated the patient is. Due to the more severe nature of the functional pyloric stenosis and a greater degree of dehydration, the packed cell volume (PCV) typically rises. Increases in the percentage of band cells, polymophonuclear cells, or both are seen in the total white blood cell count if vagal indigestion develops as a result of TRP. Hyperproteinemia and hyperfibrinogenemia are present in most animals.

Abdominal contents refluxed back into the reticulorumen as a result of abomasal reflux result in dehydration, hypochloremia, hypokalemia, metabolic alkalosis, azotemia, and a notable increase in the concentration of chloride in the ruminal fluid. Even while the rumen pH may or may not alter, refluxing abomasal contents into the forestomaches significantly reduces the ability of rumen fluid to act as a buffer.

In omasal transport failure, the ingesta builds up in the rumenoreticulum because they are unable to transit via the reticulo-omasal orifice. However, the abomasal fluid can continue into the duodenum, therefore no metabolic alkalosis is anticipated. In cattle with omasal transport failure, the plasma bicarbonate concentration does not significantly vary.

However, it has been noted that there is a decrease in sodium concentration of the rumen fluid. The chloride and potassium concentrations in the plasma and rumen fluid are unaffected by the omasal transport failure because there is no abomasal reflux. Blood urea nitrogen, creatinine, pH, and the buffering capacity of rumen fluid are not statistically significant (Constable et al. 2017).

When an abomasal reflux syndrome is suggested by elevated rumen fluid chloride concentrations; a hypochloremic, hypokalemic metabolic alkalosis; and clinical indications, mainly the papular shape of the abdomen and decreased defecation, a diagnosis of functional pyloric stenosis can be made. The degree of metabolic alkalosis, azotemia, hypochloremia, and hypokalemia can be utilized to distinguish between omasal transport failure and pyloric functional dysfunction (Braun et al. 2009).

Because of various lesions in the region, demonstrating vagal nerve injury during a postmortem investigation is challenging. Postmortem examinations of clinical patients typically indicate rumen distension with liquid or semiliquid contents. If vagal dyspepsia is caused by TRP sequelae, reticular adhesions may be detected. Peritonitis, abscess, and reticulum–diaphragm adhesions have all been reported as probable causes of omasal transport failure.

The goal of an ultrasonographic examination is to find adhesions and abscesses that could be the cause of the vagal indigestion close to the reticulum, liver, omasum, and abomasum. The distinction between proximal jejunal ileus and distal functional stenosis of the duodenum is made possible by ultrasound. A foreign object may occasionally be seen obstructing the reticulo-omasal orifice during radiography, which helps in the detection or exclusion of reticular ferro metallic foreign bodies as the cause of vagal indigestion. The diagnosis may also benefit from exploratory laparotomies and rumenotomies. If the underlying cause of vagal indigestion cannot be determined with clinical, ultrasonographic, or radiographic investigations, the prognosis is poor, and no therapy is recommended. Cattle with a mechanically blocked reticulo-omasal orifice (e.g. objects like a rope or a placenta), TRP, abscesses that involve the reticulum and liver, bronchopneumonia, or who are farther along in pregnancy should be treated (Kahn 2005).

22.4 Ruminal Impaction

Because of their indiscriminate eating habits, cattle frequently exhibit ruminal impaction. Both metallic and nonmetallic foreign bodies can be found in the rumen of cattle; however, metallic foreign bodies are more likely to induce pericarditis and TRP. The rumen was where foreign bodies were mostly found. Foreign objects that were not made of metal included plastic bags, cloth, rope, leather, and paper bags. An increased consumption of foreign objects can lead to decreased feed intake, weight loss, and abnormalities in electrolytes and the acid–base balance (Constable et al. 2017).

Emaciation, recurrent bloat, abdomen distension and symmetry, lack of feces in the rectum, foamy salivation, recumbency, and inappetence are the symptoms of ruminal impaction.

Along with the patient's medical history and clinical symptoms, biochemical data like hyperglycemia, metabolic alkalosis, hyponatremia, hypochloremia, hypocalcemia, hypoproteinemia, and hypoalbuminemia are used to diagnose ruminal impaction. A few patients may benefit from diagnostic ultrasonography. Rumenotomy and electrolyte balance restoration are the two main objectives of therapy.

22.4.1 Left-side Displacement of the Abomasum

Feed intake before and after parturition is linked to the prevalence of LDA in cattle. The highest period for LDA incidence is 2 weeks prior to and 2–4 weeks following parturition. Together, the decreased ruminal fill, decreased feed intake during the prepartum period, and increased feed intake following parturition produce LDA. Large, high yield adult dairy cows immediately following parturition are especially susceptible to LDA. Ninety percent of cases start within 6 weeks of giving birth. A few to several weeks before parturition, there are sporadic incidences.

22.4.2 Pathogenesis

In a nonpregnant animal, the abomasum often occupies the ventral region of the abdomen, more to the right of the midline than on it. In a pregnant animal, the expanding uterus gradually takes up more and more of the abdominal cavity. At the end of gestation, the uterus starts to move under the caudal portions of the rumen, which decreases its capacity by one-third. While the pylorus still extends across the belly to the right side, this also pushes the abomasum forward and somewhat to the left side of the abdomen.

Following calving, the uterus pulls caudally toward the pelvic inlet, allowing the abomasum to reposition itself. The pyloric end of the abomasum moves completely to the left side of the abdomen during LDA. The abomasum might expand and shift onto the left side of the abdomen as a result of rumen fill shortage and hypomotility. The chief dysfunctions in LDA are thought to be abomasal hypomotility and gaseous distension. After delivery, there is a decrease in plasma calcium levels, which contributes to abomasal hypomotility. Gas builds up in the abomasum when its mobility is insufficient (Constable et al. 2017).

22.4.3 Clinical Signs

Clinical signs typically appear after a few days or a week post parturition and include inappetence or complete anorexia, varied levels of ketosis, and decreased milk output. The rumen is smaller than usual and is moved medially by the abomasum, which gives the left lateral abdomen a "slab-sided" look. The animal's temperature, heart rate, and respiration rate remain unchanged. The feces are often lighter and less bulky than usual, but intermittent bouts of severe diarrhea may occur.

High-pitched tinkling sounds are audible in a region below an imaginary line drawn from the left paralumbar fossa's center to just behind the left elbow, and these sounds frequently have a gradual peristaltic nature. These sounds are abnormal. The high-pitched tympanitic noises (pings) that are typical of LDA are frequently elicited by simultaneously auscultating an area between the upper third of the ninth and twelfth ribs of the abdomen wall, while percussing with a flick of the finger (Constable et al. 2017).

22.4.4 Diagnosis

The history of a recent calving and the clinical features of a slab-sided, left lateral abdomen are used to make a diagnosis of LDA. Significant biochemical alterations typically include mild metabolic alkalosis, mild hypochloremia, and hypokalemia. There is always a moderate-to-severe ketonuria. The most frequent consequence of LDA is ketosis, and fatty liver is frequently present in severe cases of ketosis. In cattle with LDA, the abomasum can be observed between the left abdominal wall and the rumen, which aids in the diagnosis of abomasal displacements. The Liptak test, or abomasocentesis (Figure 22.2), involves taking a sample of fluid with a pH of 2 and no protozoa through the tenth or eleventh intercostal gap in the middle portion of the left abdominal wall.

The displaced abomasum is wedged between the rumen and the ventral abdominal floor and contains varying volumes of fluid and gas, according to postmortem investigations. It is occasionally held in place by adhesions, which are typically caused by a ruptured abomasal ulcer with localized peritonitis. In cows that die from LDA problems soon after giving birth or having surgery, fatty liver is frequently observed. Surgical correction is now commonly practiced to avoid the recurrence of the displacement.

22.5 Traumatic Pericarditis

The primary cause of traumatic pericarditis (TP) is the penetration of the pericardial sac by a sharp, migrant foreign body from the reticulum. The primary characteristics of TP include pericarditis, toxemia, tachycardia, development of congestive heart failure, fever, enlargement of the jugular veins, anasarca, hydrothorax and ascites, and abnormalities in heart

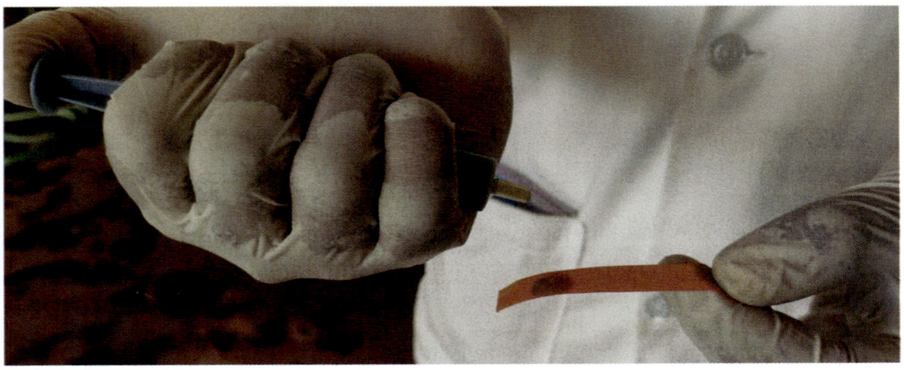

Figure 22.2 The Liptak test is used to distinguish rumen fluid from abdominal fluid.

sounds. Compared to other times, the last 3 months of pregnancy and the time right before parturition have higher prevalences of TP. TP develops in about 8% of all TRP instances. Most of the time, infected animals die or develop chronic pericarditis without ever fully recovering.

22.5.1 Pathogenesis

The pericardial sac may be penetrated by a foreign object (Figure 22.3) following the initial reticular wall breach. The development of pericarditis during late pregnancy or during parturition is possible in animals who have previously had TRP. This is most likely because the foreign object, which was initially perforated, eventually entered a sinus in the reticular wall and entered the pericardial sac. Because infections from the traumatized mediastinum can enter through the pericardium, the physical puncture of the sac by a metallic foreign body is not necessary for the development of pericarditis.

A significant local inflammation is brought on by the introduction of a mixed bacterial infection from the reticulum; the presence of the foreign body in the tissues is not necessary for the disease to progress further. Hyperemia of the pericardial surfaces and frictional sounds produced in time with heartbeats are the earliest side effects of inflammation. These two mechanisms are crucial for the appearance of the clinical symptoms: toxemia brought on by the infection and pressure on the heart from fluid buildup in the sac causes congestive heart failure. Edema and depression follow as the main features of TRP. Because of this, an infected animal may experience severe illness for several weeks before developing edema gradually or severely within 2–3 days. Edema that develops quickly is typically a sign of impending mortality.

The adherence of the pericardium to the heart restricts heart function if chronic pericarditis continues. Most often, congestive heart failure occurs, but some animals may recover. Uncommon complications following pericardial sac penetration by a foreign body include the laceration of a coronary artery by a wire or less frequently, rupture of the ventricular wall. Acute, congestive heart failure brought on by the compression of the heart by the hemopericardium typically results in sudden death (Constable et al. 2017).

22.5.2 Clinical Signs

The cow has an arched back, appears reluctant to move, and walks slowly and cautiously. The cow may groan while sleeping, standing up, urinating, and defecating. The respiration is shallow and quick, and the heart rate is normal or slightly elevated (Kahn 2005). Additionally noted signs are teeth grinding and salivation. Respiratory movements and bilateral jugular vein distension are more pronounced. With an increase in heart rate to 40–50 beats per minute frequently accompanied by grunting, abdominal and shallow breathing is noted. Both the ventral abdominal wall and the brisket region frequently exhibit edema. In extreme circumstances, there may even be conjunctival edema, with grape-like masses of edematous conjunctiva hanging over the eyelids. Typically, a noticeable jugular venous pulse is present. Early-stage pyrexia is frequently observed, the heart rate can increase by up to 100 beats per minute, the amplitude of the pulse is decreased, and there is decreased ruminal motility. When there is effusion, muffled heartbeats are audible.

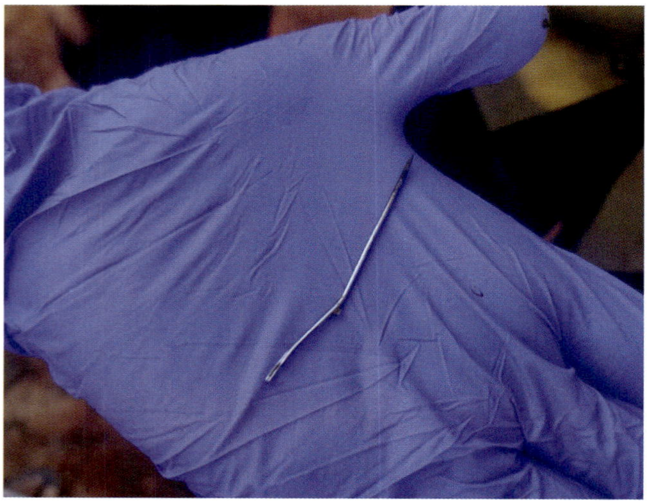

Figure 22.3 A sharp needle was discovered during the postmortem examination of a cow that had died from traumatic pericarditis.

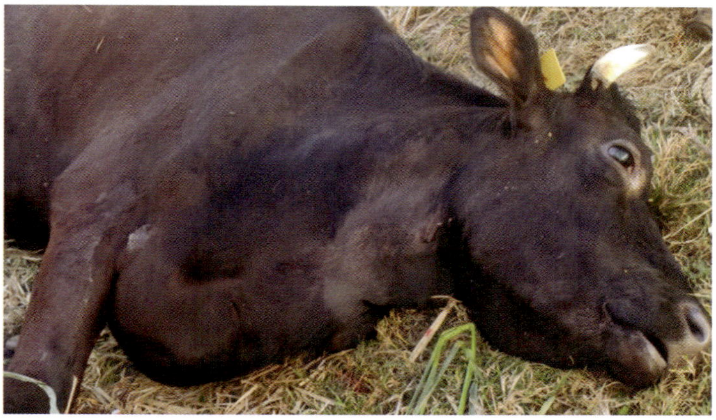

Figure 22.4 A cow with traumatic pericarditis developed severe brisket and ventral abdominal wall edema.

22.5.3 Diagnosis

The diagnosis is made based on the patient's medical history and clinical indicators such as brisket (Figure 22.4) and ventral abdominal wall edema, jugular pulsation, and abducted elbow. Leukocytosis is a major hematologic finding. When the animal is standing, lateral radiographs of the ventral thorax and cranial abdomen can aid the location of metallic foreign bodies. The diagnosis of pericardial effusion is aided by ultrasound, which is also used to guide pericardiocentesis. A 10-cm, 18-gauge needle can be used for pericardiocentesis in the fourth or fifth intercostal gap on the left side. When pericarditis is in the middle stage, the pericardial fluid has an unpleasant odor and is turbid. Only trace levels may exist in chronic pericarditis, and obtaining a sample may not be possible.

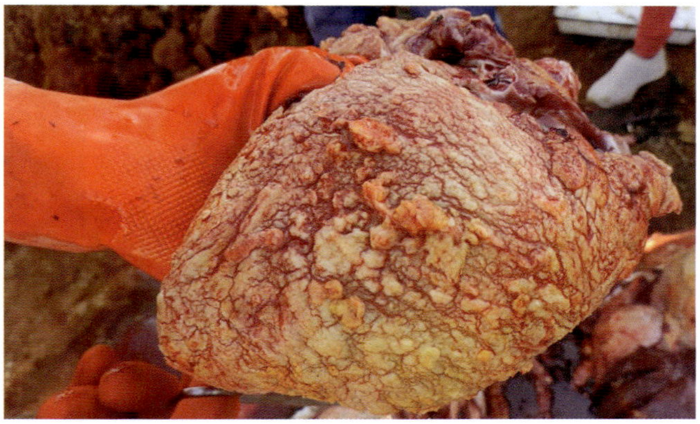

Figure 22.5 The serous surface of the sac is heavily coated with fibrin in cows that die from traumatic pericarditis.

Acute and chronic instances have different postmortem alterations. In acute cases, the pericardial sac will be grossly dilated and filled with an unpleasant-smelling, grayish fluid that contains fibrin flakes. Additionally, the serous surface of the sac will be heavily covered in deposits of freshly generated fibrin (Figure 22.5). The reticulum and pericardium are typically connected by a fibrous sinus tract. Pneumonia and pleurisy are frequently prevalent. In chronic situations, the pericardial sac is markedly enlarged, and strongly fibrous adhesions bond it to the pericardium (Constable et al. 2017).

Endocarditis, lymphosarcoma, congenital cardiac abnormalities, emaciated animals or animals with severe anemia, pasteurellosis, thoracic tumors and abscesses, thymic lymphosarcoma, and diaphragmatic hernia should be distinguished from TP. All of these have the same clinical signs as TP.

22.5.4 Treatment

Recovery may be aided by the implantation of a pericardial catheter, daily pericardial lavage with diluted iodine solutions in 0.9% NaCl, and long term systemic antibacterial therapy. The edema and respiratory discomfort may be momentarily relieved by draining the pericardial sac, but it reoccurs within a few days. Using a fifth rib excision pericardiotomy, certain cases of TP have been successfully treated. Typically, treatment outcomes are not satisfactory.

22.6 Traumatic Reticuloperitonitis/Hardware Disease

Peritonitis is an inflammation of the peritoneum that can occur when a sharp foreign body (metallic foreign body) perforates the reticulum wall. Initially, it causes local peritonitis, which progresses to diffuse peritonitis. In rare circumstances, it may remain localized and cause future harm such as vagal indigestion and diaphragmatic hernia. When a foreign body penetrates the peritoneum, it can cause pericarditis, cardiac tamponade, pneumonia, pleurisy, mediastinitis, and hepatic, splenic, or diaphragmatic abscess.

22.6.1 Etiology

TRP is brought on by metallic foreign substances that have infiltrated the reticulum after entering the body through a prepared meal. Fence wire that has been cut with a chaff cutter is one of the most common sources of TRP when fences next to feed troughs are serviced.

22.6.2 Pathogenesis

Cattle are indiscriminate feeders, and their lack of oral discrimination leads to the ingestion of foreign items that other animals reject. Foreign bodies that have been swallowed may become lodged in the upper esophagus or the esophageal groove. However, most foreign bodies will pass through the reticulum. These foreign entities infiltrate several sacs of the reticulo-rumen before reaching the reticulum. Many foreign bodies rest there without causing harm, however the honeycomb structure of the reticulum supports foreign body fixation, and reticulum contractions help force a sharp foreign body through the reticulum wall, which leads to acute local peritonitis or generalized peritonitis. Clinically observable signs will not be present if the reticulum's wall is damaged without being penetrated since, in certain animals, corrosion may cause foreign bodies to vanish within 6 weeks. However, some nails endure much longer and rarely rust (Constable et al. 2017).

22.6.2.1 Acute Local Peritonitis

The reaction to the puncture of the reticulum wall results in local peritonitis. In experimental investigations, clinical symptoms start to show 24 hours after penetration. Ruminal atony and stomach discomfort are symptoms of perforation. If the foreign body moves back to the reticulum, a spontaneous recovery occurs. The ventral portion of the reticulum adheres to the abdomen floor and diaphragm to variable degrees, depending on the intensity of the local peritonitis.

Chronic ruminal tympany, persistent mild fever, abdominal pain upon deep palpation, decreased reticulorumen motility, inappetence to anorexia, a capricious appetite (may eat hay but not concentrate), and alterations in the hemogram and feces are all symptoms of persistent local peritonitis. Immobilization of the reticulum affects the reticulum's ability to remove waste, which causes the passage of inadequately comminuted stool with a higher percentage of larger particles.

22.6.2.2 Generalized Peritonitis and Extension of Disease

Generalized peritonitis develops when the inflammation spreads and affects animals that are forced to exercise as well as cows that might calve during penetration. Because adhesions localize the peritonitis, immobility is a significant clinical feature and could represent a protective mechanism. Due to the disruption of adhesions by body movements when an animal is forced to walk or is carried across long distances, relapses are common. Toxemia, gastrointestinal tract stasis, dehydration, and shock are the outcomes of generalized peritonitis (Constable et al. 2017).

22.6.3 Clinical Findings

22.6.3.1 Acute Local Peritonitis

Acute local peritonitis is distinguished by the rapid onset of total anorexia and a significant decrease in milk production. The abrupt appearance of these alterations, which occur over a 12-hour period, is common. Most often, subacute abdominal discomfort is present. The animal moves slowly and with reluctance. Animals make a grunting noise when they walk, especially when going downhill. Most animals like to stand still for extended periods of time. The animal seems emaciated or "tucked up" due to the back's tendency to arch and the appearance of tight abdominal and back muscles. Both defecation and urination are painful, and they are only done occasionally. When an animal urinates or defecates, it makes a grunting noise. Acute local peritonitis causes constipation, sparse feces, and in rare cases, urinary retention. Acute abdominal pain with belly kicking and stretching occurs occasionally. In acute localized peritonitis, a mild systemic reaction is typical. With an elevated heart rate and respiratory rate, the temperature is between 39.5 and 40 °C (103 and 104 °F). Reticulorumen motions are severely suppressed and frequently nonexistent, and rumination is absent. Deep palpation of the abdominal wall just caudal to the xiphisternum results in pain (Constable et al. 2017).

22.6.3.2 Acute Diffuse (Generalized) Peritonitis

The presence of significant toxemia within a day or two of the onset of local peritonitis is a defining feature of acute diffuse peritonitis. In extreme cases, particularly those that happen immediately after calving, the motility of the gastrointestinal system is impaired, depression is noticeable, and the temperature is raised or subnormal. A painful groan can be heard practically everywhere over the ventral abdominal wall when deep digital palpation is applied. The heart rate rises to 100–120 beats per minute. Rapid collapse, peripheral circulatory failure, and a lack of pain sensations typically come after this stage. Depression and recumbency are frequent in the terminal stage (Constable et al. 2017).

22.6.3.3 Chronic Local Peritonitis

Despite prolonged antibiotic treatment in chronic peritonitis, milk production and appetite do not recover to normal. Typically, the body is in poor health, there are fewer feces, and there are more undigested particles. Rumination, feces, and urination can occasionally result in grunting. There is ruminal atony or some mild reticulorumen activity, the rumen is often smaller than normal, chronic moderate bloat is typical, and ruminations are not frequent.

22.6.4 Diagnosis

A diagnosis can be made based on hematologic findings. In cases with acute local peritonitis, a higher number of neutrophils will be present, and an increased number of immature neutrophils will be visible (shift to the left); in simple cases, numbers will return to normal. In chronic cases, the levels take several days or more to return to normal, and there is typically mild to severe leukocytosis, neutrophilia, and monocytosis. Leukopenia with a higher absolute number of immature neutrophils than mature neutrophils is present in acute diffuse peritonitis. An elevated plasma concentration of serum amyloid α is a sign of the acute phase response in cattle with active peritonitis brought on by TRP (Atakisi et al. 2010).

Peritonitis is diagnosed via abdominal sonography and peritoneal fluid analysis. It is best to perform the radiologic examination of the reticulum while the animal is standing to ensure an accurate diagnosis of reticuloperitonitis. For the investigation of reticular contractions in healthy ruminants and in cattle for the diagnosis of TRP, the ultrasound is an appropriate approach. Cattle with TRP almost invariably have altered reticular activity. Contractions may be aberrant in their frequency, amplitude, or velocity, either separately or in combination.

The diagnosis of TRP is aided by metal detectors. Metal detectors can find ferrous metallic foreign objects, but their utility is restricted because most dairy cows that eat chopped forages test positive for metal over their reticular region.

22.6.5 Treatment

The two main treatment options are rumenotomy and conservative medical therapy. The best course of treatment for TRP involves surgical removal of the foreign material through a rumenotomy. The conservative course of therapy includes immobilizing the animal, giving antibiotics for the infection, and giving a magnet orally to immobilize the foreign substance. About 1–4 days after administration, magnets enter the reticulum and attach to penetrating foreign bodies. For several days, the cow is restrained or chained within a box stall. The animal's immobility makes it easier for adhesions to form (Constable et al. 2017).

22.7 Subacute Ruminal Acidosis (SARA)

SARA in dairy cattle is a disorder of ruminal fermentation in dairy cattle caused by the ingestion of large amounts of concentrates and inadequate amounts of fiber that are administered to increase milk production in early lactation. SARA occurs in dairy cattle herds fed high grain, low fiber rations in early lactation. It is considered of major economic importance because of its possible association with laminitis in dairy herds.

Most metabolic disorders in dairy cows develop as they change from being pregnant and nonlactating to being nonpregnant and lactating. Because the cow switches from a diet that is high in fiber and low in concentrate feeds to one that is higher in concentrate feeds and lower in fiber, this period usually lasts from 3 weeks prior to parturition until 3 weeks following calving. Ruminal acidosis is especially dangerous for cows who have not adapted to these high grain diets.

SARA is distinguished by frequent episodes of low rumen pH between 5.2 and 5.6. The aberration is frequently caused by a high intake of rapidly fermentable carbohydrates, which causes an accumulation of organic acids in the rumen. In early to mid-lactation, up to 20% of cows on commercial dairy farms have a rumen pH less than 5.5, which indicates SARA. It is a financially significant disease that generates massive losses in the dairy business.

Periparturient cows are at risk of SARA because it takes time for the rumen microbiota and papillae to adapt to increased concentrate intakes just before parturition as well as during early lactation, when feed intake increases rapidly to meet the energy needs of high producing dairy cows. It takes a gradual transition over the course of 3–5 weeks for the ruminal microbiota and papillae to adjust from being adapted for forage to being able to use high energy lactation diets. Subacute acidosis is most likely caused by feeding animals large amounts of concentrate and minimal forage, which results in a ration lacking in fiber.

22.7.1 Pathogenesis

Not much is known about the pathogenesis of SARA in lactating dairy cows. SARA is typically brought on in early lactating dairy cows by diets high in quickly fermentable carbohydrates or low, frequently deficient, in physically active fiber. Most SARA cases have been reported in confinement herds that are fed a total mixed diet or component feeds.

In Ireland and New Zealand, where there are lush pastures with high concentrations of quickly fermentable carbs and low quantities of useful fiber, it can also happen to cattle that are fed on pasture. In SARA, nonstructural carbohydrates are fermented to produce high amounts of volatile fatty acids and lactate, which build up in the rumen and ultimately lower pH levels.

22.7.2 Clinical Signs

Laminitis-related limping, intermittent diarrhea, a poor appetite or cyclic feed intake, a loss of body condition despite appropriate calorie intake, liver abscesses, and a decrease in milk fat are the main clinical indications of SARA. It is associated with hemoptysis and epistaxis with pulmonary hemorrhage and vena cava thrombosis. It is possible for cows in their second and subsequent lactations to produce less milk than those in their first lactation. Ridges in the dorsal hoof wall, sole ulceration, white line lesions, sole hemorrhages, and deformed hooves are symptoms of laminitis. When the incidence of laminitis exceeds 10% of the herd, it is proposed that it be considered a herd concern associated with the feeding program.

22.7.3 Diagnosis and Treatment

The diagnosis is based on a history of recent calving as well as high grain and low fiber feeds. In order to diagnose SARA, rumenocentesis is frequently employed. The main approach of the treatment is to avoid abrupt changes in ration by limiting the sudden intake of rapidly digested carbs. Ruminal buffering agents can also be given. Diets high in sodium and potassium compared to chloride and sulfur have greater dietary cation–anion difference (DCAD) concentrations, promote higher ruminal pH, and improve dry matter intake and milk output.

The cow produces endogenous buffers that are secreted into the rumen via saliva. The amount of physical fiber in the diet impacts the extent to which the salivary glands produce buffers. To contribute to the creation of the intermediate mat layer, fiber particles must be at least 4 cm long. Rumination stimulates chewing action as well as the release of significant volumes of saliva into the rumen. During rumination, the pH of the rumen rises. Endogenous buffers are produced by the cow and secreted into the rumen via saliva. The amount of physical fiber in the diet determines the extent of buffer production by the salivary glands. Fiber particles must be at least 4 cm in length to contribute to mat layer formation. Rumination promotes a great deal of chewing activity and the secretion of large amounts of saliva into the rumen. Ruminal adaptation to fermentable carbohydrate diets is dependent on microbial adaptation (particularly lactate-utilizing bacteria, which grow more slowly than lactate-producing bacteria) and ruminal papillae length (longer rumen papillae promote greater volatile fatty acid absorption and thus lower ruminal pH). Ruminal adaptability to high grain diets should be carefully monitored. Ruminal pH increases during bouts of rumination.

22.8 Ruminal Tympany (Bloat)

Normal fermentation in ruminants generates gas bubbles that develop, agglomerate, and separate from the ruminal contents to form free gas, which is then expelled by eructation. Bloat is an abnormal enlargement of the rumen and reticulum brought on by an excessive retention of fermentation gases, either as free gas that is separate from the contents of the rumen or as a persistent foam mixed with those contents.

Bloat comes in two forms: foamy bloat and free gas bloat. The primary ruminal tympany, often known as foamy bloat, is distinguished by stable foam development in the rumen. A blockage that prevents gas from the rumen from escaping or an excess of gas generation by fermentation causes secondary ruminal tympany, also known as free gas bloat.

The foaming properties of the leaf protein found in legumes and other bloating forages consumed by cattle are the source of foamy bloat. Protein type matters more than protein intake when it comes to the development of frothy bloat. When nonadapted animals are given a high concentrate and low roughage feed, foamy bloat could result. Due to the high concentrate diet and extensive feeding of legumes used to increase milk production, the odds of foamy bloat are higher during the periparturient phase.

Free gas bloat is brought on by physical obstructions to eructation, which can be brought on by stenosis of the esophagus, obstruction of the cardia, obstruction of the esophagus brought on by any foreign body, or by pressure from growths outside the esophagus such as tuberculous lymphadenitis or bovine viral leukosis with involvement of the bronchial lymph nodes. Chronic ruminal tympany may result from diaphragmatic hernia and vagus indigestion interfering with esophageal groove function.

The condition also happens in cases of tetanus and poisoning from *Rhizoctonia leguminicola*, most likely as a result of esophageal muscle spasm. Less frequent causes of obstructive bloat include carcinoma, granulomatous lesions linked to *Actinomyces bovis* along the esophagus groove and in the reticular wall, and papillomata of the esophageal groove and reticulum. Secondary free gas bloat from tetanus in cattle is frequently brought on by esophageal spasm and an inability to eructate appropriately. Free gas bloat can happen at any point in an animal's life, however, during the periparturient stage, diaphragmatic hernia, tetanus, and vagus indigestion should be ruled out.

22.8.1 Pathogenesis

Gas builds up in the rumen of ruminants when eructation is affected, causing the rumen to become stretched and bloated. As pressure in the rumen rises, respiration becomes difficult because the diaphragm is unable to expand and generate the negative pressure essential for inhalation. In extreme circumstances, this inability to breathe may result in asphyxia and death.

22.8.2 Clinical Findings

In dairy animals, bloat is a frequent cause of abrupt death. In lactating dairy cattle, foamy bloat usually occurs within 1 hour of being moved to a bloat producing pasture. In primary pasture bloat, the entire abdomen expands, the rumen becomes visibly distended, and the left flank may be so distended that the paralumbar fossa protrudes above the vertebral column. The skin across the left side grows progressively tauter as the bloat worsens, and in extreme cases, it cannot be tented. Dyspnea and grunting are noticeable, and they are accompanied by frequent urination, mouth breathing, tongue protrusion, and extension of the head. The animal will collapse and die if the tympany worsens (Lehmkuhler et al. 2011).

22.8.3 Diagnosis

Rumen distension is used to diagnose bloat, although it can be challenging to distinguish between frothy bloat and free gas bloat based on rumen distension. The clinical symptom of foamy bloat on pasture is the development of stable foam, which traps and holds gases from fermentation in the rumen (Moate 2018). Free gas or foamy bloat can be definitively diagnosed by rumen content investigation, trocarization, or stomach tube insertion.

22.8.4 Treatment

Whether it is a free gas bloat or a frothy bloat, the type will determine the course of treatment. The stomach tube may be the first and only effective treatment for free gas bloating, and it also partially relieves high concentrate frothy bloating. In the event of foamy bloat, an effort should be made to administer antifoaming medications through the stomach tube after relieving the gas. Mineral and vegetable oils are equally helpful and provide a decent cure for foamy bloat. Vegetable oils prevent foaming for a shorter period of time, unless given in higher levels, because they break down in the rumen more quickly than detergents or mineral oils. (Majak et al. 2001).

Commercial remedies contain detergents and other antifoaming agents that allow the foam to disperse quickly. The trocar and cannula approach as well as emergency rumenotomy should be utilized only when the stomach tube cannot relieve animal suffering. Recently, the intraluminal injection of Alfa detergent or Anti Gaz Emulsion has been shown to be fully effective in the treatment of pasture bloat (Perry and Cecava 2015).

22.8.5 Prevention and Control

22.8.5.1 Administration of Antifoaming Agents

There are two categories of surface-active substances that are useful for preventing pasture bloat: (i) synthetic surfactants and (ii) vegetable oils, mineral oils, and animal fats. Poloxalene, a synthetic surfactant, is a very effective bloat preventive when used at the prescribed dosage of 1018 g/day split into two doses per day. When administered at the recommended doses, it has no negative effects on feed intake or animal productivity and leaves no residues in the milk or body tissues (Constable 2024). Although mineral oil decreases the likelihood of bloating, its drawbacks make it less effective as a bloat preventive.

22.8.5.2 Grazing Management

When animals are let onto pasture in the afternoon as opposed to the morning, bloat is less likely to happen. Animals need to be fully fed coarse hay before being put on a pasture with legumes. This regimen prevents them from the excessive consumption off fresh, lush, legume forage. Cattle pasture bloat can be prevented by regularly giving them grass hay before they graze lucerne (Majak et al. 2008).

22.9 Acute Carbohydrate Engorgement of Ruminants (Ruminal Lactic Acidosis)

Acute ruminal acidosis is a metabolic condition characterized by low blood pH and bicarbonate levels induced by ruminal D-lactate overproduction. It manifests when animals consume an excessive amount of nonstructural carbohydrates with little neutral detergent fiber (Hernández et al. 2014). The most prevalent cause of acute ruminal acidosis is the intake of hazardous quantities of carbohydrate-rich feed, such as grain. Engorgement caused by apples, grapes, bread, baker's dough, sugar beetroot, mangels, sour wet brewers' grain that was incompletely fermented in the brewery, and high sucrose solutions used in apiculture are among the less common causes.

22.9.1 Epidemiology

Acute ruminal acidosis can affect all ruminant cattle and sheep; however, it is more common in feedlot cattle. Cattle are particularly susceptible to ruminal lactic acidosis during the periparturient period because they are fed a high concentrate and grain diet in order to maximize milk yield in the following lactation. The condition can also be caused by inadvertently consuming an excessive amount of grain or by feeding livestock an unusually large amount of grain. When consumed in significant quantities, wheat, barley, and maize grains are the most hazardous. Oats and grain sorghum are the least toxic grains. All grains become more poisonous when coarsely ground, crushed, or even cracked, as these actions expose the starch component of the grain to the ruminal microbiota. In cattle, life-threatening feed quantities ranged from 25 to 62 g/kg body weight (BW) of maize cereal grain or maize, which causes severe acidosis.

22.9.2 Pathogenesis

When a ruminant consumes an excessive amount of highly fermentable feed, the microbial population in the rumen changes dramatically within 2–6 hours. There is an increase in the quantity of *Streptococcus bovis*, which uses glucose to make significant amounts of lactic acid. In the presence of a sufficient amount of glucose, the organism will continue to produce lactic acid, which lowers the rumen pH to 5 or below and causes the cellulolytic bacteria and protozoa to be destroyed. Initially, the concentration of volatile fatty acids rises, contributing to the drop in ruminal pH.

Because of the low pH, lactobacilli can utilize the substantial amounts of carbohydrates in the rumen to produce excessive amounts of lactic acid, which leads to ruminal lactic acidosis that significantly raises ruminal osmolality and draws water from the systemic circulation to results in hemoconcentration and dehydration.

The amplitude and frequency of rumen contractions decrease as the ruminal pH drops, and at a pH of around 5, there is ruminal atony. It produces both D- and L-lactic acids. The D-isomer, which builds up and causes severe D-lactic acidosis, is utilized much more slowly than the L-isomer. Chemical rumenitis, which is the forerunner to mycotic rumenitis in animals that survive, is brought on by the high levels of lactic acid in the rumen. *Fusobacterium necrophorum* and *Trueperella pyogenes* can penetrate directly into ruminal arteries and move to the liver, which might have also been injured by the lactic acidosis, as a common consequence of rumenitis brought on by lactic acidosis.

22.9.3 Clinical Findings

In the mild type, the affected cattle are anorexic but still relatively bright and alert, and the feces may be softer than usual. Though diminished, rumen movements still occur. Affected cattle do not ruminate for a few days but typically start eating on the third or fourth day without any specific therapy.

In the severe type, some animals will be recumbent, some may stumble, and some will stand quietly alone within 24–48 hours. Most affected cattle are anorexic, apathetic, and depressed. Cattle may engorge themselves on water if it is easily available immediately after consuming large quantities of grain, but they often do not drink water after the onset of condition.

Depression, dehydration, lethargy, weakness, stomach distension, diarrhea, and anorexia are common symptoms. Normally, the temperature ranges from 36.5 to 38.5 °C (98–101 °F), although animals that are exposed to the sun may experience temperatures as high as 41 °C (106 °F). With the severity of the acidosis and circulatory failure, the heart rate in cattle typically rises and stays elevated. Most of the time, there is diarrhea, which is often severe. The feces are pale in color and have a strong sweet-sour odor. When there is a grain overload, the feces frequently have pips and skins from eaten grapes or apples as well as an excessive number of grain kernels. Dehydration is severe and advancing.

Affected animals lie calmly, frequently with their heads inclined to the flank, and their responsiveness to any stimuli is greatly reduced, which resembles parturient paresis. A rapid development of recumbency indicates an unfavorable prognosis and the need for immediate treatment because death might occur within 24–72 hours of ingesting the meal.

22.9.4 Diagnosis

Clinical signs, physical examination findings, investigation of ruminal fluid, and blood analysis can all be used to make a diagnosis. The ruminal fluid must be evaluated right away because the pH will increase upon exposure to air. The ruminal fluid is milky green to olive-brown in color and has a strong acidic odor. A sample of ruminal fluid collected in a glass beaker will demonstrate the absence of froth. The pH of rumen fluid is usually less than 5. A few drops of ruminal fluid on a glass slide (with a coverslip) at low magnification will indicate the absence of ruminal protozoa, particularly medium- and large-sized protozoa, which is a good indicator of an aberrant state of the rumen and is generally acidosis. The rumen's gram-negative bacterial microbiota gets replaced by a gram-positive one.

The degree of hemoconcentration, as measured by hematocrit, increases as more fluid is drained from the extracellular fluid space into the rumen and is likely the best single indication of clinical severity in ruminal acidosis (Marchesini et al. 2013). There is nearly always modest hypocalcemia, which is thought to be caused by a brief decrease in feed intake and gastrointestinal motility. Serum concentrations may fall to 6–8 mg/dl.

22.9.5 Treatment

The primary goals of treatment are to rectify ruminal and systemic acidosis, stop further lactic acid production, stop fluid and electrolyte loss, maintain circulating blood volumes, and return stomach and intestine motility to normal.

Preventing further access to feed should come first when livestock are discovered engorging themselves. Monitor water intake to avoid consuming excessive amounts of water quickly. Provide a supply of high quality, palatable hay equivalent to half of the daily allowance for each head of livestock. Exercise all animals once every hour for 12–24 hours to promote the movement of food through the digestive system.

A rumenotomy is recommended in serious circumstances where the animal is recumbent, suffers from severe depression, hypothermia, obvious ruminal distension with fluid, a heart rate of 110–130 beats per minute, and a rumen pH of 5 or lower. Rumen lavage is an alternative to a rumenotomy in less severe cases where the affected cattle are still standing but are depressed, their heart rate is 90–100 beats per minute, there is considerable ruminal distension, and the rumen pH is between 5 and 6.

The use of 500 g of magnesium hydroxide per 450 kg BW or magnesium oxide in 10 l of warm water pumped into the rumen, followed by rumen kneading to enhance mixing, is typically sufficient in mildly affected instances. Magnesium hydroxide is a strong alkalinizing agent that can be used as a moderate laxative and antacid in ruminants. It should only be administered in cattle with verified ruminal acidosis since it can drastically reduce rumen microbial activity.

Intravenous sodium bicarbonate solutions, diluted to 5% at a rate of 5 l per 450 kg of animal, are administered over a period of around 30 minutes to treat systemic acidosis and dehydration. Usually, this will reverse systemic acidosis. Isotonic sodium bicarbonate (1.3%) is then administered intravenously over the course of the next 6–12 hours at a rate of 150 ml/kg BW.

Adult cattle with acute ruminal acidosis should generally receive at least 5 l of fresh rumen fluid from a healthy animal but only after rumen lavage or rumenotomy has been done. Antihistamines for laminitis, nonsteroidal anti-inflammatory medication (NSAIDs) for their anti-inflammatory and analgesic properties, thiamin or brewer's yeast to enhance lactic acid metabolism, and parasympathomimetics to increase gastrointestinal motility have all been used as ancillary treatments. Because of a slight hypocalcemia, calcium borogluconate is extensively utilized.

References

Atakisi, E., Bozukluhan, K., and Atakisi, O. (2010). Total oxidant and antioxidant capacities and nitric oxide levels in cattle with traumatic reticuloperitonitis. *Veterinary Record* 167: 908–909.

Braun, U., Rauch, S., and Hassig, M. (2009). Ultrasonographic evaluation of reticular motility in 144 cattle with vagal indigestion. *Veterinary Record* 164: 11–13.

Constable, P.D., Hinchcliff, K.W., Done, S.H., and Grünberg, W. (2017). *Veterinary Medicine: A Textbook of the Diseases of Cattle, Horses, Sheep, Pigs, and Goats*, 11e. St. Louis, MO: Elsevier Publications.

Constable, P.D. (2024). Bloat in ruminants. In: *Merck Veterinary Manual*, vol. 12. Rahway, NJ, USA: Merck and Co., Inc. https://www.msdvetmanual.com/digestive-system/diseases-of-the-ruminant-forestomach/bloat-in-ruminants (accessed 14 February 2024).

Hernández, J., Benedito, J.L., Abuelo, A., and Castillo, C. (2014). Ruminal acidosis in feedlot: from aetiology to prevention. *The Scientific World Journal* 1–8. https://doi.org/10.1155/2014/702572.

Hussain, S.A., Uppal, S.K., Singh, A., and Mahajan, S.K. (2014). Vagal indigestion in a buffalo due to obstruction of cardia by a cloth. *Buffalo Bulletin* 33 (4): 258–262.

Iggo, A. and Leek, B.F. (1967). An electrophysiology study of single vagal nerve efferent units associated with gastric movements in sheep. *Journal of Physiology* 191: 177–179.

Kahn, C.M. (2005). *The Merck Veterinary Manual*, 9e. Whitehouse Station, NJ; Great Britain: Merck & Co.

Lehmkuhler, J., Burrism, R., Arnold, M. et al. (2011). *Managing Legume-Induced Bloat in Cattle.* UK University of Kentucky College of Agriculture.

Majak, W., Hall, J., and McAllister, T. (2001). Practical measures for reducing the risk of alfalfa bloat in cattle. *Journal of Range Management* 54 (4): 490–493.

Majak, W., McAllister, T.A., McCartney, D. et al. (2008). Bloat in Cattle. Agriculture and Agri-Food Canada. Edmonton, Alberta, Canada: Alberta Agriculture and Rural Development.

Mamaghani, A., Maham, M., and Dalir-Naghadeh, B. (2013). Effects of ginger extract on smooth muscle activity of sheep reticulum and rumen. *Veterinary Research Forum* 4: 91–97.

Marchesini, G., Nardi, R.D., Gianesella, M. et al. (2013). Effect of induced ruminal acidosis on blood variables in heifers. *BMC Veterinary Research* 9: 98.

Moate, W. (2018). Pasture management systems for reducing the risk of legume bloat in cattle. *Journal of Animal Science* 73: 1493–1498.

Neal, P.A. and Edwards, G.B. (1968). Vagus indigestion in cattle. *The Veterinary Record* 82: 396–402.

Perry, T. and Cecava, J. (2015). Feedlot disease. In: *Beef Cattle Feeding and Nutrition*, 2e (ed. M.J. Cecava), 283–290. San Diego, CA: Academic Press.

Pope, D.C. and Bennett, J.B. (1961). Abomasal ulceration in a Jersey cow. *Canadian Veterinary Journal* 5: 189–191.

Rebhun, W.C., Fubini, S.L., Lesser, F.R. (1986). Clinical results of 112 cattle affected with vagal indigestion. *Fourteenth World Congress on Diseases of Cattle: Proceedings*. Dublin, Ireland, 2: 1146115.

23

Respiratory Problems

Anil Kumar[1], Sonam Bhatt[1], Ankesh Kumar[2], and Tanmoy Rana[3]

[1] *Department of Veterinary Medicine, BVC, BASU, Patna, Bihar, India*
[2] *Department of VCC, BVC, BASU, Patna, Bihar, India*
[3] *Department of VCC, F/VAS, WBUAFS, Kolkata, West Bengal, India*

23.1 Introduction

Respiratory disease in dairy cattle remains a serious issue in the dairy enterprise, despite improvements in veterinary treatment, animal husbandry, and animal welfare (Gorden and Plummer 2010). Disease of the respiratory tract is a major problem for cattle, and it continues to cause serious economic loss for producers. The name "periparturient" is derived from the words "parturition" and the prefix "peri," which literally but figuratively means "around." The dry period and the first 3–4 weeks that follow calving typically fall within this phase. (Stevenson 1987). Dairy cattle must deal with physiological, metabolic, and endocrine changes as well as a number of environmental and management-related stresses during the periparturient period, which is commonly described as the time just before and following calving (Sepúlveda-Varas et al. 2013). Respiratory diseases have a number of negative effects on cattle, including death, decreased weight gain, lower production, decreased pregnancy rate, increased treatment, immunization expenses, etc. (Peel 2020). All breeds and ages of cattle are prone to respiratory issues, and in some production environments, respiratory disease is the leading cause of morbidity and mortality in livestock. Respiratory disease affects 2.5% of adult dairy cattle annually and is responsible for 9.6% of dairy cow deaths, despite being a less significant cause of morbidity in adult dairy cows than mastitis, lameness, metabolic diseases, and reproductive disorders (Callan and Garry 2002). A dynamic network of interconnected layers – including mucociliary clearance, host defense factors like antimicrobial peptides in the epithelial lining fluid, pro-inflammatory responses of the respiratory epithelium, resident alveolar macrophages, and recruited neutrophils and monocytes – effectively protect the respiratory system from inhaled bacteria. However, stress, glucocorticoids, viral infections, abrupt exposure to cold air, and poor air quality can cause these diverse defenses to malfunction. When some of these defenses break down, the lung may become colonized by bacterial pathogens that can evade other defenses and cause pneumonia (Caswell 2014). The bovine respiratory disease complex (BRDC) is the main cause of morbidity and economic loss in wealthy nations, accounting for up to 80% in the United States (Hilton 2014). Bovine respiratory disease (BRD) complex is the name given to respiratory illnesses because they are frequently accompanied by different pathogens (McGill and Sacco 2020). It is not a single entity nor is it attributable to a single cause. They are the main causes of substantial economic loss. In addition to other stressors, including heat, cold, exhaustion, inadequate hydration or nutrition, injury, or environmental dust exposure, a number of bacteria and viruses are linked to BRD (McGill and Sacco 2020; Saif 2010). Since transportation compromises the immune system, which favors increases in pathogen prevalence and pathogen growth, it has been linked to an increased risk of BRD (Holman et al. 2017; Griebel et al. 2014). The most widely recognized pathogenesis concept assumes that the primary lung injury and/or immunological dysfunction results from an initial viral infection. As a result, the damaged lung tissue might be colonized by bacteria that are frequently commensals of the upper respiratory tract (URT), which leads to clinical disease (Horwood et al. 2014). The immune system is compromised or depressed in cows around the time of parturition, which makes the animals more vulnerable to infectious diseases. Environmental or behavioral stressors may affect

Periparturient Diseases of Cattle, First Edition. Edited by Tanmoy Rana.

periparturient cows, which results in greater immune function suppression due to elevated cortisol levels (Drackley et al. 2005). As a result, cows under stress could become more susceptible to infectious diseases (Hopster et al. 1998). Critical lymphocyte (immunoglobulin and cytokine secretion) and neutrophil (egress and phagocytic activities) functions are all compromised at this time. The disease process may be influenced by a wide range of stressors and agents (Figure 23.1). Furthermore, stressors and primary viral infections, which have been shown to impair mucociliary clearance of the URT and dysregulate tracheal antimicrobial peptides that belong to the respiratory innate defense, have been linked to BRD severity. This, in turn, increases the severity of a secondary bacterial infection (Earley et al. 2017; Guzman and Taylor 2015). Viruses that play prominent roles in the BRDC include bovine herpes virus-1, bovine respiratory syncytial virus (BRSV), bovine viral diarrhea virus (BVDV), and parainfluenza-3 virus. All of the bacterial species that cause infections implicated in BRDC can be isolated from the URTs of healthy cattle and calves. These diseases are considered widespread in cow herds because they are easily recognized in the nasopharynx of some animals in most populations, not because they can be found in every animal. In the absence of additional disease-causing factors, the presence of these bacterial pathogens does not appear to be significant. The disease complex is best described as multifactorial, developing only when a number of factors – including the animal, environment, and infectious pathogens – align (Callan and Garry 2002). Bacteria that play prominent roles in this disease complex are *Mannheimia haemolytica* and *Mycoplasma bovis*. Other bacteria that infect the bovine respiratory tract are *Histophilus somni* (*Haemophilus somnus)* and *Pasteurella multocida* (Srikumaran et al. 2007). Although bacteria and viruses account for most pneumonia outbreaks, some *Aspergillus* spp. fungus (Sorenson et al. 1992) and parasites, referred to as "lungworms" (Forbes 2018), can also cause respiratory disease. The general list of BRD impacts includes mortality (value of death loss), reduced weight gain, reduced feed efficiency, reduced salvage value of chronic animals, treatment costs, vaccination costs, and metaphylaxis costs. Early BRD symptoms include general warning indicators like anorexia, isolation, melancholy, and fever. These symptoms may progress to more serious respiratory symptoms such as nose and ocular discharge, salivation, rapid breathing, dyspnea, and a protracted cough (Gaudino et al. 2022). A number of physiological and physical factors together make cattle more susceptible to pneumonia. Housing, ventilation, and management factors may play a role in mediating the impact of heat stress on the risk for BRD. The growth of dairy calves preweaning, passive immunity, and physiology could all be negatively impacted by heat stress, which would raise their risk of respiratory disease.

Heat stress during the latter stages of pregnancy impairs placental growth, which leads to hypoxia, malnutrition, and eventually growth restriction in the fetus. Maternal heat stress may also have a lasting impact on the postnatal growth of

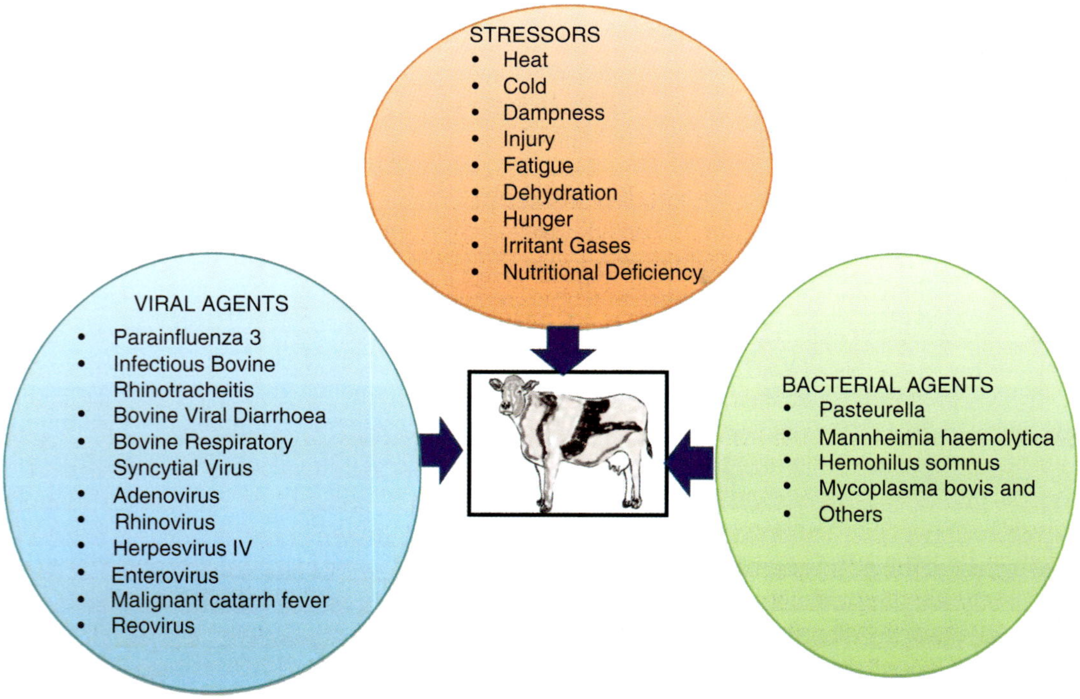

Figure 23.1 Factors that cause bovine respiratory disease.

offspring. New research reveals that compared to the offspring of cooled cows, those from prepartum heat-stressed cows have decreased passive immunity and poor cell-mediated immune activity (Tao and Dahl 2013).

The most widely recognized noninfectious risk factor for BRD is travel, which gave rise to the colloquial phrase "shipping fever." Another factor considered a potential contributor to the prevalence of BRD is the mode of transportation. Due to transport stress, the host immune system is suppressed and inflammatory responses are up- and down-regulated, which allows opportunistic infections to penetrate tissues (Padalino et al. 2017). Acute phase protein responses and cytokine-induced inflammation are consistent elements of BRD development. Through reductions in average daily gain, dry matter intake, and feed conversion, BRD-induced lung inflammation has a considerable negative impact on performance (Gifford et al. 2012). Many researchers have argued that BRD is more likely to affect cattle during abrupt and dramatic changes in weather, rather than just cold or bad weather (Taylor et al. 2010). Airborne dust also impacts BRD incidence. Close nose-to-nose contact, environmental or fomite exposure, and airborne exposure are all ways for respiratory infections to spread. Many factors influence the airborne transmission of pathogens, including ambient temperature, relative humidity, airborne particle (dust) density, ventilation, prevailing wind, and structural or geographic barriers. Pathogen dissemination is aided by increased interactions between shedding and susceptible individuals. Environmental exposure via shared spaces and equipment that involves oral or nasal contact, such as feed bunks, water troughs, and salt blocks, may pose an even bigger risk (Callan and Garry 2002). In cows, ventilation may be an important determinant of pulmonary hemodynamics during pregnancy. Pregnancy was associated with a greater rise in arterial pressure and total pulmonary vascular resistance during acute hypoxia and failed to elicit as great a ventilatory response in susceptible cows, compared to resistant (Moore et al. 1979).

The most prevalent infections linked with BRD will be covered in the following sections so that readers can better comprehend the dynamic interactions between the many cattle respiratory pathogens. For each pathogen, options for treatment and preventive measures (such as immunizations) will also be discussed.

23.2 Viral Diseases of the Respiratory Tract

Respiratory viruses can enter the lower respiratory tract and cause disease on their own, or they may suppress the immune system, which causes harm to the respiratory epithelium and defense mechanisms. Secondary bacterial species, some of which may be present in the nasopharynx, may multiply and subsequently colonize the lower respiratory tract as a result of both pathogenesis mechanisms (Figure 23.2) (Ruiz et al. 2022). The most prevalent and well-documented coinfection model of the respiratory syndrome complex applied to cattle and pigs is an initial viral infection followed by a secondary bacterial superinfection (Gaudino et al. 2022). The most frequent cause of viral disorders, including anything from the ordinary cold to potentially fatal pneumonia, is respiratory tract viral infections. The respiratory tract is used by a significant number of RNA and DNA viruses to infect their host. The trachea, bronchi, or alveoli are some examples of airway system regions that infections may be limited to or more noticeable. It is possible that some viruses only use the respiratory tract as their main point of entry before infecting other tissues or organs. These viruses all encounter the respiratory epithelium, which serves as the first line of defense or barrier against invasive pathogens. Differentiated epithelial cells with varying roles comprise this barrier. The mucociliary clearance system is an essential component of defense. While some epithelial cells have been developed to make and release mucins, other cells have cilia that allow them to assist in removing mucus from the respiratory system (Kirchhoff et al. 2014).

23.2.1 Bovine Herpesvirus Type-1 (BHV-1)

Infectious bovine rhinotracheitis (IBR) is also known as "red nose"(Peek et al. 2018) and is caused by bovine herpes virus type-1 (BHV-1), which belongs to the *Herpesviridae* family. IBR can be a mild, moderate, or severe disease. Mortality could reach 10%, and morbidity approaches 100% (Nandi et al. 2009). BHV-1 has two circulating subtypes, BHV-1.1 and BHV-1.2, both of which cause acute URT inflammation. However, it can also sporadically cause abortion in cattle as well as conjunctivitis, vaginitis, and enteritis. Cattle are susceptible to a variety of infections, including endemic abortions, infectious balanoposthitis of the male external genitalia, respiratory, conjunctival, and infectious pustular vulvovaginitis that affects the caudal reproductive tract; the neonatal septicemic form is characterized by encephalitis and focal plaque necrosis of the tongue. The respiratory form of BHV-1 is the most common and may occur alone or coupled with the conjunctival form (Gaudino et al. 2022). Cattle with

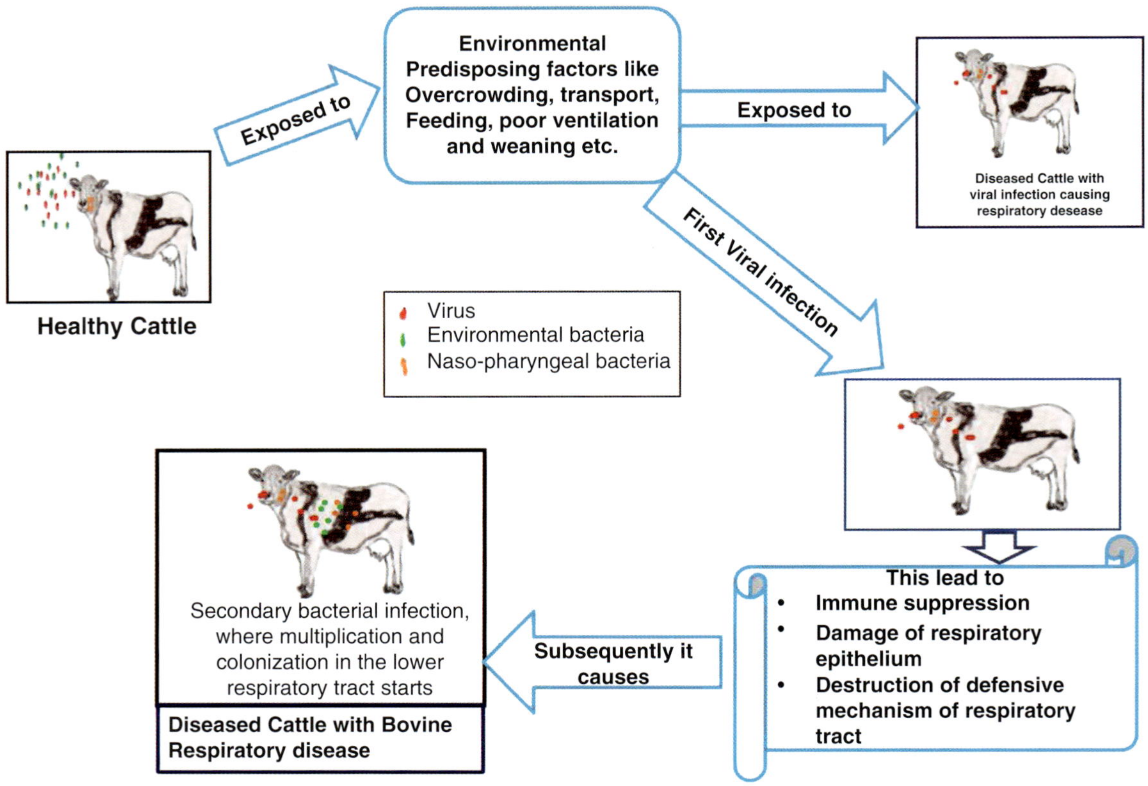

Figure 23.2 Virus-induced mechanisms that predispose cattle to bacterial infections in bovine respiratory disease.

BHV-1 infections have respiratory symptoms like conjunctivitis, mucopurulent nasal discharge that may occasionally be accompanied with mouth and nose ulcers, coughing, sneezing, and difficulty breathing (Tikoo et al. 1995). Pyrexia (40.5–42 °C), inappetence, increased respiratory rate, dyspnea, persistent harsh cough, depression, and a significant decrease in milk production in milking cows are all symptoms of classic IBR. An initial serous and later muco-purulent nasal discharge is present on both sides of the nose. The nasal mucosa is hyperemic, and the lesions progress from pustular necrosis to significant hemorrhage and ulceration, which are surrounded by a diphtheritic, cream-colored membrane (Nandi et al. 2009; Murphy et al. 1999). The underlying tissues are hyperemic if the encrustations are removed, which gives the condition the name "red nose." Primary or repeated IBR infections are rarely fatal, unless secondary bacterial bronchopneumonia – particularly with *Mann. haemolytica* – or a concomitant viral infection with BVDV or BRSV is involved (Gaudino et al. 2022). BHV-1 infections can be identified using nucleic acid–based tests that detect genomic DNA by polymerase chain reaction (PCR), nucleic acid hybridization, and sequencing as well as serologic tests that look for virus or virus components or antibodies. To protect cattle against BHV, there are four different types of vaccines available: modified live virus vaccines, inactivated vaccines, subunit vaccines, and marker vaccines (Tikoo et al. 1995).

23.2.2 Bovine Coronavirus (BCoV)

Bovine coronavirus (BCoV) is a single-stranded RNA virus that belongs to the family *Coronaviridae* and is classified within the viral species *Betacoronavirus 1* (Gaudino et al. 2022). It is known for its pneumo-enteric tropism that causes both enteric disease (especially calf diarrhea) and pneumonia outbreaks in cattle and makes it an endemic disease worldwide (Zhu et al. 2022). Colostrum-deprived calves experience coughing, nasal discharge, respiratory distress, and diarrhea after receiving an experimental BCoV inoculation (Vlasova and Saif 2021). Most enteric disease caused by BCoV infections is treated with supportive care, such as rehydration, administering electrolytes, and providing non-steroidal anti-inflammatory drugs (NSAIDs) (Constable 2009; Boileau and Kapil 2010). There are currently several vaccines against the enteric form (Maier et al. 2022). There are not yet any vaccines available to protect against respiratory diseases linked to BCoV.

23.2.3 Bovine Viral Diarrhea Virus

Bovine viral diarrhea virus (BVDV) is a member of the *Flaviviridae* family and is a single-stranded RNA virus. The genus *Pestivirus* is a member of this family. There are currently two different *Pestivirus* species in circulation: *Pestivirus A* (previously known as BVDV-1) and *Pestivirus B* (previously known as BVDV-2) (Smith et al. 2017). It is a significant pathogen associated with gastrointestinal, respiratory, and reproductive diseases in every class of cattle worldwide. All BVDV strains suppress the immune system, which makes infected cattle more susceptible to bacterial or viral pneumonia. BVDV rarely causes serious respiratory disease on its own, with the exception of type 2 infections that can cause interstitial pneumonia and acute death in naive cattle, occasionally without the typical upper gastrointestinal tract lesions. In BVDV outbreaks, type 1 strains are frequently isolated from pulmonary and lower airway macrophages and have the potential to be significant players in the BRD complex. Any strain that causes an acute BVDV infection can temporarily suppress the immune system, which predisposes cattle exposed to other respiratory pathogens to severe respiratory infections (Peek et al. 2018). An infection by BVDV mainly causes gastrointestinal and respiratory symptoms. The gastrointestinal form is associated with diarrhea and mucosal disease (when a cytopathic strain is present), especially during persistent infections (Bachofen et al. 2010; Bachofen et al. 2013). Cows and newborn calves can be protected by vaccine prophylaxis using maternally derived antibodies, but further work is needed to completely eradicate the disease (Antos et al. 2021).

23.2.4 Bovine Respiratory Syncytial Virus (BRSV)

BRSV belongs to the *Pneumovirus* genus within the family *Paramyxoviridae* and is a major cause of respiratory disease in cattle. The virus is enveloped with a nonsegmented, single-stranded, negative-sense RNA genome. It replicates predominantly in the respiratory tract (Gaudino et al. 2022). This virus is spread by nasal secretions and may survive because of the heterogeneity of its genome and low fidelity in replication. Once inhaled, the viruses infiltrate or maybe destroy the mucous – the innate immune system's first line of defense – and then enters URT epithelial cells by adhering to sialic acid residues on cell membranes. In addition to the host's pro-inflammatory reaction, the resulting tissue damage favors additional bacterial infections that aggravate the disease. (Makoschey and Berge 2021). With mild, moderate, or subclinical symptoms, BRSV has the highest harm potential of all circulating viruses in cattle. Less frequently, BRSV infections can develop into respiratory acute distress syndrome, which can worsen during late stages of the infection and includes fever, depression, decreased appetite, and dyspnea with open-mouth breathing. At necropsy, a BRSV infection is evident by emphysematous and hemorrhagic lung lesions, necrotizing bronchiolitis, and interstitial pneumonia, particularly in the cranial lobes. In acute cases, auscultation of the lungs may produce a wide range of sounds. There have been reports of increased bronchovesicular sounds, bronchial tones, fine crepitation brought on by emphysema, and rales, which are typically brought on by secondary bacterial bronchopneumonia (Peek et al. 2018). The signs of a high fever and subcutaneous emphysema in an acute BRSV infection may be suggestive of this diagnosis. In acute instances, auscultation of the lungs may be useful if the lungs sound diffusely quiet despite clear severe dyspnea. Serology can aid in the diagnosis of BRSV since the infection results in a significant humoral antibody titer. Acute BRSV infections are treated with symptomatic and supportive care. Broad-spectrum antibiotics are recommended to prevent or treat subsequent bacterial bronchopneumonia and should be started when diagnostic samples are collected. Nonsteroidal anti-inflammatory medicines (aspirin or flunixin) may be beneficial during acute BRSV infections. Antihistamines, like tripelennamine hydrochloride at 1 mg/kg intramuscularly (IM) twice daily, have also been recommended for BRSV treatment (Peek et al. 2018). In order to prevent BRSV infections, there are several vaccinations on the market (Gaudino et al. 2022).

23.2.5 Bovine Parainfluenza Type-3

The *Paramyxoviridae* family (genus *Respirovirus*, order *Mononegavirales*) contains bovine parainfluenza type-3 (BPIV-3), a single-stranded RNA virus (Ellis 2010). BPIV-3 is currently endemic, with three genetic groups circulating worldwide: A, B, and C (Kumagai et al. 2020). A BPIV-3 infection typically causes minor respiratory symptoms such as a fever, dry cough, nasal and ocular discharge, increased respiratory rate, and dyspnea (Gaudino et al. 2022). Infections of the URT can also cause transitory immunosuppression, which allows for secondary bacterial superinfections (Ellis 2010) that are a component of calf enzootic pneumonia. Several vaccinations are commercially marketed, frequently in conjunction with BRSV (Theurer et al. 2015).

23.3 Bacterial Pathogens

Common BRD-associated bacteria, such as commensals that most likely exist in healthy cattle as biofilms, include *Mann. haemolytica*, *P. multocida*, *Histophilus somni*, and *Myco. bovis* (MB). Commensal BRD-associated bacteria have the potential to become opportunistically pathogenic and colonize the deeper parts of the lung through biofilm dispersion (Mosier 2014). A dynamic network of interconnected layers – including mucociliary clearance, host defense factors like antimicrobial peptides in the epithelial lining fluid, pro-inflammatory responses of the respiratory epithelium, resident alveolar macrophages, and recruited neutrophils and monocytes – effectively protect the respiratory system from inhaled bacteria. However, stress, glucocorticoids, viral infections, rapid exposure to cold air, and poor air quality can cause these diverse defenses to malfunction. When some of these defenses break down, the lungs may become colonized by bacterial pathogens that can evade other defenses and cause pneumonia (Caswell 2014). Due to their immune-depressive effects on the affected animal, viral agents are typically considered primary or predisposing factors to bacterial agents (Headley et al. 2017).

23.3.1 *Pasteurella multocida*

A variety of domesticated birds and mammals are susceptible to infection by the gram-negative bacterium *P. multocida*. Louis Pasteur made the initial discovery of it sometime in the 1880s while studying the cause of poultry cholera (Harper et al. 2006). Scientists proposed in 1939 to group these bacterial strains under one genus and species, which they later termed *P. multocida* (Rosenbusch and Merchant 1939). This was done because the same bacterium might cause disease in several animal species. Currently, it is separated into 16 somatic serotypes (1–16) and five capsular groups (A–E). *P. multocida* A:3 is the most prevalent serotype found in cattle with BRD (Dowling et al. 2002). *P. multocida* is a likely opportunist whenever lower airway defense mechanisms are weakened. *P. multocida* may have the chance to colonize the lower airway if chemical mucociliary clearance is harmed, e.g. by ammonia fumes in poorly ventilated barns. Postpartum respiratory disease is far more likely to become a herd issue when there are frequent pen moves, excessive stocking, poor ventilation, coexisting metabolic disorders, and certain treatments and therapeutic methods employed by farmers. Fever, depression, anorexia, a moist cough, an increase in breathing rate and depth, and a decrease in milk production associated with anorexia are all symptoms of acute *P. multocida* pneumonia. In most instances, the fever is between 103.5 and 105.5 °F. Moist and dry rales auscultated in the anterior ventral lung field are classical findings in acute cases (Peek et al. 2018). *P. multocida* infections in cattle can result in a variety of bronchopneumonias, including subacute, chronic fibrinopurulent, fibrinous, and fibro-necrotizing. These bronchopneumonias can also be accompanied by varying degrees of intra-alveolar hemorrhage and mild-to-severe neutrophil and macrophage infiltration into the bronchi and bronchioles (Praveena et al. 2014). The only available treatments for *P. multocida* infection are antibiotics, whose development of drug resistance was recently documented (Cuevas et al. 2020). Various antibiotics like penicillin, ampicillin, erythromycin, and tetracycline have been used to treat pneumonia associated with *P. multocida*. Macrolides, fluoroquinolones, and florfenicol also have a wide range of actions in lung tissue that contains gram-negative bacteria. If these fail, a specific antibiotic may be selected based on the sensitivity results. Anti-inflammatory agents (e.g. aspirin and flunixin meglumine) can also be used in conjunction with antimicrobial therapy with the goal to reduce fever, block specific parts or mediators of the inflammatory cycle, and counteract endotoxins released from gram-negative bacterial cell walls as well as result in symptomatic improvement through improved appetite and attitude. Low-dose dexamethasone, a corticosteroid (10–20 mg/450 kg) may be administered once as part of the initial therapy, but it should not be administered again. Due to the abortifacient properties of dexamethasone, this medication is contraindicated in pregnant cows. When treating bacterial bronchopneumonia in cattle, nonsteroidal anti-inflammatory medications are safer than corticosteroids, but they do have some drawbacks. Apart from this, atropine may be given parenterally as a bronchodilator. Albuterol might be useful for cattle because as it acts as a bronchodilator and improves mucociliary clearance (Peek et al. 2018). Existing vaccines to prevent *P. multocida* infection are made of bacterins (killed bacteria) (Mostaan et al. 2020).

23.3.2 *Mannheimia haemolytica*

Man. haemolytica is a gram-negative rod that may be a normal inhabitant of the upper airway. Stress increases the virulence of the organism, makes it easier for the virulent strain to colonize, and weakens the host defense mechanisms, which put stressed cattle at a high risk of developing *Man. haemolytica* pneumonia. *Man. haemolytica* pathogenicity is due to its capsules that provide defense against phagocytosis, a cell wall-derived endotoxin that assists in the initiation of complement and coagulation cascades, an ability to reside in the upper airway among other nonpathogenic serotypes and transform or overgrow under stressful stimuli into a pathogenic serotype, and the production of an exotoxin (leucotoxin) lethal to alveolar macrophages, monocytes, and neutrophils (Peek et al. 2018). There are currently 12 capsular serotypes (A1, A2, A5, A6, A7, A8, A9, A12, A13, A14, A16, and A17) used to categorize *Man. haemolytica* (Rice et al. 2007). Among these, serotypes A1 and A6 are more prevalent causes of respiratory disease in cattle (Gibbs et al. 1984). Animals with an infection may first exhibit general clinical symptoms like a fever, appetite loss, and weight loss as well as respiratory symptoms including coughing, nasal discharge, and respiratory distress. Acute fibrinous pleuropneumonia, which is caused by fibrinous exudate that obstructs the bronchioles and alveoli, is the main cause of death (Singh et al. 2011). Its primary pathogenic component, *Man. haemolytica* leucotoxin, is now used in vaccines (Tucci et al. 2016). The scientific literature still lacks the necessary data to support the full efficacy of this preventive intervention (Capik et al. 2021). However, clinical trial evaluations of delivering a probiotic *Lactobacillus* strain intranasally to prevent *Man. haemolytica* colonization of the URT suggests that this approach may be used to prevent cow pneumonia in the future (Amat et al. 2020). The main therapeutic strategy for *Man. haemolytica* pneumonia is broad-spectrum antibiotics. Depending on the antibiotic employed, a minimum of 3 days of antibiotic coverage is often essential. More frequently, however, 5–7 days of continuous therapy are required, which reduces the risk of recurrence (Peek et al. 2018).

23.3.3 *Histophilus somni (Haemophilus somnus)*

Initially, thromboembolic meningoencephalitis (TEME), an infectious disease that affects the central nervous system, was recognized as the result of *Hae. somnus* infections in cattle. However, a number of additional cattle syndromes, such as weak calf syndrome, polyarthritis, tendonitis, abortion, infertility, and respiratory tract disease, have also been linked to infections by this organism (Potgieter et al. 1988). Also known as *His. somni*, it is a gram-negative bacterium associated with a disease complex (termed histophilosis) that can produce several clinical syndromes and predominantly affects cattle, but sporadic cases also occur in several species of small ruminants (Pérez et al. 2010). A major outer membrane protein (MOMP), other outer membrane proteins (OMPs), exopolysaccharide, immunoglobulin-binding proteins (as a surface fibrillar network), and lipooligosaccharide are examples of virulence factors. Additional pathogenesis factors may include quorum sensing, histamine synthesis, and biofilm formation (Corbeil 2007). Clinically, the pneumonia caused by *His. somni* cannot be distinguished from that caused by other BRD bacteria. Massive fibrin deposition is the most frequently noted finding upon a gross examination of the affected lungs, but *P. multocida* and *Man. haemolytica* have also been associated with similar findings. *His. somni, P. multocida,* and *Man. haemolytica* are frequently isolated from a single diseased lung sample, (Corbeil 2007). Due to these similarities, it can be difficult to make a firm determination of histophilosis. When it colonizes in the lungs and enters the bloodstream, the bacterium can cause systemic disease. Thus, *His. somni* infections can also cause encephalitis, myocarditis, and sudden death due to acute septicemia. Although bacterins are currently available as a preventive strategy, similar to *Man. haemolytica*, they have not proven to be an effective form of protection in vaccinated animals. Treatment options include broad-spectrum antibiotics like florfenicol (Gaudino et al. 2022). In adults and calves, ampicillin and ceftiofur have traditionally been used to treat *His. somni* pneumonia. In most cases, ampicillin is administered by injection at a dose of 11–22 mg/kg twice daily for 3–7 days (Peek et al. 2018).

23.3.4 *Mycoplasma bovis*

Myc. bovis has a worldwide distribution. It is one of the most challenging bacterial BRD pathogens. Like all other members of the *Mycoplasmataceae* family, it is the smallest known bacteria. It lacks a cell wall, which makes it naturally resistant to several classes of antibiotics (Gaudino et al. 2022). In the absence of disease, *Myc. bovis* can be isolated from the upper respiratory of cattle, which enables it to survive within herds undetected. Consequently, the most significant route of *Myc. bovis* propagation is believed to be the migration of infected animals across locations and countries. So, healthy and pneumonic cattle both have *Myc. bovis* in their upper and lower respiratory tracts (Horwood et al. 2014). It is unclear whether *Myc. bovis* is a main cause of BRDC or a secondary opportunistic pathogen because coinfections with *Myc. bovis* and other BRDC pathogens frequently occur. A synergism between BVDV-1 and *Myc. bovis* has been suggested. Fever, anorexia, nasal discharge, hyperpnea, depression, intermittent coughing, and lethargy are the nonspecific clinical symptoms (Caswell and Archambault 2007). Septic arthritis and less frequently, meningitis, tenosynovitis, decubital abscesses, and abortion are the most common side effects of *Myc. bovis* spread throughout the body. The pneumonia is characterized by peribronchiolar and peribronchial lymphoid hyperplasia as well as purulent bronchiolitis (Peek et al. 2018). Postmortem observations include fibrinosuppurative bronchopneumonia and bronchopneumonia with typical caseous necrotic lesions (Gaudino et al. 2022). Once introduced to a farm (through contaminated animals), eradication is difficult because of its high environmental resilience (McAuliffe et al. 2006) and herd spread through direct contact (Dudek et al. 2020). Because it is a persistent intracellular bacterium without a cell wall, antibiotic treatment options are limited, which poses another barrier to its eradication. Other significant obstacles are the great antigenic diversity of its surface glycoproteins and its capacity to elude the host immune system (Dudek et al. 2021). In vitro antimicrobial testing for *Mycoplasma* spp. is barely performed or available. As a result, choosing an antibiotic is based on intuition, although it is important to remember that treating *Myc. bovis* infections with antibiotics from the β-lactam class is ineffective due to the absence of a cell wall. However, the use of antimicrobials like tulathromycin (2.5 mg/kg, SC), florfenicol (20 mg/kg, IM in the neck), erythromycin (5.5 mg/kg, twice daily), and tilmicosin (10 mg/kg, SC) or other macrolides is effective. In addition to these, the fluoroquinolone group of antibiotics, like enrofloxacin, is also effective against *Mycoplasma* spp. (Peek et al. 2018). In North America, only a few vaccinations (which contain bacterins) that provide modest protection are available (Dudek et al. 2021). The United States Department of Agriculture has licensed two *Myc. bovis* vaccines, both bacterins, for use in the prevention of pneumonia in cattle: Pulmo-Guard® MpB (Boehringer Ingelheim Vetmedica, Inc., Duluth, Georgia, USA) and Myco-Bac® B (Texas Vet Lab, Inc., now Bimeda Biologicals, San Angelo, Texas, USA) (Caswell and Archambault 2007).

23.4 Preventive Measures for BRD

The prevention of respiratory disease necessitates management to both increase animal resistance and decrease pathogen exposure. The crucial issue is to emphasize the importance of various management aspects that increase animal resistance in addition to minimizing pathogen introduction, exposure, and transmission (i.e. biosecurity). It has become essential to coordinate and employ preventive management practices in tandem, because no one management procedure is successful without the support of other practices. Our inability to minimize the prevalence of respiratory disease in cattle is likely due in part to our failure to integrate many facets of respiratory disease prevention practices, including biosecurity (Callan and Garry 2002). With estimates of annual costs that exceed £100 million, BRD continues to be extremely expensive for the beef and dairy industries despite significant advancements in veterinary medicine, diagnostics, and therapeutics (Nicholas and Ayling 2003). The basic idea of biosecurity is to reduce infection transmission between animals. Effective respiratory disease prevention practices aim to reduce identified risk factors for disease development in the animal, environment, and infectious agents. Management to improve animal nutrition (with a focus on micronutrient nutrition), practices to reduce animal stress, reduced commingling of animals, improved animal transportation and feedlot receiving practices, improved preconditioning and vaccination programs that emphasize vaccination before shipment and during times of low calf stress, and improved ventilation with reduced crowding are among these practices. Existing BRD prevention strategies focus on either the individual animal or herd level and include immunization, mass antibiotic treatment, modification of the animal's habitat, and general health status (Callan and Garry 2002). Therefore, it makes sense to concentrate management strategies on preventing disease through sound management of the transitional period, along with sound immunization and biosecurity programs. The best way to control BRD, as with any disease control program, is to concentrate on the following (Chmiel and Grooms 2012):

a) Integrated vaccination programs against BRD-related viral and bacterial pathogens will increase disease resistance. An adequate nutrition plan must made with a high quality diet, particularly for calves exposed to stressful situations. The diet should be high in protein, contain a high proportion of micronutrients, and contain the right amounts of minerals like Zn, Cu, Fe, and Se as well as vitamins E, B complex, and C.
b) Reduce exposure to BRD pathogens by reducing the possibility of introducing infected animals into a herd: bring only animals from uninfected herds in; bring only animals from herds with a known effective vaccination program in; avoid the purchase of animals from sale barns; test new animals for persistent infections; isolate new animals for 30 days before allowing contact with on-farm animals; improve sanitation to reduce pathogen buildup; and isolate new animals from sales.
c) Metaphylactic use of antimicrobials can be used for the control of BRD in high risk cattle. Metaphylaxis is a treatment for animals in a population who may suffer from BRD as well as a preventive measure for other animals in a population

who are at risk of developing BRD. Metaphylaxis is typically reserved for animals at high risk of contracting BRD (Maples et al. 2022). There are now eight injectable antimicrobials (danofloxacin, enrofloxacin, tulathromycin, ceftiofur, tilmicosin, florfenicol, gamithromycin, and tildipirosin) and four oral antimicrobials (chlortetracycline–sulfamethazine, chlortetracycline, tilmicosin, and oxytetracycline) licensed for metaphylactic usage (Ives and Richeson 2015).

References

Amat, S., Alexander, T.W., Holman, D.B. et al. (2020). Intranasal bacterial therapeutics reduce colonization by the respiratory pathogen *Mannheimia haemolytica* in dairy calves. *mSystems* 5 (2): 10.1128/mSystems.00629-19.

Antos, A., Miroslaw, P., Rola, J., and Polak, M.P. (2021 Jun). Vaccination failure in eradication and control programs for bovine viral diarrhea infection. *Frontiers in Veterinary Science* 29 (8): 688911. https://doi.org/10.3389/fvets.2021.688911.

Bachofen, C., Braun, U., Hilbe, M. et al. (2010). Clinical appearance and pathology of cattle persistently infected with bovine viral diarrhoea virus of different genetic subgroups. *Veterinary Microbiology* 141 (3–4): 258–267. https://doi.org/10.1016/J.VETMIC. 2009.09.022.

Bachofen, C., Vogt, H., Stalder, H. et al. (2013). Persistent infections after natural transmission of bovine viral diarrhoea virus from cattle to goats and among goats. *Veterinary Research* 44 (1): 32. https://doi.org/10.1186/1297-9716-44-32.

Boileau, M.J. and Kapil, S. (2010). Bovine coronavirus associated syndromes. *Veterinary Clinics of North America. Food Animal Practice* 26 (1): 123–146. https://doi.org/10.1016/J.CVFA.2009.10.003.

Callan, R.J. and Garry, F.B. (2002). Biosecurity and bovine respiratory disease. *Veterinary Clinics of North America. Food Animal Practice* 18 (1): 57–77.

Callan, R.J. and Garry, F.B. (2002). Biosecurity and bovine respiratory disease. *Veterinary Clinics of North America. Food Animal Practice* 18 (1): 57–77.

Capik, S.F., Moberly, H.K., and Larson, R.L. (2021). Systematic review of vaccine efficacy against *Mannheimia haemolytica*, *Pasteurella multocida*, and *Histophilus somni* in North American cattle. *Bovpract* 55 (2): 125–133. https://doi.org/10.21423/BOVINE-VOL55 NO2P1 25-133.

Caswell, J.L. (2014). Failure of respiratory defenses in the pathogenesis of bacterial pneumonia of cattle. *Veterinary Pathology* 51 (2): 393–409. https://doi.org/10.1177/0300985813502821.

Caswell, J.L. (2014). Failure of respiratory defenses in the pathogenesis of bacterial pneumonia of cattle. *Veterinary Pathology* 51 (2): 393–409. https://doi.org/10.1177/0300985813502821.

Caswell, J.L. and Archambault, M. (2007). *Mycoplasma bovis* pneumonia in cattle. *Animal Health Research Reviews* 8 (2): 161–186.

Chmiel, R.U. and Grooms, D.L. (2012). Prevention and control of bovine respiratory disease. *Journal of Livestock Science* 3: 27–36.

Constable, P.D. (2009). Treatment of calf diarrhea: antimicrobial and ancillary treatments. *Veterinary Clinics of North America. Food Animal Practice* 25 (1): 101–120. https://doi.org/10.1016/J.CVFA.2008.10.012.

Corbeil, L.B. (2007). *Histophilus somni* host–parasite relationships. *Animal Health Research Reviews* 8 (2): 151–160. https://doi.org/10.1017/S1466252307001417.

Cuevas, I., Carbonero, A., Cano, D. et al. (2020). Antimicrobial resistance of *Pasteurella multocida* type B isolates associated with acute septicemia in pigs and cattle in Spain. *BMC Veterinary Research* 16 (1): 222. https://doi.org/10.1186/s12917-020-02442-z.

Dowling, A., Hodgson, J., Schock, A. et al. (2002). Experimental induction of pneumonic pasteurellosis in calves by intratracheal infection with *Pasteurella multocida* biotype A:3. *Research in Veterinary Science* 73 (1): 37–44. https://doi.org/10.1016/S0034-5288(02)00037-1.

Drackley, J.K., Dann, H.M., Douglas, N. et al. (2005). Physiological and pathological adaptations in dairy cows that may increase susceptibility to periparturient diseases and disorders. *Italian Journal of Animal Science* 4 (4): 323–344. https://doi.org/10.4081/ijas.2005.323.

Dudek, K., Nicholas, R.A.J., Szacawa, E., and Bednarek, D. (2020). *Mycoplasma bovis* infections – occurrence, diagnosis and control. *Pathogens* 9 (8): 640. https://doi.org/10.3390/PATHOGENS9080640.

Dudek, K., Szacawa, E., and Nicholas, R.A.J. (2021). Recent developments in vaccines for bovine *Mycoplas moses* caused by *Mycoplasma bovis* and *Mycoplasma mycoides* subsp. mycoides. *Vaccine* 9 (6): 549. https://doi.org/10.3390/vaccines9060549.

Earley, B., Buckham Sporer, K., and Gupta, S. (2017). Invited review: relationship between cattle transport, immunity and respiratory disease. *Animal* 11 (3): 486–492. https://doi.org/10.1017/S1751731116001622.

Ellis, J.A. (2010). Bovine Parainfluenza-3 virus. *Veterinary Clinics of North America. Food Animal Practice* 26 (3): 575–593. https://doi.org/10.1016/j. cvfa.2010.08.002.

Forbes, A. (2018). Lungworm in cattle: epidemiology, pathology and immunobiology. *Livestock* 23 (2): 59–66. https://doi.org/10.12968/live.2018.23.2.59.

Gaudino, M., Nagamine, B., Ducatez, M.F., and Meyer, G. (2022). Understanding the mechanisms of viral and bacterial coinfections in bovine respiratory disease: a comprehensive literature review of experimental evidence. *Veterinary Research* 53 (1): 70. https://doi.org/10.1186/s13567-022-01086-1.

Gibbs, H., Allan, E., Wiseman, A., and Selman, I. (1984). Experimental production of bovine pneumonic pasteurellosis. *Research in Veterinary Science* 37 (2): 154–166. https://doi.org/10.1016/S0034-5288(18)31898-8.

Gifford, C.A., Holland, B.P., Mills, R.L. et al. (2012). Growth and development symposium: impacts of inflammation on cattle growth and carcass merit 1,2. *Journal of Animal Science* 90 (5): 1438–1451. https://doi.org/10.2527/jas.2011-4846.

Gorden, P.J. and Plummer, P. (2010). Control, management, and prevention of bovine respiratory disease in dairy calves and cows. *The Veterinary Clinics of North America. Food Animal Practice* 26: 234–259.

Griebel, P., Hill, K., and Stookey, J. (2014). How stress alters immune responses during respiratory infection. *Animal Health Research Reviews* 15: 161–165. https://doi.org/10.1017/S1466252314000280.

Guzman, E. and Taylor, G. (2015). Immunology of bovine respiratory syncytial virus in calves. *Molecular Immunology* 66 (1): 48–56. https://doi.org/10.1016/j.molimm.2014.12.004.

Harper, M., Boyce, J.D., and Adler, B. (2006). *Pasteurella multocida* pathogenesis: 125 years after Pasteur. *FEMS Microbiology Letters* 265 (1): 1–10. https://doi.org/10.1111/J.1574-6968.2006.00442.X.

Headley, S.A., Balbo, L.C., Alfieri, A.F. et al. (2017). Bovine respiratory disease associated with *Histophilus somni* and bovine respiratory syncytial virus in a beef cattle feedlot from southeastern Brazil. *SCA* 38 (1): 283.

Hilton, W.M. (2014). BRD in 2014: where have we been, where are we now, and where do we want to go? *Animal Health Research Reviews* 15 (2): 120–122. https://doi.org/10.1017/S1466252314000115.

Holman, D.B., Timsit, E., Amat, S. et al. (2017). The nasopharyngeal microbiota of beef cattle before and after transport to a feedlot. *BMC Microbiology* 17 (1): 70. https://doi.org/10.1186/s12866-017-0978-6.

Hopster, H., van der Werf, J.T., and Blokhuis, H.J. (1998). Stress enhanced reduction in peripheral blood lymphocyte numbers in dairy cows during endotoxin-induced mastitis. *Veterinary Immunology and Immunopathology* 66 (1): 83–97.

Horwood, P., Schibrowski, M., Fowler, E. et al. (2014). Is *Mycoplasma bovis* a missing component of the bovine respiratory disease complex in Australia? *Australian Veterinary Journal* 92 (6): 185–191. https://doi.org/10.1111/avj.12184.

Ives, S.E. and Richeson, J.T. (2015). Use of antimicrobial metaphylaxis for the control of bovine respiratory disease in high-risk cattle. *Veterinary Clinics of North America. Food Animal Practice* 31 (3): 341–350. doi: 10.1016/j.cvfa.2015.05.008.

Kirchhoff, J., Uhlenbruck, S., Goris, K. et al. (2014). Three viruses of the bovine respiratory disease complex apply different strategies to initiate infection. *Veterinary Research* 45 (1): 20. https://doi.org/10.1186/1297-9716-45-20.

Kumagai, A., Kanno, T., Kawauchi, K. et al. (2020). Phylogenetic and antigenic analysis of bovine parainfluenza virus type 3 isolated in Japan between 2002 and 2019. *Veterinary Microbiology* 247: 108774.

Maier, G.U., Breitenbuecher, J., Gomez, J.P. et al. (2022). Vaccination for the prevention of neonatal calf diarrhea in cow-calf operations: a scoping review. *Veterinary and Animal Science* 15: 100238. https://doi.org/10.1016/J.VAS.2022.100238.

Makoschey, B. and Berge, A.C. (2021). Review on bovine respiratory syncytial virus and bovine parainfluenza – usual suspects in bovine respiratory disease – a narrative review. *BMC Veterinary Research* 17 (1): 261. https://doi.org/10.1186/s12917-021-02935-5.

Maples, W.E., Brorsen, B.W., Peel, D., and Hicks, B. (2022). Observational study of the effect of metaphylaxis treatment on feedlot cattle productivity and health. *Frontiers in Veterinary Science* 9: 947585. https://doi.org/10.3389/fvets.2022.947585.

McAuliffe, L., Ellis, R.J., Miles, K. et al. (2006). Biofilm formation by *Mycoplasma* species and its role in environmental persistence and survival. *Microbiology* 152 (4): 913–922. https://doi.org/10.1099/mic.0.28604-0.

McGill, J.L. and Sacco, R.E. (2020). The immunology of bovine respiratory disease. *Veterinary Clinics of North America. Food Animal Practice* 36 (2): 333–348. https://doi.org/10.1016/j.cvfa.2020.03.002.

Moore, L.G., Reeves, J.T., Will, D.H., and Grover, R.F. (1979). Pregnancy-induced pulmonary hypertension in cows susceptible to high mountain disease. *Journal of Applied Physiology: Respiratory, Environmental and Exercise Physiology* 46 (1): 184–188. https://doi.org/10.1152/jappl.1979.46.1.184.

Mosier, D. (2014). Review of BRD pathogenesis: the old and the new. *Animal Health Research Reviews* 15 (2): 166–168. 10.1017/S1466252314000176.

Mostaan, S., Ghasemzadeh, A., Sardari, S. et al. (2020). *Pasteurella multocida* vaccine candidates: a systematic review. *Avicenna Journal of Medical Biotechnology* 12 (3): 140–147.

Murphy, F.A., Gibbs, E.P.J., Horzinek, M.C., and Studdert, M.J. (1999). *Veterinary Virology*, 3e. New York: Academic Press.

Nandi, S., Kumar, M., Manohar, M., and Chauhan, R.S. (2009). Bovine herpes virus infections in cattle. *Animal Health Research Reviews* 10 (1): 85–98. https://doi.org/10.1017/S1466252309990028.

Nicholas, R. and Ayling, R. (2003). *Mycoplasma bovis*: disease, diagnosis, and control. *Research in Veterinary Science* 74 (2): 105–112. https://doi.org/10.1016/s0034-5288(02)00155-8.

Padalino, B., Raidal, S.L., Carter, N. et al. (2017). Immunological, clinical, haematological and oxidative responses to long distance transportation in horses. *Research in Veterinary Science* 115: 78–87. https://doi.org/10.1016/j.rvsc.2017.01.024.

Peek, S.F., Ollivett, T.L., and Divers, T.J. (2018). Respiratory diseases. *Rebhun's Diseases of Dairy Cattle* 94–167. https://doi.org/10.1016/B978-0-323-39055-2.00004-8.

Peel, D.S. (2020). The effect of market forces on bovine respiratory disease. *Veterinary Clinics of North America. Food Animal Practice* 36 (2): 497–508. https://doi.org/10.1016/j.cvfa.2020.03.008.

Pérez, D.S., Pérez, F.A., and Bretschneider, G. (2010). Pathogenicity of *Histophilus somni*. *Anales de Veterinaria de Murcia* 26: 5–21.

Potgieter, L.N.D., Helman, R.G., Greene, W. et al. (1988). Experimental bovine respiratory tract disease with *Haemophilus somnus*. *Veterinary Pathology* 25 (2): 124–130. https://doi.org/10.1177/030098588802500204.

Praveena, P.E., Periasamy, S., Kumar, A.A., and Singh, N. (2014). Pathology of experimental infection by *Pasteurella multocida* serotype A. *Veterinary Pathology* 51 (6): 1109–1112. doi: 10.1177/0300985813516647.

Rice, J.A., Carrasco-Medina, L., Hodgins, D.C., and Shewen, P.E. (2007). *Mannheimia haemolytica* and bovine respiratory disease. *Animal Health Research Reviews* 8 (2): 117–128. https://doi.org/10.1017/S1466252307001375.

Rosenbusch, C.T. and Merchant, I.A. (1939). A study of the hemorrhagic septicemia Pasteurellae. *Journal of Bacteriology* 37 (1): 69–89. https://doi.org/10.1128/JB.37.1.69-89.1939.

Ruiz, M., Puig, A., Bassols, M. et al. (2022). Influenza D virus: a review and update of its role in bovine respiratory syndrome. *Viruses* 14 (12): 2717. https://doi.org/10.3390/v14122717.

Saif, L.J. (2010). Bovine respiratory coronavirus. *Veterinary Clinics of North America. Food Animal Practice* 26 (2): 349–364. https://doi.org/10.1016/j.cvfa.2010.04.005.

Sepúlveda-Varas, P., Huzzey, J.M., Weary, D.M., and von Keyserlingk, M.A.G. (2013). Behaviour, illness and management during the periparturient period in dairy cows. *Animal Production Science* 53 (9): 988. https://doi.org/10.1071/AN12286.

Singh, K., Ritchey, J.W., and Confer, A.W. (2011). Mannheimia haemolytica. *Veterinary Pathology* 48 (2): 338–348. https://doi.org/10.1177/0300985810377182.

Smith, D.B., Meyers, G., Bukh, J. et al. (2017). Proposed revision to the taxonomy of the genus Pestivirus, family Flaviviridae. *Journal of General Virology* 98 (8): 2106–2112. https://doi.org/10.1099/JGV.0.000873.

Sorenson, W., Siegel, P.D., Olenchock, S.A. et al. (1992). Fungi in aerosols of hay associated with respiratory distress in dairy cattle. *International Biodeterioration & Biodegradation* 30 (4): 353–362. https://doi.org/10.1016/0964-8305(92)90039-Q.

Srikumaran, S., Kelling, C.L., and Ambagala, A. (2007). Immune evasion by pathogens of bovine respiratory disease complex. *Animal Health Research Reviews* 8 (2): 215–229. https://doi.org/10.1017/s1466252307001326.

Stevenson, J.S. (1987). Periparturient disorders in dairy cows. Kansas agricultural Experiment Station. *Research Reports* 11–18. https://doi.org/10.4148/2378-5977.3024.

Tao, S. and Dahl, G. (2013). Invited review: heat stress effects during late gestation on dry cows and their calves. *Journal of Dairy Science* 96 (7): 4079–4093. https://doi.org/10.3168/jds.2012-6278.

Taylor, J.D., Fulton, R.W., Lehenbauer, T.W. et al. (2010). The epidemiology of bovine respiratory disease: what is the evidence for predisposing factors? *The Canadian Veterinary Journal* 51 (10): 1095–1102.

Theurer, M.E., Larson, R.L., and White, B.J. (2015). Systematic review and meta-analysis of the effectiveness of commercially available vaccines against bovine herpesvirus, bovine viral diarrhea virus, bovine respiratory syncytial virus, and parainfluenza type 3 virus for mitigation of bovine respiratory disease complex in cattle. *JAVMA* 246 (1): 126–142. https://doi.org/10.2460/JAVMA.246.1.126.

Tikoo, S.K., Campos, M., and Babiuk, L.A. (1995). Bovine herpesvirus 1 (BHV-1): biology, pathogenesis, and control. *Advances in Virus Research* 45: 191–223. https://doi.org/10.1016/s0065-3527(08)60061-5.

Tucci, P., Estevez, V., Becco, L. et al. (2016). Identification of Leukotoxin and other vaccine candidate proteins in a *Mannheimia haemolytica* commercial antigen. *Heliyon* 2 (9): e00158. https://doi.org/10.1016/j.heliy on.2016.e00158.

Vlasova, A.N. and Saif, L.J. (2021). Bovine coronavirus and the associated diseases. *Frontiers in Veterinary Science* 8: 643220. https://doi.org/10.3389/FVETS.2021.643220.

Zhu, Q., Li, B., and Sun, D. (2022). Advances in bovine coronavirus epidemiology. *Viruses* 14 (5): 1109. https://doi.org/10.3390/V14051109.

24

Uterine Torsion

Rajesh Kumar, Kabir Alam, Daund S. Sakhahari, and Bhoopendra Singh

Department of Veterinary Gynaecology and Obstetrics, College Veterinary Science and Animal Husbandry, Acharya Narendra Deva University of Agriculture and Technology, Ayodhya, Uttar Pradesh, India

Uterine torsion, first documented by Boutrolle in 1766, is related to the rotation of the pregnant uterus along its longitudinal axis (Craig 1930). Uterine torsion has been documented in various domesticated species like cattle (Cergolj et al. 1999), buffaloes (Prabhakar et al. 1994), does (Dhaliwal et al. 1986), ewes (Ijaz and Talafha 1999), llamas (Hopkins et al. 1991), camels (Cebra et al. 1997), mares (Jung et al. 2008), dogs (Brown 1974), and cats (Thilagar et al. 2005). Furthermore, cases of uterine torsion have been observed in laboratory species such as rabbits (Hobbs and Parker 1990) and guinea pigs (Kunstyr 1981). This is referred to as "torsio uteri" or "torsion of the uterus." It can be defined as the "revolution or twisting of [the] uterus on its longitudinal axis." Uterine torsion is a complication of late first stage or early second stage labor (Manning et al. 1982).

24.1 Incidence

The incidence of uterine torsion is higher in pluriparous cows (Roberts 2002) and cows reared in mountainous regions (Singh 1995). Moreover, the highest frequency of occurrence is observed during the second and third calvings (Nanda 1995). Uterine torsion typically affects cows between the ages of 5–7 years (Mogha et al. 1976). Indeed, uterine torsion may occur in all species of animals; however, its incidence is uncommon in mares due to the dorsal attachment of the broad ligament, which tends to prevent torsion. Roberts (1986) noted that uterine torsion was sometimes seen as a cause of dystocia in beef cows, dogs, cats, ewes, does, and mares, but rarely in sows. It was seen more often in dairy cows than in any other species (Laven and Howe 2005). However, Srinivas et al. (2007) found that uterine torsion was the major factor in the occurrence of maternal dystocia in buffaloes. In dairy cows, various researchers (Manning et al. 1982; Laven and Howe 2005) have reported incidences of uterine torsion in 3–10.7% of dystocia cases. A wide range of incidence (13.97–27.46%) has been reported by various researchers (Karthick et al. 2015; Faria and Simoes 2015). Moreover, Roberts (1986) opined that uterine torsion was most often seen in the spring season, when cows were let out onto pasture after being kept in stalls for a long time.

24.2 Classification of Uterine Torsion

For the ease of understanding, uterine torsion can be classified based on the direction (clockwise and anticlockwise or counter-clockwise), location (precervical and post cervical), and degree (> 45°, 90°, 180°, etc.) of twist.

Periparturient Diseases of Cattle, First Edition. Edited by Tanmoy Rana.

24.2.1 Direction of Uterine Torsion

Several studies have suggested that torsion in cows is typically observed on the left side (Singla et al. 1992; Arthur et al. 1996; Roberts 2002). In contrast, other researchers have observed that torsion should occur more frequently on the right side due to the presence of the rumen on the left (Mannari 1969; Prabhakar et al. 1994; Penny 1999). Furthermore, Frazer et al. (1996) and Aubry et al. (2008) found a higher occurrence of counter-clockwise (left) torsion compared to clockwise torsion in exotic cows. Singh (1991) reported that *Bos taurus* cattle possess an extra muscular fold on the right broad ligament, which tends to prevent the downward rotation of the right horn. Indeed, several studies have reported that the predominant direction of uterine rotation is toward the right in *Bos indicus* cattle, crossbred cattle, and *Bubalus bubalis* buffaloes (Roberts and Hillman 1973; Vasishta 1983; Malhotra 1990; Singla et al. 1992; Prabhakar et al. 1994; Prasad et al. 2000; Srinivas et al. 2007; Kumar et al. 2014).

24.2.2 Site of Uterine Torsion

In uniparous animals, because of a strong intercornual ligament and distension of the uterine horns and body with placenta and fluid, both gravid and nongravid horns are involved in torsion. In multiparous animals, only a portion of one horn, usually containing one fetus, may be twisted or rotated because of the absence of a fully developed intercornual ligament. The point of rotation can be caudal to the cervix, i.e. post cervical (Deori et al. 2009), or just cranial to the cervix or anterior vagina, i.e. precervical (Kumar et al. 2014). Furthermore, Sloss and Dufty (1980) have reported that occurrences of precervical torsions are more prevalent during the final trimester. Precervical torsion has been observed to occur with a higher frequency in *Bos indicus* cattle, as documented by Roberts and Hillman (1973), Prabhakar et al. (1994), and Prasad et al. (2000). Conversely, post-cervical torsion has been found to be more prevalent in *Bos taurus* cattle, as reported by Pearson (1971), and in crossbred cattle, as indicated by Singla et al. (1992) and Sharma et al. (1995).

24.2.3 Degree of Uterine Torsion

The degree of torsion is determined by the degree of twists present on the body of uterus, which are grouped as mild (90°; mostly), moderate (90–180°; most common), and severe (180–360°). In addition, a torsion of more than 45° may lead to dystocia (Sloss and Dufty 1980). However, it typically occurs between 90° and 180° but can reach up to 360° or even 540° (Matharu and Prabhakar 2001) or 760° (Ruegg 1988). Indeed, minor torsions (45–90°) identified during routine pregnancy diagnoses were observed to undergo spontaneous correction (Roberts 1986). Most cases (approximately 75%) have a twist of less than 180° and are managed in the field, and 6–15% of torsions are managed at referral hospitals (Pearson 1971; Sloss and Dufty 1980; Manning et al. 1982; Aubry et al. 2008). Furthermore, many previous studies have reported that the prevalence of torsions ranging from 180° to 270° at referral hospitals is estimated at 57–80% (Manning et al. 1982; Frazer et al. 1996; Aubry et al. 2008).

24.3 Predisposing Factors

A number of predisposing factors have been considered to have direct or indirect effects on uterine torsion.

- Instances of uterine instability and excessive fetal or maternal movement have been documented in cases of single-horn pregnancy, which are likely the primary factors that contribute to the rotation of the uterus on its longitudinal axis (Purohit et al. 2011).
- External injury, lack of exercise, and irregular movement of animals (Selvaraju et al. 2014).
- Uterus didelphys (Singh et al. 1992).
- Geographical location (Roberts 1986).
- Husbandry practices (Ahmed et al. 1980).
- Uterine torsion was more frequent with male calves than females, and most uterine torsion was associated with the presence of a heavy fetus (Frazer et al. 1996). In a study conducted by Karthick et al. (2015), 67.57% of male fetuses and 32.43% of female fetuses in cows were affected by uterine torsion.

- Travel or accidents during late pregnancy (Brar et al. 2008).
- Secondary rolling can occur due to gastrointestinal issues or as a result of a traumatic event (Taylor et al. 1989).
- Weaker broad ligaments, a smaller quantity of fetal fluids, and a decrease in uterine tone coupled with inordinate fetal movements (Purohit and Gaur 2014).

24.4 Symptoms

The severity of symptoms is determined by the degree of torsion. The most common clinical signs are the onset of labor without the delivery of the fetus and/or fetal membranes and a subsequent regression of parturition signs (Singh et al. 1978). The cow may exhibit mild discomfort. The animal may adopt a rocking horse stance and exhibit mild abdominal pain (Jackson 1995; Mannari et al. 1976). Moreover, Pearson (1971) observed partial anorexia, dullness, and depression. Animals can exhibit restlessness, back arching, and colic. According to Pearson (1971), it has been observed that the fetal membranes frequently remain undamaged and do not manifest any visible signs, even in cases with a prolonged duration. This indicates that torsion is a contributing factor to the occurrence of partial or complete uterine inertia. Additionally, the author asserts that uterine torsion is the sole manifestation of dystocia in cattle wherein the fetus has the potential to perish while both placental membranes remain intact and the placental cotyledons are completely detached.

The authors observed severe cases of uterine torsion accompanied by complications such as uterine gangrene, uterine rupture, and fetal emphysema. The animal may exhibit toxicity symptoms such as a rapid and weak pulse, severe depression, low body temperature, weakness, prostration, cold extremities, and potentially fetid diarrhea. Hemorrhage resulting from the rupture of uterine vessels can occur in cases of uterine torsion, which leads to symptoms such as anemia, weakness, rapid breathing, a rapid pulse rate, and prostration in cows. Additionally, in severe instances, the dorsal commissure of the vulva is displaced toward either the left or right side, depending on the direction of the torsion.

24.5 Diagnosis

I) **By history:** Animal has completed a full gestation with all signs of approaching parturition, but parturition was absent and the symptoms gradually disappeared.

II) **By rectal examination:** Rectal examinations should always be performed to detect if uterine torsion is present.
   a) In right side or clockwise torsion, the right broad ligament is pulled strongly downward under the twisted uterine body or vagina and the left broad ligament is pulled tightly across the top of the cervix. The body of the uterus and the vagina are toward the right side, or a hand can extend deeply into a pouch on the right side.
   b) In left side or anticlockwise torsion, the location and direction of the two broad ligaments are reversed, with the right broad ligament crossing over the top of the twisted portion of the birth canal, or a hand can extend deeply into a pouch on the left side.
   c) Rectal examinations are preferred over vaginal examinations because occasionally the twisted portion of the genital tract may lie cranial to the cervix, in the region of the uterine body, and not extend into the vagina.

III) **By vaginal examination:** Starting from the dorsum of the vagina, if the folds spiral forward and downward to the left or counter-clockwise, left torsion is present. If the folds spiral downward and forward to the right or clockwise, it is a right torsion of the uterus. In a post-cervical torsion, spiral folds occur in the vagina and approaching the cervix is difficult.

24.6 Treatment

The choice of detorsion technique in bovine uterine torsion depends on factors such as the veterinarian's skill level, pregnancy stage, torsion severity, and the condition of the dam, uterus, and fetus. The most commonly used techniques include per vaginum fetal rotation, rolling of the dam, and cesarean section.

24.6.1 Rolling of the Dam

This is one of the simplest and oldest methods of treating uterine torsion in cows and buffaloes. The animal must roll, preferably on grass, with its head lower than its hindquarters. The animal is positioned in lateral recumbency on the same side as the torsion. A rope binds the two hindlegs together. A separate rope is also used to tie the forelegs together. The animal is suddenly rolled in the same direction as the uterine torsion on the opposite side. The rapid rotation of the body overtakes the slower-rotating gravid uterus. After the animal has been rolled to 180°, her body must be gradually returned to its original position so that it can be rolled again. Following the completion of two rotations, it is imperative to conduct an examination of the birth canal in order to ascertain the rectification or persistence of torsion. When appropriately rectified, the spiral folds and stenosis of the birth canal will cease to exist, and if the cervix is dilated, the fetus can be easily palpated. The presence of blood-stained fluid that discharges from the birth canal when the cervix is open can serve as significant evidence of torsion correction. If the torsion was not corrected, it is recommended to repeat the rolling procedure three to four times. If torsion is still not corrected after four attempts, alternative procedures should be considered to correct the torsion. This is because violent rolling can lead to uterine rupture (Prabhaker et al. 1997; Singh et al. 1998). Furthermore, several studies (Roberts and Hilman 1973; Sloss and Dufty 1980; Frazer et al. 1996; Kruse 2004) have demonstrated that rolling the dam without a plank and detorsion of the uterus has success rates that range from 18% to 100% in various cases.

24.6.2 Plank Method or Schaffer's Method (1946)

Arthur (1966) described a modified version of the rolling technique known as Schaffer's method, which has been widely recommended for detorsion of the uterus in cows and buffaloes by Sane et al. (1982) and Roberts (2002). In this method, a wooden plank, 9–12 feet long and 8–12 inches wide that has some slight flexibility, is positioned on the flank of the resting cow. The lower end of the plank is placed on the ground. An assistant stands on the plank while slowly turning over the cow by pulling the ropes. The plank secures the uterus while the cow's body is turned, and because the cow is turned slowly, less assistance is needed, and it is easier for the veterinarian to determine the correct direction of the rolling by vaginal palpation (Purohit 2006). Typically, the first roll demonstrates a high rate of success (Arthur et al. 1996). In addition, several studies (Arthur 1966; Roberts and Hilman 1973; Noakes et al. 2001; Aubry et al. 2008) have discovered that using Schaffer's method (Schaffer 1946) of rolling, which involves the placement of a 12-foot long and 10-inch wide plank on the upper paralumbar fossa during the rolling process, yields a success rate that ranges from 84% to 90%.

24.6.3 Rolling of the Fetus

Rotation of the fetus and uterus through the birth canal is probably the most common way of relieving dystocia due to torsion of the uterus in cows. Fetal rotation per vaginum is feasible only in cases of mild torsion where the obstetrician can physically reach the fetus and there is an adequate amount of amniotic fluid in the uterus (Jackson 1995). The fetus is rotated by applying force to a bony prominence, such as the elbow, sternum, or thigh, which causes it to swing from side to side. Subsequently, the fetus is pushed in the opposite direction of the torsion until resulting in a complete rotation. If both fetal limbs are palpable, they can be secured using either Cammerer's torsion fork or a Kunh's crutch, and an assistant can then rotate them. Successful manipulation results in the disappearance of torsion, the restoration of normal vaginal folds, and facilitates the delivery of the fetus with minimal complications. Adequate lubrication is necessary in the birth canal and uterus prior to using instruments for fetal rotation. Once a certain amount of time has elapsed since the problem began, the uterus will contract firmly around the fetus and make it impossible for any distortion to occur using this method.

24.6.4 Laparotomy

When the cervix is closed or there is torsion during the middle or late stages of pregnancy, a laparotomy combined with manual intra-abdominal detorsion is advised (Robert 2002). It is usually performed on the standing cow through the left or right paralumbar fossa. This is done while the animal is standing and lightly tranquilized, using either paravertebral or local infiltration anesthesia. The right flank in the cow is anesthetized by paravertebral or local anesthesia and a 6–8 inch vertical laparotomy incision is made. The omentum is pulled cranially, if it is over the uterus. If torsion of the uterus is to the right side, the hands and arms are passed downward between the uterus and abdominal wall until the bottom or ventral surface of the uterus can be felt. A portion of the fetus, usually the leg, is grasped through the uterine wall and by alternately lifting and lowering the uterus, it is made to rock up and down in an arc of 10–12 inches. Finally, by strongly lifting the uterus and pushing it toward the midline and downward, the torsion may be corrected. If the torsion is to the left side, hands and arms are passed over the top of the uterus and down between the rumen and uterus. The same procedure of rocking and then rotating to the right or laterally and downward is carried out to correct the left torsion. Then the laparotomy incision is closed.

24.6.5 Laparo-hysterotomy

A laparo-hysterotomy is recommended in cases of uterine torsion that cannot be corrected by rolling or in long-standing cases where the fetus dies and there is a high probability of uterine adhesions or rupture. The outcome of a cesarean when the fetus dies and becomes emphysematous can be serious. Before making the decision to operate, it is recommended to consider the patient's overall condition and health. Cesarean section is the preferred method for cases where the cervix is closed and there is a dead fetus with reduced signs of parturition (Dhaliwal et al. 1993). Prior to beginning the procedure, it is advisable to administer a sufficient amount of fluid therapy, antibiotics, and corticosteroids. Various operative sites for cesarean sections have been suggested in the literature. These include the right flank (Dhaliwal et al. 1988) or left flank, a midline incision along or parallel to the linea alba, a horizontal incision above the arcus cruralis (Singh et al. 1978), or an appropriate incision in the right (Dhaliwal et al. 1993) or left lower flank (Singh et al. 1998; Murty et al. 1999). Another proposed approach is an oblique ventro-lateral approach with the animal positioned in right lateral recumbency (Purohit 2006). Several studies (Pattabiraman et al. 1979; Varshney et al. 1992) have suggested that the left oblique ventro-lateral approach, with the animal positioned in right lateral recumbency, is a more favorable surgical site due to its association with reduced postoperative complications. Typically, mild sedation with local infiltration is the anesthetic modality commonly applied. Recently, the anesthetic management of cattle was reviewed (Riebold 2001), and detomidine is recommended as the drug of choice when sedation is required in pregnant cattle. An intravenous dose of 2.5–10 g/kg produces 30–45 minutes of standing sedation (Carroll and Hartsfield 1996). A higher dose (40 g/kg, intravenous) causes profound sedation and recumbency (Nanda et al. 2003). Cattle can be administered general anesthesia using xylazine (0.1–0.2 mg/kg, intramuscular) followed by ketamine (10–15 mg/kg, intramuscular). The duration of this anesthesia is 45 minutes and can be extended by administering additional ketamine intravenously at a dosage of 1–2 mg/kg. Inhalation anesthesia, using halothane and isoflurane along with tracheal intubations that use conventional human anesthetic machines, is considered adequate for animals weighing up to 200 kg (Riebold 2001). This approach is now becoming more prevalent for bovine anesthesia as cows rarely exhibit emergence delirium when administered inhalation anesthetics. During the laparo-hysterotomy procedure, the uterus is carefully brought to the incision site by gently holding a fetal extremity and making an incision. The fetus is carefully removed. Due to the occurrence of fetal death and the resulting uterine adhesions that develop after 36 hours, it is typically challenging to detort the uterus prior to removing the fetus. In rare cases, attempting to correct a uterine torsion in an animal by rolling it could lead to the rupture of the uterus. During the operation, it is important to actively search for any ruptures, and if feasible, promptly repair them. If the tear is not easily accessible, the recommended course of action is to inject 20–40 IU of oxytocin into the uterine wall at three to four or more specific locations in order to induce uterine contractions. The abdominal wound is routinely closed.

24.7 Complications of Uterine Torsion

Uterine torsion can lead to various complications, including fetal and maternal death (Das et al. 2008), uterine rupture, vaginal rupture (Dhaliwal et al. 1991; Sood et al. 2002), and reduced fertility after correcting a long-standing case of torsion. Peritonitis, or the expulsion of the fetus into the abdominal cavity after uterine rupture, can occur in some cases.

24.7.1 Prognosis

The prognosis of uterine torsion prior to parturition depends upon the degree of torsion.

i) Usually, if 90° or less, the prognosis is good.
ii) In 180–270° torsion with definite symptoms that are diagnosed and treated early, the immediate prognosis is usually good for the dam and fetus, but the torsion may occasionally recover prior to parturition.
iii) In advanced severe and neglected cases, the prognosis is poor for the life and reproductive life of the dam, and usually, the fetus is dead.

References

Ahmed, M., Choudhary, R.A., and Khan, I.H. (1980). Torsion of uterus as a cause of dystocia in the buffalo. *Pakistan Veterinary Journal* 1: 22–24.

Arthur, G.H. (1966). Recent advances in bovine obstetrics. *The Veterinary Record* 79 (22): 630–640.

Arthur, G.H., Noakes, D.E., and Pearson, H. (1996). Maternal dystocia treatment. In: *Veterinary Reproduction and Obstetrics* (ed. G.H. Arthur). Philadelphia: WB Saunders Philadelphia.

Aubry, P., Warnick, L.D., DesCôteaux, L., and Bouchard, É. (2008). A study of 55 field cases of uterine torsion in dairy cattle. *The Canadian Veterinary Journal* 49 (4): 366.

Brar, P.S., Saigal, R.P., Nanda, A.S., and Sharma, R.D. (2008). Role of broad ligament in the causation of utrine torsion in dairy buffaloes. *The Indian Journal of Animal Sciences* 78 (9): 940–942.

Brown, A.J. (1974). Torsion of the gravid uterus in a bitch. *The Veterinary Record* 94 (10): 202.

Carroll, G.L. and Hartsfield, S.M. (1996). General anesthetic techniques in ruminants. *Veterinary Clinics of North America: Food Animal Practice* 12 (3): 627–661.

Cebra, C.K., Cebra, M.L., Garry, F.B., and Johnson, L.W. (1997). Surgical and nonsurgical correction of uterine torsion in New World camelids: 20 cases (1990–1996). *Journal of the American Veterinary Medical Association* 211 (5): 600–602.

Cergolj, M., Tomaskovic, A., and Makek, Z. (1999). Diagnosis and treatment of uterine torsion during pregnancy in cattle. *Tierärztliche Umschau* 54: 79–83.

Craig, J.F. (1930). *Fleming's Veterinary Obstetrics*, 4e. Bailliere. London: Tindall and Cox.

Das, G.K., Dutt, R., Deori, S. et al. (2008). Incomplete cervical dilatation causing dystocia in a buffalo. *The Indian Journal of Veterinary Research* 17 (2): 41–43.

Deori, S., Kumar, R., Jaglan, P. et al. (2009). Post-cervical uterine torsion in a buffalo-a case study. *The Indian Journal of Animal Reproduction* 30 (1): 85.

Dhaliwal, G.S., Vashista, N.K., and Sharma, R.D. (1986). Uterine torsion in a goat – a case report. *Indian Journal of Animal Reproduction* 7 (2): 90–91.

Dhaliwal, G.S., Sharma, R.D., Singla, V.K., and Prabhakar, S. (1988). Torsion of didelphic uterus in a cow. *Indian Journal of Animal Reproduction* 9: 71–72.

Dhaliwal, G.S., Prabhakar, S., and Sharma, R.D. (1991). Spontaneous rupture of vagina in buffalo heifers. *Indian Journal of Animal Reproduction* 12: 98–101.

Dhaliwal, G.S., Prabhakar, S., and Sharma, R.D. (1993). Torsion of pregnant horn in a cow-a case report. *The Indian Journal of Animal Reproduction* 14: 129.

Faria, N. and Simões, J. (2015). Incidence of uterine torsion during veterinary-assisted dystocia and singleton live births after vaginal delivery in Holstein-Friesian cows at pasture. *Asian Pacific Journal of Reproduction* 4 (4): 309–312.

Frazer, G.S., Perkins, N.R., and Constable, P.D. (1996). Bovine uterine torsion: 164 hospital referral cases. *Theriogenology* 46 (5): 739–758. https://doi.org/10.1016/s0093-691x(96)00233-6.

Hobbs, B.A. and Parker, R.F. (1990). Uterine torsion associated with either hydrometra or endometritis in two rabbits. *Laboratory animal science* 40 (5): 535–536.

Hopkins, S.M., Althouse, G.C., Jackson, L.L., and Evans, L.E. (1991). Surgical treatment of uterine torsion in a llama (Lama glama). *The Cornell Veterinarian* 81 (4): 425–428.

Ijaz, A. and Talafha, A.Q. (1999). Torsion of the uterus in an Awassi ewe. *Australian Veterinary Journal* 77 (10): 652–653.

Jackson, P.G.G. (1995). Dystocia in the cow. In: *Hand Book of Veterinary Obstetrics* (ed. P.G.G. Jackson), 30–69. Philadelphia: W.B. Saunders Co. Ltd.

Jung, C., Hospes, R., Bostedt, H., and Litzke, L.F. (2008). Surgical treatment of uterine torsion using a ventral midline laparotomy in 19 mares. *Australian Veterinary Journal* 86 (7): 272–276.

Karthick, C., Selvaraju, M., Napolean, R.E., and Doraisamy, K.A. (2015). Incidence of uterine torsion and its occurrence in relation to various factors in cows and buffaloes. *Indian Journal of Animal Reproduction* 36 (2): 60–63.

Kruse M. (2004). 'Genetic and environmental influences on the occurrence of torsio uteri in dairy cows.' Doctoral dissertation. University of Veterinary Medicine Hannover.

Kumar, R., Singh, B., Srivastava, S., and Singh, K.D. (2014). Management of pre-cervical uterine torsion in a buffalo. *Intas Polivet* 5 (2): 239–240.

Kunstyr, I. (1981). Torsion of the uterus and the stomach in guinea pigs. *Zeitschrift fur Versuchstierkunde* 23 (1): 67–69.

Laven, R. and Howe, M. (2005). Uterine torsion in cattle in the UK. *Veterinary Record* 157: 96.

Malhotra, P. (1990). Some studies on the cervical changes in the uterine torsion cases with special reference to cervical filtration in buffaloes. M.V.Sc. Thesis, Punjab Agriculture University, Ludhiana, India.

Mannari, M.N. (1969). Cervical non-dilation in buffaloes. *Gujarat Veterinarian* 3: 37–38.

Mannari, M.N. and Tadkod, D.M. (1976). Uterine torsion in buffaloes. *Indian Journal of Animal Sciences* 10: 83.

Manning, J., Marsh, P., Marshall, F. et al. (1982). Bovine uterine torsion: a review illustrated by cases from the Western College of Veterinary Medicine Large Animal Clinic. *The Bovine Practitioner* 17: 94–98.

Matharu, S.S. and Prabhakar, S. (2001). Clinical observations and success of treatment of uterine torsion in buffaloes. *The Indian Journal of Animal Reproduction* 22 (1): 45–48.

Mogha, I.V., Das, S.C., Bhattacharya, A.R. et al. (1976). Bovine uterine torsion-a case report [India]. *Indian Veterinary Journal* 53: 373–376.

Murty, K.K., Prasad, V., Murty, R.K., and P. (1999). Clinical observations on uterine torsion in buffaloes. *Indian Veterinary Journal* 76 (7): 643–645.

Nanda, A.S. (1995). *Recent Advances in Animal Reproduction and Gynaecology*. Ludhiana: USG Publishers and Distributors.

Nanda, A.S., Brar, P.S., and Prabhakar, S. (2003). Enhancing reproductive performance in dairy buffalo: major constraints and achievements. Reproduction (Cambridge, England). *Supplement* 61: 27–36.

Noakes, D.E., Parkinson, D.J., and England, G.C.W. (2001). *Maternal Dystocias. Arthurs Veterinary Reproduction and Obstetrics* (ed. D.E. Noakes). India: Saunders Harcourt.

Pattabiraman, S.R., Singh, J., Rathor, S.S., and Dhablania, D.C. (1979). Non-surgical method of correction of bovine uterine torsion-a clinical analysis. *Indian Veterinary Journal (India)* 56: 424–428.

Pearson, H. (1971). Uterine torsion in cattle: a review of 168 cases. *Veterinary Record* 89 (23): 597–603.

Penny, C.D. (1999). Uterine torsion of 540 in a mid-gestation cow. *The Veterinary Record* 145 (8): 230.

Prabhakar, S., Singh, P., Nanda, A.S., and Sharma, R.D. (1994). Clinico-obstetrical observations on uterine torsion in bovines. *Indian Veterinary Journal* 71 (8): 822–824.

Prabhakar, S., Dhaliwal, G.S., Sharma, R.D., and Nanda, A.S. (1997). Success of treatment and dam survival in bovines with precervical uterine torsion. *The Indian Journal of Animal Reproduction* 18 (2): 121–123.

Prasad, S., Rohit, K., and Maurya, S.N. (2000). Efficacy of laparohysterotomy and rolling of dam to treat uterine torsion in buffaloes. *Indian Veterinary Journal* 77: 784–786.

Purohit, G.N. (2006). Maternal causes of dystocia in cows and buffaloes. In: *Veterinary Obstetrics: A Practical Guide* (ed. S.H. Suresh and M.K. Tandle), 16–25. New Delhi: Jaypee Brothers Medical Publishers.

Purohit, G.N. and Gaur, M. (2014). Uterine torsion in buffaloes: A critical analysis. *Buffalo Bulletin* 33: 363–378.

Purohit, G.N., Barolia, Y., Shekhar, C., and Kumar, P. (2011). Maternal dystocia in cows and buffaloes: a review. *Open journal of Animal sciences* 1 (02): 41.

Riebold, T.W. (2001). Anaesthetic management of cattle. In: *Recent Advances in Anaesthetic Management of Large Domestic Animals* (ed. E.P. Steffy). Ithaca: International Veterinary Information Service.

Roberts, S.J. (1986). *Veterinary obstetrics and genital diseases: theriogenology*, 3e, 230–352. Woodstock: VT Published by the author.

Roberts, S.J. (2002). Diagnosis and treatment of dystocia. In: *Veterinary Obstetrics and Genital Diseases*, Indian edition (ed. S.J. Roberts), 274–299. New Delhi: CBS Publishers.

Roberts, S.J. and Hillman, R.B. (1973). An improved technique for the relief of bovine uterine torsion. *The Cornell Veterinarian* 63 (1): 111–116.

Ruegg, P.L. (1988). Uterine torsion of 720 degrees in a midgestation cow. *Journal of the American Veterinary Medical Association* 192 (2): 207–208.

Sane, C.R., Luktuke, S.N., and Deshpande, B.R. (1982). *Reproduction in Farm Animals*. Bombay, India: Varghese Publishing House.

Selvaraju, M., Manokaran, S., Prakash, S. et al. (2014). Bovine Obstetrical management in field practice. *Proceedings of Kerela Veterinary Science Congress* 175–179.

Sharma, S.P., Agrawal, K.B.P., and Singh, D.P. (1995). Torsion of gravid uterus and laparohysterektomy in bovine—a report on 72 clinical cases. *Indian Veterinary Journal* 72: 1180–1182.

Singh, P. (1991). Studies on broad ligament in relation to uterine torsion in buffaloes. Thesis, Punjab Agriculture University, Ludhiana, India.

Singh, P. (1995). Recent observations on etiology and treatment of uterine torsion in buffaloes. In: *Recent Advances in Animal Reproduction and Gynaecology* (ed. A.S. Nanda), 137–141. Ludhiana: USG Publishers and Distributors.

Singh, J., Prasad, B., and Rathor, S.S. (1978). Torsio uteri in buffaloes (Bubalus bubalis). An analysis of 65 cases. *Indian Veterinary Journal* 55: 161–165.

Singh, M., Singh, M., and Kumar, V. (1998). Rupture of uterus following uterine torsion in a buffalo-a case report. *Indian Journal of Animal Reproduction* 19: 71.

Singla, V.K., Sharma, R.D., Dhaliwal, G.S. et al. (1992). Uterine torsion in cows-an analysis of 34 cases. *Indian Veterinary Journal* 69 (3): 281–282.

Sloss, V. and Dufty, J.H. (1980). Obstetrical physiology. Obstetrical pathology. Obstetrical procedures. In: *Handbook of Bovine Obstetrics*, vol. 39(105), 108–111. Baltimore: Williams and Wilkins.

Sood, P., Singh, M., and Vasistha, N.K. (2002). Uterine torsion in a goat. *Indian Journal of Animal Reproduction* 23: 203.

Srinivas, M., Sreenu, M., Rani, N.L. et al. (2007). Studies on dystocia in graded Murrah buffaloes: A retrospective study. *Buffalo Bulletin* 26 (2): 40–45.

Taylor, T.S., Varner, D.D., Martin, M.T. et al. (1989). Management of dystocia in mares: uterine torsion and cesarean section. *Compendium of Continuing Education for Practicing Veterinarian* 11: 1265–1273.

Thilagar, S., Yew, Y.C., Dhaliwal, G.K. et al. (2005). Uterine horn torsion in a pregnant cat. *Veterinary Record* 157 (18): 558.

Varshney, A.C., Kumar, A., Singh, H. et al. (1992). Studies on hematological and biochemical-alterations following cesarean-section in cows. *Indian Veterinary Journal* 69 (7): 632–636.

Vasishta, N. K. (1983). Torsion of uterus in buffaloes in relation to incidence, etiology and treatment. M.V.Sc. Thesis, Punjab Agriculture University, Ludhiana, India.

25

Genital Prolapse and Its Management in Cows

Sabarinathan Akambaram[1] *and Chhavi Gupta*[2]

[1] *Veterinary Clinical Complex, Veterinary College and Research Institute, TANUVAS, Tirunelveli, Tamil Nadu, India*
[2] *Department of Veterinary Gynaecology and Obstetrics, Veterinary College and Research Institute, TANUVAS, Tirunelveli, Tamil Nadu, India*

25.1 Introduction

Genital prolapse can be defined as the eversion of part or all of a genital organ, namely the vagina, cervix, and uterus, away from its anatomical position through the vulva (Fielden 1980). The word prolapse originates from the Latin "prolapi," which means "to fall before" (Watts 1954). Genital prolapses are mostly seen in ruminants, especially cattle, buffalo, sheep, and goats (Patra et al. 2014). The pathophysiology of pelvic organ prolapse is multifactorial, which includes hereditary predisposition, atypical or abnormal connective tissue in the perineal region, hormones, and many other risk factors (Adams 1990; Couri et al. 2012; Kahn 2005; Sobiraj 1990).

Among all prolapses, uterine and vaginal prolapses are frequently observed in the reproductive tracts of cows (Ward and Powell 2007). Vaginal prolapses extend up to and include the cervix. Prolapse of the cervix as a result of vaginal displacement is considered an extension of a pre-existing vaginal prolapse (Cox 1987). It is more appropriate to refer such a condition as a cervico-vaginal prolapse (CVP). Uterine prolapse is a complication associated with the postpartum period. Spontaneous uterine prolapse in cows is an occasionally encountered, post parturient complication that requires immediate attention. Uterine prolapse is a nonhereditary complication that occurs immediately postpartum and occasionally up to several hours afterwards (Roberts 1971). Uterine prolapse is a common complication of the third stage of labor in the cow (Joseph et al. 2001). It happens within 12–24 hours of calving. Occasionally, the occurrence is delayed until days after calving and is complicated by a partial cervical involution (closure) that creates additional difficulty when replacing the uterus. It is considered an emergency condition and should be managed before excessive edema, mucosal trauma, contamination, and fatal hemorrhage lead to a grave prognosis (Miesner and Anderson 2008).

In ruminants, the prolapse is generally a complete inversion of the gravid cornual (Arthur et al. 1996). A uterine prolapse can vary in size from about 18 inches to 3–4 feet in a large cow. In crossbred cattle, prolapse of the uterus is usually associated with a mineral deficiency such as hypocalcemia. Uterine prolapse occurs during the third stage of labor at after the fetus has been expelled and the fetal cotyledons have separated from the maternal caruncles (Noakes et al. 2001).

Among obstetrical emergency conditions, a genital prolapse can be diagnosed with ease; the real challenge lies with treating a recurrent, long standing, complicated case of genital prolapse. Early intervention, treatment, proper management, follow up, and client advice are essential for better outcomes. The prompt assessment and selection of appropriate obstetrical management techniques based on the individual case is of primary importance to achieve an acceptable outcome.

25.2 Etiological or Predisposing Factors

Contributing factors in the occurrence of cervico-vaginal genital prolapses are any of the following, either alone or in combination, which includes increased intra-abdominal pressure in late pregnancy, excessive relaxation and edema of the pelvic ligaments, extreme cold weather, unfavorable environmental conditions, excess perivaginal fat, prior injury to the perivaginal tissues, consumption of large volumes of poorly digestible roughage, poor vaginal conformation, persistence of

Periparturient Diseases of Cattle, First Edition. Edited by Tanmoy Rana.

the medial walls of the mullerian ducts and changes in hormonal secretions, increased estrogen as observed in late pregnancy, imbalance of the estrogen–progesterone ratio, and deficient mineral and electrolyte levels. Incompetence of the constrictor vestibule and constrictor vulvae muscles may also have a role in etiology (Augustine 2014). It has been suggested that increased concentrations of estrogens found during pregnancy can contribute to the excessive relaxation and edema of pelvic ligaments that support the vagina. The condition is more often observed in multiple ovulation and embryo transfer technology (MOET) cattle when they are exposed to frequent superovulation, during which the estrogen–progesterone ratio is altered. Other contributing factors include hypocalcemia due to an imbalance in the calcium–phosphorus ratio.

Bovine uterine prolapse typically happens after calving when the cervix is dilated, and the uterus is atonic. The predisposing factors for a uterine prolapse are long mesometrial attachment; violent or strong tenesmus; flaccid, relaxed, and tympanic uterus (Hanie 2006); retention of fetal membranes at the ovarian pole of the gravid horn in cows and the non-gravid horn in mares (Causey et al. 2007); prolonged relaxation of the perineal and pelvic musculatures and surrounding structures; confined or stabled cows without any exercise; forced extraction of the fetus in dystocia; an animal under the low plane of nutrition; increased numbers of calving or parity (Patterson et al. 1981); and a deficiency or imbalance in a macromineral ratio, such as calcium and phosphorus.

25.3 Prevalence

Among all prolapses, uterine and vaginal prolapses are frequently observed in the reproductive tracts of cows (Powell 2007). The incidence of reproductive tract prolapses in cattle ranges between 1% and 2% (Patterson et al. 1981). Vaginal prolapses mostly occur in crossbreed cattle before calving, usually in the last trimester of pregnancy (Roberts 1971). Uterine prolapse was observed in 95.45% of the animals within 6 days of parturition (Bhattacharyya et al. 2012). Uterine prolapse commonly occurs within 2–24 hours of calving, yet it rarely occurs up to 72 hours post calving (Patil 2014). Uterine prolapse has been recorded in all animal species, although it is most commonly seen in pluriparous dairy cows (Roberts 1986). Uterine prolapse is a fairly common condition on dairy farms, and it may involve the complete prolapse of the uterus, vagina, and cervix (Augustine 2014). CVP is a common reproductive disorder of ruminants in late gestation and rarely occurs in postpartum animals. A variable incidence of prolapse between breeds suggests heritable differences for this characteristic (Milne 1954). *Bos indicus* breeds are predisposed to CVP, and the diameter of the CVP varies from 8 to 20 cm, depending on the condition and duration of the disorder (Scott 2017).

25.4 Pathophysiology

Irritability and discomfort due to a vaginal prolapse, with or without the cervix, leads to progressively increased straining or tenesmus and increases the size of the extensive prolapse (Kahn 2005). The size of the CVP also increases as it becomes more swollen due to both edema and urine retention inside the occluded urinary bladder (Kennedy 2013). A relaxed, atonic, flaccid uterus; tympany and retention of the placenta, especially at the ovarian pole of the gravid horn in cows; and low serum calcium levels enhance the chances of a uterine prolapse. Decreased myometrial tone is a logical predisposing mechanism for its occurrence, which leads to the proposed risk factors of hypocalcemia and dystocia that cause myometrial fatigue and trauma (Murphy and Dobson 2002). The hormonal changes that occur during the last trimester of gestation cause a relaxation of the sacroischiatic and sacroiliac pelvic ligaments as well as the surrounding soft tissues (Wolfe 2009), which may lead to instability of the genital tract. This concurrent relaxation, along with the increased intra-abdominal pressure caused by the weight of the gravid uterus, is considered the most important predisposing factor for CVP (Kahn 2005).

Various studies have reported that dietary and/or metabolic diseases such as hypocalcemia and grazing on phytoestrogen rich pastures also contribute to the occurrence of CVPs (Adams 1990; Miesner and Anderson 2008; Sobiraj 1990). Manual extraction of the calf and retained fetal membranes may initiate uterine eversion of the gravid horns followed by complete uterine prolapse after delivery. Uterine prolapse facilitates the accumulation of excessive edema, contamination, mucosal trauma, and cervical closure.

Manual extraction of the calf and retained fetal membranes may initiate uterine eversion of the gravid horns followed by complete uterine prolapse after delivery. Excessive movement after genital prolapse may lead to the rupture of blood vessels that cause fatal hemorrhage. Some animals may experience hypovolemic shock as a result of significant internal bleeding, an organ prolapse, or the incarceration of abdominal viscera (Potter 2008). Systemic clinical parameters such as pale or blanched conjunctival mucous membranes, prolonged capillary refill time, abdominal respiration, and tachycardia are frequently indicative of systemic involvement, which leads to a poor prognosis.

25.5 Classification of Cervico-vaginal Prolapse

According to the severity of eversion, the extent of injury, and the duration of vaginal and cervix exposure, vaginal eversions are classified into four grades (Augustine 2014).

Grade 1 prolapse: A small intermittent protrusion of the vaginal mucosa through the vulvar lips that occurs when the animal lies down. A grade 1 eversion is readily repaired by applying vulval retention sutures. If the condition is not treated, the tissue becomes dehydrated and traumatized, which may lead to a grade 2 eversion.

Grade 2 prolapse: Vaginal mucosa continuously protrudes through the vulval lips with the possibility of the urinary bladder becoming trapped in the everted organ. If left untreated, a grade 2 progresses to a grade 3 eversion.

Grade 3 prolapse: The entire vaginal mucosa and cervix protrude continuously through the vulval lips with a trapped urinary bladder and an exposed cervical mucus plug. The cervical seal may liquefy (Figure 25.1), which allows bacterial contamination of the uterus that can lead to placentitis and fetal death. Often these fetuses become emphysematous and cervical dilation is insufficient for a vaginal delivery. This condition is often referred to as a cervical eversion but is more correctly referred to as a cervico-vaginal eversion.

Grade 4 prolapse: A chronic eversion, the entire vaginal mucosa becomes necrotic and fibrosed with vascular compromise (Figure 25.2), which leads to an unfavorable prognosis. Untimely and delayed intervention when treating the prolapsed mass may cause irreparable damage to the reproductive organs, which leads to infertility and economic loss to the farming community (Augustine 2014).

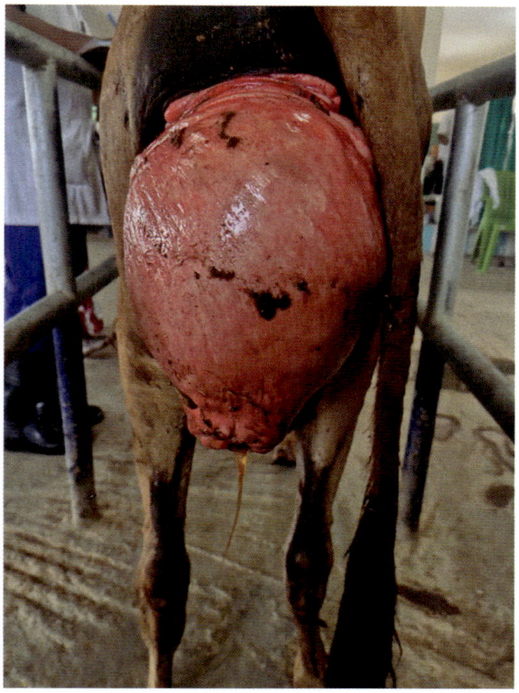

Figure 25.1 A prepartum cervico-vaginal prolapse with cervical seal liquefaction.

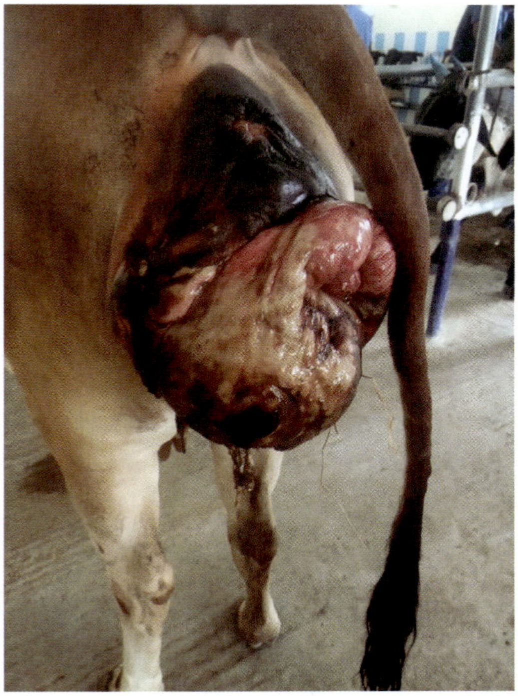

Figure 25.2 A grade 4 cervico-vaginal prolapse.

25.6 Diagnostic Approaches

Diagnosis involves visual observation and physical examination to confirm the protrusion of a portion of the floor, lateral walls, and roof of the vagina through the vulva along with the cervix and uterus, with the exposure of mucosa and movement caudally. The condition occurs sporadically, is easily recognized, and yet, is sometimes not so easily repaired.

25.7 Differential Diagnosis

Genital prolapses are sometimes misdiagnosed as a condition like Gartner's duct cysts or Bartholin's gland cysts. To rule out such conditions, one should perform a thorough per vaginum examination to check for the presence of a retained cystic structure base to confirm the enlarged cystic fluid. Further, a Gartner's duct cyst should be differentiated from a Bartholin's gland cyst based on the location of the cystic accumulation and its origin. In the reproductive passage, Gartner's ducts are located on the submucosal layer of the floor of the vaginal passage, whereas the Bartholin's gland is located on the lateral aspect of the external urethral orifice.

25.8 Treatment and Management

Repairing, replacing, and retaining the prolapsed genital tract in the original anatomical location are the primary aims of genital prolapse management. In longstanding, potentially complicated cases with irreversible damage to the uterus, amputation of the uterus is indicated. Obstetrical approaches should be followed after a thorough examination of the prolapsed mass for the extent of injury to the prolapsed mass and presence of strangulation of pelvic organs. Repairing should be initiated before the accumulation of excessive edema, contamination, mucosal trauma, and cervical closure occurs (Miesner and Anderson 2008).

The affected animal should be restrained properly to avoid undue damage to the animal, prolapsed mass, and obstetrician. If the animal is fractious for handling, rope casting restraining methods can be applied. It provides great relief to the obstetrician if animal is casted on a height-adjustable hindquarter elevator. The exposed genital mass should be thoroughly cleaned with water and a mild antiseptic solution, and a further prolapsed mass should be doused with a hypertonic solution to reduce the edema and swelling. The topical application of osmotic agents, such as salts or sugar, has proven effective at reducing and preventing the edema that rapidly accumulates within the prolapsed tissue. It is also recognized that these products can amplify existing trauma; to avoid endometrial trauma caused by the application of salt or sugar, one can use a saturated salt or sugar solution as a topical application (Roberts 1986).

The cow should be administered lignocaine 2% in an epidural at the sacrococcygeal or intercoccygeal space at a dose rate of 0.22 mg/kg body weight for the standing restraining procedure to reduce straining or tenesmus, which will help ease of the handling of the prolapsed mass and improve comfort for both the animals and handlers. Low epidural or caudal epidural anesthetic protocols can be advocated for to prevent straining or tenesmus, which facilitate the repositioning of the prolapsed genital tract (Miesner and Anderson 2008). It is important to confirm the proper infiltration of lignocaine into the epidural space with a hanging drop technique. Following epidural anesthesia, involvement of the urethral passage or urinary bladder or entrapment of abdominal viscera should be ruled out, and the bladder should be emptied with the use of urinary catheters. The prolapsed mass can be washed with mild antiseptic solutions like a potassium permanganate solution (1:1000 dilution).

The uterus should be lifted to relieve the pressure on the external urinary meatus to facilitate passage of urine. To reduce swelling or edema, osmotic agents like sugar and salt are beneficial (Roberts 1986). Reducing edema with cold ice packs or hypertonic salt solutions is suggested before replacement (Kumar et al. 2013). Handling-induced trauma is common, and this can be minimized by the prior reduction of uterine edema and enclosing the everted uterus in a plastic or porous fabric bag (Miesner and Anderson 2008).

Delayed and complicated cases of uterine prolapse may have full-thickness lacerations that should be repaired before repositioning of the prolapsed mass, or if there is a prolapsed uterine horn with vascular compromise, necrotic changes in the endometrium and maternal caruncles (Figure 25.3) indicate a poor prognosis. The incomplete repositioning and rough handling of a total uterine prolapse may lead to recurrent eversion with perineal lacerations (Figure 25.4). It is often

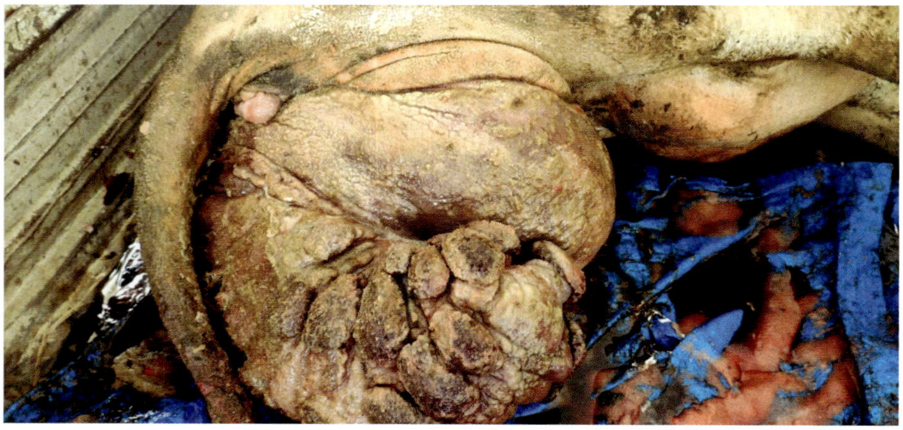

Figure 25.3 A uterine prolapse with necrotic changes.

suggested that repair can be forgone if lacerations are less than 2–3 inches and dorsal, because the defect closes sufficiently with oxytocin therapy and uterine involution (Hopper 2007). When tears occur in the uterine wall, they are easily repaired by suturing with absorbable suture material. The intrauterine administration of oxytocin into the uterine musculature has been suggested to reduce the size of the uterus. The uterine damage can be alleviated by physically massaging the prolapsed mass with lubrication (Youngquist 1989).

A prolapsed uterus should be lifted up to the ischial arch because in genital prolapse the urethra is often positioned at an acute angle, which prevents urination, further aggravates the tenesmus, and causes discomfort. To straighten the urethra, urinary catheterization may be indicated to allow urination as well as relieve undue strain on the blood vessels and genital tissue to provide additional cow comfort and further reduce straining.

It is useful to raise the hindquarters to minimize abdominal pressure if the animal is recumbent. A very efficient means of positioning is with the cow in sternal recumbency and "frog legged," which means stifles down and the pelvic limbs stretched out behind the cow. Approaches to raise the hindquarters in cows include the use of a commercially available cow lift or by tying the hindlegs together at the upper part of the enarthrodial joints with a soft rope and raising the rear part of the cow mechanically with a tractor or a chain block about 1 m in height (Ishii et al. 2010).

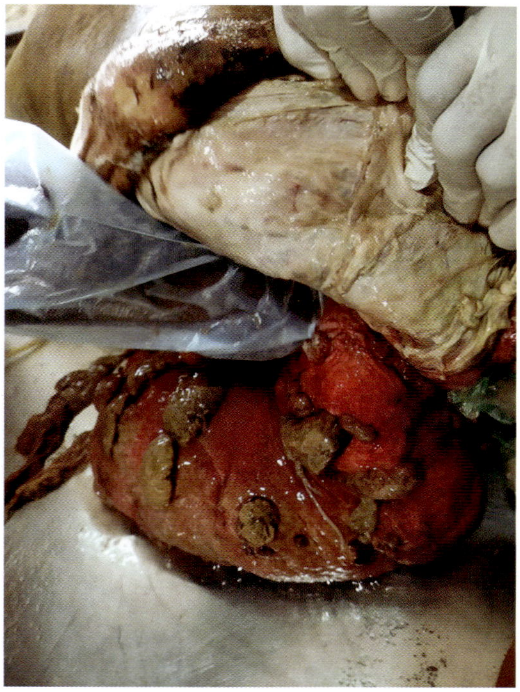

Figure 25.4 A uterine prolapse with a perineal laceration.

25.8.1 Hindquarter Elevation

The replacement of a fully prolapsed uterus in a cow causes considerable damage to the animal. Chronic and delayed cases of uterine prolapse that lead to swollen, hardened, friable conditions in turn lead to more difficult repositioning. In such conditions, it is essential to raise the rear end of the cow to facilitate the ease of repositioning. The method of raising the rear end of the cow using a tractor was reported as a quick, easy, and essentially practical method of dealing with a prolapsed uterus (White 2007). The recovery rate in the hindquarter-raising group was significantly higher than the lying group (Ishii et al. 2010). It was reported that the replacement of the uterus should be done with the cow in sternal recumbency with "frog-legged positioning" (Potter 2008), "New Zealand methods" (Jackson 1995), or with the aid of hindquarter elevators.

The hindquarter elevation technique (Figure 25.5) is a great boon for the animal and obstetrician for the successful management of the genital prolapse. Thus, hindquarter raising reduces abdominal pressure on the cow and makes it easy

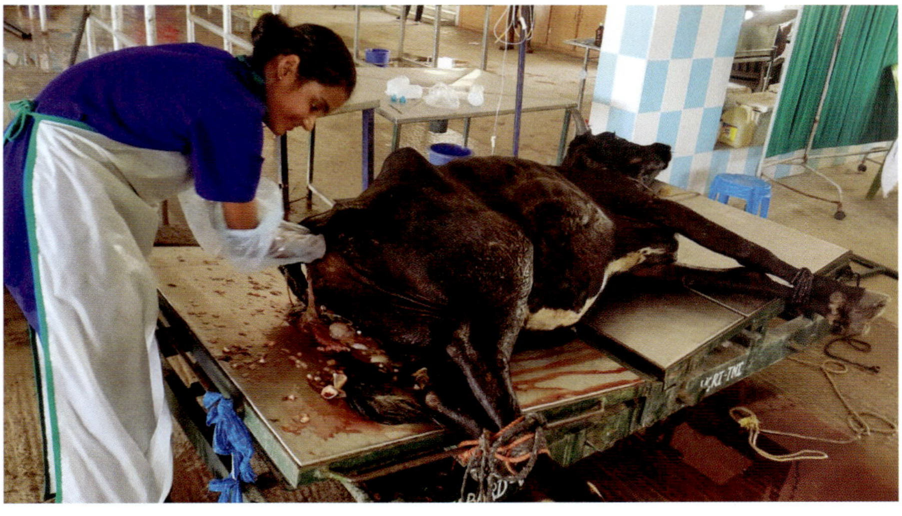

Figure 25.5 The hindquarter elevation technique.

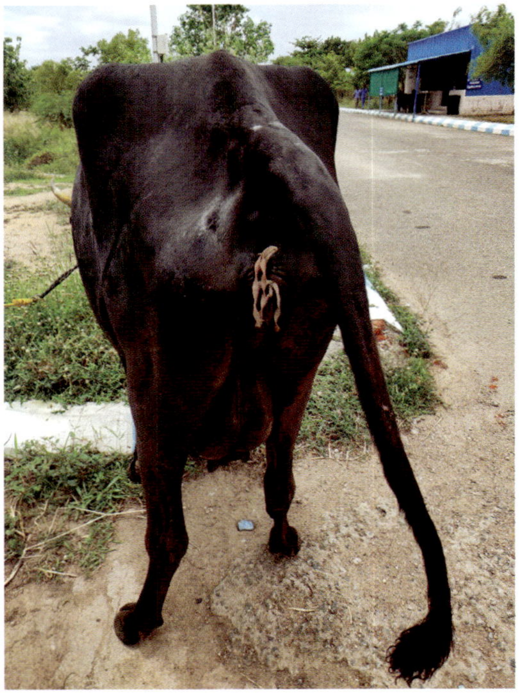

Figure 25.6 A vulvar tape retention suture for a total uterine prolapse.

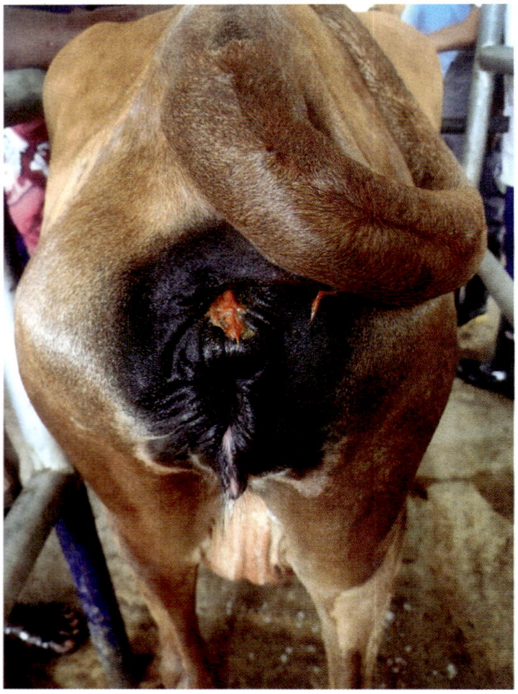

Figure 25.7 Buher's suture for the retention of a cervico-vaginal prolapse.

to replace a prolapsed uterus. This technique is safe and has no adverse effect on the treated animals. Putting excessive pressure on the uterus while replacing a prolapsed uterus might cause unrecoverable damage to the uterus. Similarly, it is important to choose a posture in which it is possible to replace the uterus under weak pressure. Replacing the prolapsed uterus is considered to be a technique that requires considerable physical strength in large animal medical treatments. On the other hand, in many cases, large animal clinicians may be physically unfit to treat more than one case at the same time. Therefore, replacing the prolapsed uterus with hindquarter-raising postures will benefit the clinicians' performance by requiring less physical strength, and this method of replacing the uterus by raising the hindlegs was found to cause only slight damage to the uterus (Ishii et al. 2010).

Various treatment regimens have been described to treat genital prolapse that include the vulvar tape retention suture (Figure 25.6), Buhner's suture, bootlace sutures, paravaginal stents, Caslick's suture, rope slings, and a rope truss. Buhner's suture and other described methods give temporary relief from vaginal prolapse whereas chronic and recurrent vaginal prolapses require more invasive techniques to stabilize the vagina in its original anatomical position. The available permanent stabilization techniques are the Johnson button and Minchev suture techniques, which are appropriate procedures for chronic genital prolapse associated with excessive redundancy of the dorsal vaginal wall (Augustine 2014). Limitations of these invasive and traumatic techniques include tearing of the vagina into the abdomen because of chronic straining or tenesmus after surgery as well as damage to the sciatic nerve or internal pudendal artery.

25.8.2 Temporary Fixation Techniques

25.8.2.1 Buhner's Technique

Buhner's technique is a type of purse string suture pattern applied around the vulvar region to hold the genital tract in position (Figure 25.7). In this technique, the vulva is thoroughly washed with detergent and a 1-cm stab incision is made on the midline below the vulva and as far forward as practical. A second incision is made midway between the anus and dorsal commissure of the vulva. The Buhner needle is then passed deeply from the ventral incision up one side of the vulva and out through the dorsal incision. The Buhner's tape is passed through the eye of the needle and the needle retracted through the ventral incision along with the tape. The same pattern followed for the other side, and Buhner's tape is pulled either through the dorsal or ventral incision site, tightened around the vulvar region, and knotted with a two to three finger gap to hold the genital tract in position without affecting urination.

25.8.2.2 Caslick's Technique

This technique should be reserved for only nonirritated grade 1 vaginal eversions that occur during the prepartum period and when tenesmus is not expected to be a concern. Unfortunately, a simple Caslick's suture in many cases is insufficient. As intra-abdominal pressure increases, tenesmus begins and either the sutures are torn away or the vagina begins to evert below the sutures. During the first stage of labor, the vulval softening and stretching that occurs close to parturition contributes to suture disturbance. A Caslick's suture may suffice in animals that are not pregnant and have a grade 1 eversion during estrus. This is often the case with embryo donor animals whose ovaries are frequently superstimulated with hormones for the sole purpose of increasing the number of ovulations (Augustine 2014).

25.8.2.3 Bootlace Technique

The bootlace technique is not a preferred technique as the vulval lips are inverted and the suture placement is tedious. However, the advantage of this technique is that it is a bit stronger than the Caslick's suture technique. Following an epidural anesthetic procedure and disinfecting of the vulva and perineal area, four to five small eyelets are made with umbilical tape or hognose rings on either side of the vulva in a dorsal to ventral line at the hair to hairless junction on the vulval lips. After placing the eyelets, umbilical or Buhner's tape is used to "lace up" the vulva, much like a boot. As the pattern is tightened, the vulval lips invert. Again, the bootlace must be loosened prior to calving to avoid serious trauma to the vagina (Augustine 2014).

25.8.2.4 Deep Vertical Mattress Technique

The difference here is that a vertical mattress suture pattern is used, and stents are recommended to disperse tension on the vulval lips. This replacement method can also have serious consequences if assistance is not available at the onset of parturition.

25.8.3 Permanent Stabilization Techniques

Two common methodologies are advocated as providing permanent stabilization of the genital tract, namely the Johnson button technique, in which an indwelling needle is utilized, and the Minchev suture technique, in which umbilical tapes are applied from the dorso-lateral vaginal wall through the sacrotuberous ligament, gluteal musculature, and skin. These permanent fixation technique sutures are left in place for 2–6 weeks to allow extensive fibrous adhesions to form between the vagina and the sacrosciatic ligaments, which serve as anchors for the vaginal shelf. Vaginal prolapses associated with the involvement of the ventral vaginal wall can be treated with cervicopexy through a transvaginal approach or by flank laparotomy.

25.8.3.1 Minchev's Technique

There are two Minchev techniques described that differ only in the location of needle insertion. In the original Minchev technique, epidural anesthesia is administered through the sacrococcygeal or intercoccygeal epidural space, then the gluteal areas are shaved and disinfected; a large S-shaped needle is threaded with 0.95-cm umbilical tape, and a gauze bandage or large plastic or metal plate is attached at the end of the tape, which is then passed through the lesser sciatic foramen. The needle is then taken in vaginally, and the lesser sciatic foramen is located on the dorso-lateral wall of the vagina. The needle is then pushed through the dorsal area of the foramen in order to avoid the pudendal nerve. The needle is pushed through the skin in the gluteal area, the suture is pulled up snug, and another button, plate, or gauze is tied onto the suture (Augustine 2014). This is repeated on the other side. This technique is an excellent prepartum method that aims to retain the vagina in the correct pelvic location by adhesion formation between the submucosa of the vagina and surrounding fascia. The Minchev technique can be difficult to perform if the tissue has severe edema.

25.8.3.2 Modified Minchev Vaginopexy

This technique involves a more cranial fixation of the vaginal wall and is similar, except the stay sutures are placed anterior to the lesser sciatic foramen, about 5 cm lateral to the midline, and just posterior to the shaft of the ilium.

After repositioning a prolapsed uterus, an infusion of 2–5 l of warm saline into the uterus helps return the organ to its normal position through gravity (Gnanasubramanian et al. 2000). The administration of antibiotics, fluid replacements, antihistamines, and uterine motility stimulants (20–40 IU oxytocin or ergometrine intramuscularly) is suggested. Oxytocin injections (20–40 IU) given within 2–4 hours of birth may help in uterine involution (Hopper 2007). An intravenous infusion of calcium borogluconate helps to increase myometrial motility and thus increases the likelihood of the uterus to regain its normal size and contour.

Delay in repositioning sometimes makes it difficult to repair, and when coupled with trauma and shock, it may culminate in death (Singhal et al. 2011). The mortality rates in large studies on dairy cows varied from 20% to 25% (Murphy and

Dobson 2002). The high mortality was attributed to shock, blood loss, refractory downer-cow syndrome, and other complications. In extreme cases of long-duration uterine prolapses with severe necrosis, circumferential lacerations, and closure of cervix that means replacement is not possible, amputation of the prolapsed uterus must be considered. After the successful repositioning and stabilization of the prolapsed genital tract, the client should be advised to restrict animal movement to reduce the chances of uterine artery or venous rupture, which may lead to fatal hemorrhage and hypovolemic shock.

Complications and a poor prognosis in genital prolapses due to delayed or improper interventions include severe tenesmus due to increased intra-abdominal pressure, difficulty in urination caused by strangulation of the urethral passage, hardening of the prolapsed genitalia wall, and occasionally, rupture of the vaginal wall through which viscera such as the intestines or urinary bladder may eviscerate. A rupture of the vaginal wall with evisceration of the intestines, bladder, or even uterus is also a severe complication of untreated CVP (Veeraiah and Srinivas 2010).

In extreme conditions, there is a long-duration uterine prolapse with severe necrosis, circumferential lacerations, and closure of the cervix wherein replacement is not possible. Complications develop when lacerations, necrosis, and infections are present or when treatment is delayed. Shock, hemorrhage, and thromboembolism are potential sequelae of a prolonged prolapse (Noakes et al. 2001).

The recovery rate and conception percentage after treatment were 72.4% and 81.25%, respectively (Gardner et al. 1990). The recovery rate and conception percentage after treatment were 81.9% and 84.7%, respectively (Carluccio et al. 2020). The insemination rate of cows that survived a treated uterine prolapse was 77.5% (31 of 40). The conception rate of inseminated cows was 80.6% (25 of 31), whereas the pregnancy rate of surviving cows was 62.5% (25 of 40). The calving-to-conception interval was 50 days longer for rebred prolapse cases compared with matched controls (Murphy and Dobson 2002). In the recumbent cow, the recovery rate decreased gradually with increasing parity (first: 64.7%; second: 50.0%; third or more: 45.8%) (Ishii et al. 2010).

25.9 Summary

Genital prolapses are obstetrical emergencies that require intervention at the earliest possible opportunity in order to assess the type of genital protrusion, if concurrent protrusion of pelvic structures is involved, vascular compromise, duration of exposure, extent of damage, and systemic signs. The corrective procedure should be carried out promptly after restraining, assessing, and stabilizing the animal.

The approach to take should be selected based on the individual case. The use of hindquarter elevators is a great support for both the animals and obstetricians. The prognosis for survival is dependent on timely interventions, parity, calf viability, and the lack of secondary metabolic or musculoskeletal disease. Client communication is of primary importance post-correction procedure to overcome post-operative complications. Restricting the animal's movement before and after obstetrical procedures will enhance the prognosis in terms of avoiding or reducing the chances of uterine arterial and venous damage.

References

Adams, N.R. (1990). Permanent infertility in ewes exposed to plant oestrogens. *Australian Veterinary Journal* 67: 197.

Arthur, G.H., Noakes, D.E., Peterson, H., and Parkinson, T.J. (1996). *Veterinary Reproduction and Obstetrics*, 7e. London: WB Saunders Company Ltd.

Augustine, T.P. (2014). Vaginal, cervical and uterine prolapse of cow. In: *Bovine Reproduction*, 1e (ed. R.M. Hopper). Willey Blackwell https://doi.org/10.1002/9781118833971.ch43.

Bhattacharyya, H.K., Fazili, M.R., Buchoo, B.A., and Akand, A.H. (2012). Genital prolapse in crossbred cows: prevalence, clinical picture and management by a modified Bühner's technique using infusion (drip) set tubing as suture material. *Veterinarski Arhiv* 82 (1): 11–24.

Carluccio, A., De Amicis, I., Probo, M. et al. (2020). Prevalence, survival and subsequent fertility of dairy and beef cows with uterine prolapse. *Acta Veterinaria Hungarica* 68 (1): 91–94.

Causey, R., Ruksznis, D., and Miles, R. (2007). Field management of equine uterine prolapse in a Thorough bred mare. *Equine Veterinary Education* 19 (5): 254–259.

Couri, B.M., Lenis, A.T., Borazjani, A. et al. (2012). Animal models of female pelvic organ prolapse: lessons learned. *Expert Review of Obstetrics and Gynecology* 7 (3): 249–260.

Cox, J.E. (1987). *Surgery of the Reproductive Tract in Large Animals*, 3e, 1–208. England: Liverpool University Press.

Fielden, E.D. (1980). Vaginal prolapse. In: *Current Therapy in Theriogenology* (ed. D.A. Morrow), 914. Philadelphia, U.S.A.: W.B. Saunders and Co.

Gardner, I.A., Reynolds, J.P., Risco, C.A., and Hird, D.W. (1990). Patterns of uterine prolapse in dairy cows and prognosis after treatment. *Journal of the American Veterinary Medical Association* 197 (8): 1021–1024.

Gnanasubramanian, T., Balasubramanian, S., Joseph, C., and Kathiresan, D. (2000). Vagino-cervical prolapse with partial uterine prolapse in a she buffalo. *The Indian Journal of Animal Reproduction* 21 (2): 161.

Hanie, E.A. (2006). Prolapse of the vaginal and uterus. In: *Large Animal Clinical Procedures for Veterinary Technicians* (ed. E.A. Hanie), 218–221. Mosby: Elsevier.

Hopper, R.M. (2007). Surgical correction of abnormalities of genital organs of cows: management of uterine prolapse. In: *Current Therapy in Large Animal Theriogenology*, 2e (ed. R.S. Youngquist and W.R. Threlfall), 470–471. Philadelphia: Saunders, Elsevier.

Ishii, M., Aoki, T., Yamakawa, K. et al. (2010). Uterine prolapse in cows: effect of raising the rear end on the clinical outcomes and reproductive performance. *Veterinární Medicína* 55 (3): 113–118.

Jackson, P.G. (1995). postparturient problems in large animals. In: *Handbook of Veterinary Obstetrics*, 2e (ed. P.G. Jackson), 209–232. London: WB Saunders.

Joseph, C., Kulasekar, K., Balasubramanian, S. et al. (2001). An unusual complication of post-partum uterine prolapse in a she buffalo-a case report. *The Indian Veterinary Journal* 78: 57–58.

Kahn, C. (2005, 2005). *Merck Veterinary Manual*, 9e. Rahway, NJ: Merck.

Kennedy, G.F. (2013). Prolapse vagina and/or uterus. *Ask-a-Vet Sheep*. https://askavetsheep.wordpress.com/2013/02/02/prolapse/ (accessed 3 January 2024).

Kumar, S., Bhatt, P., and Dhama, K. (2013). Post-Partum complete uterine prolapse in buffalo–a case report. *Veterinary Practioner* 14: 70.

Miesner, M.D. and Anderson, D.E. (2008). Management of uterine and vaginal prolapse in the bovine. *Veterinary Clinics of North America. Food Animal Practice* 24 (2): 409–419.

Milne, E.J. (1954). Efocaine an aid in the treatment of bovine vaginal prolapse. *Journal of the American Veterinary Medical Association* 124: 108.

Murphy, A.M. and Dobson, H. (2002). Predisposition, subsequent fertility, and mortality of cows with uterine prolapse. *The Veterinary Record* 151 (24): 733–735.

Noakes, E.D., Parkinson, T.J., and England, G.C.W. (2001). Post parturient prolapse of the uterus. In: *Arthur's Veterinary Reproduction and Obstetrics*, 8e, vol. 19 (ed. D.E. Noakes, T.J. Parkinson, G.C.W. England, and G.H. Arthur), 333–338. New Delhi: Harcourt (India) Pvt. Ltd.

Patil, A.D. (2014). Management of postpartum uterine prolapse a report of 16 buffaloes. *Intas Polivet* 15: 405–407.

Patra, B.K., Nahak, A.K., Dash, S.K. et al. (2014). Cervico vaginal prolapse in a pregnant cow and its management – a case report. *International Journal of Livestock Research* 4 (5): 55–59.

Patterson, D.J., Bellows, R.A., and Burfening, P.J. (1981). Effects of caesarean section, retained placenta and vaginal or uterine prolapse on subsequent fertility in beef cattle. *Journal of Animal Science* 53 (4): 916–921.

Potter, T. (2008). Prolapse of the uterus in the cow. *UK Veterinary Journal* 13: 1–3.

Roberts, S.J. (1971). *Veterinary Obstetrics and Genital Disease (Theriogenology)*, 2e. India: CBS Publishers and Distributors.

Roberts, S.J. (1986). Injuries and diseases of the puperal period. In: *Veterinary Obstetrics and Genital Diseases (Theriogenology)*, 3e (ed. S.J. Roberts), 364. Woodstock (VT): Roberts, S.J. publisher.

Scott, P. (2017). Lambing part 3 vaginal and uterine prolapse: Vaginal prolapse. *NADIS Animal Health Skills*. Haverfordwest, United Kingdom: National Animal Disease Information Service. https://www.nadis.org.uk/disease-a-z/sheep/lambing/lambing-part-3-vaginal-and-uterine-prolapse/ (accessed 3 January 2024).

Singhal, S., Srivastava, N., and Srivastava, R. (2011). Post partum uterine prolapse in buffalo – a report of two cases. *Veterinary Practioner* 12: 34.

Sobiraj, A. (1990). Ante partum vaginal prolapse in the sheep: a unsolved problem. *Tierärztliche Praxis* 18 (1): 9–12.

Veeraiah, G. and Srinivas, M. (2010). Spontaneous extrusion of the intestines and uterus as a squeal to vaginal prolapse in a buffalo heifer: a case report. *Buffalo Bulletin* 29 (1): 60–64.

Ward, H. and Powell, J. (2007). Reproductive prolapses of cattle (FSA3102). In: *Livestock Health Series*. University of Arkansas Division of Agriculture Research and Extension https://www.uaex.uada.edu/publications/PDF/FSA-3102.pdf.

Watts, R.E. (1954). Periparturient prolapse of the vaginal wall. *Proceedings 91st Annual Meeting of the American Veterinary Medical Association,* Seattle, Washington, USA (23–26 August 1954). Ithaca, NY, USA: American Veterinary Medical Association.

White, A. (2007). Uterine prolapse in the cow. *UK Veterinary Journal* 12: 1–3.

Wolfe, D.F. (2009). Medical and surgical management of vaginal prolapse in cattle. Eighty-first Western Veterinary Conference, Auburn, Alabama (15 February 2009).

Youngquist, R.S. (1989). Bovine uterine prolapse. In: *Theriogoenology Handbook*, vol. 3 (ed. R.S. Youngquist), 79–81. Society for Theriogenology.

26

Postpartum Hemorrhage

Somu Yogeshpriya[1,4], *Subramaniam Sivaraman*[2,4], *and Sengodan Raja*[3,4]

[1] *Department of Veterinary Medicine, Veterinary College and Research Institute, Orathnadu, Thanjavur, Tamil Nadu, India*
[2] *Department of Clinics, Veterinary College and Research Institute, Namakkal, Tamil Nadu, India*
[3] *Department of Veterinary Gynecology and Obstetrics, Veterinary College and Research Institute, Orathnadu, Thanjavur, Tamil Nadu, India*
[4] *Tamil nadu Veterinary and Animal Sciences University, Chennai, Tamil Nadu, India*

26.1 Introduction

Postpartum hemorrhage (PPH) is a significant concern in the field of veterinary medicine, particularly among cattle. It refers to the excessive loss of blood that occurs in the aftermath of calving and poses a serious threat to both the health of the mother cow and the overall productivity of the herd (Smith and Risco 2005). PPH in cattle can lead to a range of complications, including uterine atony, a retained placenta, and increased susceptibility to infections (Purohit 2012). The timely recognition, accurate diagnosis, and appropriate management of this condition are vital to ensure the well-being of the animal and to maintain the profitability (Jeyakumari et al. 2006) and sustainability of cattle operations.

The process of calving, while natural, places substantial physiological demands on the cow's body. The intricate orchestration of hormonal changes, uterine contractions, and physical adaptations is aimed at facilitating the safe delivery of a healthy calf (Mandali et al. 2004). However, these processes do not always unfold seamlessly, and PPH can arise when the uterus fails to contract effectively after calving. This condition can be triggered by a variety of factors that include hormonal imbalances, uterine exhaustion, malnutrition, and the strain of multiple births (Purohit 2012).

The consequences of PPH can be dire. Profuse bleeding can lead to anemia, weakness, and even shock in the affected cow, which jeopardizes her ability to care for her calf and recover her own health (Mandali et al. 2004). Furthermore, the loss of valuable blood and nutrients can have long term implications for milk production, reproductive performance, and the overall profitability of dairy and beef operations.

In this context, it becomes imperative to understand the causes, signs, and potential complications of PPH in cattle. Equally important is the knowledge of appropriate management strategies that range from uterine massage and the administration of oxytocin to potential surgical interventions (Purohit 2012). By promptly addressing PPH and its underlying causes, veterinarians and livestock producers can significantly improve the chances of a cow's recovery and minimize the impact on the entire herd.

In the subsequent sections, we will delve deeper into the various aspects of PPH in cattle, exploring its causes, clinical manifestations, diagnostic approaches, and the diverse strategies available for effective management (Smith and Risco 2005). It is through a comprehensive understanding of this condition that veterinarians and cattle producers can work collaboratively to safeguard the health and productivity of their herds.

Periparturient Diseases of Cattle, First Edition. Edited by Tanmoy Rana.

26.2 Causes of Postpartum Hemorrhage in Cattle

26.2.1 Uterine Atony

Uterine atony and subsequent PPH in cattle are interrelated conditions that can have significant impacts on the health and productivity of both individual cows and the entire herd. Uterine atony refers to the failure of the uterus to contract properly after calving, which leads to inadequate hemostasis (cessation of bleeding) and an increased risk of excessive postpartum bleeding (Jeyakumari et al. 2006). Understanding the underlying causes of uterine atony is crucial for preventing and managing the subsequent PPH.

26.2.1.1 Causes of Uterine Atony

- Hormonal imbalances
- Fatigue and uterine exhaustion
- Retained placenta
- Malnutrition and mineral deficiencies
- Twin calves
- Dystocia (difficult calving)
- Stress and disturbances
- Age and parity
- Genetics
- Hypocalcemia (milk fever)

Proper uterine contraction is orchestrated by hormonal changes that particularly involve oxytocin. Hormonal imbalances can disrupt the normal contraction and retraction of the uterine muscles, which leads to atony (Sheldon et al. 2008). When the uterus fails to contract effectively, blood vessels remain open and result in bleeding and potential PPH. Prolonged or difficult labor can exhaust the uterine muscles, reducing their ability to contract adequately post calving (Jeyakumari et al. 2006). This exhaustion hampers the ability of the uterus to constrict and close off blood vessels, which contributes to atony and subsequent bleeding. When the placenta is not expelled within the expected time frame, it can cause inflammation and irritation of the uterine lining (Abuom et al. 2012). This irritation disrupts normal contractions, which leads to atony and a heightened risk of PPH. Inadequate nutrition, especially during late pregnancy, can weaken uterine muscles and hinder proper contraction (Mandali et al. 2004).

Mineral deficiencies, such as calcium and magnesium, can also negatively impact muscle function, including uterine contractions (Sharma 2006). Carrying and delivering twin calves can stretch the uterus extensively, which causes uterine fatigue and reduced contractility. This stretching can lead to atony and increased bleeding after calving (Jeyakumari et al. 2006). Difficult calving can strain the uterine muscles, which leads to uterine exhaustion and impaired contraction. Dystocia can result from various factors that include calf size, positioning, and maternal factors. High-stress conditions, such as transportation, sudden environmental changes, or disturbances during calving, can interfere with normal hormonal responses and disrupt uterine contractions, which contributes to uterine atony.

Older cows or those with multiple calvings may experience reduced uterine contractility due to factors such as muscle tone changes and tissue wear and tear. Genetic factors can influence muscle tone and the ability of the uterus to contract effectively (Jeyakumari et al. 2006). Some breeds or genetic lines may be more prone to uterine atony. Low blood calcium levels, commonly associated with hypocalcemia (milk fever), can lead to muscle weakness and affect uterine contractions, potentially leading to atony.

The combination of these factors can lead to uterine atony, which in turn increases the likelihood of PPH. Prompt recognition, appropriate management, and veterinary intervention are essential to address uterine atony and minimize the risk of PPH (Abuom et al. 2012). Measures such as providing proper nutrition, managing calving conditions, administering oxytocin, and closely monitoring cows during and after calving can all contribute to preventing and managing these conditions effectively.

26.2.1.2 Treating Uterine Atony

The treatment for uterine atony in cattle involves a combination of medical interventions and management strategies aimed at stimulating uterine contractions, promoting the expulsion of fetal membranes, and preventing or addressing complications like PPH (Jeyakumari et al. 2006). Timely and appropriate management is essential to ensure the cow's recovery and prevent further complications.

1) **Oxytocin administration:** Oxytocin is a hormone that stimulates uterine contractions. Its administration is a common first step in treating uterine atony. Oxytocin helps the uterus contract and expel any remaining fetal membranes. It can be given at 20–50 U intramuscularly. Careful dosage and timing are crucial to avoid overstimulation or potential side effects.
2) **Uterine massage:** Gentle massage of the uterus can help stimulate contractions and encourage the expulsion of fetal membranes. This technique can be performed by a trained veterinary professional. Uterine massage is often used in conjunction with oxytocin administration.
3) **Intravenous fluids:** Intravenous fluids may be administered to the cow to help stabilize her condition and support overall health. Fluid therapy helps restore electrolyte balance and improves blood circulation, which aids in uterine contraction.
4) **Calcium supplementation:** If hypocalcemia is suspected as a contributing factor to uterine atony, calcium supplements may be administered. Calcium supports muscle function, including uterine contractions (250–500 ml of calcium borogluconate is often helpful).
5) **Antibiotics:** Antibiotics may be prescribed to prevent or treat infections that could arise due to retained placental tissues or other complications associated with uterine atony.
6) **Surgical intervention:** In severe cases or if conservative methods fail, a veterinarian may need to perform a manual removal of retained fetal membranes (Sheldon et al. 2008). This procedure involves physically removing any remaining placental tissues from the uterus. It is typically done under sterile conditions and with proper sedation or anesthesia.
7) **Hormonal therapy:** In some cases, additional hormonal therapies may be considered, such as prostaglandins, to promote uterine contractions.
8) **Monitoring and support:** Close monitoring of the cow's vital signs, overall health, and uterine contractions is essential during treatment (Sheldon et al. 2008). Providing a clean and comfortable environment, along with proper nutrition, helps support the cow's recovery.
9) **Prevention of complications:** Treating uterine atony should include measures to prevent complications such as PPH. If excessive bleeding occurs, it should be promptly addressed through additional interventions like blood transfusions.

26.2.2 Retained Placenta

Retained placentas and subsequent PPH are significant concerns in cattle reproduction. Retained placenta refers to the failure of the placenta (fetal membranes) to be expelled from the uterus within a normal timeframe after calving. This condition can lead to various complications, including PPH, which is excessive bleeding following calving (Abuom et al. 2012). Understanding the causes of retained placentas and the association with PPH is crucial for effective management and prevention.

The placenta is a vital organ that develops during pregnancy and serves as a connection between the dam (mother) and the fetus that provides nutrients, oxygen, and waste elimination (Jeyakumari et al. 2006). After calving, the placenta should normally detach and be expelled from the uterus due to uterine contractions. When this process does not occur as expected and the placenta remains attached, it can lead to various complications for the cow's health and subsequent fertility, including PPH.

26.2.2.1 Causes of Retained Placenta-associated Postpartum Hemorrhage

- Hormonal imbalance
- Stress and nutritional factors
- Breed predisposition and age
- Previous cases of retained placentas
- Twin pregnancies

26.2.2.2 Clinical Signs

When the placental membranes are not expelled within the expected timeframe, they can continue to release blood and fluids into the uterus. This can lead to PPH, which is excessive bleeding after calving (Abuom et al. 2012). The retained

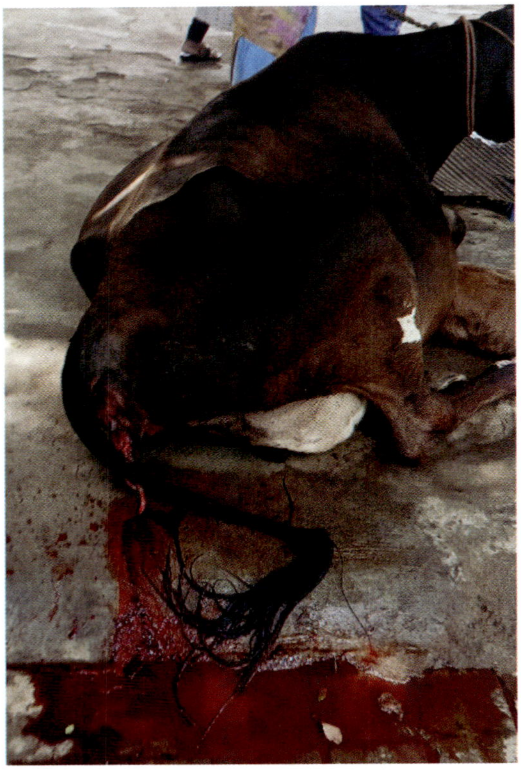

Figure 26.1 Cow with a retained placenta and hemorrhage.

placenta prevents the uterus from contracting properly, which hinders the closure of blood vessels that were attached to the placenta. As a result, the cow may experience prolonged and heavy bleeding (Figure 26.1).

Cattle with retained placentas and PPH may exhibit the following signs (Sheldon et al. 2008):

- Continued vaginal discharge beyond the normal timeframe.
- General weakness and lethargy.
- Anemia due to blood loss.
- Increased heart rate and respiratory rate.
- Reduced appetite.
- Dehydration.

26.2.2.3 Effects and Complications

- Metritis
- Reduced fertility
- Reduced milk production
- Delayed estrus
- Cystic ovarian follicles

26.2.2.4 Treatment for Retained Placenta

The treatment of PPH associated with retained placentas in cattle involves a combination of medical interventions and supportive care. It is important to note that guidance should be sought for proper diagnosis and treatment (Purohit 2012).

- **Manual removal of retained placenta:** If the placenta is not expelled naturally within the expected timeframe (usually within 12 hours of calving), it may need to be manually removed. This procedure should only be performed by a skilled professional to prevent injury or infection (Sheldon et al. 2008).
- **Antibiotics:** In cases of retained placentas, there is an increased risk of uterine infections (metritis). Antibiotics may be prescribed to prevent or treat infections. Commonly used antibiotics include:
  1) <u>Penicillin:</u> Effective against a wide range of bacteria.
  2) <u>Ceftiofur:</u> A commonly used cephalosporin antibiotic.
  3) <u>Tetracyclines:</u> Broad-spectrum antibiotics that are effective against various bacterial infections (Jeyakumari et al. 2006).
- **Oxytocin and other hormones.**
- **Fluid therapy and nutritional support.**
- **NSAIDs (nonsteroidal anti-inflammatory drugs):** NSAIDs can help reduce inflammation, pain, and fever associated with uterine infections or other complications (Abuom et al. 2012). Examples of NSAIDs used in veterinary medicine include flunixin meglumine (Banamine®, Merck and Company, Inc., Rahway, New Jersey, USA) and meloxicam.
- **Calcium supplementation.**
- **Uterine lavage.**

26.2.3 Uterine Rupture

Uterine rupture is a serious and potentially life-threatening condition that can lead to PPH in cattle (Sheldon et al. 2008). It occurs when there is a tear or rupture in the wall of the uterus, often during or after calving (Jeyakumari et al. 2006). Uterine rupture is considered a rare but severe complication, and it requires immediate attention.

26.2.3.1 Causes and Risk Factors

- **Dystocia (difficult calving):** Excessive force or prolonged labor during calving can weaken the uterine wall and increase the risk of rupture.

- ➢ **Trauma:** Physical trauma during calving, such as rough handling or improper assistance, can lead to uterine injury (Njenga and Tsuma 2004).
- ➢ **Uterine distension:** Overstretching of the uterus due to excessive fetal size, multiple pregnancies, or retained fetuses can increase the likelihood of rupture.
- ➢ **Uterine abnormalities:** Congenital or acquired uterine abnormalities can make the uterine wall more susceptible to rupture.
- ➢ **Previous uterine surgery:** Cattle that have undergone previous cesarean sections or other uterine surgeries may have weakened uterine walls, which increases the risk of rupture.

26.2.3.2 Clinical Signs and Symptoms

Uterine rupture can lead to profound PPH and other serious clinical signs that include (Abuom et al. 2012):

- **Severe hemorrhage:** Rapid and excessive bleeding from the vulva.
- **Shock:** The cow may exhibit signs of shock, including pale mucous membranes, rapid heart rate, and a weak pulse.
- **Abdominal pain:** Cows may display signs of discomfort, such as restlessness and kicking at the abdomen.
- **Depression and weakness:** The cow may appear lethargic, weak, and reluctant to move (Njenga and Tsuma 2004).
- **Reduced milk production:** Uterine rupture can lead to reduced milk production and signs of systemic illness.

26.2.3.3 Diagnosis

- ❖ **Physical examination:** Assess the cow's overall condition, vital signs, and the extent of hemorrhage (Purohit 2012).
- ❖ **Ultrasonography:** Ultrasonographic examinations can be a valuable diagnostic tool for assessing uterine rupture and its associated complications, such as PPH, in cattle (Abuom et al. 2012). While ultrasonography may not be the primary method of diagnosing uterine rupture, it can provide valuable information about the condition of the uterus and surrounding tissues (Figure 26.2).
  - ❖ Confirming uterine rupture: Ultrasonography may help when confirming the presence of uterine rupture by visualizing the following:
    1) *Fluid accumulation:* Uterine rupture can lead to the accumulation of fluid within the abdominal cavity (Jeyakumari et al. 2006). Ultrasonography can detect the presence of free fluid or blood in the abdomen, which can be indicative of a ruptured uterus.
    2) *Uterine wall integrity:* Ultrasonography can help assess the integrity of the uterine wall (Njenga and Tsuma 2004). A rupture may appear as a disruption in the normal uterine wall layers.
  - ❖ Assessing PPH: Ultrasonography can provide insights into the extent of PPH and its effects on the reproductive tract (Njenga and Tsuma 2004):
    1) *Blood clots and fluids:* Ultrasonography may reveal the presence of blood clots or fluids within the uterus or abdominal cavity.
    2) *Uterine contractility:* Ultrasonography can be used to monitor the contraction of the uterus, which can help assess its ability to expel remaining fetal membranes and manage PPH (Abuom et al. 2012).

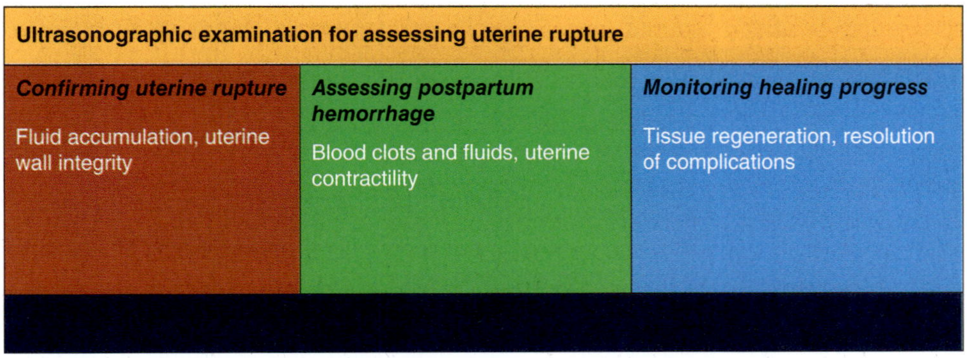

Figure 26.2 Use of ultrasonograms for assessing uterine rupture.

- Monitoring healing progress: After treatment and intervention for uterine rupture and PPH, ultrasonography can be used to monitor the healing process (Jeyakumari et al. 2006):
  1) *Tissue regeneration:* Ultrasonography can track the healing of the uterine wall and the reduction of fluid accumulation within the abdominal cavity.
  2) *Resolution of complications:* Ultrasonography can help assess the resolution of any complications (Purohit 2012), such as uterine infection or inflammation.
- Guiding interventions: Ultrasonography can guide veterinarians during certain interventions related to uterine rupture and PPH (Sheldon et al. 2008):
  1) *Surgical planning:* If surgical intervention is required, ultrasonography can assist in guiding the placement of incisions and sutures.
  2) *Fluid drainage:* Ultrasonography can guide the placement of drainage catheters if fluid accumulation needs to be addressed.

26.2.3.4 Treatment

The treatment approach aims to stabilize the cow, manage shock, address PPH, and repair the uterine rupture if possible.

1) **Stabilization and support:**
   a) Fluid therapy: Intravenous fluid administration is essential to restore fluid balance and combat shock caused by severe blood loss.
   b) Blood transfusion: If the cow is severely anemic due to significant hemorrhage, a blood transfusion may be necessary to replace lost blood volume and improve oxygen-carrying capacity (Abuom et al. 2012).
   c) Pain management: Appropriate pain relief medication, such as NSAIDs, can help alleviate pain and discomfort.
2) **Surgical intervention:** Surgery is often the primary treatment option for uterine rupture (Njenga and Tsuma 2004). The goal of surgery is to repair the uterine tear and prevent further complications. The surgical procedure may involve:
   a) Exploratory laparotomy: An abdominal incision is made to access the abdominal cavity and examine the extent of the rupture and associated damage.
   b) Uterine repair: If the rupture is identified and is amenable to repair, the veterinarian will carefully suture the torn uterine wall layers to promote healing.
   c) Hysterectomy: In cases of severe uterine damage or extensive rupture, a partial or complete hysterectomy (removal of the uterus) may be performed to control bleeding and prevent further complications (Sheldon et al. 2008).
3) **Antibiotics:** Broad-spectrum antibiotics are typically administered to prevent or treat uterine infections that can arise from uterine rupture. Infections can exacerbate the cow's condition and delay healing.
4) **Monitoring and post-operative care:**
   a) Uterine healing: Post surgery, the cow will need careful monitoring to ensure proper uterine healing and prevent complications like infection or dehiscence (re-opening of the surgical site).
   b) Wound care: Careful wound management and hygiene are crucial to prevent infections at the surgical site.
   c) Fluid and nutritional support: Continued fluid therapy and nutritional support help the cow recover from shock and blood loss.
5) **Prognosis and decision making:** The prognosis for uterine rupture depends on factors such as the severity of the rupture, the promptness of treatment, the cow's overall health, and the success of surgical intervention (Jeyakumari et al. 2006). Uterine rupture is a serious condition, and the outcome can be guarded, especially in cases of extensive damage or severe hemorrhage (Njenga and Tsuma 2004).

26.2.3.5 Prevention

Preventing uterine rupture involves proper management during calving and pregnancy.

- **Assisted calving:** Timely and proper assistance during difficult calvings can help reduce the risk of uterine rupture.
- **Nutrition:** Adequate nutrition during pregnancy helps prevent excessive fetal growth and uterine distension.
- **Avoid trauma:** Minimize physical stress and trauma during calving and handling.

It is important to emphasize that uterine rupture is a critical emergency, and prompt intervention is essential for a positive outcome (Mandali et al. 2004). If you suspect uterine rupture in a cow, immediate care is crucial to maximize the chances of saving the animal's life and minimizing complications.

26.2.3.6 Prognosis

The prognosis for a cow with uterine rupture depends on the severity of the rupture, the promptness of veterinary care, and the cow's overall health (Sheldon et al. 2008). In many cases, uterine rupture is a life-threatening condition, and the outcome can be guarded, particularly if there is extensive hemorrhage or other complications.

26.2.3.7 Prevention

Preventing uterine rupture involves the careful management of calving and minimizing risk factors (Mandali et al. 2004). Proper nutrition, appropriate assistance during calving, and maintaining a clean and stress-free calving environment can help reduce the likelihood of uterine rupture (Abuom et al. 2012). If you suspect uterine rupture or notice severe PPH in a cow, it is crucial to seek immediate assistance to maximize the chances of a positive outcome.

26.3 Conclusion

In conclusion, PPH in cattle is a significant and potentially life-threatening complication that can occur after calving. It is characterized by excessive bleeding from the reproductive tract following the birth of a calf (Mandali et al. 2004). Retained placentas and uterine rupture are common underlying causes of PPH, both of which can result in severe blood loss, shock, and systemic complications.

Effective management and treatment of postpartum hemorrhaging requires a multidimensional approach that involves prompt veterinary intervention, proper diagnosis, and appropriate therapeutic strategies (Sheldon et al. 2008). The timely recognition of clinical signs, such as prolonged vaginal discharge, weakness, and anemia, is crucial for early intervention.

References

Abuom, T.O., Njenga, M.J., Wabacha, J.K. et al. (2012). Incidence and risk factors of periparturient conditions in smallholder dairy cattle herds in Kikuyu Division of Kiambu District, Kenya. *Ethiopian Veterinary Journal* 16 (2): 85–102.

Jeyakumari, M., Thirunavukkarasu, M., and Kathivaran, G. (2006). Factors influencing the incidence of postpartum reproductive disorders in bovines Tamil Nadu. *Journal of Veterinary and Animal Sciences* 2 (5): 188–190.

Mandali, G.C., Patel, P.R., and Joshi, R.S. (2004). Techno-economics of periparturient disorders in dairy buffaloes of rural Gujarat. *Indian Journal of Veterinary Medicine* 24: 84–89.

Njenga, J.M. and Tsuma, V.T. (2004). Sudden death following rupture of mid uterine artery, in a bovine dystocia. *Kenya Veterinary* 26: 27–28.

Purohit, G.N. (2012). Postpartum complications in large animals. In: *Domestic Animal Obstetrics* (ed. G.N. Purohit), 551–603. Germany: Lambert Academic Publishers.

Sharma, N., Gautam, A., and Upadhyay, S.R. (2006). Role of antioxidants in udder health: a review. *Indian Journal of Field Veterinarians* 2: 73–76.

Sheldon, I.M., Williams, E.J., Miller, A.N. et al. (2008). Uterine diseases in cattle after parturition. *Veterinary Journal* 176 (1): 115–121. https://doi.org/10.1016/j.tvjl.2007.12.031.

Smith, B.I. and Risco, C.A. (2005). Management of periparturient disorders in dairy cattle. *The Veterinary Clinics of North America. Food Animal Practice* 21: 503–521.

27

Nutritional Hemoglobinuria

Suman Biswas[1], *Shubhamitra Chaudhuri*[2], *and Tanmoy Rana*[2]

[1] *Department of Avian Science, West Bengal University of Animal & Fishery Sciences, Kolkata, West Bengal, India*
[2] *Department of Veterinary Clinical Complex, West Bengal University of Animal & Fishery Sciences, Kolkata, West Bengal, India*

27.1 Introduction

Nutritional hemoglobinuria (NH) is a metabolic disease of high yield dairy cattle, usually occurs in late pregnancy to 30 days post calving during their third to sixth lactation (Radostits et al. 2007), and is characterized by intravascular hemolysis, anemia, and hemoglobinuria (Sharma et al. 2020). The disease has been documented as sporadic in nature, affecting one or two animals in a herd at a time. NH has also been recorded in sheep, Egyptian and Indian buffaloes, and goats, along with many other similarities (Macwilliams et al. 1982). This disease has been documented worldwide with different names like parturient hemoglobinemia or hemoglobinuria (Madsen and Nielsen 1939), red water (Schofield 1933), and rakthmutna (Resum et al. 2017) that have been used synonymously with post-parturient hemoglobinuria (PPH) in many publications (Farquharson and Smith 1938). Even though the precise etiology of NH is unknown, phosphorus depletion or hypophosphatemia, copper deficiency, and maybe the hemolyzing chemicals present in some feed have all been identified as potential causes or risk factors (Radostits et al. 2007). Due to the low milk production, high costs of treatment, and high case-fatality rates, the disease is very important economically (Sharma et al. 2014). This chapter includes NH etiology, epidemiology, risk factors, etiopathogenesis, clinical findings, clinical pathology, diagnosis, treatment, and prevention strategies with a summary and conclusion.

27.2 Etiology

NH is caused by a variety of underlying variables, many of which are poorly understood. Hypophosphatemia and phosphorous insufficiencies have been listed as potential causes of the NH syndrome (Gocher et al. 2018). However, diets lacking in phosphorus or feeds without phosphorous supplements are frequently linked with this disease in dairy cows in several nations, including the United States, India, Pakistan, and other Asian countries (Rahmati et al. 2021). The deficiency of copper (Cu) in soil or supplemented feed causes NH in dairy cattle (Radostits et al. 2007). Copper supplementation of feed has been found to reduce the incidence of NH in dairy cattle (Resum et al. 2017). The lack of copper (Cu) and selenium (Se), according to some literature, is another factor in the high incidence of one form of NH in New Zealand (Ellison et al. 1986). According to several reports, the ingestion of certain plants through feed, like cruciferous vegetables, is connected to the occurrence of NH in cattle (Freudenberg 1955). A chronic calcium deficiency may lead to the development of NH in lactating cattle (Goff 2000).

27.3 Epidemiology and Risk Factors

NH typically affects lactating cattle herds sporadically, and its occurrence in the animal population is relatively rare (Senthil Kumar et al. 2014). NH in dairy cattle has been reported from Iraq (SaedAlbayati and Luaibi 2020), India (Bhikane and Syed 2014), North America, and Australia (Macwilliams et al. 1982). The incidence of NH in cattle is very high during the

Periparturient Diseases of Cattle, First Edition. Edited by Tanmoy Rana.

third to sixth lactations, with a case-fatality rate from 10% to 50% (Resum et al. 2017). In Europe and North America, PPH is more frequent after a long period of housing, although in regions with severe phosphorous deficiency, it can happen when cattle are feeding in the pasture (Rahmati et al. 2021).

There are numerous potential risk factors for NH, including age, number of lactations, pregnancy stage, postpartum period, previous history of hemoglobinuria, and the consumption of cruciferous and/or poisonous plants (Mahmood et al. 2013; Khan and Akhtar 2007). In dairy cattle, an exposure to cold temperatures and drinking cold water can also result in NH (Radostits et al. 2007). The application of lime or molybdate fertilizer to pastureland increases the concentration of molybdenum (Mo) in the soil and decreases copper (Cu) concentrations. These conditions lead to the development of NH in grazing lactating cattle, especially during the months of July, August, September, and October. It mostly occurs due to excess molybdenum that interferes with the absorption of copper from the gastrointestinal tract of cattle (Smith 1978). There are several reports suggesting that some other minerals like iron (Fe) and aluminum (Al) also interfere with the availability of phosphorus (P) to animals (Payne 1989). This relationship is known as a "conditioning factor." Insufficient phosphorus levels in the soil, caused by rain-induced leaching or human activities like continuous crop removal, lead to phosphorus deficiency in the grown plants, which in turn causes NH in cattle when consumed (Shupe et al. 1988).

From calving until 3–4 weeks after parturition, which is the transition between late pregnancy and early lactation, is a time when the disease in dairy cows is most likely to occur (Mahmut et al. 2009). During the advanced gestational period, more phosphorus and calcium are required by the growing fetus and hypophosphatemia or NH develops if supplementation is not provided in the proper ratio (Digraskar et al. 1991). Hypophosphatemia may be caused by impaired phosphorus absorption from the gut as a result of a high Ca : P ratio, vitamin D deficiency, or gastrointestinal diseases (Bhikane and Syed 2014). Hypophosphatemia may result from excessive phosphorus loss through milk, especially in high milk producing animals (Bhikane et al. 1995). Lactational stress conditions and calcium deficiency increase the activities of the parathyroid hormone, which increases the excretion of phosphorus through renal and salivary secretions and ultimately leads to phosphorus deficiency in cattle (Goff 2000; Gocher et al. 2018). But some researchers have also reported that high milk production is not related to NH (Akhtar et al. 2008; Mahmood et al. 2012).

27.4 Etiopathogenesis

NH is caused by a phosphorous shortage, even though its etiology and pathophysiology are not completely understood. As a result, its incidence may rise in high yield dairy animals at the start of lactation. It has been noted by some researchers that most animals with phosphorous deficiencies do not experience intravascular hemolysis (Gocher et al. 2018). Although, the precise mechanism of intravascular hemolysis in NH is as yet unknown, the severe hypophosphatemia seen in affected animals clearly suggests a role for phosphorus in this condition. The following describes one possible method of hemolysis in NH.

The energy requirement of erythrocytes is provided by extracellular glucose. Glucose absorption by erythrocytes is facilitated by inorganic phosphorus. Therefore, hypophosphatemia affects the glycolytic pathway in bovine erythrocytes, causing ATP depletion (Malik and Samad 1996). The phosphorylation of numerous cytoskeletal proteins, including spectrin and actomysin, and the production of membrane phospholipids within erythrocytes are significant functions of ATP that contribute to the regulation of erythrocyte shape and deformability. As a result, erythrocytes with low ATP levels are less pliable and more susceptible to hemolysis (Ogawa et al. 1987). Lowered ATP within the red blood cell (RBC) causes the pentose phosphate shunt to function less efficiently, which in turn causes NADPH, NADH, and glutathione (GSH) to decrease. While NADPH is required for the regeneration of reduced GSH from its oxidized (glutathione disulfide [GSSG]) form, NADH is required for the conversion of methemoglobin to oxyhemoglobin (Ogawa et al. 1989). Reduced glutathione provides protection to erythrocytes against free radicals. Hence, lowering GSH, NADPH, and NADH results in increased oxidative stress and decreased reducing potential (Mata and Bhardwaj 1985). This leads to the precipitation of hemoglobin as Heinz bodies and intravascular hemolysis.

27.5 Clinical Findings

The first notable clinical symptom in affected dairy cows is a change in the color of their urine from red to brown (Resum et al. 2017), which is followed by anemia, depression, inappetence, or a reduction in milk production (Madsen and Nielsen 1939). Mucous membranes become pale and may turn icteric as the anemia progresses. Breathing becomes shallow and fast as the heart rate rises (80–130 beats per minute). Affected cows are emaciated and frequently found lying down. The feces of the affected animal are usually dry and firm but may also be bile stained or fetid and diarrheic (Macwilliams et al. 1982). An elevated body temperature (103–104 °F) is noticed in the early stage of the disease with a variable feature of increased thirsts.

Acute disease (3–5 days) may lead to the death of the animals or be followed by a prolonged convalescence (2–8 weeks). Recovered animals may show ketonuria with a depraved appetite (Radostits et al. 2007). The body condition and milk production of recovered animals gradually returns to normal. Some animals may show common sequelae, i.e. gangrene and sloughing of the digits, tails, and teats (Macwilliams et al. 1982).

27.6 Clinical Pathology

A serum analysis of the affected animals reveals low phosphorus concentrations (1.6–3.0 mg/dl) with typical symptoms of NH (Kumar et al. 2021). But some animals may have moderately low concentrations of phosphorus (>4 mg/dl) without any proper clinical sign and symptoms (Rahmati et al. 2021). Hematologically, NH exhibits the characteristics of an acute intravascular hemolytic anemia. About 4–9 days after hemoglobinuria first appears, the packed cell volume (PCV) rapidly decreases (16%) to its lowest point (Kumar et al. 2021; Macwilliams et al. 1982). The plasma and visible mucous membranes initially become hemoglobinemic, but as the massive RBC destruction progresses, they turn yellow. Polychromasia, anisocytosis, macrocytosis, basophilic stippling, reticulocytosis, and an increase of metarubricytes are all seen on a stained blood smear. Swollen erythrocytes with dimpled centers result in the increased osmotic fragility of RBCs. The RBC concentration, hemoglobin (Hb), and PCV levels of affected animals were significantly lower than normal, which demonstrates a positive correlation between the total RBC count and both Hb and PCV that resulted in severe anemia. According to several studies, the elevated levels of creatinine, bilirubin, blood sugar, and serum ALP suggest that the affected animals may have developed jaundice as a result of intravascular hemolysis (Bradford 2002; Akhtar et al. 2008). According to Zhang et al. (2017), NH is associated with a notable reduction in RBC count, a rise in mean corpuscular volume (MCV), and a drop in mean corpuscular hemoglobin level (MCH).

27.7 Diagnosis

The affected animal's past clinical history, clinical symptoms, including coffee-colored urine (Figure 27.1), pale mucous membranes, and straining during feces, as well as laboratory results like the activity of lecithin cholesterol acyltransferase (LCAT), are commonly used to diagnose NH (Ghanem and El-Deeb 2010). Serum phosphorus levels in the affected cattle are also used as an important diagnostic and prognostic marker of NH (Ogawa et al. 1987). The benzidine test can be used to determine whether there is hemoglobin in the urine, and it is also useful for diagnosing NH (Senthil Kumar et al. 2014). A low PCV, low serum phosphorus, and hemoglobinuria have all been reported as diagnostic indicators of NH.

27.7.1 Necropsy Findings

The common features of necropsy observed in cattle include a visibly pale mucous membrane, hepatomegaly, a huge amount of red-colored urine in the bladder, and renomegaly with congestion (Figure 27.2) (Radostits et al. 2007). Hemosiderin deposition is also observed in the liver and kidneys.

27.7.2 Urine Analysis

In NH, the simplest and most crucial diagnostic technique is a urine analysis of the affected cattle. The visible color of the urine of the cattle varies from a dark red to coffee colored (Khan and Akhtar, 2007). The affected NH cattle had 100% hemoglobin positivity and 95% albumin positivity in their urine (Akhtar et al. 2008). A high urine pH is also observed in cattle. The pH range varies from 8 to 9 (Gocher et al. 2018).

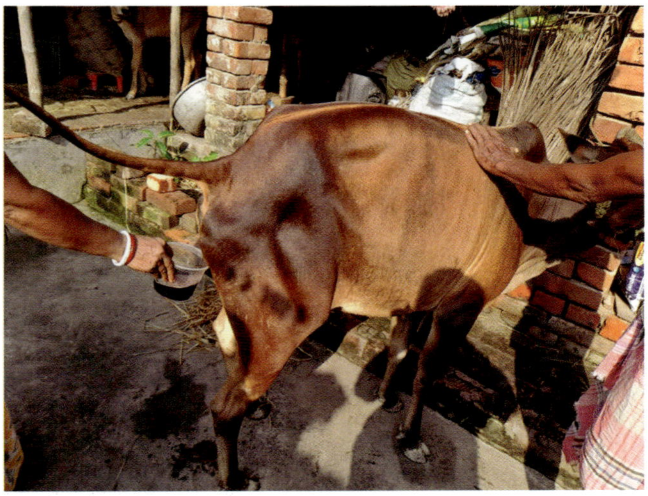

Figure 27.1 Nutritional hemoglobinuria in a cow.

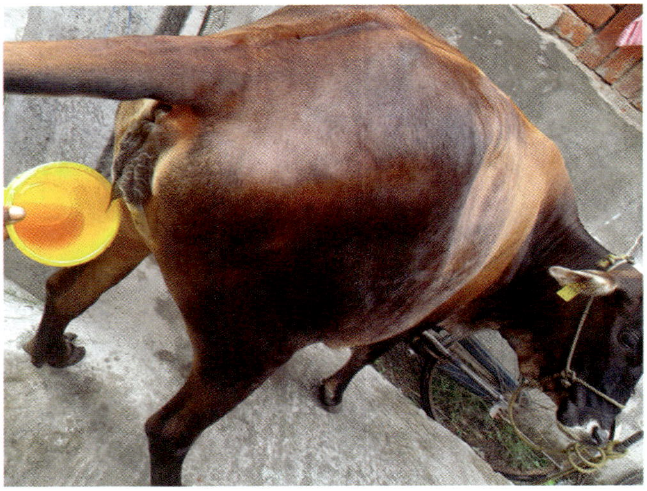

Figure 27.2 Red urine from a cow.

27.7.3 Hematology

Hematologically, NH resembles an acute, intravascular, hemolytic anemia. The anemia is characterized morphologically by indications of increased erythrogenesis. On stained blood films, polychromasia, anisocytosis, macrocytosis, basophilic stippling, reticulocytosis, and an increase in metarubricytes are frequently observed (Macwilliams et al. 1982). About 4–9 days following the commencement of hemoglobinuria, the PCV decreases quickly and reaches its lowest level. When compared to healthy animals, NH-affected animals have higher erythrocyte sedimentation rates, while having reduced mean erythrocyte counts, hemoglobin concentrations, and hematocrit levels (Durrani et al. 2010).

27.7.4 Biochemical Analysis

Severe hypophosphatemia has been reported from NH-affected cattle. Low levels of phosphorus are responsible for the development of NH in cattle (Mahmut et al. 2009). In acute cases, the serum phosphorus levels were reduced to 0.5–1.5 mg/dl (Karapınar et al. 2006). Animals with NH had lower serum levels of phosphorus (1.8 mg/dl) and copper (63.4 μg/dl) but greater levels of molybdenum (185.2 μg/dl) (Durrani et al. 2010). Whereas healthy animals were reported to have higher levels of copper (118.4 μg/dl) and phosphorus (5.41 mg/dl) with low serum molybdenum (54.8 μg/dl) concentrations. Sulfides are generally produced by rumen microbes through the reduction of sulfate and degradation of sulfur-containing amino acids. These sulfides combine with molybdate to form thiomolybdates, which bind to copper and form insoluble complexes that prevent copper from being used by the animal, which results in copper deficiency. This insoluble complex is resistant to acidic conditions, does not release copper, and ultimately, results in hemoglobinuria (Durrani et al. 2010). High urea and creatinine in NH-affected animals have been reported by many authors (Durrani et al. 2010; Tewari et al. 2014). This may be due to renal cell damage that results from anemic hypoxia and extensive hemolysis during the disease process (Digraskar et al. 1991).

27.8 Treatment

There are a variety of NH therapy options available that can save the lives of affected animals and reduce the severity of their anemia. A diagnosis concurrent with immediate specific treatment is an important factor in NH therapy. In the case of hemoglobinuria in cattle, parenteral phosphorus supplementation and routine hematologic assessments can be helpful in determining the prognosis and effectiveness of treatment. The different therapeutic options are:

a) Through the intravenous method, 60 g of sodium dihydrogen orthophosphate ($NaH_2PO_4 \cdot 2H_2O$) mixed in 5% dextrose solution (D_5) was administered, followed by oral administration of the same dose twice daily for 3 days (Pandey and Misra 1987).
b) Animals with hemoglobinuria can be effectively and safely treated with a buffered solution of sodium acid phosphate, inosine, and sodium pyruvate administered intravenously at a dose of 50 ml on the first day and 25 ml on the subsequent 2–3 days (Bhikane et al. 2011). Being a buffered preparation, it does not exacerbate the acidosis that occurs in cases of hemoglobinuria. Inosine and sodium pyruvate are also added, which promotes ATP synthesis in RBC cells, reduces high oxidative stress, and eliminates Heinz bodies from the circulatory system.
c) As a standard treatment for hemoglobinuria in dairy animals, sodium acid phosphate at 60–80 g through an intravenous route as a 20% solution in dextrose or distilled water, daily for 2–4 days, has been utilized (Chugh et al. 1996).
d) In situations where copper insufficiency is thought to be the underlying cause of NH, 60 g of sodium acid phosphate administered intravenously is advised, followed by copper glycinate at 1.5 mg/kg body weight (BW) in 500 ml of normal saline solution administered intravenously as a single dosage (Radostits et al. 2007).

e) Supportive therapy with vitamin C at 15–20 mg/kg BW through an intravenous route is also recommended (Bhikane and Syed 2014). As an antioxidant, ascorbic acid helps minimize intravascular hemolysis and RBC oxidative stress (Soren et al. 2014).
f) Supportive therapy with dexamethasone, the parental administration of vitamin B complex, calcium borogluconate, and oral liver tonic supplementation are also recommended (Rahmati et al. 2021). To replenish lost blood, parental iron injections or oral hematinic preparations are also encouraged.

27.9 Prevention

For the prevention of NH, especially during late pregnancy and early lactation, a sufficient intake of phosphorus should be ensured in accordance with maintenance and milk production needs (Gocher et al. 2018). As it is a multifactorial metabolic disorder of cattle, along with an adequate supplementation of daily phosphorus needs, other mineral and vitamin supplementations should also be ensured. It is advised to supplement a source of phosphorous in rations or drinking water when the serum inorganic phosphorous level is below 5 g/dl (Muhammad et al. 2001). Other minerals like Ca, Zn, Cu, iodine, Mn, and Mg should be supplemented as per recommended doses to maintain normal mineral homeostasis in dairy cattle. Vitamins D and E in the form of a composite injection should be used once a month as per the BW of the animals. Phosphorous and calcium absorption from the small intestine can be improved by parenteral vitamin D therapy. It is recommended to eliminate lucerne, berseem, sugar beets, and other cruciferous plants from the diets of dairy and pregnant cattle. In copper deficient areas, ensure adequate supplementation or consumption of dietary phosphorous and copper.

27.10 Summary and Conclusion

NH, which is characterized by acute intravascular hemolysis, hemoglobinuria, anemia, and hypophosphatemia, is mainly caused by a phosphorus insufficiency. The third to sixth lactational postpartum period are crucial time periods in high yielding dairy cows. Dietary phosphorus deficits and/or diets high in cruciferous vegetables or beetroot products are thought to be the root causes of NH. Once all other potential causes of intravascular hemolysis have been ruled out, a diagnosis of NH can be made based on the environmental and ration history, clinical presentation, and laboratory results. It may be possible to prevent PPH by providing mineral supplements throughout the final trimester of pregnancy or the first few months of the lactational period.

References

Akhtar, M.Z., Khan, A., Khan, M.Z., and Javaid, A. (2008). Patho-biochemical changes in buffaloes (*Bubalus bubalis*) suffering from parturient hemoglobinuria. *Pakistan Veterinary Journal* 28: 139–143.

Bhikane, A.U. and Syed, A.U. (2014). Recent trends in management of metabolic disorders of transition cows and buffaloes. *Intas Polivet* 15 (II): 485–496.

Bhikane, A.U., Ali, M.S., Narladkar, B.W., and Kawitkar, S.B. (1995). Post parturient hemoglobinuria in a crossbred cow and its treatment. *Indian Veteterinaty Journal* 72: 734–736.

Bhikane, A.U., Ghoke, S.S., Masare, P.S. et al. (2011). A new approach in clinical management of phosphorous deficiency haemoglobinuria in buffaloes. *Intas Polivet* 12: 56–58.

Bradford, P.S. (2002). *Large Animal Internal Medicine*, 303–304. London: Mosby.

Chugh, S.K., Mata, M.M., and Malik, K.S. (1996). Epidemiological observations in post-parturient haemoglobinuria in buffaloes. *The Indian Journal of Animal Sciences* 66: 1123–1125.

Digraskar, S., Singh, B., and Deshpande, B.B. (1991). Epidemiology and clinico-pathology of hemoglobinuria in buffalo (*Bubalus bubalis*). *Livestock Advisor.* 16: 32–38.

Durrani, A.Z., Kamal, N., Shakoori, A.R., and Younus, R.M. (2010). Prevalence of post parturient hemoglobinuria in buffalo and therapeutic trials with toldimfos sodium and tea leaves in Pakistan. *Turkish Journal of Veterinary and Animal Sciences* 34: 45–51.

Ellison, R.S., Young, B.J., and Read, D.H. (1986). Bovine postparturient hemoglobinuria: two distinct entities in New Zealand. *New Zealand Veterinary Journal* 34: 7–10.

Farquharson, J. and Smith, K.W. (1938). Post-parturient hemoglobinuria of cattle. *Journal of the American Veterinary Medical Association* 93: 37–39.

Freudenberg, F. (1955). Incidence and causes of haemoglobinuria in cows in central Germany. *Deutsche Tierärztliche Wochenschrift* 62: 422–429.

Ghanem, M.M. and El-Deeb, W.M. (2010). Lecithin cholesterol acyltransferase (LCAT) activity as a predictor for ketosis and parturient hemoglobinuria in Egyptian water buffaloes. *Research in Veterinary Science* 88: 20–25.

Gocher, P.T., Chaudhary, A.K., Arora, A.S. et al. (2018). Perspectives of parturient hemoglobinuria (Pph) in buffaloes. *International Journal of Development Research* 8: 23513–23520.

Goff, J.P. (2000). Pathology of calcium and phosphorous disorders. *Veterinary Clinics of North America: Food Animal Practice* 16: 319–337.

Karapınar, T., Dabak, M., and Kırbas, A. (2006). İkiinekte tespit edilen puerperel hemoglobinüri ve tedavisi. *Dogu Anadolu Arastırma Dergisi, Türkiye.* 2: 7–10.

Khan, A. and Akhtar, M.Z. (2007). Hemato-biochemical and clinico-epidemiological aspects of parturient hemoglobinuria in Nili-Ravi buffaloes. *Italian Journal of Animal Science* 6 (2): 953–956.

Kumar, G.S., Kumar, T.A., and Dharmaceelan, S. (2021). Postparturient hemoglobinuria and its medical management in a Buffalo. *Indian Journal of Veterinary Medicine* 41 (1): 89–90.

Macwilliams, P.S., Searcy, G.P., and Bellamy, J.E. (1982). Bovine postparturient hemoglobinuria: a review of the literature. *The Canadian Veterinary Journal* 23 (11): 309–312.

Madsen, D.E. and Nielsen, H.M. (1939). Parturient hemoglobinemia of dairy cows. *Journal of the American Veterinary Medical Association* 94: 577–586.

Mahmood, A., Khan, M., Younus, M. et al. (2012). Case-control study of parturient hemoglobinuria in buffaloes. *Pakistan Veterinary Journal* 32 (3): 375–377.

Mahmood, A., Khan, M.A., Younus, M. et al. (2013). Haematological and biochemical risk factors of parturient hemoglobinuria in buffaloes. *Journal of Animal and Plant Sciences* 23: 364–368.

Mahmut, O.K., Guzelbektes, H., Ismail, S. et al. (2009). Post-parturient hemoglobinuria in three dairy cows. A case report. *Bulletin of the Veterinary Institute in Pulawy* 53: 421–423.

Malik, H.U. and Samad, A. (1996). Study on the utilization of glucose by erythrocytes and its dependence on inorganic phosphorus. *Buffalo Journal* 1: 94–97.

Mata, M.M. and Bhardwaj, R.M. (1985). Possible alterations in erythrocyte metabolism and integrity in post-parturient hemoglobinuria. *Indian Journal of Veterinary Medicine* 5 (2): 67–72.

Muhammad, G., Saqib, M., and Athar, M. (2001). A rational approach to diagnosis, treatment and control of parturient haemoglobinuria (red water) in buffaloes and cattle. *Pakistan Veterinary Journal* 21: 214–219.

Ogawa, E., Koboyashi, K., Yoshiura, M., and Mukai, J. (1987). Bovine post-parturient haemoglobinuria: hypophosphataemia and metabolic disorder in red blood cells. *American Journal of Veterinary Research* 48: 1300–1303.

Ogawa, E., Kosaky, K., Yoshiura, N., and Mukai, J. (1989). Haemolytic anaemia and red cell metabolic disorder attributable to low phosphorus intake in cows. *American Journal of Veterinary Research* 50: 388–392.

Pandey, N.N. and Misra, S.K. (1987). Clinico-biochemical studies of nutritional haemoglobinuria in buffaloes and its therapy. *The Indian Veterinary Journal* 64: 39–43.

Payne, J.M. (1989). *Metabolic and Nutritional Diseases of Cattle*. London: Blackwell Scientific Publishers.

Radostits, O.M., Gay, C.C., Hinchcliff, K.W., and Constable, P.D. (2007). *Veterinary Medicine: A Textbook of the Diseases of Cattle, Horses, Sheep, Pigs and Goats*, 10e, 1682–1683. Philadelphia: WB Saunders Co. Ltd.

Rahmati, S., Aziz, A., Tawfeeq, M.M. et al. (2021). Clinical features of post-parturient hemoglobinuria in dairy cattle and buffaloes: a review. *Open Journal of Veterinary Medicine* 11: 143–155.

Resum, N.S., Kour, P., Singh, H., and Sharma, N. (2017). Post-partum hemoglobinuria (PPH) in bovine. *Theriogenology Insight* 7 (1): 51–59.

SaedAlbayati, O.A.S. and Luaibi, O.K. (2020). Study of hemato-biochemical changes in post-parturient hemoglobinurea in Iraqi local cows. *Plant Archives* 20: 584–588.

Schofield, F.W. (1933). Bovine hemoglobinuria associated with an intestinal infection caused by the Cl. welchii. *Report of the Ontario Veterinary College*, 1933: 42–61.

Senthil Kumar, A., Sri Balaji, N., and Uma Rani, R. (2014). Acute post-parturient hemoglobinuria in a cross bred dairy cow. *International Journal of Agricultural Sciences and Veterinary Medicine* 2: 1–3.

Sharma, S.K., Joshi, M., Singh, D., and Khosa, J.S. (2014). A hemato-biochemical and therapeutic study of postpartum hemoglobinuria in buffaloes. *Intas Polivet* 15 (2): 523–525.

Sharma, V., Kumar, H., Kumar, S., and Yadav, M. (2020). Therapeutic management of post-parturient haemoglobunuria in buffalo: a case report. *The Pharma Innovation Journal* 9: 299–301.

Shupe, J.L., Butcher, J.E., Call, J.W. et al. (1988). Clinical signs and bone changes associated with phosphorus deficiency in beef cattle. *American Journal of Veterinary Research* 49 (9): 1629–1636.

Smith, R.H. (1978). S-methylcysteine sulphoxide, the brassica anaemia factor. *Veterinary Science Communications* 2: 47–61.

Soren, S., Srivastava, M., Kachhawa, J.P., and Soren, P. (2014). Clinical study on postpartum hemoglobinuria in buffaloes. *Intas Polivet* 15 (2): 518–522.

Tewari, D., Singh, V.K., and Gautam, S. (2014). Clinical Management of Parturient Hemoglobinuria in a Buffalo (*Bubalus Bubalis*). *Intas Polivet.* 15 (2): 528–530.

Zhang, Z., Bi, M., Yang, J. et al. (2017). Effect of Phosphorus Deficiency on Erythrocytic Morphology and Function in Cows. *Journal of Veterinary Science* 18: 333–340.

28

Infertility

Abhijeet Fernandes[1], Gitesh Saini[1], and Neeti Lakhani[2]

[1] *Department of Veterinary Gynaecology and Obstetrics, COVS, Rampura Phul, Guru Angad Dev Veterinary and Animal Sciences University, Bathinda, Punjab, India*
[2] *Department of Animal Nutrition, COVS, Rampura Phul, Guru Angad Dev Veterinary and Animal Sciences University, Bathinda, Punjab, India*

28.1 Introduction

Fertility plays a pivotal role in achieving the ultimate reproductive objective of "one calf per cow per year," thereby augmenting the overall lifetime productivity of a cow (Dijkhuizen et al. 1985). To accomplish this goal, livestock must be bred consistently, necessitating a well-functioning and physiologically proficient reproductive system that includes the demonstration of estrus behavior, successful ovulation, facilitation of fertilization, and support for embryonic development. Determining the underlying cause of decreased fertility is challenging since fertility is a multifactorial attribute that is influenced by a complex interplay of various agents (Figure 28.1). Any physiological deviation in environmental and management elements will hinder the reproductive ability of livestock.

Cattle infertility is an important economic factor in cattle farming (Kastelic 2013), which is interpreted as a decline in the annual calf weaning rate per cow (Titterington et al. 2017); infertility is the temporary loss of fertility or reduced fertility, and sterility is the complete inability of a female to become pregnant and give birth to live offspring. Infertility not only curtails reproductive efficiency but also leads to significant economic loss, including increased veterinary expenses, calf mortality, production declines, and ultimately, necessitates the culling of animals. Understanding the significance of cattle infertility is vital for farmers, veterinarians, and policymakers as it directly influences the profitability and productivity of cattle farming operations. Addressing this issue necessitates a comprehensive approach that includes improved management practices, enhanced genetic selection, and a focus on preventing and managing infectious causes of infertility.

28.2 Causes of Infertility

Infertility, a multifaceted and complex concern, presents substantial hurdles in cattle production on a global scale. A range of factors can contribute to reproductive difficulties, which impact fertility rates and jeopardize the overall efficiency of breeding programs. Causes of infertility in cattle are diverse and can stem from infectious diseases, nutritional imbalances, management practices, and environmental factors. Identifying and understanding these underlying causes are crucial for implementing effective strategies to address infertility, improve reproductive performance, and sustain a productive and profitable cattle industry. Causes of infertility can be grossly divided into four categories (Figure 28.2):

I) Nutritional causes
II) Management causes
III) Infectious causes
IV) Functional causes

Periparturient Diseases of Cattle, First Edition. Edited by Tanmoy Rana.

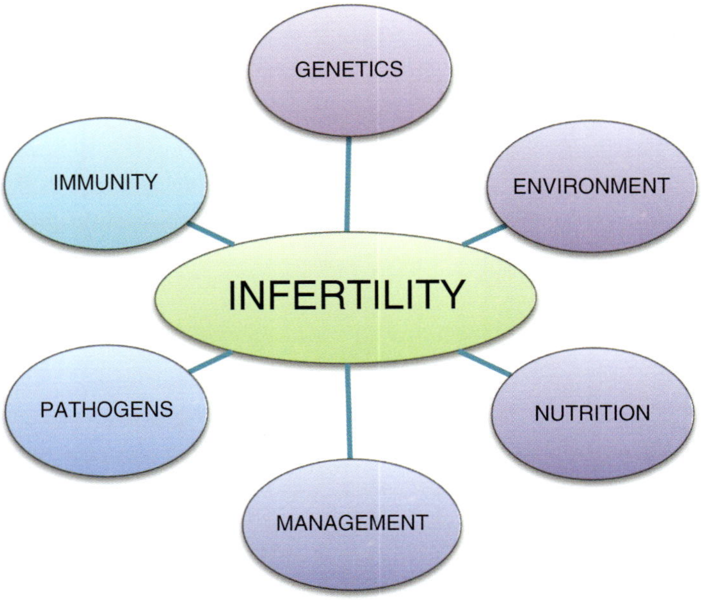

Figure 28.1 Factors that affect fertility in cattle.

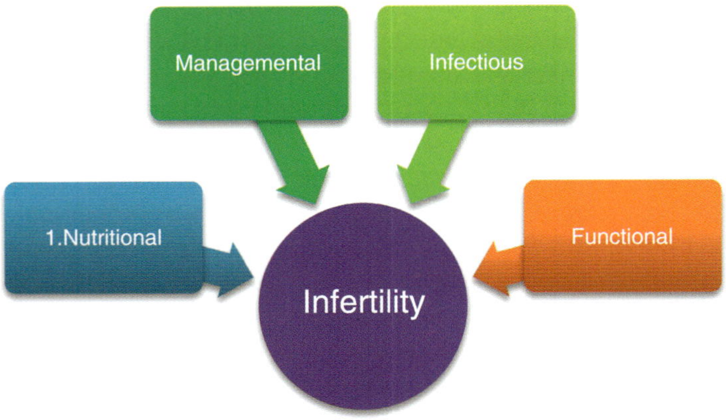

Figure 28.2 Causes of infertility in cattle.

28.2.1 Nutritional Causes

Clinical symptoms of infertility in cattle develop after a deficiency has persisted for a while, therefore it is practically impossible to pinpoint the precise nutritional cause of infertility (Fathalla et al. 2001). Nutritional stress alters the body's state and impairs reproductive capacity, including the peripubertal stage, breeding season, and postpartum period. Deficiencies of various trace minerals, inadequate vitamin intake, and energy protein imbalances (Salem et al. 2006) are mentioned as contributors to infertility and poor reproductive performance. Nutrition and reproduction have a complex interaction starting from birth to first lactation that is important in terms of body weight gain and mammary gland development. A higher growth rate with optimum mammary gland development is required for raising replacement dairy heifers profitably. A decline in reproductive performance with increasing milk yield is not a result of genetic selection for lower breeding efficiency but rather due to unsatisfied nutrient demands.

28.2.1.1 Role of Energy in Diet

In high yielding dairy cows, particularly during early lactation, the substantial energy required to maintain body tissues and support milk production necessitates an increased consumption of nutrients to accommodate the sharp rise in energy demand. These needs are partially met by increased feed consumption and the remaining requirement is fulfilled by mobilizing body reserves, which results in a state of negative energy balance (NEB) (Evans and Walsh 2012). A variety of risk factors like metabolic, hormonal, and environmental factors influence the individual cow response to an NEB and associated adverse health, reproductive, and productive consequences (Youngquist and Threlfall 2006). During an NEB there is a metabolic and hormonal shift because of the increased concentration of non-esterified fatty acids (NEFAs) and lowered concentrations of glucose, insulin, and insulin-like growth factor (IGF)-1 that affect the hypothalamic–pituitary–gonadal (HPG) axis; reducing gonadotropin release impairs steroidogenesis, folliculogenesis, and luteal function as well as interfering with pregnancy maintenance and causing the cessation of cyclical activity, silent estrus, fertilization failure, and early embryonic death (Wodaje and Mekuria 2016). To combat the energy deficiency and improve reproductive status, provision to feed a total of 6% fat in the rations of high yielding animals.

28.2.1.2 Role of Protein in Diet

Dietary protein is a crucial component in the diet that can influence fertility in animals, depending on their concentration in the diet. When excessive amounts of protein are ingested, rumen microorganisms convert it to urea, which modifies the uterine pH and makes it unsuitable for embryonic development as well as hazardous to oocytes and sperm (Hansen 2007). A lower conception rate is observed when blood urea nitrogen (BUN) exceeds 18 mg/dl (Chakurkar et al. 2008). Other consequences include a reduced energy balance in the body due to the utilization of energy in the metabolism and excretion of excess protein. Feeding excess rumen degradable protein (RDP) has a negative effect on fertility as it delays the first ovulation or estrus, reduces the conception rate at first insemination, increases days open, and causes an overall reduction in conception rate (Mulligan et al. 2008). Feeding a high protein diet (23% dry matter [DM]) decreases the uterine concentrations of phosphorus, magnesium, and potassium compared to a low protein diet. All these negative effects can be reduced by restricting the crude protein (CP) content in the diet to less than 19% and limiting RDP to less than 10% of the diet DM (Hansen 2007).

28.2.1.3 Deficiency of Micronutrients

Micronutrient deficits (Table 28.1) affect reproduction by inhibiting ruminal microbial activity and decreasing enzymatic activity, which affects energy, protein metabolism, hormone synthesis, and the integrity of rapidly reproducing cells within the reproductive system (England 2005). Furthermore, a lower antioxidant activity causes a decrease in free radical defense activity.

Table 28.1 Deficiency symptoms of micronutrients.

Nutrient	Deficiency symptoms	References
Energy	Delayed puberty, suppressed estrus and ovulation, suppressed libido, and spermatozoa production	Lucy (2003)
Protein	Suppressed estrus, low conception, fetal resorption, premature parturition, weak offspring	Anderson and Barton (1988), Rhoads et al. (2004), and Wodaje and Mekuria (2016)
Manganese	Impaired steroidogenesis, anestrus, poor follicular development, delayed ovulation and puberty, silent estrus	Kendall and Bone (2006)
Iodine	Fetal goiter, congenital defect, prolonged gestation in horse and sheep, poor libido and estrus behavior, embryonic death	Radostits et al. (2006)
Cobalt	Anemia, silent estrus, irregular inter-estrus interval, altered folliculogenesis	Gagnon et al. (2015)
Copper	Reduction in first service conception rate, silent estrus, impaired embryonic survival	Phillippo et al. (1987)
Phosphorus	Anestrus, subestrus, acyclicity, reduced conception rate, delayed puberty, delayed ovulation	Morris (1976)
Selenium and vitamin E	Retained fetal membranes, delayed uterine involution, metritis, cystic ovarian degeneration, oxidative stress, embryonic loss, fertilization failure	Harrison et al. (1986)
Vitamin A and β-carotene	Delayed puberty, low pregnancy rate, extended follicular phase, delayed ovulation, silent estrus, follicular cysts, congenital blindness, decreased progesterone secretion	Lotthammer et al. (1978) and Radostits et al. (2006)
Zinc	Impaired spermatogenesis, steroidogenesis, prostaglandin synthesis, early embryonic death	Corah 1996
Vitamin D	Suppresses the signs of estrus, delayed ovulation	Chakurkar et al. (2008)

Table 28.2 Phytotoxic plants and their effects on the reproductive system.

Poisoning/toxic plants	Toxic substance	Signs	References
Nitrate	Nitrite (hemoglobin is oxidized to methemoglobin)	Anoxia, abortions, stillbirths, and the birth of weak calves approximately 3–7 days or more following maternal toxic exposure	Evans, (2011) and Cockburn et al. (2013)
Pinus ponderosa	Isocupressic acid	Abortion, premature parturition, retained fetal membranes, and metritis	Gardner et al. (1999), Wang et al. (2004), and Knight and Walter (2003)
Broom snakeweeds	Saponins, furano diterpene acids, terpenoids, steroids, and flavones	Abortion, retained fetal membranes, and metritis	Panter et al. (2018)
Sweet clover	Dicoumarol	Fetal hemorrhage, abortion	Blakley (1985) and Knight and Walter (2003)
Locoweed (*Astragalus* and *Oxytropis*)	Swainsonine	Embryonic loss, abortion, and occasional birth defects like brachygnathia	Molyneux and Panter (2009)
Lupine	Alkaloid	Arthrogryposis of hindlimbs (crooked calf), cleft palate	Panter and Stegelmeier (2011)
Conium maculatum	Alkaloid	Abortion, fetal malformation	Vetter (2004)
Veratrum californicum	Alkaloid	Cleft palate, harelip, brachygnathia, metacarpal and metatarsal defects	Evans (2018)

28.2.1.4 Reproductive Phytotoxicant

Exposure to various plant toxins (Table 28.2) will adversely impair sexual behavior, gametogenesis, conception, embryonic development, and parturition in cattle. Certain plants that contain phytoestrogens cause anestrus, cystic conditions, and cervical and vulvar enlargement upon ingestion in large quantities (Evans 2011). Normally, animals avoid eating poisonous plants, but under unfavorable seasonal conditions (dry season/drought), they might accidentally consume such plants as they are more succulent and green, which makes them more appealing to starving animals (Youngquist and Threlfall 2006; McDonagh et al. 2010).

28.2.2 Environment Factors

28.2.2.1 Heat Stress

In tropical nations, summer stress is a significant factor that reduces fertility (López-Gatius 2018). Heat stress is any confluence of environmental elements that causes conditions to worsen compared to those that are most conducive to an animal's thermal comfort (Fuquay 1981). Dairy animals are more prone to this due to production stress (Hansen 2007). The animal first attempts to restore the thermal balance by reducing feed intake and metabolism while increasing water intake, salivation, and sweating with the redistribution of blood toward peripheral circulation (Wakayo et al. 2015). Reproductive characteristics significantly decrease when the temperature humidity index (THI) exceeds 72 (De Rensis and Scaramuzzi 2003). Heat stress affects reproduction by disturbing the synchrony of the hypothalamus-pituitary-gonadal axis, which impairs luteinizing hormone (LH) and progesterone release, impairs folliculogenesis with lower estradiol release, causes ovulation aberrations, aberrations in dominant follicle hierarchy due to the removal of the negative effect of inhibin on follicle-stimulating hormone (FSH), and finally, luteal defects (Pavani et al. 2017; Schüller et al. 2017) (Figure 28.3). In addition, it induces a state of oxidative stress that damages cellular organelles and DNA in follicular somatic cells, which lowers the quality of oocytes and results in poor embryonic development as well as mortality due to hampered endometrial and protein synthesis during early cleavage division. Thus, a variety of management measures, including the provision of shade, water sprays, sprinklers, adequate ventilation, nutritional (provision of antioxidant rich feed supplements, energy dense feed, herbal plants, buffers), and hormonal (estrus synchronization protocols with fixed-time artificial insemination [FTAI] like Ovsynch as well as progesterone- and melatonin-based protocols) can be taken to reduce stress (Garcia-Ispierto et al. 2013; De Rensis et al. 2015).

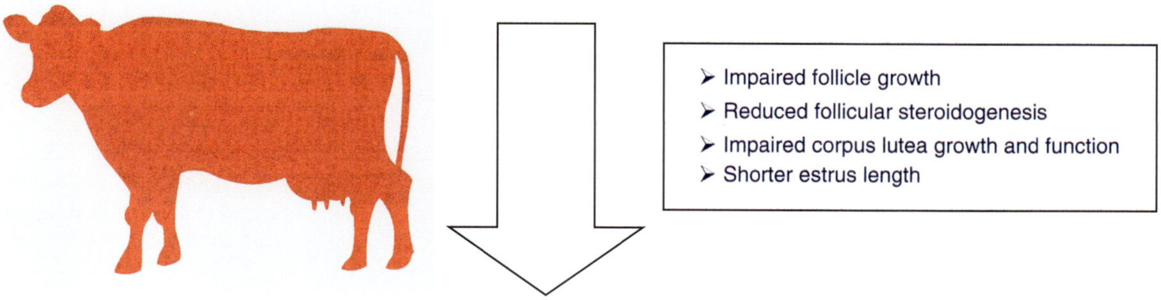

Figure 28.3 Heat stress effects on the fertility of cattle.

28.2.3 Management Causes

Estrus detection is a critical aspect of dairy herd management for attaining good reproductive efficiency. The length and intensity of estrus expression varies with environment, management practices, and selective breeding. In a naturally mated herd, estrus detection is less important and mostly limited to the nonreturn rate after service. Herd size also affects estrus detection, as a larger herd size reduces the accuracy and efficiency of detection (Wood 1976). Animals were unlikely to show estrus behaviors in a collecting yard, milking barn, or while feeding and moving due to crowding. Tie stall housing has a significant adverse effect on displays of estrus (Felton et al. 2012) without any diminution of accuracy. Management systems where animals were continuously kept in tie stalls throughout part or all of the year are on the verge of poor estrus detection (Abeygunawardena et al. 2000). The kind of flooring has an impact on the estrus behavior presentation as well (Vailes and Britt 1990). In order to maximize the effectiveness and precision of estrus detection, management levels should be very precise (Kerbrat and Disenhaus 2004). Manual observation for 30 minutes, four times a day can be conducted to improve the precision and effectiveness of the detection method (Van Vliet and Van Eerdenburg 1996). Moreover, a trained staff and incentive-based approach should be followed to improve the farm's economics (O'Connor 2007). Several estrus detection aids (Table 28.3) have been used in addition to human observation to increase the detection rate, which reduces human error, lessens the intensity of behavioral estrus indicators, and addresses the lack of specialized labor.

28.2.4 Infectious Causes

Infectious microorganisms can negatively impact fertility through two main pathways: (i) direct effects on the reproductive system and semen quality and (ii) indirect effects on other systems, which then interfere with semen production, libido, mating ability, and can prolong reaction time (Foote, 1978). In the first case, these microorganisms directly attack and compromise the reproductive system, which leads to issues with fertility and semen quality. This can result in reduced sperm counts, impaired sperm motility, and abnormal sperm morphology, all of which significantly affect the chances of successful fertilization.

In the second case, these infectious agents may affect other body systems, causing general debility or an increase in body temperature (Parkinson et al., 2010). As a consequence, semen production can be hindered due to the overall weakened state of the individual (Perumal et al. 2013) (Figure 28.4).

28.2.4.1 Brucellosis: Bang's Disease/Malta Fever/Rock Fever/Gibraltar Fever/Undulant Fever

It is caused by the intracellular organism *Brucella abortus* and is characterized by abortion in third trimester of gestation, infertility, mastitis, retained placentas, stillbirths, increasing calving intervals, and arthritis (Radostits et al. 2007). Immediately following an abortion, the organism leaves the uterus and becomes localized in the supramammary, retropharyngeal, external, and internal iliac lymph nodes. It is spread by the ingestion of contaminated pasture, feed, and water; through injured or intact skin and conjunctiva; licking aborted fetuses or genital exudates; and consuming milk from recently aborted cows or carrier cattle that have calved normally (Degefa et al. 2011). Increased herd sizes, age, sex of the animal, husbandry practices, and keeping multiple breeds in a herd are some of the risk factors (Mekonnen et al. 2010; Tolosa et al. 2010). It has a preference for placental tissues because they contain erythritol, which enhances bacterial growth. *B. abortus* causes endometritis; a thickened, cracked placenta covered in yellowish exudates in the intercotyledonary area; necrotic cotyledons; orchitis; epididymitis; and degeneration of the male testes. Various techniques such as

Table 28.3 Various estrus detection aids.

Based on mounting behavior			
Method	**Use**	**Advantages**	**Disadvantages**
Tail paint	Paint/capsule/patch is applied over the tailhead that is removed upon mounting by other animals	Improves visual detection	Considerable experience is needed to detect actual estrus in an animal with slightly erased paint
Heat mount detectors (Kamar®, Kamar Products, Inc., Zionsville, Indiana, USA; Bulling Beacon®, Beacon Automation Pty Ltd., Muswellbrook, New South Wales, Australia)		Better than tail paint, more precise	Capsule can burst by rubbing or incomplete and multiple mount attempts
Estrus detection patches			Missed estrus can occur when the device is not checked or rubbed in cubicle
Electronic heat mount detector	Electronically records mounting activity when applied to tailhead	More accurate in detecting standing to be mounted animals	Expensive
Teaser bulls	Chin bull marker shows which cows have been mounted	Positive indication of estrus	Bulls become disinterested with time
Based on activity monitoring			
Pedometers Neck mounted activity	Track physical activity as an indicator of estrus	Improved results compared to visual observation	Expensive, equipment or software used for this should have good sensitivity and specificity
Based on physiological changes			
Milk progesterone	Monitor cycle and use fixed-time artificial insemination (FTAI) when the concentration falls	Very accurate	Expensive
Vaginal mucus resistance	Daily monitoring of vaginal resistance (decreases during estrus)	Independent of estrus behavior	Invasive
Milk composition and temperature	Inline measurement during milking	Fully automated, no human error	Highly expensive

modified acid-fast staining, culture, molecular techniques, and serological tests, such as the serum agglutination test, rose bengal test, buffered plate agglutination test, fluorescence polarization assay, and enzyme-linked immunosorbent assay (ELISA) are often used. Limitations to the use of serological tests are false positives from vaccinated animals and cross-reactivity with other gram-negative bacteria; low serological tests like the serum agglutination test, rose bengal test, buffered plate agglutination test, fluorescence polarization assay, and ELISA are frequently used. At the herd level, a milk ring test is performed for diagnosis. It can be prevented and controlled by keeping the farm clean, eliminating infected animals, and immunizing calves with the *B. abortus* strain S19 and strain RB51 vaccines at 4–8 and 4–12 months, respectively.

28.2.4.2 Campylobacteriosis (Vibriosis)

It is a venereal disease caused by the gram-negative, flagellated, microaerophilic bacteria *Campylobacter fetis*. Bulls serve as a vector and permanent carrier for this disease and transmit it to females during coitus. Bull-to-bull transmission may occur through mounting when kept in close confinement (Wagner et al. 1965). It is characterized by fertilization failure; early embryonic mortality; endometritis; mid-gestation abortion; mucopurulent vaginal discharge (Dekeyser and Butzler 1984); placentitis; edematous, leather-like, thickened intercotyledons; and hemorrhagic cotyledons. It is self-limiting in females, and the bull acts as an asymptomatic carrier. When maiden heifers are bred to an

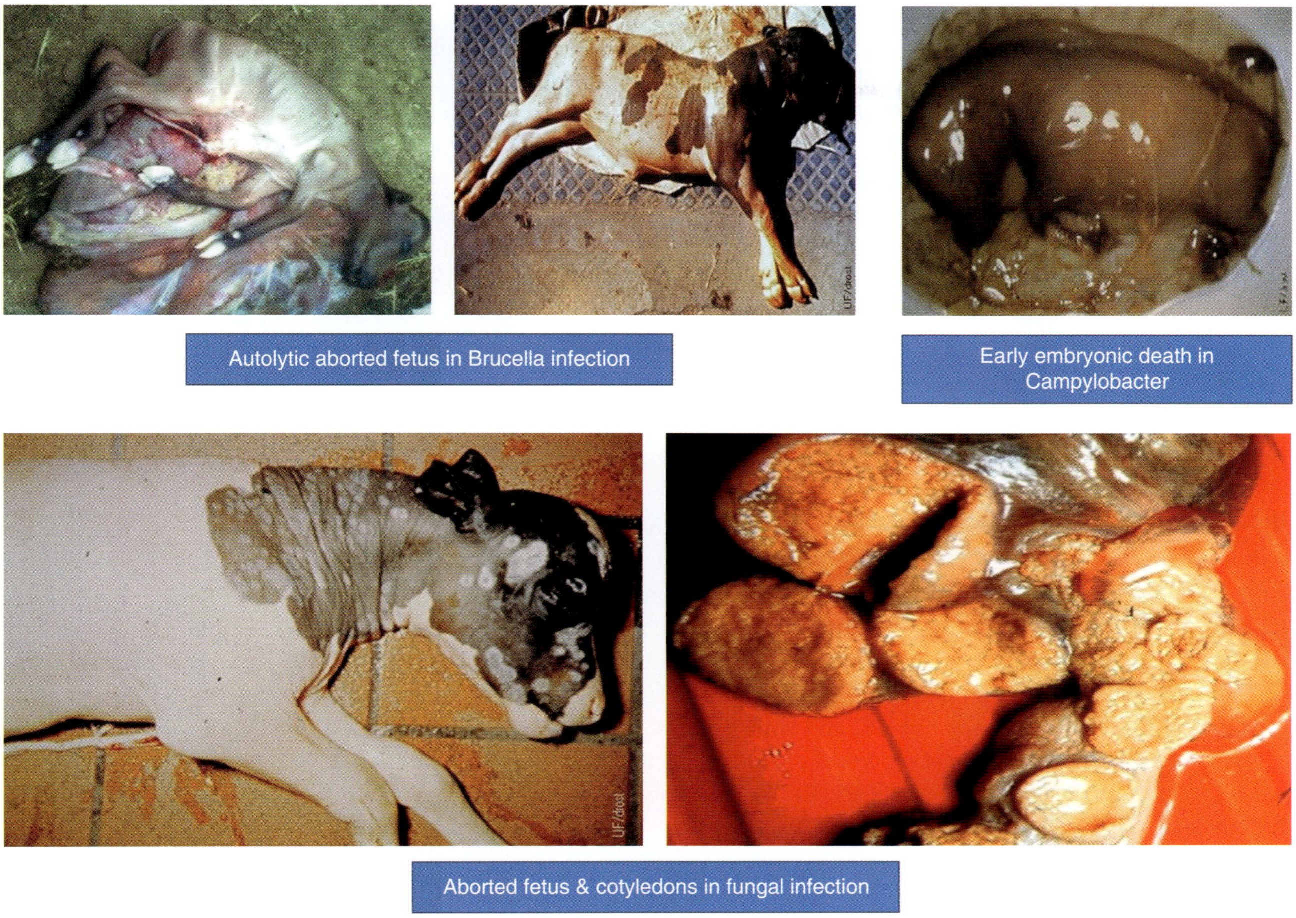

Figure 28.4 Clinical symptoms during infectious causes of infertility.

infected bull, they exhibit low conception rates and irregular returns to estrus that are characteristic of campylobacteriosis. A direct culture of bulls' preputial smegma, vaginal secretions from infected females, or tissue from an aborted fetus is required for the diagnosis in order to isolate and identify the organism. The test of preference for a diagnosis is ELISA. Immunofluorescence can be applied to identify the organism by direct technique. The herd screening is done using a vaginal mucus agglutination test. The fluorescent antibody test (FAT) is commonly used for antigen detection in preputial washing. Preventive management aims to ensure the nonintroduction of infected animal into a susceptible herd. Some preventive measures include not sharing bulls, replacing them with virgin bulls, avoiding sharing grazing areas with other animals, isolation and antibiotic treatment (dihydrostreptomycin), and vaccination prior to the beginning of the breeding season (30–90 days).

28.2.4.3 Trichomoniasis

This is a classical venereal disease transmitted to cows from asymptomatic carrier bulls during coitus. It is caused by a flagellate protozoan *Tritrichomonas foetus* that is characterized by sterility, early abortion, and pyometra. It lives in the crypts and folds of penile integument, preputial mucosa, and stratified squamous epithelial surface of the vagina. It causes early embryonic mortality, irregularly extended estrus cycles, early abortion (first trimester), post-coital pyometra, and infertility. Diagnosis is based on the demonstration of live organisms from preputial washings as well as aborted fetal and placental tissues by a microscopic agglutination test (MAT), in vitro culture on Diamond's trichomonad medium, InPouch TF® test (Biomed Diagnostics, White City, Oregon, USA), and polymerase chain reaction (PCR). Eliminating bulls, replacing natural service with artificial insemination (AI), and either tryptaflavin, iodine-based compounds or acriflavine for local application to the penis and prepuce can be practiced.

28.2.4.4 *Neospora caninum*

This is an obligate, cyst-forming, intracellular, coccidian parasite that causes abortion or stillbirth and neuromuscular paralysis (Weston 2010) in neonatal calves. It is transmitted vertically from the infected pregnant dam to the fetus (Marugan-Hernandez 2017) and horizontally by the ingestion of contaminated feed; it is characterized by fetal loss, retained fetal membranes (RFMs), fetal mummification, stillbirth, multiple hemorrhagic necrotic foci in cotyledons (Marugan-Hernandez 2017), and abortion that mostly occurs in the last trimester (Dubey 2005). A moderate or severely autolyzed fetus is the characteristic feature (Abbitt and Rae 2007). Different serological tests, such as the direct agglutination test, ELISA, and indirect fluorescent antibody test (IFAT), can be performed to provide a diagnosis. A recent abortion is indicated by an IFAT titer of more than 1 : 2000, whereas a titer greater than 1 : 200 indicates a pre-existing infection. A definitive diagnosis is made using a combination of immunohistochemistry (IHC) or PCR in fetal tissues and a histological examination of bovine fetal tissue (brain tissue should be fixed in 10% buffered neutral formalin). In order to minimize transmission, dogs should be kept out of feeding sites, silage pits, calving regions, and feed depots. Vertical transmission should also be minimized through breeding control, testing, culling of infected animals, and the rapid disposal of abortus materials.

28.2.4.5 Bovine Chlamydial/Foothill/Epizootic Bovine Abortion

This is caused by a gram-negative, obligate, intracellular parasite *Chlamydia psittaci,* and it is characterized by abortion in the last trimester of pregnancy, a leathery intercotyledonary area, and a reddish-white, opaque discoloration of the placenta. Infection spreads through ingestion or inhalation; however, a venereal infection (Storz et al. 1976) followed by colonization and replication in the endometrium causes endometritis (Bowen et al. 1978) and embryonic death (Yaeger and Holler 2007). The aborted fetus has enlarged lymph nodes, spleen, and liver; a reduced thymus; and petechial hemorrhaging in the mouth, tongue, thymus, and lymph nodes. The fetus may have a pot-bellied appearance due to ascites and subcutaneous edema. A histology-based diagnosis, bacterial cultures from aborted fetuses and discharges, Giemsa staining to identify elementary bodies, CFT, ELISA-based antigen detection, immune staining, and PCR are all methods for detection.

28.2.4.6 Bovine Viral Diarrhea (BVD)

Bovine viral diarrhea (BVD) is caused by a member of the *Pestivirus* genus that is related to border disease and classical swine fever. It is characterized by pyrexia, watery diarrhea, nasal discharge, buccal ulcerations, and lameness. It has two main biotypes: cytopathic and noncytopathic strains, where noncytopathic strains can spread the illness both vertically and horizontally by direct contact with the saliva, feces, semen, urine, tears, and milk of infected calves (Radostits et al. 2007). Infection in the first trimester results in early embryonic mortality and repeat breeding. After 5–6 months of gestation, there may be an abortion or birth of calves with congenital abnormalities of the central nervous system and eyes. Infection in the second trimester is frequently associated with an increased risk of birth abnormalities, calves with poor growth rates, and an increased average age at first calving (Heuer et al. 2007). The virus is known to suppress ovarian function in infected heifers by interfering with gonadal steroidogenesis (Altamarand et al. 2013). Virus isolation in bovine tissue culture (kidney, lung, testis, and turbinate cells), IHC, PCR to identify nucleic acids, and serological tests like virus neutralization and ELISA are techniques to identify the virus. Some management strategies that can be used include maintaining strong biosecurity measures to prevent infection from entering the herd, testing infected animals, following the quarantine of a newly purchased bull, and immunizing the entire herd (Brownlie 2005).

28.2.4.7 Infectious Bovine Rhinotracheitis (IBR)

This is caused by bovine herpes virus type-1 (BHV-1) and results in infectious pustular vulvovaginitis (IPV), vesicular venereal disease, and coital vesicular exanthema. BHV-1 also causes abortion and infertility in heifers and cows. The genital form is transmitted by coitus, contaminated bedding, and mutual licking. The corpus luteum is the major predilection site (Chase et al. 2017). After the first infection or after recovery, the virus spreads due to its latent residence within the Gasserian ganglion of the fifth cranial nerve. Serological methods for diagnosis include indirect ELISA and virus neutralization tests. The identification of healthy animals that are serologically positive offers a clear picture of the herd's infection due to virus latency. Diagnosis is typically made using histological lesions, IHC of the afflicted tissue, and PCR tests (Crook et al. 2012). Infected animals should be isolated. Heifers should be vaccinated with live attenuated vaccines at 6 months of age and before mating, to be followed by annual vaccination.

28.2.4.8 Leptospirosis

This is an important zoonotic disease caused by pathogenic spirochaetes of the genus *Leptospira* (*Leptospira* Hardjo serovars and *Leptospira pomona*) (Parthiban et al. 2015). It is a significant cause of reproductive failure that results in enormous economic loss in tropical and subtropical countries. The virus is excreted in the urine and in aborted or stillborn fetuses as well as in normal fetuses or vaginal discharges after calving (Levett 2001). Abrasions of the skin, mucous membranes of the eyes, mouth, or nose, and semen after natural service are all possible entry points for infection (Ellis et al. 1986). After establishing an infection, the bacteria localize inside renal tubules, cotyledons, and the fetus. There may be signs of hepatitis, nephritis, icterus, hemoglobinuria, mastitis, and abortion in the last trimester. A diagnosis is made by isolation of the causative agent and the detection of antigens in tissue and body fluids using methods such as immunofluorescence staining, immunochemistry, immune peroxidase staining, silver staining, and various PCR methods. Serological tests like ELISA, indirect immunofluorescence, the spot agglutination test, or MAT can be used (OIE 2017). Fluorouracil-containing selective medium (EMJH base) is useful for isolating organisms from urine. Leptospirosis can be prevented or treated using vaccination, safe AI, rodent control, the prophylactic antibiotic treatment of exposed cattle (streptomycin/dihydrostreptomycin at 25 mg/kg), quarantining of newly introduced cattle, and regular serological testing (Himani et al. 2013).

28.2.4.9 Listeriosis

This is caused by the zoonotic intracellular pathogen *Listeria monocytogenes*. Consuming substandard feed or grass silage that has undergone insufficient fermentation and been contaminated with an infected fetus, placenta, or uterine discharge is the cause of the infection. Vertical transmission is the usual source of infection in ruminants, and it can be transmitted transplacentally. The organism gains entry through ingestion or the mucus membranes of the conjunctiva or respiratory system and has a predilection for the placenta that can cause placentitis, death of the fetus, metritis, retention of the fetal membranes, and abortion in the last trimester. Gross lesions are tiny pinpoint yellow foci in the liver, lungs, myocardium, kidneys, spleen, and brain. The bacteria can be demonstrated in the center of these focal areas (Quinn et al. 2002). A diagnosis depends on the isolation of the organism from fetal tissues, placenta, vaginal discharge, and brain of infected animals. Agglutination and complement fixation tests can be used but titers remain high in clinically normal animals and may return to normal within one month. Farm management practices, such as improving the nutritional status of animals and their housing conditions, can be of some value in preventing disease (Dhama et al. 2015).

28.2.4.10 *Histophilus somni*

This is a common inhabitant of the genital tract in male and female cattle. The organism can be routinely isolated from the mucosal surface of the urogenital tract in normal healthy cattle. It can lead to a variety of disorders in cattle, including endometritis, vulvovaginitis, cervicitis, early embryonic mortality, testicular degeneration, orchitis, epididymitis, and abortion (Stephens et al. 1986; Ruegg et al. 1988; Barber et al. 1994). The placenta and the aborted fetus both have nonspecific lesions that resemble nonsuppurative placentitis in the cotyledons (Jubb et al. 1993).

28.2.4.11 Mycotic Causes

Aspergillus fumigatus accounts for approximately 75% of mycotic abortion cases, with the remaining 25% caused by *Candida* and *Phycomycetes*. Winter is the most frequent time of year for abortions. Fungi enter the body by the oral or respiratory systems and spread hematogenously to the placenta. Severe necrotizing placentitis, a leathery and thickened intercotyledonary region, and large, necrotic cotyledons with turned-in borders are common features. The fetus is rarely autolyzed, and 30% of them have a gray, ringworm-like lesion that primarily affects the head and shoulders. The presence of fungal hyphae linked to necrotizing placentitis, dermatitis, or pneumonia serves as the basis for this diagnosis. Additionally, fungi can be isolated from the placenta, skin lesions, and stomach contents.

28.2.4.12 *Ureaplasma diversum*

This is a typical resident of the genital tract in cows that can be detected in the vestibule and vagina. It also affects male animals, which results in seminal vesiculitis, granular balanoposthitis, and impaired semen morphology (Marques et al. 2009). In females, it produces granules around the clitoral region and the lateral walls of the vagina, hyperemia of the vulva, profuse mucopurulent vaginal discharge, and granular vulvovaginitis (Gaeti et al. 2014). For the diagnosis of vulvovaginitis, samples should be taken from the area of active inflammation. Samples for abortion should contain amniotic fluid, lung, placentome, and stomach contents (Yaeger and Holler 2007). Endometritis, salpingitis with a mononuclear inflammatory infiltrate, fibrosis, intestinal necrosis, and nonsuppurative alveolitis are among the conditions that might occur during pregnancy. Abortion usually occurs in the last trimester of pregnancy. Macroscopic lesions include a thickening of the amnion and intercotyledonary zones of the allantochorion; it is detected by PCR or isolated by culture (Marques et al. 2011).

28.2.5 Functional Causes

Functional causes of infertility typically affect individual animals within a herd but have the tendency to become prevalent among a specific subgroup, which indicates underlying issues of nutrition and management. Functional abnormalities primarily result from endocrinological irregularities, which are challenging to identify accurately, especially with limited hormone assay methods that rely on single, spot samples of blood or milk. Other factors include inherited traits, imbalances in nutrition, and social influences that stem from modern husbandry practices, such as grouping large numbers of cows, that disrupt the establishment of a stable social hierarchy. It encompasses various conditions, including:

I) Cystic ovarian degeneration (CyOvD)
II) Anestrus
III) Silent estrus
IV) Delayed ovulation
V) Anovulation
VI) Persistent corpus luteum

28.2.5.1 Cystic Ovarian Degeneration/Disease (CyOvD)

CyOvD is defined as the presence of one or more follicles with a diameter of at least 20 mm, present on one or both ovaries (for at least 10 days) in the absence of any active luteal tissue that clearly interferes with normal ovarian cyclicity (Jeengar et al. 2018). It is a major contributor to infertility, particularly in dairy cattle, and it is associated with anovulation and suboptimal fertility by increasing service periods, reduced productivity (Silvia et al. 2002), prolonged calving intervals, higher veterinary aids, and higher culling rates. The incidence ranges from 10% to 20% in cattle, with a higher occurrence in lactating animals aged 4–6 years and a peak between 15 and 45 days after calving. There are three types of cysts associated with CyOvD, depending on inconsistent follicular wall thickness (Kahn and Line, 2010): (i) a large, thin-walled, anovulatory follicular cyst with high estradiol and nymphomania; (ii) a thick-walled, anovulatory luteal or luteinized cyst with elevated progesterone; and (iii) cystic corpus luteum (nonpathological).

Factors Contributing to CyOvD

- **Hereditary predisposition:** Differences in CyOvD incidence among breeds, families, and sires suggest a genetic influence.
- **Breed:** Holstein–Friesians have a higher prevalence of CyOvD compared to other dairy breeds, while beef breeds rarely experience it.
- **Age:** CyOvD is most common between the second and fifth lactation.
- **Milk yield and nutrition:** CyOvD is genetically correlated with milk production (Fleischer et al. 2001) with higher yielding cows being more susceptible. High milk production mobilizes fat, which leads to elevated levels of NEFA and β-hydroxybutyrate (BHBA), as well as reduced insulin, glucose, and IGF-I concentrations (Buckley et al. 2003).
- **Stress, metabolic disturbances, and an NEB:** These also play a role in cyst development.
- **Season:** CyOvD is more common during autumn and winter.
- **Intercurrent disease:** Conditions like ketosis, dystocia, stress, twin births, RFMs, milk fever, and postpartum uterine infections are considered risk factors.
- **Hypothyroidism:** Reduced thyroxine (T_4) levels affect the structure of granulosa cells.

Etiology and Pathogenesis CyOvD etiology is multifactorial, involving genetic, phenotypic, and environmental factors (Vanholder et al. 2006). The most widely accepted hypothesis is based on neuroendocrinological dysfunction of the hypothalamic–pituitary–gonadal axis. In cows with CyOvD, the preovulatory LH surge is absent or reduced, which leads to the failure of ovulation and results in the persistence of a follicle as a cystic structure. The absence of the normal positive feedback from an LH surge indicates a reduced sensitivity of the hypothalamic surge-generating center to estradiol and a failure of gonadotropin-releasing hormone (GnRH) release, either as a consequence of abnormal follicular production or increased metabolism (Wiltbank et al. 2002; Brito and Palmer 2004). Normal postpartum cows experience follicular waves

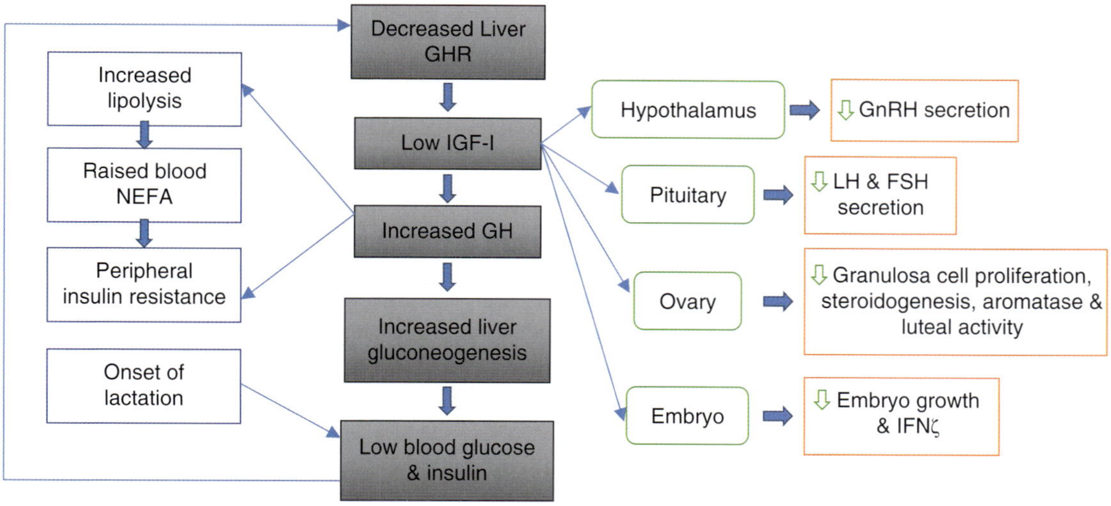

Figure 28.5 The inter-relationship between growth hormone (GH), insulin-like growth factor (IGF)-1, insulin, a negative energy balance (NEB), and its effect on reproduction. *Source:* adapted from Zulu et al. (2002) and Butler (2005).

after calving with ovulation of the dominant follicle from one of the early waves, and any dysfunction in this process causes CyOvD. Stress can further attenuate the LH surge. Biochemical alterations within the follicle play a significant role in CyOvD (Singh et al. 2018). An NEB, commonly associated with CyOvD, and elevated NEFA levels directly affect follicular function (Figure 28.5).

Clinical Signs and Diagnosis Abnormal estrus behavior patterns like persistent estrus; shortened estrus intervals; failure to cycle; persistent bulling behavior accompanied by masculinization of head and neck; bellowing; relaxation of the vulva, perineum, and pelvic ligaments; and an elevated tail head (sterility hump) occur in chronic cases. The affected ovaries are generally enlarged and rounded with a variable size that depends on size and number of cysts present. The uterus undergoes a palpable change in the first week, the uterine wall is thickened, edematous, and sponge-like toward the end of first week. In chronic conditions, atony and atrophy of the uterine wall along with mild to moderate mucoid to mucopurulent vaginal discharge is common. Histologically, there is marked hyperplasia of the uterine lining along with cystic dilatation of the endometrial glands that gives the appearance of "Swiss cheese." Luteal cysts cause the cessation of cyclical activity and function, which results in the animal becoming heavier and coarser, with a thick and heavy neck. This condition is referred to as adrenal virilism, and it is accompanied by increased levels of 17-ketosteroids in the urine from the adrenal gland. A progesterone (P_4) assay and ultrasonography (USG) help to accurately differentiate ovarian abnormalities like follicular cysts, luteal cysts, and ovarian inactivity. The cyst wall thickness is less than 3 mm in follicular cysts and greater than 3 mm in luteal cysts (Brito and Palmer 2004). Animals with follicular cysts fail to ovulate a preovulatory follicle and the uterus lacks tone. Measuring plasma P4 detects the degree of luteinization. During rectal examinations, a cystic corpus luteum appears similar to a normal corpus luteum, but it has a slightly softer consistency.

Treatment and Control Spontaneous recovery occurs in early postpartum for animals with lower production. Treatment must be initiated as soon as the condition is diagnosed in multiparous animals. Treatment regimens include the aspiration of cystic fluid or ultrasound guided cyst ablation (Lievaart et al. 2006) and exogenous hormone application (Chorulon®, Merck and Company, Inc., Rahway, New Jersy, USA; for follicular cysts) at a dose of 3000–5000 IU intramuscularly or buserelin acetate (Gynarich®, Intas Pharmaceuticals, Ltd., Metoda, Gujarat, India) at a dose of 5 ml intramuscularly, and prostaglandins for luteal cyst. Ovulation synchronization protocols like Ovsynch or CO-Synch + CIDR® (InterAg, Hamilton, New Zealand; to decrease LH secretion, result in cyst regression, and facilitate the emergence of new follicular wave) followed by FTAI have been used successfully (Singh et al. 2017).

28.2.5.2 Anestrus

Anestrus refers to the absence of overt signs of estrus that manifest either due to a lack of expression of estrus or failure of its detection, while acyclicity denotes the absence of ovarian cyclic activity. True anestrus occurs when there is a prolonged period of cessation in cyclic activity, which is typically associated with smooth ovaries and the absence of palpable follicles and corpus luteum (CL). False anestrus can be either physiological, such as pubertal, lactational, or gestational (5–10%), or occur during the postpartum period when caused by conditions like pyometra and chronic metritis. A higher incidence is reported in adult cattle and buffalo. Anestrus causes huge economic loss due to increased intercalving intervals, poor net calf crops, production loss, treatment expenses, and replacement costs.

Factors Responsible for Anestrus

- Congenital abnormalities like ovarian agenesis or hypoplasia, freemartinism, and intersexuality.
- Retention of the CL due to uterine pathological conditions like pyometra, chronic metritis, or fetal mummification.
- Malnutrition can lead to delayed puberty or ovarian atrophy in heifers. The genitalia may be poorly developed or infantile, and lactating animals may have small and smooth ovaries.
- Hormonal imbalances that result from the inadequate production of hormones from the hypothalamus, pituitary, and ovaries can contribute to anestrus. Genitalia appear properly developed upon rectal examination, but the ovaries are smooth and no CL is present.
- Luteal cysts.
- Heat stress, which is particularly common in buffaloes during the summer, can diminish the external signs of heat. Heat stress increases the secretion of the adrenocorticotropic hormone (ACTH) and reduces the secretion of LH.

Diagnosis A diagnosis of anestrus involves considering the animal's history and clinical signs, performing per rectum examination to identify smooth ovaries without luteal structures, using an ultrasound to confirm the absence of a CL and dominant follicle, and measuring progesterone (P4) levels at 8–10 day intervals in the blood. In true anestrus, P4 levels are consistently lower than 1 ng/ml. Follicles may develop up to the prematuration stage and become atretic (Ghuman et al. 2010). Functional CL can be palpated per rectally in cases of silent estrus or anestrus due to persistent CL.

Treatment

1) **Physical examination:** A thorough examination of the animal and culling if congenital abnormalities are present.
2) **Lugol's iodine paint:** Painting Lugol's iodine solution (0.5–1.0%) on the posterior part of the cervix irritates the uterine mucosa, which can lead to enhanced circulation and iodine absorption from the uterus as well as stimulate the anterior pituitary to secrete gonadotrophins, thereby inducing cyclicity.
3) **Herbal therapies:** Curry leaves, kalonji, methi, bamboo, asparagus, jute plant, etc. either alone or in combination, have shown variable responses for estrus induction.
4) **Hormonal treatment:**
   a) Progesterone supplementation (intravaginal devices, ear implants).
   b) Gonadotrophins.
   c) Combination protocols like Ovsynsch and CIDR-based Ovsynch protocols.
   d) Pregnant mare's serum gonadotropin (PMSG; 500 IU) combined with the subcutaneous injection of insulin (0.25 IU/kg).
   e) Melatonin implants (one implant per 50 kg) has proved to be efficacious in estrus induction and ovulation within 4–36 days.

28.2.5.3 Silent Estrus

Silent heat refers to a condition where signs of estrus are exhibited but are not easily observed or are expressed poorly. This phenomenon is common in buffaloes, especially during the summer season due to altered endocrine milieu that disrupts the HPG axis. While the animal may be experiencing normal cyclic activity, the external signs of heat are not prominent due to low levels of estrogen, which is responsible for these external manifestations. A slight vaginal discharge may be present, and upon rectal examination, either a follicle or CL is observed on the ovary. In such cases, the owner should be asked about the day of vaginal discharge, and prostaglandin (PG)F2α should be administered 10–12 days after the discharge. Alternatively, if the CL can be palpated, PGF2α should be given. The animal typically comes enters heat within 72 hours of PGF2α administration. A double shot of PGF2α injections can be given at a 10-day interval when the history of the animal is not sufficient.

28.2.5.4 Delayed Ovulation

Delayed ovulation is characterized by the detection of a single follicle in the same ovary on two consecutive examinations, one during peak estrus and another 24–36 hours later. The underlying mechanism behind delayed ovulation is a delay in the LH surge. The diagnosis of this condition can be challenging as it requires sequential rectal palpation of the ovaries. Delayed ovulation is often considered a cause of conception failure in cyclic nonbreeders. If ovulation has not occurred within 24 hours of mating, the cow should be re-inseminated. The administration of a GnRH agonist can induce a rapid rise in FSH and LH concentrations, with peak levels occurring within 30–60 minutes and returning to preinjection values within 4 hours. The pattern of LH release observed in this scenario resembles the preovulatory surge seen during late estrus in normal cyclic animals.

28.2.5.5 Anovulation

Anovulation, the absence of ovulation, can be a cause of conception failure in cyclic breeders. A diagnosis of anovulation can be made retrospectively by noting upon rectal palpation or ultrasonography that a follicle persists longer than expected. Treatment aims to ensure that ovulation occurs normally during the subsequent estrus. In such cases, the administration of GnRH, as described for delayed ovulation, is indicated.

28.2.5.6 Persistent Corpus Luteum

Persistent CL occurs when there is interference with the production or release of endogenous luteolysin (PGF2α) that results in the persistence of the CL. Pregnancy is the most common condition associated with a persistent CL, but uterine infections and inflammation can also interfere with luteolysin production or release. Evidence suggests that a persistent CL can occur even in the absence of uterine lesions. In such cases, a single injection of synthetic or natural PGF2α is the preferred treatment to induce lysis of the CL and restore cyclicity.

28.2.5.7 Repeat Breeding Syndrome

A normal adult female animal (3–10 years of age) with regular reproductive cycles and normal genitalia that fails to conceive after mating with a fertile bull or undergoing AI in three or more consecutive estrus is referred to as a repeater or cyclic nonbreeder. Multiple factors are associated with this condition, which is known as repeat breeding syndrome. Hormonal insufficiency and dysfunction contribute to about 40% of repeat breeding causes. A prolonged duration of estrus, extended follicular phase, delayed LH release and ovulation, and suprabasal P4 are considered the most prominent risk factors.

A repeat breeder cow must meet the following criteria:

1) It has been bred at least three times without achieving pregnancy.
2) It exhibits a normal estrous cycle.
3) There are no palpable abnormalities.
4) There is no abnormal vaginal discharge.
5) The cow has calved at least once.
6) The cow is under 10 years old.

The factors that contribute to repeat breeding syndrome include:

- **Male factors:** An infertile bull, high abnormalities in the sperm, and low sperm motility.
- **Female factors:** Delayed ovulation, anovulation, fertilization failure, luteal insufficiency, endometritis, ovario-bursal adhesions, tubal blockage or occluded oviducts, early embryonic death, urovagina, and pneumo-vagina.
- **Management factors:**
  a) Improper heat detection, which can be addressed by observing animals closely for heat symptoms and recording heat dates.
  b) Environmental stress, including high temperatures or fever, can cause early embryonic death. Rest before and after AI is advised to reduce cortisol levels and avoid physical stress.
  c) Nutritional deficiencies, such as deficiencies in vitamin E, selenium, or specific nutrients, can affect reproductive performance. Providing a balanced mineral mixture and ensuring a positive nutritive energy balance is important.
  d) Improper timing of AI, which can be corrected by following the a.m.–p.m. method based on heat observation.
  e) Untrained inseminators or faulty AI techniques. AI should be performed by trained professionals, and the semen should be deposited in the body of the uterus.
  f) Unhygienic conditions during AI, which can introduce infections. Strict hygiene measures should be followed.
  g) Improper thawing of semen straws. Thawing should be done in a water bath at the appropriate temperature to maintain sperm viability.

28.3 Conclusion

The prevalence of infertility in cattle can be influenced by various factors, including functional causes that affect individual animals within a herd. However, when infertility becomes more widespread among a specific subgroup of cattle it may indicate underlying issues such as infectious diseases, management practices, or nutritional deficiencies. Identifying and addressing these underlying factors are essential to effectively managing and improving reproductive performance in the cattle herd as well as ensuring optimal fertility and overall herd health. Regular monitoring, veterinary care, and proper management strategies are crucial to minimizing infertility and promoting successful breeding outcomes in cattle populations.

References

Abbitt, B. and Rae, D.O. (2007). Protozoal Abortion in Cattle. In: *Current Therapy in Large Animal Theriogenology*, 2e (ed. R.S. Youngquist and W.R. Threlfall), 409–413. St Louis, MO: Saunders-Elsevier.

Abeygunawardena, H., Alexander, P.A.B.D., Abeygunawardena, I.S., and Perera, B.M.A.O. (2000). Use of milk progesterone RIA to determine factors affecting the success rate of artificial insemination services in cattle in mid-country small-holder farms in Sri Lanka. *Tropical Agricultural Research and Extension* 3: 75.

Altamarand, E.A., Kaiser, G.G., Mucci, N.C. et al. (2013). Effect of bovine viral diarrhoea virus on the ovarian functionality and in-vitro reproductive performance of persistently infected heifers. *Veterinary Microbiology* 165: 326–332.

Anderson, G.W. and Barton, B.A. (1988). Reproductive efficiency: potential nutrition-management interactions. *Proceedings of Winter Dairy Management Schools*, 107. Ithaca, New York, USA: Cornell University.

Barber, J.A., Momont, H., Tibary, A., and Sedgwick, G.P. (1994). Recovery from severe dysspermatogenesis in a bull: a case report. *Theriogenology* 41: 353–363.

Blakley, B.R. (1985). Moldy sweet clover (dicoumarol) poisoning in Saskatchewan cattle. *The Canadian Veterinary Journal* 26: 357.

Bowen, R.A., Spears, P., Storz, J., and Seidel, G.E. Jr. (1978). Mechanisms of infertility in genital tract infections due to *Chlamydia psittaci* transmitted through contaminated semen. *Journal of Infectious Diseases* 138: 95–104.

Brito, L.F.C. and Palmer, C.W. (2004). Cystic ovarian disease in cattle. *Large Animal Veterinary Rounds* 4 (10): 1–4.

Brownlie, J. (2005). Bovine virus diarrhoea virus -Strategic directions for diagnosis and control, *Proceedings of the Dairy Cattle Veterinarians of the NZVA*, Volume Proceedings of a BDVD Symposium (FCE Publication No. 241). Massey University, Palmerston North, Wellington, New Zealand (January 2005), 1-19. Wellington, NZ: New Zealand Veterinary Association.

Buckley, F., O'sullivan, K., Mee, J.F. et al. (2003). Relationships among milk yield, body condition, cow weight, and reproduction in spring-calved Holstein-Friesians. *Journal of dairy science* 86 (7): 2308–2319.

Butler, W.R. (2005). Nutrition, negative energy balance and fertility in the postpartum dairy cow. *Cattle Practice* 13: 13–18.

Chakurkar, E.B., Barbuddhe, B., and Sundaram, R.N.S. (2008). Infertility in farm animals: Causes and remedies. Goa, India: ICAR Research Complex for Goa. *Technical Bulletin No. 15.*

Chase, C.C., Fulton, R.W., O'Toole, D. et al. (2017). Bovine herpesvirus 1 modified live virus vaccines for cattle reproduction: balancing protection with undesired effects. *Veterinary Microbiology* 206: 69–77.

Cockburn, A., Brambilla, G., Fernández, M.L. et al. (2013). Nitrite in feed: from animal health to human health. *Toxicology and Applied Pharmacology* 270: 209–217.

Corah, L. (1996). Trace mineral requirements of grazing cattle. *Animal Feed Science and Technology* 59: 61–70.

Crook, T., Benavides, J., Russell, G. et al. (2012). Bovine herpesvirus 1 abortion: current prevalence in the United Kingdom and evidence of hematogenous spread within the fetus in natural cases. *Journal of Veterinary Diagnostic Investigation* 24: 662–670.

De Rensis, F. and Scaramuzzi, R.J. (2003). Heat stress and seasonal effects on reproduction in the dairy cow – a review. *Theriogenology* 60: 1139–1151.

De Rensis, F., Garcia-Ispierto, I., and López-Gatius, F. (2015). Seasonal heat stress: clinical implications and hormone treatments for the fertility of dairy cows. *Theriogenology* 84: 659–666.

Degefa, T., Duressa, A., and Duguma, R. (2011). Brucellosis and some reproductive problems of indigenous Arsi cattle in selected Arsi zones of Oromia regional state, Ethiopia. *Global Veterinaria* 7: 45–53.

Dekeyser, J. and Butzler, J.P. (1984). *Campylobacter Infections in Man and Animals*, 181–191. Florida: CRC Press Inc.

Dhama, K., Karthik, K., Tiwari, R. et al. (2015). Listeriosis in animals, its public health significance (food-borne zoonosis) and advances in diagnosis and control: a comprehensive review. *Veterinary Quarterly* 35: 211–235.

Dijkhuizen, A.A., Stelwagen, J., and Renkema, J.A. (1985). Economic aspects of reproductive failure in dairy cattle. I. Financial loss at farm level. *Preventive Veterinary Medicine* 3 (3): 251–263.

Dubey, J.P. (2005). Neosporosis in cattle. *Veterinary Clinics: Food Animal Practice* 21: 473–483.

Ellis, W.A., Songer, J.G., Montgomery, J., and Cassells, J.A. (1986). Prevalence of *Leptospira interrogans* serovar hardjo in the genital and urinary tracts of nonpregnant cattle. *The Veterinary Record* 118: 11–13.

England, G.C. (2005). *Fertility and Obstetrics in the Horse*. Blackwell.

Evans, T.J. (2011). Diminished reproductive performance and selected toxicants in forages and grains. *Veterinary Clinics: Food Animal Practice* 27: 345–371.

Evans, T.J. (2018). Reproductive toxicity and endocrine disruption. In: *Veterinary Toxicology: Basic and Clinical Principles*, 3e (ed. R.C. Gupta), 273–316. Academic Press.

Evans, A.C. and Walsh, S.W. (2012). The physiology of multifactorial problems limiting the establishment of pregnancy in dairy cattle. *Reproduction, Fertility and Development* 24: 233–237.

Fathalla, M., Williamson, N.B., and Parkinson, T.J. (2001). A case of bovine placental mole associated with twin embryonic death and resorption. *New Zealand Veterinary Journal* 49: 119–120.

Felton, C.A., Colazo, M.G., Ponce-Barajas, P. et al. (2012). Dairy cows continuously-housed in tie-stalls failed to manifest activity changes during estrus. *Canadian Journal of Animal Science* 92: 189–196.

Fleischer, P., Metzner, M., Beyerbach, M. et al. (2001). The relationship between milk yield and the incidence of some diseases in dairy cows. *Journal of dairy science* 84 (9): 2025–2035.

Foote, R.H. (1978). Reproductive performance and problems in New York dairy herds. *Cornell University Agricultural Experiment Station Memoir*, 8: 1.

Fuquay, J.W. (1981). Heat stress as it affects animal production. *Journal of Animal Science* 52: 164–174.

Gaeti, J.G.L., Lana, M.V., Silva, G.S. et al. (2014). *Ureaplasma diversum* as a cause of pustular vulvovaginitis in bovine females in Vale Guapore, Mato Grosso state, Brazil. *Tropical Animal Health and Production* 46: 1059–1063.

Gagnon, A., Khan, D.R., Sirard, M.A. et al. (2015). Effects of intramuscular administration of folic acid and vitamin B12 on granulosa cells gene expression in postpartum dairy cows. *Journal of Dairy Science* 98: 7797–7809.

Garcia-Ispierto, I., Roselló, M.A., De Rensis, F., and Lopez-Gatius, F. (2013). A five-day progesterone plus eCG-based fixed-time AI protocol improves fertility over spontaneous estrus in high producing dairy cows under heat stress. *Journal of Reproduction and Development* 59: 544–548.

Gardner, D.R., Panter, K.E., and James, L.F. (1999). Pine needle abortion in cattle: metabolism of isocupressic acid. *Journal of Agricultural and Food Chemistry* 47: 2891–2897.

Ghuman, S.P.S., Honparkhe, M., and Singh, J. (2010). Optimizing ovarian and reproductive events of anestrous buffaloes using intravaginal progesterone, GnRH, and PGF2α. *Proceedings of the International Buffalo Conference*, New Delhi, India, (1–4 February 2010), 82–83.

Hansen, P.J. (2007). Hidden factors affecting fertility. *WCDS Advances in Dairy Technology, Proceedings of the Twenty-fifth Western Canadian Dairy Seminar*, Red Deer, Alberta, Canada (6–9 March 2007), 19: 339–349. Edmonton, Canada: Western Canadian Dairy Seminar.

Harrison, J.H., Hancock, D.D., Pierre, N.S. et al. (1986). Effect of prepartum selenium treatment on uterine involution in the dairy cow. *Journal of Dairy Science* 69: 1421–1425.

Heuer, C., Healy, A., and Zerbini, C. (2007). Economic effects of exposure to bovine viral diarrhea virus on dairy herds in New Zealand. *Journal of Dairy Science* 90: 5428–5438.

Himani, D., Suman, M.K., and Mane, B.G. (2013). Epidemiology of leptospirosis: an Indian perspective. *Journal of Foodborne and Zoonotic Diseases* 1: 6–13.

Jeengar, K., Chaudhary, V., Kumar, A. et al. (2018). Ovarian cysts in dairy cows: old and new concepts for definition, diagnosis and therapy. *Animal Reproduction (AR)* 11 (2): 63–73.

Jubb, K.V.F., Kennedy, P.C., and Palmer, N. (1993). *Pathology of Domestic Animals*, 4e. San Diego, CA: Academic Press.

Kahn, C.M. and Line, S. (2010). *The Merck veterinary manual*, vol. 2825. Kenilworth, New Jersy, USA: Merck and Company, Inc.

Kastelic, J.P. (2013). Male involvement in fertility and factors affecting semen quality in bulls. *Animal Frontiers* 3 (4): 20–25.

Kendall, N.R. and Bone, P. (2006). Fertility and trace elements - an underestimated problem. *Cattle Practice* 14: 17.

Kerbrat, S. and Disenhaus, C. (2004). A proposition for an updated behavioural characterisation of the oestrus period in dairy cows. *Applied Animal Behaviour Science* 87: 223–238.

Knight, A.P. and Walter, R.G. (2003). *A Guide to Plant Poisoning of Animals in North America, 2001*, 194–197. Jackson, Wyoming: Teton New Media.

Levett, P.N. (2001). Leptospirosis. *Clinical Microbiology Reviews* 14: 296–326.

Lievaart, J.J., Parlevliet, J.M., Dieleman, S.J. et al. (2006). Transvaginal aspiration as first treatment of ovarian follicular cysts in dairy cattle under field circumstances. *Tijdschrift voor Diergeneeskunde* 131 (12): 438–442.

López-Gatius, F. (2018). Approaches to increase reproductive efficiency in artificially inseminated dairy cows. *Animal Reproduction* 10: 143–147.

Lotthammer, K.H., Schams, D., and Scholz, H. (1978). Untersuchungen uber einespezifische Vitamin A-unabhangigeWirkung des β-Carotene auf die Fruchtbarkeit von laktierendedKuhen. *Zuchthygiene* 13: 76.

Lucy, M.C. (2003). Mechanisms linking nutrition and reproduction in postpartum cows. *Reproduction (Cambridge, England) Supplement* 61: 415–427.

Marques, L.M., Buzinhani, M., Neto, R.L. et al. (2009). Detection of *Ureaplasma diversum* in bovine semen straws for artificial insemination. *The Veterinary Record* 165: 572.

Marques, L.M., Buzinhani, M., Guimarães, A.M.S. et al. (2011). Intraspecific sequence variation in 16S rRNA gene of *Ureaplasma diversum* isolates. *Veterinary Microbiology* 152: 205–211.

Marugan-Hernandez, V. (2017). *Neospora caninum* and bovine neosporosis: current vaccine research. *Journal of Comparative Pathology* 157: 193–200.

McDonagh, P., Griffin, J., and White, P. (2010). *Veterinary Pharmacology and Toxicology*, 1e, 98. University of Sydney.

Mekonnen, H., Kalayou, S., and Kyule, M. (2010). Serological survey of bovine brucellosis in barka and arado breeds (*Bos indicus*) of Western Tigray, Ethiopia. *Preventive Veterinary Medicine* 94: 28–35.

Molyneux, R.J. and Panter, K.E. (2009). Alkaloids toxic to livestock. *The Alkaloids. Chemistry and Biology* 67: 143–216.

Morris, R.S. (1976). Diagnosis of infertility in larger dairy herds. In: *Refresher Course in Mastitis Issue 28 of Proceedings* (ed. F.H. Dodd and D.E. Jasper), 83–194. Sydney, Australia: University of Sydney, Post-Graduate Committee in Veterinary Science.

Mulligan, F.J., O'Grady, L., Gath, V.P. et al. (2008). Nutrition and fertility in dairy cows. *Irish Veterinary Journal* 60: 312–314.

O'Connor, M.L. (2007). Estrus detection. In: *Current Therapy in Large Animal Theriogenology*, 2e (ed. R.S. Youngquist and W.R. Threlfall), 270–278. WB Saunders.

Panter, K.E. and Stegelmeier, B.L. (2011). Effects of xenobiotics and phytotoxins on reproduction in food animals. *Veterinary Clinics: Food Animal Practice* 27: 429–446.

Panter, K.E., Welch, K.D., Gardner, D.R. et al. (2018). Poisonous plants of the United States. In: *Veterinary Toxicology: Basic and Clinical Principles*, 3e (ed. R.C. Gupta), 837–889. Academic Press.

Parkinson, T.J., Vermunt, J.J., and Malmo, J. (2010). *Diseases of Cattle in Australasia: A Comprehensive Textbook*. New Zealand Veterinary Association Foundation for Continuing Education.

Parthiban, S., Malmarugan, S., Murugan, M.S. et al. (2015). Review on emerging and reemerging microbial causes in bovine abortion. *International Journal of Nutrition and Food Sciences* 4: 1–6.

Pavani, K.C., Rocha, A., Baron, E. et al. (2017). The effect of kinetic heat shock on bovine oocyte maturation and subsequent gene expression of targeted genes. *Zygote* 25: 383–389.

Perumal, P., Chamuah, J.K., Srivastava, N. et al. (2013). Infectious causes of infertility in buffalo bull (*Bubalus bubalis*). *International Journal of Bio-resource and Stress Management* 4 (1): 84–90.

Phillippo, M., Humphries, W.R., Atkinson, T. et al. (1987). The effect of dietary molybdenum and iron on copper status, puberty, fertility and oestrous cycles in cattle. *The Journal of Agricultural Science* 109: 321–336.

Quinn, P.J., Markey, B.K., Carter, M.E. et al. (2002). *Veterinary Microbiology and Microbial Disease*. Blackwell Science.

Radostits, O.M., Gay, C., Hinchcliff, K.W., and Constable, P.D. (2006). *Veterinary Medicine E-Book: A Textbook of the Diseases of Cattle, Horses, Sheep, Pigs and Goats*. Elsevier Health Sciences.

Radostits, O.M., Gay, C.C., Blood, D.C., and Hinchliff, K.W. (2007). *Veterinary Medicine. A Textbook of the Diseases of Cattle, Sheep, Goats and Horses*, 10e, 963–985.

Rhoads, M.L., Gilbert, R.O., Lucy, M.C., and Butler, W.R. (2004). Effects of urea infusion on the uterine luminal environment of dairy cows. *Journal of Dairy Science* 87: 2896–2901.

Ruegg, P.L., Marteniuk, J.V., and Kaneene, J.B. (1988). Reproductive difficulties in cattle with antibody titers to *Haemophilus somnus*. *Journal of the American Veterinary Medical Association* 193: 941–942.

Salem, M.B., Djemali, M., Kayouli, C., and Majdoub, A. (2006). A review of environmental and management factors affecting the reproductive performance of Holstein-Friesian dairy herds in Tunisia. *Livestock Research for Rural Development* 18: 123–129.

Schüller, L.K., Michaelis, I., and Heuwieser, W. (2017). Impact of heat stress on estrus expression and follicle size in estrus under field conditions in dairy cows. *Theriogenology* 102: 48–53.

Silvia, W.J., Hatler, T.B., Nugent, A.M., and Da Fonseca, L.L. (2002). Ovarian follicular cysts in dairy cows: an abnormality in folliculogenesis. *Domestic animal endocrinology* 23 (1-2): 167–177.

Singh, M., Honparkhe, M., Kumar, A., and Singhal, S.G.S. (2017). Comparative efficacy of cystic ovarian follicle ablation and CIDR based Ovsynch in dairy cattle. *International Journal of Livestock Research* 7 (5): 175–182.

Singh, M., Honparkhe, M., Kumar, A., and Singhal, S. (2018). Comparison of metabolites in the follicular fluid of bovine preovulatory and cystic ovarian follicles using nuclear magnetic resonance. *Indian Journal of Animal Sciences* 88 (3): 290–294.

Stephens, L.R., Slee, K.J., Poulton, P. et al. (1986). Investigation of purulent vaginal discharge in cows, with particular reference to *Haemophilus somnus*. *Australian Veterinary Journal* 63: 182–185.

Storz, J., Carroll, E.J., Stephenson, E.H. et al. (1976). Urogenital infection and seminal excretion after inoculation of bulls and rams with chlamydiae. *American Journal of Veterinary Research* 37: 517–520.

Titterington, F.M., Lively, F.O., Ashfield, A. et al. (2017). Impacts of on farm management factors on herd fertility of commercial beef breeding herds in Northern Ireland. *The Journal of Agricultural Science* 155 (6): 1005–1021.

Tolosa, T., Bezabih, D., and Regassa, F. (2010). Study on seroprevalence of bovine brucellosis and abortion and associated risk factor. *Bulletin of Animal Health and Production in Africa* 58: 236–247.

Vailes, L.D. and Britt, J.H. (1990). Influence of footing surface on mounting and other sexual behaviors of estrual Holstein cows. *Journal of Animal Science* 68: 2333–2339.

Van Vliet, J.H. and Van Eerdenburg, F.J.C.M. (1996). Sexual activities and oestrus detection in lactating Holstein cows. *Applied Animal Behaviour Science* 50: 57–69.

Vanholder, T., Opsomer, G., and De Kruif, A. (2006). Aetiology and pathogenesis of cystic ovarian follicles in dairy cattle: a review. *Reproduction Nutrition Development* 46 (2): 105–119.

Vetter, J. (2004). Poison hemlock (*Conium maculatum* L.). *Food and Chemical Toxicology* 42: 1373–1382.

Wagner, W.C., Dunn, H.O., and Vanvleck, L.D. (1965). Incidence of vibriosis in an AI stud. *The Cornell Veterinarian* 55: 209–220.

Wakayo, B.U., Brar, P.S., and Prabhakar, S. (2015). Review on mechanisms of dairy summer infertility and implications for hormonal intervention. *Open Veterinary Journal* 5: 6–10.

Wang, S., Panter, K.E., Gardner, D.R. et al. (2004). Effects of the pine needle abortifacient, isocupressic acid, on bovine oocyte maturation and preimplantation embryo development. *Animal Reproduction Science* 81: 237–244.

Weston, J.F. (2010). Reproduction and disorders of the reproductive system. In: *Diseases of Cattle in Australasia* (ed. T.J. Parkinson, J.J. Vermunt, and J. Malmo), 414–496. Palmerston North, New Zealand: VetLearn, Palmerston North.

Wiltbank, M.C., Gümen, A.H.M.E.T., and Sartori, R. (2002). Physiological classification of anovulatory conditions in cattle. *Theriogenology* 57 (1): 21–52.

Wodaje, H.B. and Mekuria, T.A. (2016). Risk factors of repeat breeding in dairy cattle. *Advances in Biology Research* 10: 213–221.

Wood, P.D.P. (1976). A note on detection of oestrus in cattle bred by artificial insemination, and the measurement of embryonic mortality. *Animal Science* 22: 275–278.

World Organisation for Animal Health (OIE) (2017). Leptospirosis. In: *OIE Terrestrial Manual*, 26e. Paris, France: Office International des Epizooties.

Yaeger, M.J. and Holler, L.D. (2007). Bacterial causes of bovine infertility and abortion. In: *Current Therapy in Large Animal Theriogenology*, 2e (ed. R.S. Youngquist and W.R. Threlfall), 389–399. St Louis, MO: Saunders-Elsevier.

Youngquist, R.S. and Threlfall, W.R. (2006). *Current Therapy in Large Animal Theriogenology*. Elsevier Health Sciences.

Zulu, V.C., Nakao, T., and Sawamukai, Y. (2002). Insulin-like growth factor-I as a possible hormonal mediator of nutritional regulation of reproduction in cattle. *Journal of Veterinary Medical Science* 64: 657–665.

29

Ulcerative Mammillitis

Rajesh Kumar[1], Aakanksha Bhoker[1], Bhavna Priya[2], and Anil Kumar[3]

[1] Department of Veterinary Surgery and Radiology, Bihar Veterinary College, Patna, Bihar, India
[2] Department of Veterinary Gynaecology, Bihar Veterinary College, Patna, Bihar, India
[3] Department of Veterinary Medicine, Bihar Veterinary College, Patna, Bihar, India

29.1 Introduction

Ulcerative mammillitis is a viral disease seen on an irregular basis in dairy cows and buffaloes with a high incidence in temperate parts of the world (Firyal et al. 2019). It is caused by the bovine herpes virus type (BHV)-2 and is characterized by the development of erosive, ulcerative, self-limiting lesions on the udder and teats. Various designations are used to describe bovine herpes mammillitis in cattle and buffaloes including ulcerative mammillitis (Rao et al. 2003), bovine ulcerative mammillitis (Shridhar et al. 2014), ulcerative thelitis (Abd-El-Hady 2015), necrotic thelitis (Kathirvel and Dharmaceelan 2016), bovine herpes mammillitis (Bitsch 2011), and mammillitis (Sundaresh and Janaki 1997). Bovine herpes mammillitis (BHM) is also known as gulwaddee (a Punjabi term with literal meaning "neck cutter") because of the occurrence of a deep, nonhealing, ulcerative lesion at the neck of the teat, i.e. at the junction of the teat with the udder. Mastitis, the most common and dangerous disease in dairy cows, may develop during the chronic phase of ulcerative mammillitis. BHV-2 is also responsible for pseudolumpy skin disease (PLSD), which causes generalized, superficial, cutaneous nodules with central depressions over the entire body of affected animals (Gibbs 1977). It is a relatively uncommon disease that causes significant pain in the udder and teats with discomfort to the animal. It causes severe economic loss for dairy farmers due to the loss of milk production, and in chronic stages, the disease converts into a most devastating disease, mastitis (Kachhawa et al. 2017). A sudden onset of inflammation, papules, skin sloughing, vesicular growth, scab formation, and ulceration on the udder and teats can occur.

The disease often has a seasonal association with cold weather, rather than other seasons. The disease generally occurs sporadically; however, clinical outbreaks are also reported. It is more prevalent in primiparous bovines, i.e. in their first lactation (Sharma et al. 1998; Sharma and Singh 2006). Most clinical cases occur within the first 2 months of lactation (Sharma et al. 1998). Calving stress, particularly the change of hormones during parturition and udder edema, activates the BHM virus, and the development of clinical signs ensues (Kemp et al. 2008). It may be transmitted by the milker's hand, milking equipment, biting insects, semen, and air (Kemp et al. 2008). The teats of the hindquarter are more frequently involved than the forequarter teats (Mouli 1992). Generally, one teat or most commonly, two teats, are affected at a time.

29.2 Etiology

Ulcerative mammillitis is caused by BHV-2, a virus of the genus *Simplexvirus*, subfamily *Alphaherpesvirinae*, and the family *Herpesvirales*. The viral genome is linear double-stranded DNA. The virus produces intranuclear inclusion bodies and syncytia formation in infected cells. BHV-2 has close antigenic relation to human herpes simplex virus 1. However, the virus is unrelated to BHV-1, which is the causative agent of bovine rhinotracheitis. The virus was first isolated in South Africa from the generalized skin infections of cattle and was named the Allerton virus.

Periparturient Diseases of Cattle, First Edition. Edited by Tanmoy Rana.

29.3 Epidemiology

Ulcerative mammillitis is generally sporadic in nature, however, outbreaks have been reported (Bitsch 2011). An outbreak of the disease lasts 6–15 weeks; however, immunity lasts for up to 2 years after the outbreak. Outbreaks of the disease are generally not reported from the same dairy farm within 2–3 years of each other. In a susceptible dairy farm, ulcerative mammillitis spreads very quickly and infects nearly all cows within 2 months. The incubation period varies between 5 and 10 days, and there is generally systemic illness observed in the animals. It is comparatively more prevalent in temperate regions of the world. Ulcerative mammillitis has been reported from south, west, and east Africa, Asia, the United States, several European countries, and Australia. Outbreaks are mainly reported in the autumn and early winter seasons; however, in Australia, outbreaks are more often reported in the spring. Irrespective of seasonal incidence, dairy farms are randomly affected. There is considerable variation in the prevalence within areas from year to year. A cow on several dairy farms within several kilometers may become affected at the same time. The virus is present at high concentrations in the exudate and the skin lesion, therefore lateral spread may occur. The transmission of ulcerative mammillitis by natural modes is not clear, but it is suggested that mechanical vectors, particularly the milking machine, or dermal inoculation by biting flies, such as *Stomoxys calcitrans,* are responsible for transmission (Watanabe et al. 2017). Interspecies transmission of the virus from sheep and goats to buffaloes or vice versa has also been reported, and hence, sheep or goats may also serve as reservoir hosts of mammillitis in buffaloes (Lechmann et al. 2021). Calves that receive milk from the infected teats of a cow may become infected with BHV-2 and may carry the virus as a latent infection.

The prevalence of ulcerative mammillitis is higher for primiparous bovines. Heifers may become infected before calving; the reason is unclear but may be attributed to calving stress associated with udder edema and hormonal changes that activate the virus (Gibbs 1984; Kemp et al. 2008). Intact teat skin prevents penetration of the virus; however, any form of teat trauma precedes infection (Maudlin and Peters-Kennedy 2016). Healing usually occurs within 3 weeks, although ulcerated lesions may persist for months (Sandrucci et al. 2014). Abd-El-Hady (2015) reported that only buffaloes were infected, and cattle dwelling in the same areas were spared.

29.4 Pathogenesis

The incubation period of the disease ranges from 3 to 7 days. BHV-2 can cause two distinct, well-defined clinical conditions: (i) a generalized benign skin infection that somewhat mimics lumpy skin disease (LSD), referred to as pseudolumpy skin disease (PSLD), and (ii) a localized ulcerative mammillitis, also known as BHM. The disease is generally more severe than either cowpox or pseudo cowpox, and the lesions are ulcerative rather than proliferative. Vesicle formation is characteristic of the early stages of BHM in cows but remains absent (Sharma et al. 1998, 2005) or occurs rarely in buffaloes (Lokanadhamu et al. 2005). In buffaloes, BHM lesions mostly occurred at the udder–teat junction of the hind quarter teats (Sharma et al. 1998).

Experimental incubation in laboratory animals yielded three distinct observations. First, the lesion develops on the site of subcutaneous or intradermal inoculation; however, dissemination of the lesion into other parts of the skin is not observed. Second, generalized benign skin infections, i.e. PSLD, develop following intravenous inoculation of BHV-2. Third, viruses replicate to higher titers and produce more severe lesions, particularly in the cooler part of the skin.

The temperature of the skin on the teats and udder is lower than that of the body, and the interferon produced locally in the BHM virus-affected area is not only low in quantity but also has a low specific activity. That is why the BHM virus mostly produces lesions in cooler skin areas (i.e. the skin on the teats and udder where the temperature is lower than the rest of the body due to low blood circulation).

29.5 Clinical Signs

The disease remains latent and subclinical in most infected cows and buffaloes. Systemic signs of illness like a rise in body temperature, pulse, and respiration rates are generally not present (Sharma et al. 1998). Clinical signs develop in only a few infected animals, with a wide range of variation. The infected animals may become hard milkers without showing any physical abnormalities. Others may have minor teat lesions. Inflammation of the teats and udder is a typical clinical sign of ulcerative mammillitis in bovines. Inflammation results from the production of immune complexes of the virus with specific

IgM and IgG antibodies (Bitsch 2011). The affected teat(s) may increase up to two to three times its normal size and have a glossy appearance (Rao et al. 2003). Severe inflammation causes tenderness and a loss of flexibility in the teats. A small percentage of infected animals may suffer from severe teat lesions (Abd-El-Hady 2015; Sandrucci et al. 2014). The animals may develop ulceration, necrosis, or sloughing of the teat that leaves only tissue around the teat. Thickening of the wall of the affected teat may result in narrowing of the teat canal, which causes pain and difficulty when milking (Abd-El-Hady 2015). Sometimes the entire teat becomes necrotic. Calves suckling the affected teats may develop lesions in their mouths (George et al. 2008).

The disease onset initially starts with a characteristic, painful, raised, edematous teat (Sandrucci et al. 2014; Shearer et al. 2008). Initial lesions are followed by the development of a irregularly shaped vesicles (0.5–5.0 cm in diameter). Within 24 hours, the vesicles rupture, leaving an ulcerated surface that exudes copious serum. Upon drying the exudate, a thick, dark reddish-brown scab is formed on the teats. In the absence of a secondary infection, healing is completed within 3 weeks by granulation and regrowth of the epithelium. However, ulcerated lesions may persist for months (Sandrucci et al. 2014). Lesions on the udder may coalesce with those of the teat and extend to the perineum, which results in vulvovaginitis as a sequela to the infected skin of the mammary gland.

Sharma et al. (2005) described an unusual form of the disease in dairy buffaloes; the sudden appearance of multiple flattened nodules (1–4 cm in diameter) on the perineum and other parts of the body that later became necrotic and sloughed off. The perineum lesions later extended to the teats and udder. Some affected buffaloes also showed systemic signs of illness like salivation and nasal and lacrimal discharge. In the BHM-affected buffaloes, milk production was reduced by up to 31.54%.

Vesicle formation is a characteristic clinical sign of the early stages of BHM in cows, which is either absent (Sharma et al. 2005) or occurs rarely in buffaloes (Lokanadhamu et al. 2005). Mammary gland neoplasms are very common in dogs but are not generally found in mares, ewes, sows, cattle, and buffaloes. It is paradoxical that cattle, with a highly developed mammary gland, have the lowest incidence of mammary neoplasms. Cows rarely develop mammary tumors. A few cases of neoplasms in the mammary glands of buffaloes have been observed (Table 29.1).

Table 29.1 Common clinical signs of ulcerative mammillitis in bovines (Shridhar et al. 2022).

Hard milkers
Swelling of the teat and udder
Ulceration of the teat and udder surface with exudation
Formation of scabs on lesions
Systemic signs of illness like salivation and nasal and lacrimal discharge
In later stages, necrosis of the teat and udder

29.5.1 Milk Sample Status

Most studies indicate that milk samples collected during ulcerative mammillitis are normal (Shridhar 2020). Milk from the affected teats is usually negative for mastitis (Purohit et al. 2014) and remains negative for the presence of any pathogenic bacteria (Thilagar et al. 2000; Kachhawa et al. 2017; Purohit et al. 2014).

29.6 Diagnosis

A diagnosis of ulcerative mammillitis is based on the composite of clinical signs, epidemiologic features, electron microscopy, and serologic tests like the agar gel precipitation test and the neutralization test in rabbits (Janett et al. 2000; Lokanadhamu et al. 2005; Rao et al. 2003).

29.6.1 Electron Microscopy

Electron microscopy has emerged as a very accurate and useful test for the diagnosis of ulcerative mammillitis. The advantages of electron microscopy include a rapid diagnosis, the ability to detect nonviable virus, and the detection of combined viral infections.

29.6.2 Virus Isolation and Tissue Culture

Isolation of the virus using tissue culture is an effective, alternative method, particularly if electron microscopy is not available. The virus can be isolated from circulating leukocytes, skin lesions (early scabs, vesicular fluid, or scrapings from the raw surfaces of lesions), superficial and deep lymph nodes, cutaneous nerve, spinal ganglia, and central nervous system. The virus can also be isolated from nasal fluid and the milk of infected teats. Only in a generalized infection with the Alterton strain of BHV-2 can the virus also be isolated from urine, feces, and semen.

29.6.3 Histopathological Examination

Histopathologic examinations of biopsy samples taken from the lesions may reveal intranuclear inclusion bodies. The occurrence of multiple syncytia (multinucleated cells that result from the fusion of single cells) in the stratum spinosum layer with basophilic or eosinophilic intranuclear inclusions is the characteristic and diagnostic histological feature of naturally occurring BHM-2 infections in buffaloes (Sharma et al. 1998), cows (Rweyemamu et al. 1969), and experimentally inoculated rabbits (Rao et al. 2003; Lokanadhamu et al. 2005). The condition may resemble pseudo cowpox, but in pseudo cowpox, inclusion bodies are seen inside the cytoplasm, not in the nucleus (George et al. 2008). Moreover, pseudo cowpox lesions are ring shaped (Sandrucci et al. 2014).

29.6.4 Intradermal Inoculation

The rabbit is a very important laboratory animal for the confirmation of BHM. When a bacteria-free whey filtrate prepared from the milk of an infected teat is injected intradermally in rabbits, about 48 hours after inoculation, mild erythematous lesions are produced on the skin that persist for another 48 hours. However, similar reactions upon inoculation were not observed in mice (Rao et al. 2003).

29.6.5 Paired Serum Samples

In ulcerative mammillitis, paired serum samples collected (i) during the acute stage of the infection and (ii) 14 days later provide a diagnosis of BHV-2. A fourfold rise in serum antibodies is observed in cowpox and BHM, but pseudo cowpox generally does not elicit a serological response. A primary problem with this test is that the cow may already be past the acute stage of the illness by the time she is tested. This is especially true of BHM, for which acute stage serum samples must be taken within 2 days of the appearance of lesions. However, a clinical diagnosis of BHM may be made by detecting high BHV-2 antibody titers in a single sample.

29.7 Differential Diagnosis

Primary differential diagnoses include other viral diseases that produce similar lesions on the teat and udder, like pseudo cowpox (genus *Parapoxvirus*), cowpox (genus *Orthopoxvirus*), and foot-and-mouth disease (FMD). Bacteria, like staphylococci, *Fusobacterium necrophorum,* and *Borrelia burgdorferi*, as well as parasitic infections, such as stephanofilariasis, can also produce similar lesions on the teat and udder. Some noninfectious diseases like photosensitivity reactions, allergies, chemical irritation, and trauma may also produce ulcerative lesion on the teat, so these diseases should also be considered.

29.7.1 Pseudo Cowpox

- No incidence of marked seasonal fluctuation like BHV-2.
- Initially, it appears as small, red, raised sores on the teats and udders.
- Progresses to vesicles, scabs, and nodules.
- May form a “ring” or “horseshoe” of scabs over the course of several weeks.
- In humans, pseudo cowpox can cause localized skin lesions, whereas BHV-2 has no zoonotic potential.
- The inclusion bodies are seen inside the cytoplasm, not in the nucleus (George et al. 2008).

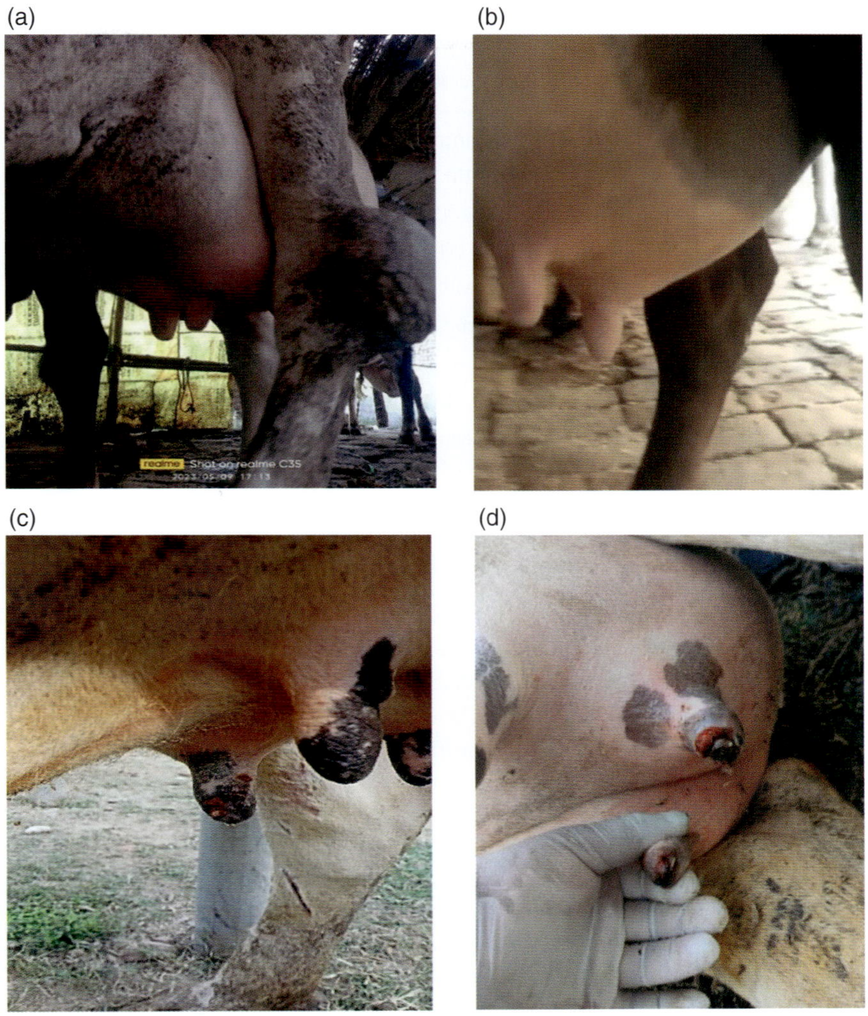

Figure 29.1 (a) and (b) Inflammation of the teat with vesicle formation. (c) and (d) Teat ulcers.

29.7.2 Cowpox

- Udder lesions are primarily proliferative, whereas they are ulcerative in BHV (Figure 29.1).
- No incidence of seasonal fluctuation like BHV-2.
- Cowpox has zoonotic potential, unlike BHV-2.

29.7.3 Foot-and-mouth Disease

- Teat lesions along with characteristic vesicles, bullae, and ulcerated areas on the muzzle, tongue, and coronary bands that causes profuse salivation and lameness.
- Affected animals are anorexic and pyretic.

29.8 Treatment

In the management of ulcerative mammillitis in bovines, a combination of different types of drugs (antibiotics, antihistamines, and anti-inflammatory drugs) (Table 29.2) along with autoimmune therapy has been suggested to hasten recovery and prevent secondary bacterial complications like mastitis (Abd-El-Hady 2015; Bentz et al. 2006; Lokanadhamu et al. 2005; Purohit et al. 2014; Purohit and Markandeya 2015). Most cases recover normally after completing the treatment protocol. Teat edema and hyperemia gradually return to normal. However, animals with necrotic rings on the teat generally do not respond well to treatment. The conventional treatment also fails to treat ulcerative mammillitis, particularly if there is an ulcer at the junction of the teat and udder (Lokanadhamu et al. 2005). Many cases in buffaloes do not respond to routine treatment for up to 3 months.

Table 29.2 Common drugs used to treat ulcerative mammillitis.

Drug	Dose (per kg body weight)
Ceftriaxone	10 mg, intramuscularly (IM)
Amoxicillin–sulbactam	10 mg, IM
Enrofloxacin	5–10 mg, IM
Meloxicam	0.1 mg, IM
Ketoprofen	2 mg, IM
Chlorpheniramine maleate	05–1.0 mg, IM
Levamisole	3–5 mg, subcutaneously (SC)
Acyclovir	1–2 mg, slow intravenous (IV)
Lithium antimony thiomalate	2 mg, deep IM
Ivermectin	0.1 µg, SC

29.8.1 Conventional Treatment (Antibiotics, Antihistamines, and Anti-inflammatories)

Antibiotics are not very effective in treating buffalo mammillitis since the milk remains free from bacterial infection. However, antibiotics may be used, when a secondary infection develops, which follows the necrosis of the teat lesion (Shridhar 2020; Shridhar et al. 2022). Syed et al. (2009) successfully treated ulcerative mammillitis in cows by giving ceftriaxone (3 g daily, intramuscularly [IM]), along with chlorpheniramine maleate (10 ml, IM) and meloxicam (10 ml, IM) for 5 days. Chlorpheneramine maleate (antihistamine, H1-receptor antagonist) is an antiallergy medicine used to treat a variety of allergic conditions in cattle and buffaloes that can be helpful in the early stages of buffalo mammillitis (Shridhar et al. 2014; Shridhar 2020; Lokanadhamu et al. 2005; Vardanyan and Hruby 2006; Sharma et al. 2007). Meloxicam is a nonsteroidal anti-inflammatory drug (NSAID) with analgesic and anti-inflammatory properties that has good efficacy in the inflammatory stage of the condition (Shridhar et al. 2014; Shridhar 2020; Syed et al. 2009). It has a low ulcerogenic property because of its preferential cyclooxygenase (COX)-2 inhibition (Mathews 2002; Breen 2017). However, in some buffaloes, the same treatment protocol was ineffective and necrosis developed in the affected teat, which later fell from the udder, as per Shridhar (2020). The necrotic tissues do not have active cells to respond to the infection. Kachhawa et al. (2017) reported complete recovery in five clinical cases treated with amoxicillin–sulbactam at 10 mg/kg body weight, IM; ketoprofen at 2 mg/kg body weight, IM; and ascorbic acid at 5 g intravenously (IV) with 500 ml normal saline.

29.8.2 Acyclovir

Acyclovir has antiherpes activity against BHV-2 (Watson 1989). Acyclovir converts to its triphosphate form, acyclovir triphosphate (ACV-TP), which incorporates into and terminates the growing viral DNA chain, thus inactivating/inhibiting the viral DNA polymerase. In cell culture studies, acyclovir was able to eliminate BHV-1 virus titers and stop the progression of the cytopathic effect (Enan et al. 2012). There are no data on the pharmacokinetics of acyclovir in cows and buffaloes (Bentz et al. 2006). Lokanadhamu et al. (2005) investigated the efficacy of oral and topical acyclovir in buffalo mammillitis. However, oral acyclovir did not achieve the required plasma concentration. Therefore, parenteral administration of acyclovir is preferred to ensure an effective plasma concentration for better antiviral activity (Watson 1989; Rollinson 1992; Firyal et al. 2019). The oral administration of acyclovir (20 mg/kg) remained ineffective for treating horses suffering from equine herpes virus (EHV-1) infections (Bentz et al. 2006). However, its prodrug, valacyclovir, attained effective plasma concentration after IV administration. Valacyclovir, thus, may be an appealing and valuable candidate for treating EHV-1 infections in horses.

29.8.3 Immunopotentiation

Since the cows and buffaloes that suffer from BHM are in a state of immunosuppression (Bitsch 2011), immunity enhancing agents such as levamisole (at about 80 ml per cow or buffalo per day for 4 days, orally [PO]), injected vitamin E, selenium, and zinc sulfate (2–3 g per cow or buffalo per day for 10 days) can be used to improve the immune response against the herpes virus.

The conventional treatment protocol that uses antibiotic, antiallergy, and anti-inflammatory drugs had a cure rate of only 12.5% in 24 buffaloes after 35 days of treatment. The addition of oral acyclovir improved the cure rate to 37.5% within 24 days. The further addition of lysine tablets and the topical application of acyclovir ointment improved the cure rate to 62.5% in 12 days (Lokanadhamu et al. 2005). Lysine has been shown to reduce the severity of herpes simplex infections in humans (Griffith et al. 1987).

29.8.4 Local Applications

The local application of 10% zinc oxide ointment along with anti-inflammatory enzymes and antibiotics can prevent ulceration, necrosis, and the sloughing of teats during the early treatment of ulcerative thelitis (Abd-El-Hady 2015). Propolis, a resinous mixture collected by honeybees from tree buds, sap flows, or other botanical sources, is used as a sealant for unwanted open spaces in their hives. The application of propolis to the affected ulcerative teat speeds up healing and restores milk yield within 2 weeks. The use of a 1% solution of potassium permanganate ($KMnO_4$) is effective for the local treatment of teats and udder in cows suffering from mammillitis. $KMnO_4$ is used as a teat dip for the prevention, treatment, and control of bovine mastitis, and in general, teat dipping is categorized among the most highly recommended mastitis control programs (Oliver et al. 2001). Chlorhexidine is also said to be effective against the herpes virus. A local application or teat dipping in chlorhexidine solution has prophylactic and therapeutic affects against the herpes virus and is useful in the therapy of bovine mammillitis (Bailey and Longson 1972; Shridhar et al. 2022). The external application of povidone-iodine is also said to be effective, along with other palliative treatments such as antihistamines and anti-inflammatories (Syed et al. 2009). A paste of *Breynia patens* and *Sclerophyllum wallichianum* moderately cures mammillitis in buffaloes (Sundaresh and Janaki 1997; Misra 1991). Different parts of these plants, which are known to have anti-inflammatory and antihistamine properties, may have played an important role in overcoming mammillitis and preventing further damage to the affected teats in these animals.

29.8.5 Lithium Antimony Thiomalate

Shridhar (2020) used lithium antimony thiomalate at 2 mg/kg, deep IM, along with chlorpheniramine maleate, meloxicam, acyclovir, and the external application of acyclovir ointment to the affected teats of buffaloes. Lithium antimony thiomalate is used for a better cure rate of ulcerative mammillitis. The probable mechanism of lithium antimony thiomalate in curing the condition might be due to its antifibrosis activity.

29.8.6 Drug Repurposing

An ivermectin injection at a dose of 0.1 μg/kg, subcutaneously, two injections 10 days apart, is said to be effective in treating bovine mammillitis.

29.8.7 Surgical Management

The ulcerative lesions present at the junction of the teat and udder should be properly debrided and cauterized until blood starts oozing from the surface. Large, chronic, indolent ulcers with scabs can be debrided using a sterile scalpel blade. The small lesions can be cauterized using handheld silver nitrate sticks or copper sulfate. Debridement or cauterization should be repeated two to three times at weekly intervals or as needed (Sharma and Singh 2006). After debridement, the affected area may be rinsed with chloroform (the herpes virus is sensitive to chloroform). Later, the local application of an antibiotic cream or an insect-repellant wound spray may be applied.

29.8.8 Temperature Regulation

Assembly and maturation of the BHV are inhibited at higher body temperatures as an elevated temperature stimulates local production of the highly active form of interferon that inhibits BHV viral replication (Letchworth and Carmichael 1984; Kathirvel and Dharmaceelan 2016). The temperature of the ulcerative teat and udder lesions can theoretically be raised using an infrared lamp. However, the practical use of this lamp to treat buffalo mammillitis has not been reported.

29.9 Control and Prevention

The treatment of individual cows suffering from teat lesions is necessary; it is also important to institute prevention and control strategies within the herd. Ideally, newly purchased animals should be quarantined for at least 14 days before their introduction into the herd. BHM-affected cows or buffaloes should not be purchased and introduced to a healthy herd. The presence of depigmented skin area on the teat may be used as an indication that the cows and buffaloes have been exposed to the BHM virus, as the mark is left after the healing process (Gibbs et al. 1970; Yager and Scott 1992). It is recommended that such animals should never be purchased.

Since ulcerative mammillitis is a contagious disease (Bitsch 2011), the affected animals should be isolated immediately and milked after healthy animals. Usually, the entire herd will be affected (Shridhar et al. 2022). Milking hygiene and post-milking antiseptic teat dipping are very important, particularly where an outbreak of BHM has occurred (Bitsch 2011). Calves should not be allowed to suckle the affected teat because suckling and forced milking could causes further damage to the teat (Firyal et al. 2019). All milking equipment should be thoroughly disinfected by boiling or with disinfectants after their use on an infected cow (Kemp et al. 2008). Milkers should wear gloves in the milking parlor and disinfect the gloves between cows. All other biosecurity measures should be implemented. In severe cases of thelitis (teat inflammation), a sterile teat siphon or Dr. Larson's® Teat Tube (Mai Animal Health, Elmwood, Wisconsin, USA) may be used to milk the affected teat(s) (Abd-El-Hady 2015). Post-milking antiseptic teat dipping should be performed on all animals in the herd to prevent the spread of disease and support the healing of lesions on affected animals.

Latent infections reactivated by stress are regarded as the most likely source of spread within a herd. Latency is characteristic of herpes virus diseases, and the reactivation of experimental BHV-2 infections after the application of corticosteroids was demonstrated. Since calving stress and udder edema are very important predisposing factors to BHM (Bitsch 2011), all measures should be taken to reduce calving stress and prevent the occurrence of parturient udder edema. If udder edema develops, appropriate therapy should be provided for its management. Insects should be controlled in the dairy farm, as they have been documented to transmit BHV.

Currently, no commercial vaccines are available for immunization against BHV.

References

Abd-El-Hady, A.A.A. (2015). Clinical observations on some surgical udder and teat affections in cattle and buffaloes. *Scholars Journal of Agriculture and Veterinary Sciences* 2 (4A): 270–281.

Bailey, A. and Longson, M. (1972). Virucidal activity of chlorhexidine on strains of Herpes virus hominis, poliovirus, and adenovirus. *Journal of Clinical Pathology* 25 (1): 76–78.

Bentz, B.G., Maxwell, L.K., Erkert, R.S. et al. (2006). Pharmacokinetics of acyclovir after single intravenous and oral administration to adult horses. *Journal of Veterinary Internal Medicine* 20 (3): 589–594.

Bitsch, V. (2011). Epidemiology and pathogenesis of the bovine herpesvirus 2 infection. In: *Disease in Response to Initial Antibody Production*, 2–13. Beder, Denmark.

Breen, J. (2017). The importance of non-steroidal anti-inflammatory drugs (NSAIDs) in mastitis therapeutics. *Livestock* 22 (4): 182–185.

Enan, G., Abdallah, F.M., and Sobhy, H. (2012). Effect of acyclovir on bovine herpes virus type 1 infection in in vitro cultured cells. *International Journal of Virology* 8 (4): 307–312.

Firyal, S., Ali, M.M., Muhammad, G. et al. (2019). Bovine herpes mammillitis (Gulwaddee) – a less known disease of cows and buffaloes in Pakistan. *Buffalo Bulletin* 38 (4): 571–578.

George, L.W., Divers, T.J., Ducharme, N., and Welcome, F.L. (2008). Diseases of the teats and udder. In: *Rebhun's Diseases of Dairy Cattle* (ed. T.J. Divers and S.F. Peek), 328–394. St. Louis, Missouri, USA: Saunders Elsevier.

Gibbs, E.P.J. (1977). Bovine herpes viruses. Part I. Bovine herpes virus 1. *Veterinary Bulletin* 47: 317–318.

Gibbs, E.P. (1984). Viral diseases of the skin of the bovine teat and udder. *The Veterinary Clinics of North America. Large Animal Practice* 6 (1): 187–202.

Gibbs, E.P.J., Johnson, R.H., and Osborne, A.D. (1970). The differential diagnosis of viral skin infections of the bovine teat. *Veterinary Record* 87 (20): 602–609.

Griffith, R.S., Walsh, D.E., Myrmel, K.H. et al. (1987). Success of L-lysine therapy in frequently recurrent herpes simplex infection. *Dermatology* 175 (4): 183–190.

Janett, F., Stäuber, N., Schraner, E. et al. (2000). Bovine herpes mammillitis: clinical symptoms and serologic course. *Schweizer Archiv fur Tierheilkunde* 142 (7): 375–380.

Kachhawa, J.P., Sharma, A., Tanwar, T.K. et al. (2017). Bovine ulcerative mammillitis and its therapeutic management. Ruminant. *Science* 6 (1): 193–194.

Kathirvel, S. and Dharmaceelan, S. (2016). The litis in buffaloes-review of 12 clinical cases. *Indian Veterinary Journal* 93 (10): 73–74.

Kemp, R.P.F.N., Holliman, A., and Nettleton, P.F. (2008). Atypical bovine herpes mammillitis affecting cows and calves. *Veterinary Research* 163: 119–120.

Lechmann, J., Ackermann, M., Kaiser, V., and Bachofen, C. (2021). Viral infections shared between water buffaloes and small ruminants in Switzerland. *Journal of Veterinary Diagnostic Investigation* 33 (5): 894–905.

Letchworth, G.J. and Carmichael, L.E. (1984). Local tissue temperature: a critical factor in the pathogenesis of bovid herpes virus 2. *Infection and Immunity* 43 (3): 1072–1079.

Lokanadhamu, M., Sreedevi, B., and Reddy, T.V. (2005). Studies on etiology, symptomatology, diagnosis and therapy in ulcerative the litis of buffaloes in Andhra Pradesh (India). *Buffalo Bulletin* 24 (3): 56–69.

Mathews, K.A. (2002). Non-steroidal anti-inflammatory analgesics: a review of current practice. *Journal of Veterinary Emergency and Critical Care* 12 (2): 89–97.

Maudlin, E.A. and Peters-Kennedy, J. (2016). Integumentary system. In: *Pathology of Domestic Animals* (ed. K.V.F. Jubb, P.C. Kennedy, and N.C. Palmer), 625–626. St. Louis: Elsevier.

Misra, S.K. (1991). Inflammation and anti inflammatory ingredients of Teeburb. *Indian Journal of Indigenous Medicine* 7: 1–4.

Mouli, S.P. (1992). A note on the incidence of necrotic the litis in buffalos. *Indian Veterinary Journal* 69 (8): 758–759.

Oliver, S.P., Gillespie, B.E., Lewis, M.J. et al. (2001). Efficacy of a new premilking teat disinfectant containing a phenolic combination for the prevention of mastitis. *Journal of Dairy Science* 84 (6): 1545–1549.

Purohit, G.N. and Markandeya, N.M. (2015). *Postpartum Complications in the Buffalo. Bubaline Theriogenology*. Ithaca, New York: International Veterinary Information Service.

Purohit, G.N., Gaur, M., and Shekher, C. (2014). Mammary gland pathologies in the parturient buffalo. *Asian Pacific Journal of Reproduction* 3 (4): 322–336.

Rao, U.M., Sreedevi, B., and Reddy, T.V. (2003). Studies on ulcerative mammillitis of buffaloes in Andhra Pradesh (India). *Buffalo Bulletin* 22 (4): 80–90.

Rollinson, E.A. (1992). Prospects for antiviral chemotherapy in veterinary medicine: 2. Avian, piscine, canine, porcine, bovine and equine virus diseases. *Antiviral Chemistry and Chemotherapy* 3 (6): 311–326.

Rweyemamu, M.M., Osborne, A.D., and Johnson, R.H. (1969). Observations on the histopathology of bovine herpes mammillitis. *Research in Veterinary Science* 10 (2): 203–211.

Sandrucci, A., Bava, L., Zucali, M., and Tamburini, A. (2014). Management factors and cow traits influencing milk somatic cell counts and teat hyperkeratosis during different seasons. *Revista Brasileira de Zootecnia* 43: 505–511.

Sharma, S. and Singh, K.B. (2006). Ischaemic necrosis of the teat base in cattle and buffaloes. *The Veterinary Record* 158 (1): 32.

Sharma, S., Singh, K.B., Oberoi, M.S., and Sood, N. (1998). Studies on the occurrence of bovine herpes mammillitis in buffaloes. *Buffalo Bulletin* 17: 79–81.

Sharma, S., Singh, K.B., Bansal, B.K., and Sharma, D.K. (2005). Clinical symptomatology and epidemiological observations on teat skin lesions in buffaloes. *Buffalo Bulletin* 24 (1): 12–16.

Sharma, N., Gupta, S.K., Sharma, U., and Hussain, K. (2007). Treatment of clinical mastitis in a buffaloes: a case report. *Buffalo Bulletin* 26 (2): 56–58.

Shearer, J.K., Townsend, J.K., and Gibbs, E.P.J. (2008). Skin infection of the bovine teat and udder and their differential diagnosis. In: *Bovine Medicine: Diseases and Husbandry of Cattle* (ed. A.H. Andrews, R.W. Blowey, H. Boyd, and R.G. Eddy), 363–372. London, UK: Wiley.

Shridhar, N.B. (2020). Lithium antimony thiomalate and acyclovir therapy for buffalo mammillitis. *The Pharma Innovation* 9: 49–52.

Shridhar, N.B., Santhosh Kumar, C.N., and Kadagi, M. (2014). Therapeutic management of mammillitis - a case report of 5 buffaloes. *Intas Polivet* 15 (1): 83–84.

Shridhar, N.B., Vinay, P.T., Santhosh Kumar, C.N. et al. (2022). Buffaloe mammillitis: a systematic review. *International Journal of Current Microbiological Applied Science* 11 (5): 267–277.

Sundaresh, N.R. and Janaki, S. (1997). Mammilities in buffaloes - a report. *Indian Veterinary Journal* 74: 785.

Syed, A.M., Halmandge, S.C., Kasaralikar, V.R., and Ganesh, U.K. (2009). A successful treatment of bovine ulcerative mammillitis. *Veterinary World* 2 (1): 33.

Thilagar, S., Rameshkumar, B., Chandran, N.D.J., and Paul, W.M. (2000). Clinical studies on obstructive the litis in buffaloes. *Indian Veterinary Journal* 77 (3): 240–241.

Vardanyan, R. and Hruby, V. (2006). Synthesis of essential drugs. In: *Antihistamine Drugs* (ed. R.S. Vardanyan and V.J. Hruby), 669–715. University of Arizona Tucson, Elsevier, 219–230.

Watanabe, T.T.N., Moeller, R.B. Jr., Crossley, B.M., and Blanchard, P.C. (2017). Outbreaks of bovine herpes virus 2 infections in calves causing ear and facial skin lesions. *Journal of Veterinary Diagnostic Investigation* 29 (5): 686–690.

Watson, C.A. (1989). *Study of Selected Antiviral Compounds on Bovine Herpes Mammillitis Virus (BHV-2)*, 6–7. Belgium: European Society for Veterinary Virology Liege.

Yager, J.A. and Scott, D.W. (1992). Bovine herpes mammillitis. In: *Pathology of Domestic Animals*, 4e (ed. K.V.F. Jubb, P.C. Kennedy, and N. Palmer). San Diego, California, USA: Academic Press.

30

Physiological Edema

Ankesh Kumar[1], *Ravi S. K. Mandal*[2], *Sonam Bhatt*[2], *and Anil Kumar*[2]

[1] *Department of Veterinary Clinical Complex, Bihar Veterinary College, Bihar Animal Sciences University, Patna, Bihar, India*
[2] *Department of Veterinary Medicine, Bihar Veterinary College, Bihar Animal Sciences University, Patna, Bihar, India*

30.1 Introduction

Approximately 60% of the total body mass in a nonobese subject is made up of water, two-thirds of which is found inside cells. Of the one-third confined to the extracellular space, 70% is distributed in the interstitium, 20% in the vasculature, and 10% in the central nervous system, eyes, serous cavities, and intestinal lumen (Figure 30.1) (Walker et al. 1990). Interstitial fluid confers a degree of turgor that the practiced examiner recognizes as normal. Although a modest expansion of interstitial fluid volume may not be detected, an excess of several liters causes visible and palpable swelling. The term “edema” refers to a discernible excess of interstitial fluid. Pitting edema gives way upon palpation, leaving persistent impressions in the skin; brawny edema offers resistance and leaves no impressions (Walker et al. 1990). The point of focus is swelling of the extracellular matrix or interstitial edema, which may occur as a result of aberrant changes in the pressures (hydrostatic and oncotic) that act across the microvascular walls and alterations in the molecular structures that comprise the barrier to fluid and solute flux in the endothelial wall that manifest as changes in hydraulic conductivity and the osmotic reflection coefficient for plasma proteins or alterations in the lymphatic outflow system (Scallan et al. 2010; Jerome et al. 1994).

The excessive accumulation of interstitial fluid is generally viewed as detrimental to tissue function because edema formation increases the diffusion distance for oxygen and other nutrients, which may compromise cellular metabolism in the swollen tissue. For the same reason, edema formation limits the removal of potentially toxic metabolic byproducts through diffusion (Jerome et al. 1994; Bhave and Neilson 2011).

30.2 Pathophysiology

Edema formation occurs into two fundamental steps. First, an alteration in capillary hemodynamics is responsible for the movement of fluids from the vascular space into the interstitial spaces, which consequently reduces plasma volume and reduces tissue perfusion. Initially, fluid moves from the vascular space into the interstitial, which reduces plasma volume and reduces tissue perfusion. To respond to these changes, the kidney retains sodium and water. The retention of dietary or intravenously administered sodium and water by the kidneys can also develop edema. There is some fluid that stays in the vascular space, and the plasma volume returns to normal. However, this change in capillary hemodynamics leads to retained fluid entering the interstitial space, which results in edema (Bhave and Neilson 2011).

Edema can also form as a response to elevated capillary hydraulic pressures, increased capillary permeability, disruption of the endothelial glycocalyx, decreased interstitial compliance, lower plasma oncotic pressure, or a combination of these factors. Lymphatic obstruction can also lead to fluid buildup because under normal conditions filtered fluids do not return to the systemic circulation (Reed and Rubin 2010). Edema can be generalized or localized, and gravity plays a critical role in fluid accumulation; thus, the lower extremities are particularly prone to fluid collection. Anything that raises capillary pressures, reduces oncotic pressure, increases endothelial permeability, or impairs lymphatic drainage will result in edema.

Periparturient Diseases of Cattle, First Edition. Edited by Tanmoy Rana.

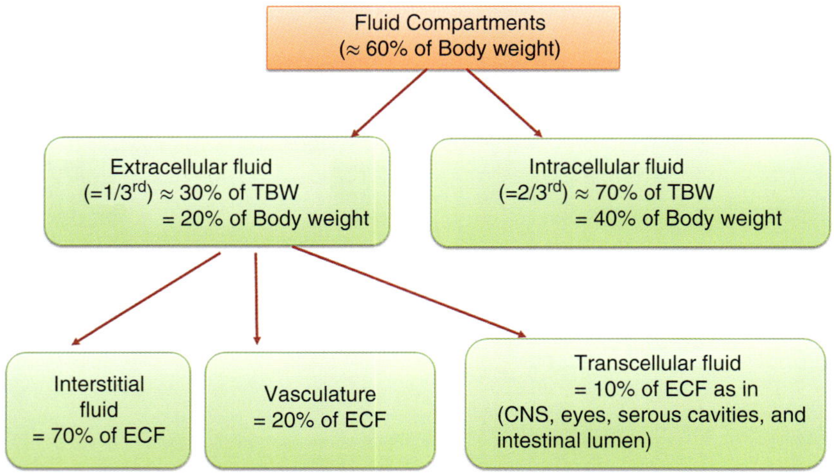

Figure 30.1 The distribution of fluid in bodily compartments.

Raised capillary pressure is a common cause of edema, including cardiac failure. Capillary hydraulic pressure has an autoregulatory capacity that allows changes in resistance at the precapillary sphincter and thus, determines the arterial pressure forced into the capillary. In contrast, the venous end of the capillary has poor regulation, and as a result, venous pressure changes lead to parallel changes in capillary hydraulic pressure. Venous pressure can increase in two settings: (i) when blood volume is expanded and (ii) when there is obstruction at the venous end. Heart failure and renal disease lead to volume expansion, while cirrhosis or right heart failure leads to venous obstruction; both instances ultimately result in edema (Jerome et al. 1994; Reed and Rubin 2010; Woodcock and Woodcock 2012; Wiig et al. 2013). Venous obstruction can also cause increased capillary pressure such as deep vein thrombosis, external compression, and superior vena cava obstruction.

Increased capillary permeability, typically due to vascular injury, results in edema for several reasons. When vessels become injured, the porosity of the capillary walls increases, and consequently, net filtration increases. Furthermore, the coefficient of proteins across the capillary wall decreases, thus narrowing the difference between the oncotic pressure of the capillary and the oncotic pressure below the endothelial glycocalyx. The oncotic pressure gradient reduces, and edema results.

30.3 Periparturient Udder Edema in Cows

Physiological udder edema is a noninfectious metabolic disorder that may be present at a higher percentage in the dairy industry. The welfare of a dairy cow has a direct effect on her production ability (von Keyserlingk et al. 2009). Udder edema is the result of lymphatic fluid accumulation in the interstitial space of the mammary gland and surrounding tissues (Al-Ani and Vestweber 1984; Tucker et al. 1992; Kojouri et al. 2015; Morrison et al. 2018).

Designated as a metabolic disorder (Kojouri et al. 2015), physiologic udder edema has been associated with excessive salt in the diet, a greater age at first calving (AFC) (Malven et al. 1983), above-ideal body condition scores (BCS), genetic traits (Ruegg 2015), physiological changes during maturation and udder development (Dyce and Wensing 1971; Robbins and Cotran 1979; Tyler and Ensminger 2006), oxidative stress (Mueller et al. 1989), increased stress from pen movements when removing or adding new animals to the group, and overcrowding (Fustini et al. 2017; Tao and Dahl 2013).

Udder edema usually occurs at the time of parturition, sometime developing to a serious degree before parturition occurs. Parity is negatively associated with the prevalence of edema (Morrison et al. 2018). It affects first-calf heifers as well as older cows, with animals of higher production potential tending to be more susceptible, especially cows with a pendulous udder. During pregnancy, the increase of fetal pressure in the pelvic area causes blood and lymphatic fluid circulation to be impaired, which results in fluid buildup in the udder tissues (Al-Ani and Vestweber 1986). This excess fluid leads to deterioration of the support structures in the udder (Dentine and McDaniel 1983), which causes misshapen quarters and teats, an increased risk of udder cleft dermatitis, and an increased risk of mastitis (Morrison et al. 2018). Tenderness of the udder and malformed teats disrupt milk letdown, increase the difficulty of attaching the milking machine due to kicking, and negatively affect production potential throughout an animal's lifetime (Vestweber and Al-Ani 1983; Melendez et al. 2006; Medrano-Galarza et al. 2012).

It has been stated that udder edema occurs more severely in Holstein and Guernseys than Jersey, Ayrshires, or Brown Swiss. Udder edema is common in Holstein dairy operations, with 66% of cows having udder edema at least once (Morrison et al. 2018).

The exact cause of udder edema is unknown. However, recent physiological and pathological studies have shown that udder edema at parturition results from decreased mammary blood flow associated with increased venous blood pressure in the cranial superficial epigastric veins. The occurrence of udder edema could be hereditary.

30.4 Physiological Udder Edema

As a pregnant heifer transitions to the milking string, her body goes through substantial physiological changes. Although the mammary system is already in place, it develops significantly in the last stages of gestation. The animal's internal anatomy begins to change, and physiologically, the demand of blood for mammary gland development is the precursor to udder edema in primiparous heifers. Mature dairy cows have a subcutaneous abdominal vein, also known as the milk vein, whereas this vein is not present in heifers. Young cattle have a cranial epigastric vein that flows anterior to the mammary gland and a caudal epigastric vein that flows posterior to the mammary gland. In the latter stages of gestation, a heifer's cranial epigastric and caudal epigastric veins merge through anastomosis, creating the milk vein (Dyce and Wensing 1971). The caudal and cranial mammary veins come together and form the subcutaneous abdominal vein. The creation of the subcutaneous abdominal vein allows for an increase in the amount of blood flow from the mammary gland. Two types of edema occur: generalized and local (Moroni et al. 2018). Generalized edema involves the whole body. It is most common in the ventral sides such as the barrel, limbs, and udder. Venous stasis due to decreased blood flow in the veins from an increase in capillary pressure or impaired lymphatic drainage causes localized edema (Robbins and Cotran 1979). Brisket edema (high altitude disease) is a prime example of localized edema, where fluid collects in a specific anatomic location instead of involving the whole body (Hecht et al. 1962). Due to the increased amount of blood needed for mammary gland development, the blood flow will reverse in direction. It is exactly the opposite of the blood flow in a young heifer. With this increase in flow, the veins respond by increasing in size (Linzell 1960). The blood must travel throughout the body to provide proper oxygen, fluid, and nutrient levels to maintain body tissues. Two forces that control fluid movement across blood supply membranes are hydrostatic pressure and osmotic pressure. Osmosis is the diffusion of water across a semipermeable membrane to balance different concentrations of solutes (salt being a primary one) on the two sides of the membrane. Osmotic pressure prevents water from moving across the capillary membrane, whereas hydrostatic pressure pulls water across the membrane (Stillwell 2013). Proteins in blood plasma draw water from interstitial spaces. When functioning properly, capillaries bring in extravascular fluid to maintain interstitial fluid levels. Without the ability to drain these tissues due to a pressure imbalance, fluid builds up in the interstitial tissues, which results in udder edema. The same result can occur with the obstruction of lymphatic drainage, but this is more localized. Another important variable in fluid movement is capillary permeability. Udder edema has a "snowball effect," whereby increased blood flow increases hydrostatic pressure (Tyler and Ensminger 2006). Greater hydrostatic pressure increases capillary permeability, which then causes the leakage of fluid into the interstitial tissues. With more blood proteins in the tissues, more fluid will be drawn to the tissue space. As fluid accumulates, the surrounding tissues become inflamed, which obstructs blood and lymph vessels and disrupts fluid movement into and out of the vessels (University of Idaho 2018). Histamine released by cells in response to inflammatory reactions is higher in the colostrum and plasma of animals with udder edema (Zarkower 1967). Higher than normal histamine concentrations in the udder tissue can lead to the self-destructive behavior of licking the udder tissue and teats until they become raw, which creates significant lesions that can lead to dermatosis (Eyre and Burka 1978; Yeruham and Markusfeld 1996). Another study found periparturient udder edema to be associated with an increased risk of clinical mastitis (Slettbakk et al. 1995).

Increased blood flow, decreased fluid movement between the tissues and capillaries, and increased histamine levels are physiological changes that present a challenge for dairy farmers. The best approach is prevention before udder edema becomes severe. Due to the natural physiological, metabolic, and vascular functions that change throughout the last stage of gestation, the farmer needs to manage nutrition, genetic, and calving factors such as body condition and age at calving to provide an optimal scenario for minimizing udder edema. Suggestions such as massaging the udder during milking and the use of diuretics have been shown to have some effects on reducing edema (Alhadrami and Faye 2016).

Mammary blood flow increases during the periparturient period and changes in mammary blood flow could be a factor in the development of udder edema at calving (von Keyserlingk et al. 2009). Udder edema is a buildup of lymphatic fluid in and around the interstitial spaces of the udder (Kojouri et al. 2015). The pressure from the developed fetus in the pelvic area hinders blood and lymphatic fluid circulation, which leads to fluid buildup during the periparturient period. Cows with udder edema have an increased risk for the development of mastitis. First-calf heifers are more susceptible to developing udder edema because even though the mammary system is already in place, significant development occurs during the last stage of gestation. The increased demand of blood for the continued development of the mammary system is a precursor to udder edema. The milk vein (subcutaneous abdominal vein) on mature cows allows for proper blood flow, whereas the milk vein is not yet present in heifers. Cows with a high milk yield have an increased genetic potential to develop udder edema compared to cows with lower milk production (Van Dorp et al. 1998). The stasis of milk in the udder, commonly observed in heifers due to the failure of milk "letdown," is considered one of the causes.

Several investigators have found a relationship between udder edema and dietary salt intake. An association was observed between chronic udder edema in milking cows and heifers with excess dietary sodium chloride (Jones et al. 1984).

Factors that contribute to a greater risk of developing udder edema include AFC, gestation length, genetics, nutritional management, over conditioning, and a lack of exercise in the late prepartum period (Hillerton 2022). A greater AFC and increased gestation length have been correlated with an increased risk of developing udder edema (Malven et al. 1983). This could be due to these animals being over conditioned at the time of calving. One researcher has reported that Jersey heifers are more susceptible to developing udder edema compared to Holstein heifers (Nestor et al. 1988). This has been attributed to the smaller body frame of Jersey cows compared to Holstein cows. This area of research has not been thoroughly studied since the 1980s, therefore, more current research is necessary to validate these results. Udder depth and udder support are conformation traits that have been correlated with an increased occurrence of udder edema. Cows with udder edema experience the deterioration of udder support structures that leads to low hanging udders (Dentine and McDaniel 1983). With low hanging, pendulous udders cows have a greater risk of injuring a teat and acquiring environmental mastitis-causing pathogens on the teat end opening from stall surfaces or walkways.

30.5 Cellular Level

Edema is believed to be the outward filtration that predominates the arterial end of the capillary, and as hydrostatic pressures fall, fluid reverts to the capillary from the interstitial space, driven by the oncotic pressure gradient. However, further investigation shows that in most capillary beds, there is a net filtration that continues throughout the capillary length, and many Frank–Starling relationships are invalid (Levick and Michel 2010). Stasis of venous blood or lymph flow during gestation due to pressure by the gravid uterus has been proposed as a cause of udder edema (Joshi et al. 1978).

30.6 Genetic Factors

The genetic correlation between milk yield and edema severity is 0.40 (Norman et al. 1974). High yielding cows have an increased genetic potential to develop udder edema due to the substantial genetic correlation (Van Dorp et al. 1998). Cows with high production pedigrees had an 11% higher incidence of edema compared to those with low production pedigrees, and 19% more daughters from high production sires were diagnosed with udder edema compared to daughters from average sires (Shanks et al. 1978). Calf birth weight is proportional to increased udder edema development. Both edema and calving ease had significant and positive estimates of genetic correlation with stature (0.42 and 0.61) and strength, which is how well the body shape supports production and longevity (0.28 and 0.85) (Malven et al. 1983; Lawstuen et al. 1988).

30.7 Periparturient Nutrition

During the transition period, a cow's endocrine system prepares the body for parturition and lactogenesis, and the cow shifts from late gestation to early lactation. In this period, growth hormones increase and plasma insulin decreases. Acute surges of both hormones occur in the plasma at parturition (Kunz et al. 1985). These changes in the endocrine system, in conjunction with decreased dry matter intake (DMI), affects metabolism, which leads to the mobilization of fat from adipose tissue and glycogen from the liver. DMI decreases occur in dairy heifers nearing parturition (Rabelo et al. 2003; Hayirli et al. 2003). A low DMI during the last week of gestation causes impairment of the liver, which results in decreased total proteins (Figure 30.2), triglycerides, cholesterol, and lipid and lipoprotein concentrations in serum, a causative factor in the development of udder edema (Kojouri et al. 2015).

Dietary programs that adjust for changes in DMI and protein needs and include anionic salts to provide the complete nutritional requirements for cows during the transition period decreases the prevalence and severity of udder edema. A reduction in udder edema severity can be achieved through salt restriction (Randall et al. 1974).

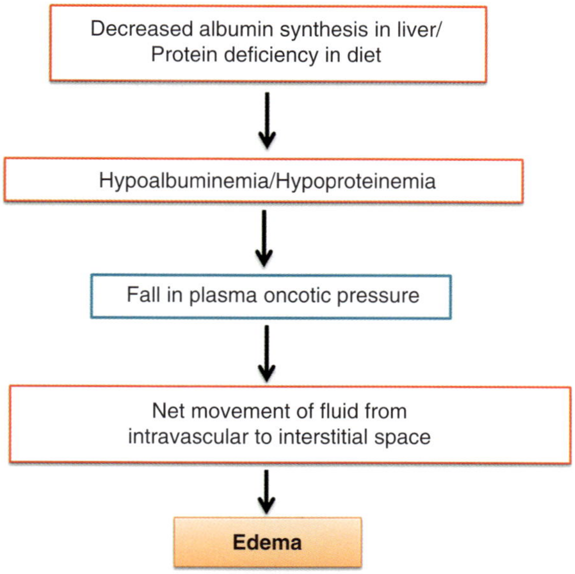

Figure 30.2 Mechanism of edema due to hypoproteinemia.

30.8 Oxidative Stress

Oxidative stress occurs when oxygen is not reduced to water during metabolic processes and partially reduced oxygen becomes a free-radical superoxide ($O_2^{\bullet -}$) (Levine and Kidd 1985). Superoxide is reduced to hydrogen peroxide (H_2O_2). Both of these occur naturally during the metabolic process and are not harmful when broken down properly. Damage from these compounds is suspected to be from their conversion into free radicals and the release of catalytic transition elements, such as iron, which have harmful effects (Gutteridge and Halliwell 1994). The release of catalytic iron becomes more likely under conditions of dietary imbalance, trauma, or stress, which often accompany calving (Madsen 1990). When reactive oxygen species surpass the defense capability of antioxidants, free radicals inflict damage on the DNA, proteins, and lipids involved in fundamental metabolic processes (Gagné 2014). These damaged cellular components result in cytotoxicity, genotoxicity, and carcinogenesis when damaged cells proliferate (Gutteridge and Halliwell 1994). Oxidative stress suppresses the production of androgens and estrogens, which impairs reproduction mechanisms, increases the occurrence and severity of milk fever, increases the amount of placental retention, and increases sodium and water retention to lead to udder edema (Miller et al. 1993). Providing a diet with adequate exogenous antioxidant molecules and amino acids counteracts this disorder (Hou et al. 2015). During oxidative stress, animals also have decreased immunity, which increases the risk of infections such as mastitis. Eliminating oxidative stress reduces the risk of periparturient disorders, reproductive failure, mastitis, and udder edema.

Udder edema usually resolves within a week of calving, but researchers have reported that this metabolic disorder can have negative effects on productivity, health and wellness, and longevity of dairy cows. Pain is a pillar of welfare assessments, along with health, productivity, and the ability to exhibit natural behaviors (von Keyserlingk et al. 2009). Dairy cows with swollen udders from mastitis exhibit behaviors such as spending less total time lying, less time lying on the affected quarter or quarters, increased standing time, and increased stepping behavior (Siivonen et al. 2011). When milking was performed by the first author, cows with udder edema exhibited greater kicking behavior during milking. Physiological changes such as tenderness of the teats and the swelling of udder tissues usually present as painful. Pain has been associated with mastitis in udders (Siivonen et al. 2011). The swollen udder tissues caused by edema have not been investigated for painfulness or as a welfare concern in dairy operations. These behaviors indicate that cows with udder edema may be experiencing pain due to tenderness of the teats and the swelling of udder tissues.

Another concern that comes along with udder edema is the increased risk for udder cleft dermatitis (Beattie and Taylor 2000). This is also referred to as "udder rot" or necrotic dermatitis – a skin lesion that appears in areas of tightly adjacent skin. For example, if there is severe swelling of the udder, friction in the pit between the leg and udder can lead to chafing and dermatitis. This area is sometimes hard to see and can be difficult to keep clean and dry. These sores typically have pus present with inflamed skin, a strong "infection" odor, and bleed easily. Udder cleft dermatitis is more commonly seen in cows with two or more lactations and is associated with a greater risk for mastitis, which is the most common disease manifested in the dairy farm industry (Slettbakk et al. 1995; Gröhn et al. 1989; Waage et al. 2001). Along with udder edema, other risk factors associated with udder cleft dermatitis on a herd level include high yearly milk production, a mean somatic cell count (SCC) greater than 200 000 cells/ml, and a prevalence of digital dermatitis (Persson Waller et al. 2014).

References

Al-Ani, F.K. and Vestweber, J.G.E. (1984). Mammary blood flow measurements associated with the development of bovine udder oedema. *American Journal of Veterinary Research* 45: 339–341.

Al-Ani, F. and Vestweber, J.G.E. (1986). Udder oedema: an updated review. *The Veterinary Bulletin* 56: 763–769.

Alhadrami, G.A. and Faye, B. (2016). Animals that produce dairy foods: camel. In: *Reference Module in Food Science*. Elsevier https://doi.org/10.1016/B978-0-08-100596-5.00620-X.

Beattie, K.G. and Taylor, D.J. (2000). An investigation into intertrigo (necrotic dermatitis or 'foul udder') in dairy cows. *Cattle Practice* 8: 377–380.

Bhave, G. and Neilson, E.G. (2011). Body fluid dynamics: back to the future. *Journal of the American Society of Nephrology* 22: 2166–2181.

Dentine, M.R. and McDaniel, B.T. (1983). Variation of oedema scores from herd-year, age, calving month, and sire. *Journal of Dairy Science* 66: 2391–2399.

Dyce, K.M. and Wensing, C.T.G. (1971). *Essentials of Bovine Anatomy*. Lea and Febiger.

Eyre, P. and Burka, J.F. (1978). Hypersensitivity in cattle and sheep: a pharmacological review. *Journal of Veterinary Pharmacology and Therapeutics* 1: 97–109. https://doi.org/10.1111/j.1365-2885.1978.tb00313.x.

Fustini, M., Galeati, G., Gabai, G. et al. (2017). Overstocking dairy cows during the dry period affects dehydroepiandrosterone and cortisol secretion. *Journal of Dairy Science* 100: 620–628. https://doi.org/10.3168/jds.2016-11293.

Gagné, F. (2014). Oxidative stress. In: *Biochemical Ecotoxicology: Principles and Methods* (ed. F. Gagne), 103–115. Cambridge, MA, USA: Academic Press.

Gröhn, Y.T., Erb, H.N., McCulloch, C.E., and Saloniemi, H.S. (1989). Epidemiology of metabolic disorders in dairy cattle: association among host characteristics, disease, and production. *Journal of Dairy Science* 72: 1876–1885. https://doi.org/10.3168/jds.S0022-0302(89)79306-1.

Gutteridge, J.M.C. and Halliwell, B. (1994). *Antioxidants in Nutrition, Health, and Disease*. Oxford University Press.

Hayirli, A., Grummer, R.R., Nordheim, E.V., and Crump, P.M. (2003). Models for predicting dry matter intake of Holsteins during the prefresh transition period. *Journal of Dairy Science* 86: 1771–1779. https://doi.org/10.3168/jds.S0022-0302(03)73762-X.

Hecht, H.H., Kuida, H., Lange, R.L. et al. (1962). Brisket disease. III. Clinical features and hemodynamic observations in altitude-dependent right heart failure of cattle. *The American Journal of Medicine* 32: 171–183. https://doi.org/10.1016/0002-9343(62)90288-7.

Hillerton, E.J. (2022). *Physiologic Disorders of the Udder in Cows*. Merck Veterinary Manual.

Hou, R., Jiang, C., Zheng, Q. et al. (2015). The AreA transcription factor mediates the regulation of deoxynivalenol (DON) synthesis by ammonium and cyclic adenosine monophosphate (cAMP) signaling in *Fusarium graminearum*. *Molecular Plant Pathology* 16: 987–999. https://doi.org/10.1111/mpp.12254.

Jerome, S.N., Akimitsu, T., and Korthuis, R.J. (1994). Leukocyte adhesion, oedema, and development of postischemic capillary no-reflow. *The American Journal of Physiology* 267: H1329–H1336.

Jones, T.O., Knight, R., and Evans, R.K. (1984). Chronic udder oedema in milking cows and heifer. *Veterinary Record* 115: 218–219.

Joshi, B.P., Saxena, S.C., and Rai, P. (1978). Udder edema in a goat: Clinico-therapeutic report. *Veterinary Research Bulletin.* 1 (1): 80–81.

von Keyserlingk, M.A., Rushen, J., de Passille, A.M., and Weary, D.M. (2009). Invited review: the welfare of dairy cattle – key concepts and the role of science. *Journal of Dairy Science* 92: 4101–4111. https://doi.org/10.3168/jds.2009-2326.

Kojouri, G.A., Mosavi Pouryeganeh, M., Nekouei, S., and Nazifi, S. (2015). Udder oedema and association with some serum biochemical measurands and dietary factors in first calving cows. *The Iranian Journal of Veterinary Research* 16: 345–349.

Kunz, P.L., Blum, J.W., Hart, I.C. et al. (1985). Effects of different energy intakes before and after calving on food intake, performance and blood hormones and metabolites in dairy cows. *Animal Science* 40: 219–231. https://doi.org/10.1017/S0003356100025320.

Lawstuen, D.A., Hansen, L.B., Steuernagel, G.R., and Johnson, L.P. (1988). Management traits scored linearly by dairy producers. *Journal of Dairy Science* 71: 788–799. https://doi.org/10.3168/jds.S0022-0302(88)79619-8.

Levick, J.R. and Michel, C.C. (2010). Microvascular fluid exchange and the revised Starling principle. *Cardiovascular Research* 87 (2): 198–210.

Levine, S.A. and Kidd, P.M. (1985). *Antioxidant Adaptation: Its Role in Free Radical Pathology*. Allergy Research Group.

Linzell, J.L. (1960). Valvular incompetence in the venous drainage of the udder. *The Journal of Physiology* 153: 481–491. https://doi.org/10.1113/jphysiol.1960.sp006549.

Madsen, F.C. (1990). Effect of disease on the metabolism of essential trace elements: a role for dietary coordination complexes. *Feed Management* 41: 20.

Malven, P.V., Erb, R.E., D'Amico, M.F. et al. (1983). Factors associated with oedema of the mammary gland in primigravid dairy heifers. *Journal of Dairy Science* 66: 246–252.

Medrano-Galarza, C., Gibbons, J., Wagner, S. et al. (2012). Behavioral changes in dairy cows with mastitis. *Journal of Dairy Science* 95: 6994–7002. https://doi.org/10.3168/jds.2011-5247.

Melendez, P., Hofer, C.C., and Donovan, G.A. (2006). Risk factors for udder oedema and its association with lactation performance on primiparous Holstein cows in a large Florida herd, U.S.A. *Preventive Veterinary Medicine* 76: 211–221. https://doi.org/10.1016/j.prevetmed.200.05.004.

Miller, J.K., Brzezinska-Slebodzinska, E., and Madsen, F.C. (1993). Oxidative stress, antioxidants, and animal function. *Journal of Dairy Science* 76: 2812–2823. https://doi.org/10.3168/jds.S0022-0302(93)77620-1.

Moroni, P., Nydam, D.V., Ospina, P.A. et al. (2018). Diseases of the teats and udder. In: *Rebhun's Diseases of Dairy Cattle*, 3e (ed. S.F. Peek and T.J. Divers), 389–465. Elsevier.

Morrison, E.I., DeVries, T.J., and LeBlanc, S.J. (2018). Short communication: associations of udder oedema with health, milk yield, and reproduction in dairy cows in early lactation. *Journal of Dairy Science* 101: 9521–9526. https://doi.org/10.3168/jds.2018-14539.

Mueller, F.J., Miller, J.K., Ramsey, N. et al. (1989). Reduced udder oedema in heifers fed vitamin E prepartum. *Journal of Dairy Science* 72: 2211. (Abstr.).

Nestor, K.E. Jr., Hemken, R.W., and Harmon, R.J. (1988). Influence of sodium chloride and potassium bicarbonate on udder oedema and selected blood parameters. *Journal of Dairy Science* 71: 366–372.

Norman, H.D., Powell, R.L., and Van Vleck, L.D. (1974). Genetic relationships among dairy cattle type appraisal traits and milk yield. *Journal of Dairy Science* 57 (Suppl. 1): 647. (Abstr.).

Persson Waller, K., Bengtsson, M., and Nyman, A.K. (2014). Prevalence and risk factors for udder cleft dermatitis in dairy cattle. *Journal of Dairy Science* 97: 310–318. https://doi.org/10.3168/jds.2013-7186.

Rabelo, E., Rezende, R.L., Bertics, S.J., and Grummer, R.R. (2003). Effects of transition diets varying in dietary energy density on lactation performance and ruminal parameters of dairy cows. *Journal of Dairy Science* 86: 916–925. https://doi.org/10.3168/jd.S0022-0302(03)73674-1.

Randall, W.E., Hemken, R.W., Bull, L.S., and Douglas, L.W. (1974). Effect of dietary sodium and potassium on udder oedema in Holstein heifers. *Journal of Dairy Science* 57: 472–475. https://doi.org/10.3168/jds.S0022-0302(74)84916-7.

Reed, R.K. and Rubin, K. (2010). Transcapillary exchange: role and importance of the interstitial fluid pressure and the extracellular matrix. *Cardiovascular Research* 87 (2): 211–217.

Robbins, S.L. and Cotran, R.S. (1979). *Pathologic Basis of Disease*. W. B. Saunders Co.

Ruegg, P. L. (2015). Diseases of bovine teat and skin. In: *Merck Veterinary Manual*. New Jersey, USA: Merck and Co., Inc. https://www.merckvetmanual.com/reproductive-system/udder-diseases/diseases-of-bovine-teats-and-skin (accessed 7 Mar 2020).

Scallan, J., Huxley, V.H., and Korthuis, R.J. (2010). *Capillary Fluid Exchange: Regulation, Functions, and Pathology*. San Rafael, CA: Morgan & Claypool Life Sciences.

Shanks, R.D., Freeman, A.E., Berger, P.J., and Kelley, D.H. (1978). Effect of selection for milk production and general health of the dairy cow. *Journal of Dairy Science* 61: 1765–1772. https://doi.org/10.3168/jds.S0022-0302(78)83800-4.

Siivonen, J., Taponen, S., Hovinen, M. et al. (2011). Impact of acute clinical mastitis on cow behaviour. *Applied Animal Behaviour Science* 132: 101–106. https://doi.org/10.1016/j.applanim.2011.04.005.

Slettbakk, T., Jorstad, A., Farver, T.B., and Holmes, J.C. (1995). Impact of milking characteristics and morphology of udder and teats on clinical mastitis in first and second lactation Norwegian cattle. *Preventive Veterinary Medicine* 24: 235–244. https://doi.org/10.1016/0167-5877(95)00490-N.

Stillwell, W. (2013). *An Introduction to Biological Membranes*, 2e. Elsevier.

Tao, S. and Dahl, G.E. (2013). Invited review: heat stress effects during late gestation on dry cows and their calves. *Journal of Dairy Science* 96: 4079–4093. https://doi.org/10.3168/jds.2012-6278.

Tucker, W.B., Adams, G.D., Lema, M. et al. (1992). Evaluation of a system for rating oedema in dairy cattle. *Journal of Dairy Science* 75: 2382–2387. https://doi.org/10.3168/jds.S0022-0302(92)77999-5.

Tyler, H.D. and Ensminger, M.E. (2006). *Dairy Cattle Science*, 4e. Pearson Prentice Hall.

University of Idaho (2018). Anatomy and lactation physiology lecture slides. http://www.webpages.uidaho.edu/avs472/Word/Mastitis%20and%20Milking/Mammary%20Udder%201%20[Compatibility%20Mode].pdf (accessed 9 April 2020).

Van Dorp, T.E., Dekkers, J.C., Martin, S.W., and Noordhuizen, J.P. (1998). Genetic parameters of health disorders, and relationships with 305-day milk yield and conformation traits of registered Holstein cows. *Journal of Dairy Science* 81: 2264–2270.

Vestweber, J.G. and Al-Ani, F.K. (1983). Udder oedema in cattle. *The Compendium on Continuing Education for the Practicing Veterinarian*. 5: S5–S12.

Waage, S., Odegaard, S.A., Lund, A. et al. (2001). Case-control study of risk factors for clinical mastitis in postpartum dairy heifers. *Journal of Dairy Science* 84: 392–399. https://doi.org/10.3168jds.S0022-0302(01)74489-X.3168/jds.S0022-0302(01)74489-X.

Walker, H.K., Hall, W.D., and Hurst, J.W. (1990). *Clinical Methods: The History, Physical, and Laboratory Examinations*, 3e. Boston: Butterworths.

Wiig, H., Schröder, A., Neuhofer, W. et al. (2013). Immune cells control skin lymphatic electrolyte homeostasis and blood pressure. *The Journal of Clinical Investigation* 123 (7): 2803–2815.

Woodcock, T.E. and Woodcock, T.M. (2012). Revised Starling equation and the glycocalyx model of transvascular fluid exchange: an improved paradigm for prescribing intravenous fluid therapy. *British Journal of Anaesthesia* 108 (3): 384–394.

Yeruham, I. and Markusfeld, O. (1996). Self-destructive behaviour in dairy cattle. *The Veterinary Record* 138: 308. https://doi.org/10.1136/vr.138.13.308.

Zarkower, A. (1967). Histamine in the cow: pre- and postparturition histamine concentrations in plasma, milk, and tissue. *American Journal of Veterinary Research* 28: 1751–1755.

31

Nerve Paralysis

Abhishek Pathak[1], Kanika Tiwari[2], Varun Asediya[3], and Pranav Anjaria[4]

[1] *Apollo College of Veterinary Medicine, Rajasthan University of Veterinary and Animal Sciences, Bikaner, Jaipur, Rajasthan, India*
[2] *Department of Veterinary Pharmacy and Toxicology, College of Veterinary and Animal Sciences, G.B. Pant University of Agriculture & Technology, Pantnagar, Uttarakhand, India*
[3] *MB Veterinary College, Rajasthan University of Veterinary and Animal Sciences, Bikaner, Dungarpur, Rajasthan, India*
[4] *College of Veterinary Science and Animal Husbandry, Kamdhenu University, Anand, Gujarat, India*

31.1 Introduction

Paralysis is a common and serious condition that affects the health and welfare of bovines. It can result from various causes, such as trauma, infection, toxins, or congenital defects, and can impair the function of different nerves and muscles. Paralysis can have significant economic and social impacts on the livestock industry and the rural communities that depend on it. Therefore, it is important to understand the etiology, pathophysiology, diagnosis, prognosis, and treatment of paralysis in bovines. In this chapter, we will provide a comprehensive overview of the different forms and manifestations of paralysis in bovines. We will first define the term paralysis and classify it into four types: local, hemiplegia, paraplegia, and quadriplegia. We will then discuss the various causes and mechanisms of nerve damage that can lead to paralysis. Next, we will describe the clinical signs, diagnosis, and treatment of specific nerve paralyses that affect bovines, such as facial nerve paralysis, suprascapular nerve injury, radial paralysis, sciatic paralysis, obturator paralysis, femoral nerve paralysis, and tibial/peroneal nerve paralysis (Abutarbush, 2011). Finally, we will summarize the main points of the chapter and highlight the importance of informed decision making in veterinary paralysis management. We hope that this chapter will serve as a useful reference for veterinarians, researchers, students, and anyone interested in learning more about paralysis in bovines. We also hope that this chapter will stimulate further research and innovation in this area and contribute to improved animal health and welfare.

31.2 Classification of Paralysis

I) **Local paralysis:** When only a single muscle or group of muscles in a particular body part is affected, then the paralysis is termed local paralysis.
II) **Hemiplegia:** When one side of the body is affected, then the paralysis is termed hemiplegia.
III) **Paraplegia:** When the hindquarter is affected, then the paralysis is termed paraplegia.
IV) **Quadriplegia:** When all four limbs are affected, the paralysis is termed quadriplegia.

31.3 Etiology

- **Traumatic injury:** This can occur due to open wounds, contusions, overstretching of the nerve, or fractures. These injuries can cause direct damage to the nerves that control muscle movement, which leads to paralysis.
- **Inflammation:** Inflammation of the nerves, also known as neuritis, can interfere with nerve function and lead to paralysis.

Periparturient Diseases of Cattle, First Edition. Edited by Tanmoy Rana.

- **Hemorrhage:** Bleeding around the nerve can put pressure on it, disrupting its ability to transmit signals effectively. This can result in paralysis.
- **Neoplasm:** Tumors or growths around the nerve can exert pressure on it, which leads to nerve damage and subsequent paralysis.
- **Toxins:** Certain toxins can damage nerves or muscle fibers directly, which leads to paralysis. These toxins may be produced by bacteria during infections, like botulism, or they may be ingested or inhaled, as with certain poisons or drugs.
- **Muscular lesions:** Some conditions can cause lesions in the muscle itself, which leads to the destruction of muscle fibers and results in paralysis.
- **Rheumatism:** Rheumatic diseases are autoimmune and inflammatory diseases that can also affect the nerves and lead to paralysis.
- **Onset of paralysis:** Paralysis that occurs suddenly is usually of a traumatic or toxic origin. Paralysis that is slow in onset is chronic in nature and could be due to progressive neurological diseases like multiple sclerosis or amyotrophic lateral sclerosis (Constable, 2023).

31.4 Symptoms

The symptoms of paralysis due to nerve damage can be quite varied, depending on the specific nerves involved. Here is a more detailed and scientific explanation.

- **Muscle state:** The affected muscles may remain in a relaxed state or in spasmodic contraction. This is due to the disruption of nerve signals that regulate muscle tension and movement.
- **Characteristic symptoms:** When major nerves are involved, characteristic symptoms are noticed.
  - Radial nerve damage: This can cause symptoms such as wrist drops, numbness on the back of the hand and arm, and difficulty straightening the arm.
  - Facial nerve damage: This can result in facial paralysis, causing an inability to control facial muscles on the affected side.
  - Sciatic nerve damage: This can cause sciatica, characterized by pain, numbness, or weakness that radiates along the path of the sciatic nerve in the lower back, buttock, and leg.
  - Paralysis symptoms: Paralysis feels like you cannot move part of your body the way you want to, no matter how hard you try. It may involve an arm or a leg, or it may involve the hand, foot, or face. Symptoms that commonly occur alongside paralysis include:
    - Numbness or tingling in the weak part of the body.
    - Loss of sensation in the weak part of the body.
    - Floppiness of the weak area of the body.
  - Peripheral neuropathy: Peripheral neuropathy happens when the nerves outside the brain and spinal cord (peripheral nerves) are damaged. This condition often causes weakness, numbness, and pain, usually in your hands and feet. It also can affect other areas and body functions including digestion and urination.

31.5 Diagnosis

A diagnosis of paralysis involves assessing the degree of sensitivity, tendinous reflexes, and electrical contractility of the affected muscles. Sensitivity is tested by pricking the affected muscle(s) with a needle or pin, and diminished sensitivity indicates nerve damage. Tendinous reflexes, such as the patellar reflex or the Achilles reflex, are elicited by tapping on the tendon and observing muscle contraction. Normal or diminished reflexes suggest various levels of spinal cord injury. Electrical contractility is measured by applying an electrical stimulus to the muscle and recording its response. The absence of electrical contractility indicates severe muscle degeneration and has a poor prognosis.

31.6 Prognosis

The prognosis of a condition that resulted in paralysis depends on many factors. The cause of the condition is a significant determinant. For instance, paralysis due to a stroke or spinal cord injury may have a different prognosis compared to paralysis caused by peripheral nerve disorders. The severity of the lesion in the muscle or nerve also plays a crucial role.

A minor lesion may result in temporary paralysis and have a better prognosis, while a severe lesion could lead to permanent paralysis. The duration of the paralysis is another crucial factor. Short-term paralysis may not result in significant muscle atrophy and may have a better prognosis. However, long term paralysis can lead to pronounced muscle atrophy, which reduces the chances of recovery. The degree of degeneration undergone by the muscle is also critical. Muscular atrophy, which refers to the wasting away of muscle tissue, can significantly impact prognosis. If muscular atrophy has occurred, it indicates that the muscle has not been used for an extended period and lead to its degeneration. This makes recovery more challenging and thus, the prognosis becomes unfavorable.

However, it is important to note that advancements in medical technology and rehabilitation therapies have improved the outlook for individuals with paralysis. Early intervention, appropriate treatment, and dedicated rehabilitation can enhance muscle function, limit muscle atrophy, and improve overall quality of life.

31.7 General Treatment of Paralysis

- If the paralysis is due to a callus or tumor pressing on the nerve, it is desirable to remove the cause.
- If the paralysis is temporary in nature and is due to minor injury, the local application of counterirritants may accelerate the recovery. Potassium iodide may be given internally to promote the absorption of inflammatory exudate pressing on the nerve.
- Nerve supplements such as vitamin B1 (thiamine), phospholecithin, etc. are advisable. They help improve the blood supply to the nerves and promote regeneration.
- Administration of calcium.
- Nerve stimulants may also be beneficial.
- Mild exercises, massage, and the application of liniments or blisters are indicated for inducing activity of the paralyzed muscles and thereby preventing muscular atrophy.
- Electrotherapy accelerates recovery and prevents muscular atrophy. The recommended voltage and current are 50–60 V and 3–20 mA for about 5–20 minutes. At the beginning of the treatment, the duration may be about 5 minutes daily or 10 minutes on alternate days. However, amperage and time may vary depending on the area involved and the individual tolerance of the patient.
- Infrared rays are also beneficial as they are hot rays that can penetrate deeper tissues and stimulate regenerative processes by favoring hyperemia.
- If the cause of paralysis is rheumatism, sodium salicylate is indicated.
- In some cases, corticosteroid preparations may be effective in quickening the recovery.
- Nerve paralysis in cattle includes facial nerve paralysis, sciatic paralysis, femoral paralysis, peroneal paralysis, suprascapular paralysis, and radial paralysis.

31.8 Facial Nerve Paralysis

The facial nerve is the chief motor nerve of the face. It is also called the nerve of expression.

31.8.1 Anatomy

The facial nerve, also known as the seventh cranial nerve, is a key player in the nervous system. It originates from the pons in the brainstem and is responsible for controlling the muscles that allow us to express our emotions on our faces. Additionally, it plays a role in transmitting taste sensations from the front two-thirds of the tongue. The journey of the facial nerve is complex. It navigates through the facial canal of the petrous temporal bone and exits through the stylomastoid foramen. After leaving the skull, it runs just in front of the outer ear. It then passes close to a major salivary gland, the parotid gland, and crosses over to the side of the mandible just below where the jaw articulates with the skull. Upon reaching its destination, the face, it splits into superior and inferior buccal nerves. These nerves are crucial as they supply the lips and muzzle. The facial nerve also provides innervation to other parts of the face such as the eyelids, ear, and cheeks. Beyond its motor functions, the facial nerve has sensory and parasympathetic components. It carries taste sensations from the front two-thirds of the tongue and provides parasympathetic innervation to various glands in the head and neck. Throughout its course, the facial nerve is associated with several important branches. Within the facial canal, it gives rise to branches such as the greater petrosal nerve, nerve to stapedius muscle, and chorda tympani. Each of these branches has specific functions related to sensation, taste, and motor control. A thorough understanding of the intricate anatomy and diverse functions of the facial nerve is crucial in clinical practice. Damage or injury to this nerve can lead to conditions like Bell's palsy or other types of facial paralysis. Therefore, preserving its integrity during surgical procedures in and around the face is paramount (Venugopalan, 2020).

31.8.2 Etiology

- Injury to the nerve may cause paralysis. Severe injury to the nerves may degenerate the nerve fibers and cause paralysis.
- External pressure on the nerve from the surroundings may also cause paralysis. Inflammation of the middle ear, inflammation of petrous temporal bone, and a tumor within the facial canal or in the parotid region may put pressure on the surrounding nerves and causes paralysis of the nerves.
- Exposure to extreme cold desensitizes the surrounding tissues and nerves, which may paralyze the nerves.
- Rheumatism.

31.8.3 Symptoms and Treatment

Facial paralysis, whether it affects one side (unilateral) or both sides (bilateral), can significantly impact an animal's daily activities. In unilateral paralysis, the lips are drawn toward the unaffected side, which leads to the accumulation of feed between the teeth and cheek. This condition may also result in quidding, a phenomenon where food is dropped from the mouth while chewing. In bilateral paralysis, both lips are paralyzed, causing the lower lip to appear pendulous. The animal may struggle to use its lips for prehension, or the grasping of food. To drink water, the animal must dip its muzzle beyond the level of the angles of the mouth. The nostrils may appear constricted, which can interfere with respiration. This can make respiration noisy during exercise. The animal may also be unable to completely close its eyelids. In some cases, the branch that supplies the ear and eyelids are also involved, which leads to drooping of the upper eyelid (ptosis) and ear. A loss of sensation in the inner surface of concha may also be observed. Facial paralysis can be classified into two types based on which portion of the facial nerve is affected: peripheral and central paralysis. Peripheral paralysis affects only the superficial portion of the nerve after it crosses over the mandible. Central paralysis involves the intratemporal portion of the nerve and affects the branches that supply the ear and eyelids. The treatment for facial paralysis depends on its underlying cause. For instance, if it is a result of a stroke, veterinarians will focus on treating stroke. If it is due to a tumor, options to remove the tumor will be discussed. If Bell's palsy is identified as the cause, medications may be prescribed along with facial strengthening exercises. Rehabilitation with physical therapy and speech and swallow therapy can also be beneficial (Lorenz et al., 2011).

31.9 Suprascapular Nerve Injury

31.9.1 Anatomy

The suprascapular nerve courses laterally, passing superior to the brachial plexus and through the posterior triangle of neck. It then traverses the scapular notch (inferior to the superior transverse scapular ligament) into the supraspinous region of the scapula. Here, it gives off a branch to the supraspinatus muscle and continues through the greater scapular (spinoglenoid) notch between the root of the spine of the scapula and the glenoid cavity, to reach the infraspinous fossa. This nerve's main function is to provide motor innervation for two muscles, the supraspinatus and infraspinatus. These muscles are part of the muscle group called the rotator cuff muscles. The supraspinatus muscle initiates abduction (lifting) of the forelimbs, while the infraspinatus muscle is responsible for lateral rotation of the forelimb. In addition to its motor functions, the suprascapular nerve provides a sensory supply for the joints of the scapula (glenohumeral and acromioclavicular joints). This sensory innervation plays a crucial role in proprioception, which is the sense of the relative position of body parts and strength of effort being employed in movement.

31.9.2 Etiology

- Trauma caused to the nerve and prescapular area directly due to a fall on the ground.
- Nerve compression in and around vertebrae, either due to abscess or fracture.

31.9.3 Symptoms

There is difficulty in extending the shoulder joint. When the animal bears weight on the affected limb, the shoulder joint markedly bulges outward. The shoulder joint appears to slip outward at each step. This condition is called shoulder slip or sweeny. Several days after the injury in the nerve, the supraspinatus and infraspinatus muscles may show signs of wasting, i.e. neurogenic atrophy, which indicates the possibility of permanent damage.

31.9.4 Treatment

General treatment for paralysis is followed. In case of an injury localized to the nerve, immediate treatment with corticosteroids or anti-inflammatory drugs is appropriate. If the trauma is severe and complex, primary treatment must be given to resolve the immediate condition. Recovery may take place in 4–6 weeks. In case there is rapid muscular atrophy, then the prognosis is unfavorable. Sometimes, blistering over the shoulder region and over the affected muscles is also effective (Lorenz et al., 2011).

31.10 Radial Paralysis

The radial nerve is the largest nerve that arises from the brachial plexus. Paralysis of the radial nerve is termed radial paralysis.

31.10.1 Anatomy

The radial nerve arises from the brachial plexus and passes downward and outward along the musculospiral groove of the humerus. It supplies the triceps brachii, extensor of the carpus and digits, i.e. triceps brachii, anconeus, extensor carpi radialis, common extensor of the digit, ulnaris lateralis, lateral extensor of the digit, and extensor carpi obliquus.

31.10.2 Etiology

- Overstretching of the nerve.
- Injury to the nerve along with fracture of the first rib.
- Compression of the nerve between the shoulder and thorax while casting the animal on the hard ground.

31.10.3 Symptoms

In complete paralysis of the radial nerve, all the branches of the nerve are affected. All the joints below the elbow are in a flexed state and the point of the elbow gets dropped. The condition is called a dropped elbow. The limb appears longer and the toe of the foot rests on the ground. When the animal is moved forward, the toe is dragged. While standing, the limbs bear weight by supporting the knee from the front with a hand. In partial paralysis of the radial nerve, the branches that supply the triceps muscles are affected or the branches that supply the extensors of the digit and carpus are affected. If the branches supplying the extensors of the digit are affected, the animal uses the limb normally when walking on level ground but stumbling and dragging of the foot is observed on uneven ground. If the branches supplying the triceps muscle are affected, the affected animal cannot extend the elbow and bear weight on the affected limb. There is an abnormal appearance of the affected limb as the point of the elbow is dropped and the knee is semiflexed. However, the planter surface of the foot touches the ground almost normally.

31.10.4 Treatment

Nonsteroidal anti-inflammatory drugs (NSAIDs) and corticosteroids may be helpful in cases of radial nerve paralysis. Recovery may take place in 10 days to 6 weeks. In some severe cases, it may take months to recover.

31.11 Ischiatic/Sciatic Paralysis

This is the paralysis of the sciatic nerve. Sciatic nerve damage is primarily seen immediately after calving but can be seen with hip fractures or faulty injections. Persistent knuckling of the fetlock and a slight "dropping" of the hock is observed as the sciatic nerve innervates the muscles of the lower limb and is important in proprioception.

31.11.1 Anatomy

The sciatic nerve supplies all muscles of the hindlimbs, except the quadriceps extensor cruris and quadriceps femoris muscles.

31.11.2 Etiology

- Overstretching of the nerve.
- Injury to the nerve by falling on the corresponding quarter.
- Toxemia in disease conditions such as pneumonia, purpura hemorrhagica, etc.
- Compression due to the presence of a tumor in the area surrounding the nerve.

31.11.3 Symptoms

The hindlimb hangs loosely as all muscles of the hindlimbs are affected except the quadriceps femoris muscle. When forced to move, the animal drags the limb with the toe of the foot. The fetlock joint of the affected limb of the animal is dragged along the ground. Persistent knuckling of the fetlock and a slight "dropping" of the hock are also observed in sciatic nerve paralysis. The stifle joint of the affected animal is lifted forward and upward at each step due to the action of the quadriceps muscle. Weight bearing is variably affected in animals with sciatic nerve damage.

31.11.4 Treatment

A general treatment of paralysis is preferred. Stall confinement with deep bedding is effective for these animals. Sand is a good base as it is soft and provides stable footing. Along with this, corticosteroids and NSAIDs are administered. Dexamethasone at a dose rate of 0.05 mg/kg body weight, intramuscularly every 1–2 days, or flunixin meglumine at a dose rate of 1 mg/kg body weight, intramuscularly every 12 hours, provide temporary relief to the animals.

31.12 Obturator Paralysis

This is the paralysis of the obturator nerve. It commonly occurs in animals during the act of parturition.

31.12.1 Anatomy

The obturator nerve is formed from the lumbar plexus. It receives fibers from the anterior divisions of L_2, L_3, and L_4. After that, it descends and emerges from its medial border. It then travels posterior to common iliac arteries and laterally along the pelvic wall toward the obturator foramen of the pelvis. It enters the medial thigh through the obturator canal. It then divides into anterior and posterior branches. Basically, the obturator nerve supplies the adductor muscle of the hindlimb. The anterior branch of the obturator nerve supplies the adductor longus, adductor brevis, gracilis, and pectineus muscles. The posterior division of the obturator nerve supplies the obturator externus and adductor magnus muscles.

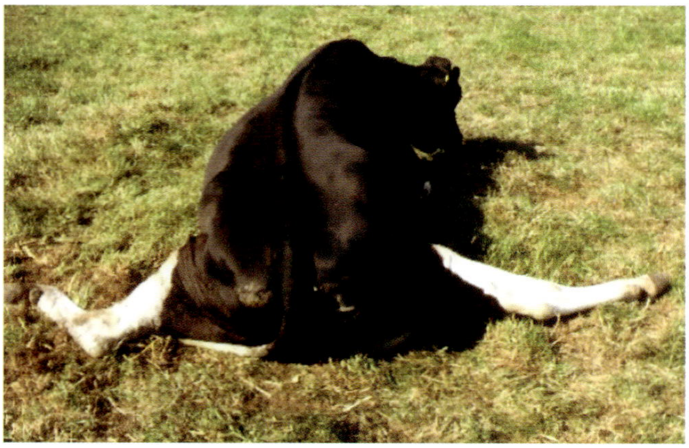

Obturator nerve paralysis.

31.12.2 Etiology

Trauma is caused to the nerve during the act of parturition. Nerves may either get damaged or compressed during parturition, which may predispose the animal to obturator nerve paralysis.

A fracture in the pelvis may also predispose the animal to obturator nerve damage. An animal that has met with an accident or fallen from a height may receive a fracture in the pelvis that affects the obturator nerve.

31.12.3 Symptoms

Animals fail to adduct the affected limb following the act of parturition. Affected animals are prone to limb abduction, particularly on slippery surfaces. When sitting, the hindlimbs are often extended forward. Obturator paralysis can also lead to hip dislocation.

31.12.4 Treatment

The animal should be moved to an area with good footing. Treatment may include hobbling the back legs to prevent the animal from doing the splits (use hobbles placed above the fetlocks). There is an elevated risk of permanent damage due to ongoing damage to the muscles and nerves. Stall confinement with deep bedding is effective for these animals.

31.13 Femoral Nerve Paralysis

The femoral nerve is one of the major peripheral nerves of the lower limb. It is the largest branch of the lumbar plexus. Paralysis of the femoral or crural nerve is termed femoral paralysis or crural paralysis.

31.13.1 Anatomy

The femoral nerve arises from the L_3–L_6 segments of the spinal cord. Then it travels inferiorly through the psoas major muscle, iliacus, and pectineus muscles before entering the thigh region. Afterward, the nerve passes underneath the inguinal ligaments to enter the femoral triangle (femoral artery, vein, and nerve). The femoral nerve divides into the anterior and posterior division just 4 cm below the inguinal ligament. The anterior division of the femoral nerve supplies the sartorius and pectineus muscles, and the posterior division of the nerve supplies the saphenous and quadriceps femoris muscle. The quadriceps femoris muscle consists of four muscles, viz. the vastus medialis, vastus lateralis, rectus femoris, and vastus intermedius muscles. The sartorius muscle adducts the limb and provides some flexion to the hip. A saphenous branch of the femoral nerve provides sensory function to the medial thigh of the hindlimb.

31.13.2 Etiology

- Overstretching of the nerve.
- Injury to the nerve by falling on the corresponding quarter or during dystocia.
- Toxemia in disease conditions such as pneumonia, purpura hemorrhagica, etc.
- Compression due to the presence of a tumor in that area.

31.13.3 Symptoms

When there is paralysis of the femoral nerve, the quadriceps femoris muscle of the affected animal becomes functionless. Due to the loss of function of the quadriceps femoris muscles, the animal cannot extend the limb for weight bearing. There is a sudden flexion of the stifle and then the hock joint. The stifle joint of the affected limb of the animal remains dropped. The patella is slack. The loose, powerless appearance of the limb may resemble some fractures upon inspection. Muscles of the affected limb may atrophy rapidly.

31.13.4 Treatment

Stall confinement along with deep bedding is recommended. NSAIDs and corticosteroids may be helpful in cases of femoral nerve paralysis. A general treatment of paralysis is preferred.

31.14 Tibial/Peroneal Nerve Paralysis

Tibial/peroneal nerve paralysis is seen primarily in cattle immediately after parturition or after a prolonged recumbency in any disease condition. It is also due to pressure ischemia over the lateral stifle region. It is a slightly milder version of sciatic nerve damage (Malone, 2015).

31.14.1 Anatomy

The peroneal nerve is the cranial division of the sciatic nerve. It passes superficially over the lateral condyle of the femur and the head of the fibula, which makes it susceptible to injury. It supplies the extensor muscles of the digit and flexor metatarsi muscles.

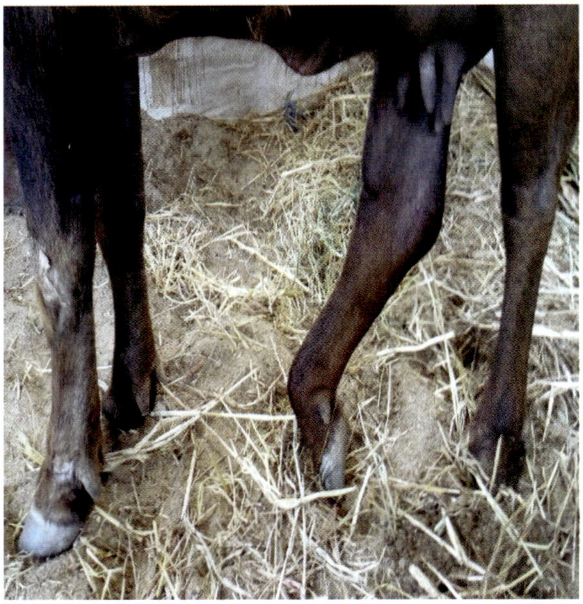

Peroneal nerve paralysis

31.14.2 Etiology

- Trauma caused to the nerve during parturition.
- Prolonged recumbency on a solid surface such as concrete, particularly during parturition with concurrent periparturient hypocalcemia.
- Due to pressure ischemia over the lateral stifle region.

31.14.3 Symptoms

Peroneal nerve paralysis results in paralysis of the muscles that flex the hock and extend the digits. Affected animals stand with the digit knuckled over onto the dorsal surface of the pastern and fetlock (metatarsophalangeal joint). The fetlocks are hyperflexed with some animals walking on the dorsum of the fetlock. The animal can bear weight on the limb, but the hock is overextended and the digit cannot be extended. Both hindlimbs are typically involved when it is related to prolonged labor. In mild cases, the fetlock tends to knuckle over intermittently during ambulation. In severe cases, the dorsal surface of the hoof may be dragged along the ground and sensation to the dorsum of the fetlock is often decreased. Testing reflexes may demonstrate that hock flexion is absent but stifle and hip joint flexion are normal.

31.14.4 Treatment

Stall confinement with deep bedding is advantageous for animals affected with tibial or peroneal nerve paralysis. Most cases of peroneal nerve paralysis involve neurapraxia that will resolve with conservative management. However, if there is an extended period of recumbency, care must be taken to avoid exacerbation of the initial injury.

References

Abutarbush, S.M. (2011). Bovine laminitis and lameness – A hands-on approach. *The Canadian Veterinary Journal* 52 (1): 73.

Constable, P.D. (2023). Lameness of cattle. In: *Musculoskeletal System. MSD Veterinary Manual*. Rahway, NJ, USA: Merck & Co., Inc.

Lorenz, M.D., Coates, J.R., and Kent, M. (2011). Paresis of one limb. In: *Handbook of Veterinary Neurology*, vol. 5, 93–108.

Malone, E. (2015). *Large Animal Surgery – Supplemental Notes*. University of Minnesota Libraries Publishing.

Venugopalan, A. (2020). *Essentials of Veterinary Surgery*. India: Oxford & IBH Publishing Company Pvt. Limited.

32

Lameness

Apoorva Mishra, Apra Shahi, Randhir Singh, and Babita Das

College of Veterinary Science and Animal Husbandry, Nanaji Deshmukh Veterinary Science University, Jabalpur, Madhya Pradesh, India

Lameness is a clinical condition that affects the gait, stride, and overall locomotor system of the animal. It is an animal health and welfare concern as well as a production issue. Pain due to lameness often limits growth because animals may be reluctant to eat or drink. It is still a significant issue for the welfare of dairy cattle across the globe. Most causes of lameness in cattle (70–90%) involve hoof lesions. Hoof lesions are commonly categorized according to their etiology, as either infectious (e.g. digital dermatitis, foot rot, heel horn erosion, interdigital dermatitis) or noninfectious (e.g. sole hemorrhages, sole ulcers, or white line disease [collectively termed "hoof horn disruption lesions"] as well as thin soles, toe ulcers and toe necrosis, corkscrew claw, fissures, interdigital hyperplasia, and deep digital sepsis). Lameness that does not come from the hoof can be brought on by injury, rheumatoid arthritis, muscle tears, and neurological conditions. In beef cattle, foot rot commonly accompanies musculoskeletal injuries because of handling, restraint, and transportation. In dairy cattle, the most common hoof lesions are digital dermatitis, sole ulcers or hemorrhages, and white line disease (Whay and Shearer 2017).

In cattle with laminitis, diagnostic imaging techniques like radiography, computed tomography, and especially, angiography have been used to examine vascular alterations in the digital and hoof tissues (Blowey 2002). This chapter deals mainly with hoof affections that are the chief causes of lameness, a better understanding of which starts with the basic anatomical structure of the foot.

32.1 Structure of the Foot/Hoof

The outer or lateral claw and the inner or medial claw are the two digits that make up the foot/hoof. The primary surface for bearing weight on the hindfeet is the lateral claw, which is larger than the medial claw. When compared to back feet, the inner claw is bigger and more weight bearing. Most lesions are assumed to develop in the inner claw of the front feet and the outer claw of the back feet for this reason. The embryonic mesoderm and ectoderm that make up the claw are used to create its dermal and epidermal tissues. In integumental tissues, interactions between these tissues appear to be crucial for the appropriate growth and operation of epidermal cells (Whay and Shearer 2017).

Each claw consists of three tissue components, namely the hoof, corium, and bone.

- **The hoof:** Subdivided into the wall, the white line, the sole, and the heel. It provides the hard outer casing of the foot.
- **The corium**: Also known as the "quick," the corium is a support tissue that provides nutrients for the hoof and bones of the foot. The papillary corium, which produces hoof horn, is present at the coronary band and over the sole; the laminar corium covers the lower half of the wall; and at the heel, the corium is modified to form the digital cushion.
- **The bone:** The pedal bone and the navicular bone.

From the hoof/skin intersection of the coronary band down to the first half of the wall, the hoof wall protrudes from the papillary corium. It moves slowly, at a rate of around 5 mm per month, over the laminar corium. The papillary creates the sole, which is a distinct structure. The "white line" refers to the cemented juncture where the sole and the wall meet (Mulling and Lischer 2002) (Figure 32.1).

Periparturient Diseases of Cattle, First Edition. Edited by Tanmoy Rana.

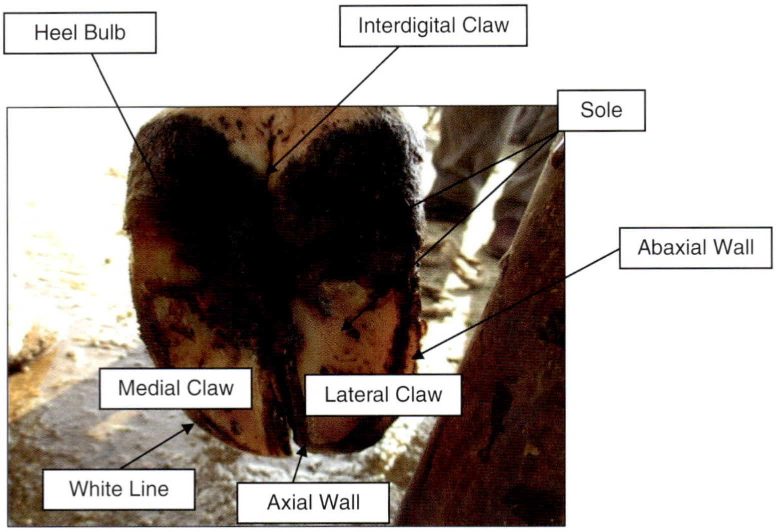

Figure 32.1 A line diagram of the hoof in cattle.

While the white line merely contains cellular cement, the hoof wall and sole are made of tubular horn and incorporate reinforcing bars. The white line, which is a cemented junction, is a point of weakness, and once damaged, it frequently serves as a point of entry for stones and other foreign objects. Heifers and cows have different digital cushions in terms of anatomy. Therefore, it is crucial to give heifers ample time to adjust to new dairy cow living arrangements.

32.2 Hoof Overgrowth

Despite being frequently omitted from texts on lameness, hoof overgrowth is arguably one of the most frequent causes of discomfort. Most overgrowth happens at the toe. As a result, the toe is raised, and the claw rotates backward. The front wall's angle shifts from its usual slope of 45° to a slope of 30°, which puts more weight on the heel. Compared to animals with well-trimmed hooves, cows with overgrown claws/digits have a worse gait and move with considerable difficulty. The artery in the underlying dermis (corium) supplies nourishment and oxygen to the horn-producing and proliferating epidermal basal cells (Ossent and Lischer 2000).

At the dermal–epidermal junction, the basal cell layer degenerates first. The suspensory mechanism of the claw fails as a result of degeneration of the dermal–epidermal connection. The entire foot sinks into the horn capsule as the connection starts to split (Blowey 2002). Additionally, excessive weight bearing on the back edge of the pedal bone may increase the risk of developing sole ulcers (Blowey and Weaver 1991) (Figure 32.2).

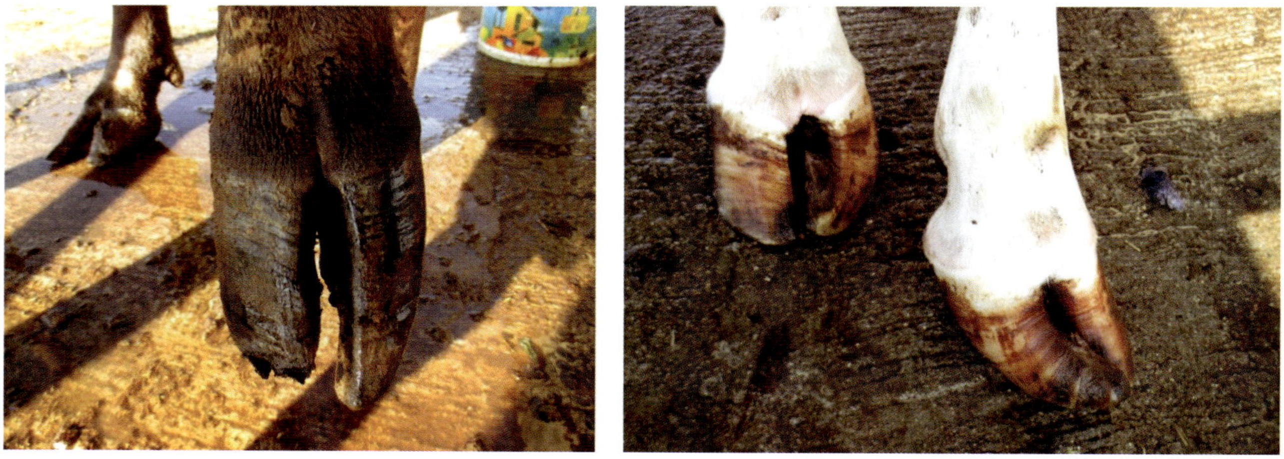

Figure 32.2 Hoof overgrowth and a corkscrew hoof.

32.3 Sole Ulcers

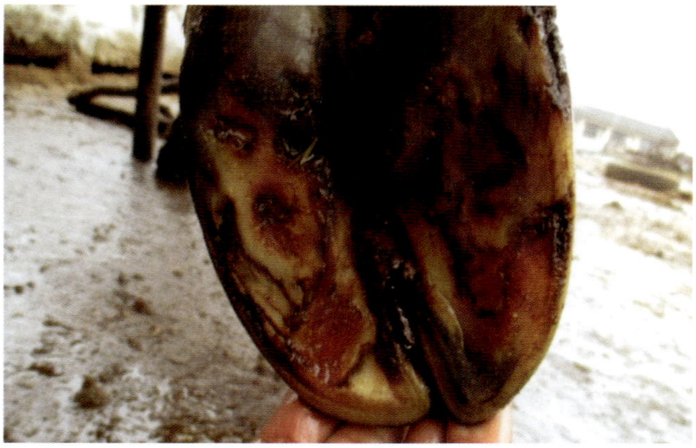

Figure 32.3 Sole ulcer.

A sole ulcer is a persistent hole in the sole horn that exposes the corium. The usual location is the middle portion of the rear sole that corresponds to the back of the pedal bone. The state of the outer claw and the degree of injury to the horn-producing tissue determine the prognosis for sole ulcers. The flexor tuberosity of the pedal bone above and the hard horn of the sole beneath place pressure on the corium, which is the main cause of a sole ulcer. When the corium is pinched, bleeding results, and blood mixed with horn weakens the strength of the hoof.

Since the average hoof is 10-mm thick, hemorrhage is not visible on the sole's surface until 2–3 months later because hooves grow at a rate of 5 mm every month. Bruising is a common term for this. The corium may occasionally be subjected to such severe compression and injury that the development of horns is wholly obstructed. This results in a sole ulcer by creating a "hole" through the hoof and onto the sole underneath. The laminae in a normal foot suspends the pedal bone within the hoof. This suspension is lost if the corium is injured or if laminitis develops, which causes the pedal bone to descend to the bottom of the hoof (Dehghani and Sadeghi 2006). The corium in the sole and heel are compressed when the distal phalanx sinks, which leads to additional bouts of capillary injury, hemorrhage, thrombosis, cellular inflammatory reaction, and ultimately, ischemic necrosis. Chronic edema, mixed with the compression caused by the animal's weight, will put the animal in danger comparable to sinkage.

Additionally, it explains why cows with sole ulcers or white line disease are at least three times more likely to experience lameness in following lactations. Therefore, it is crucial to take care of heifers as they join the dairy herd (Figure 32.3).

32.4 Toe Ulcers

Occurs when the toe of the sole is mistakenly trimmed too thin, when laminitis causes the toe to drop into the horn, or when the sole is very worn at the toe. Orthopedic blocks must always be placed on the opposing claw for toe ulcers.

32.5 White Line Disease

White line disease begins with cracks brought on by bleeding and inadequate horn development. The white line denotes the intersection of the hoof sole and the wall, which is cemented. The sole and the wall are both made of reinforced tubular horn, but the white line is just "cement," which makes it inherently weak. Aspects of administration, housing, feeding, and particularly calving can reduce the white line even further. A stone or piece of earth can easily be struck into the white line cement if it becomes weak. The foreign object could serve as a "wedge" and enlarge the gap within the white line until it breaks through the corium. Bacteria will multiply in the corium, and the pressure from the pus is what causes lameness. By choosing the route of least resistance, infection leaves the corium. Usually, this causes a discharge via the heel's softer horn. Sometimes, pus drains from the coronary band along the wall's laminae (Campbell et al. 1996).

Due to the lack of a drainage path, lameness can be particularly severe if the infection has built up in the toe. In order to treat the abscess, the underrun horn must be completely removed in order to reveal the corium beneath. Then, a fresh horn will emerge from that corium. A block should be placed on the damaged claw to prevent it from bearing weight (Dacosta Gomez et al. 1998) (Figure 32.4).

32.6 Sole and White Line Hemorrhages

These originate from corium injury, with the blood being integrated into the horn as it develops. Depending on the sole thickness and growth rate, hemorrhages will start to show several weeks after the injury. Also, if the hemorrhage becomes infected, an abscess or white line abscess may develop (Dehghani 2008) (Figure 32.5).

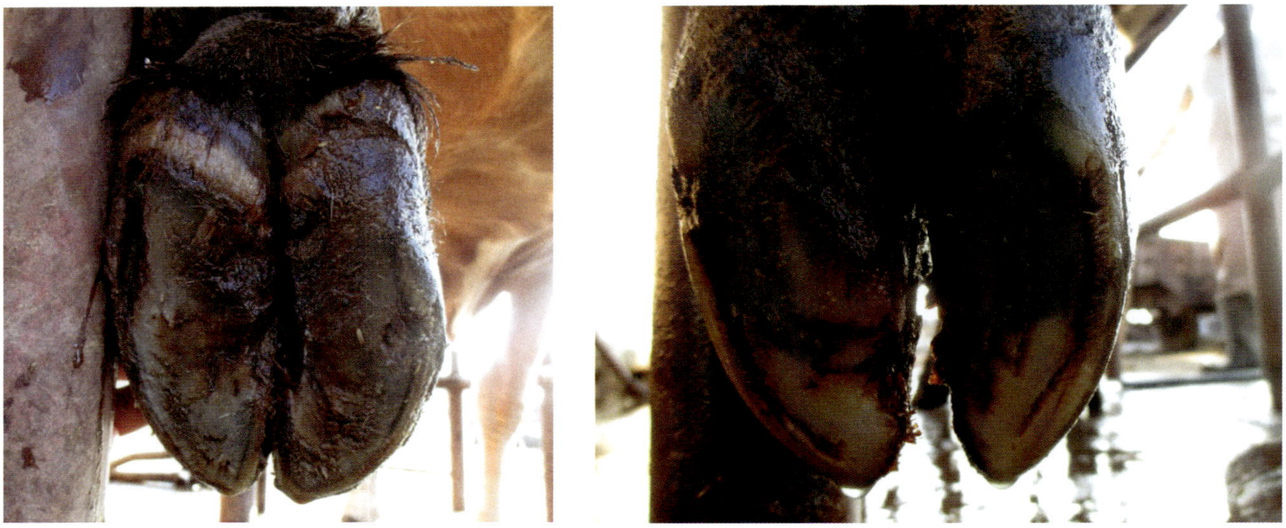

Figure 32.4 White line separation.

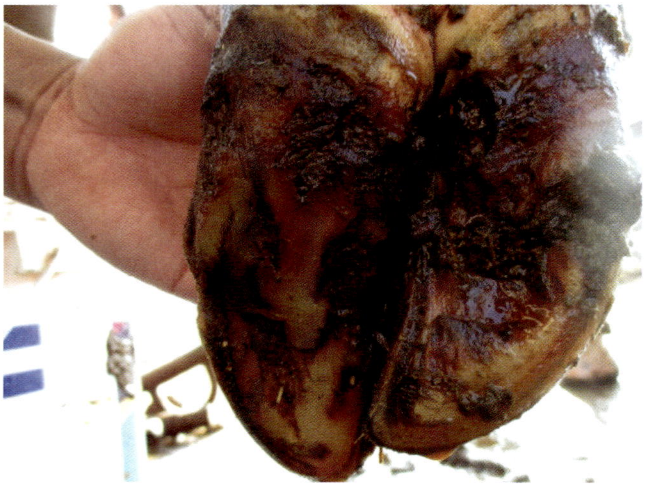

Figure 32.5 Sole hemorrhage.

32.7 Digital Dermatitis (Hairy Warts)

The commissure of the interdigital region, which is where digital dermatitis (DD) most frequently develops, is located close to the heels. It is believed to be a multifactorial illness caused by microorganisms. On the feet of dry cows, low-grade DD lesions are frequently apparent as persistent regions of hyperkeratotic skin near the interdigital cleft. Even though they do not cause lameness during the dry period, these lesions turn into open, raw sores in the early stages of lactation with normal clinical symptoms. Therefore, controlling DD must focus on preventing the emergence of these "subclinical" lesions, which can be done by maintaining good foot cleanliness, including regular hoof disinfection hygiene (Laven et al. 2000).

After calving, the incidence of DD is known to rise sharply. This is probably caused by periparturient immune suppression and increased standing, the latter of which results in damp and filthy hooves. The regular hoof disinfection required to treat DD is simply not practiced in many farms, despite the fact that the condition can be almost completely suppressed by frequent foot bathing.

Clinical cases should be managed with a topical antibiotic or disinfectant and should be dressed until they have healed. If we do not adopt this strategy, cows with hairy warts will continue to be a source of infection for the whole herd, and the issue will never be solved. The amount of environmental difficulty will determine how frequently bathing is necessary, although schedules like 4 days/week or 9 days on and 5 days off are becoming more popular. Numerous farmers foot bathe cows every day and are happy with the outcomes. The foot bath should be placed in the typical cow flow path following the parlor exit, but not so near that it impedes access or slows milking. Anything that slows milking is not likely to be carried out frequently. In order to minimize any disturbance to milking, there should ideally be space for at least one complete side of the parlor to escape before the foot wash is reached (Rodriguez-lainz et al. 1999).

Cows should exit into a clean and scraped yard. Two foot baths arranged in sequence, the first to wash the feet and the second with the active chemical, are perfect. Make sure the bath's floor is a pleasant place to walk. The presence of high ridges will make the cows reluctant to join the bath, which will increase fecal contamination and increase the likelihood that the teats will be sprayed with disinfection. Some people use foot baths with a foam rubber foundation or something similar. The liquid chemical inside the rubber mat begins to pool around the cow's foot as it steps on it, serving as a bath when it does so.

The method is simple to use, but it cannot be as effective as a conventional foot bath since the cow moves on to the next step as the depression created by the cow's foot begins to fill with the disinfectant. As a result, the foot does not receive as effective a soaking as with the plain water bath (Figure 32.6).

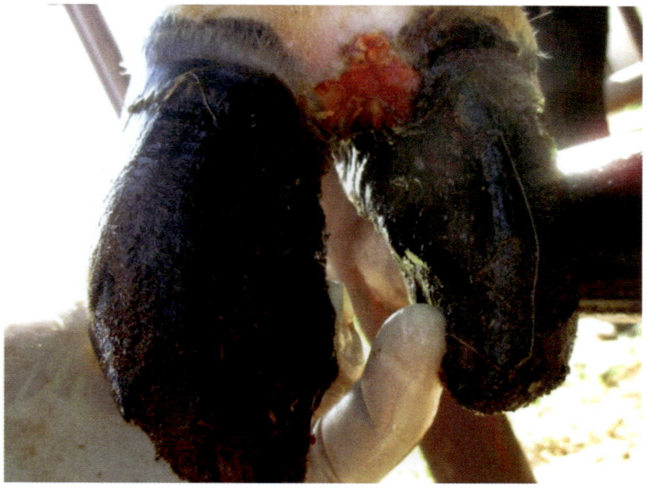

Figure 32.6 Interdigital dermatitis.

32.8 Interdigital Phlegmon (Foot Rot) and Hyperplasia

Phlegmon is a bacterial disease typically brought on by the interaction of two different bacteria. It causes necrosis in the skin between the fingers and has a distinctive scent. If antibiotic treatment is not given promptly, it may infiltrate deeper tissues (Nowrouzian 1991, 1992). Another disease related to interdigital space is hyperplasia. It is a fold of fibrous tissue that protrudes into the interdigital space. It may occur secondary to dermatitis of phlegmon. It is common in the hindlimbs of bulls and leads to spreading of the digits, which causes lameness (Figure 32.7).

32.9 Increased Movement of the Pedal Bone Within the Hoof

It has been established that the pedal bone is suspended within the hoof via attachments to the laminar corium on the axial and particularly the abaxial wall as well as by a pedal suspensory mechanism within the hoof that supports the back of the bone. During the 2 weeks prior to and 2 weeks following calving, hoof levels have been measured as being higher, which causes the suspensory system to be more flexible, the pedal bone to move more, and ultimately, increases the risk of corium bruising. The coffin bone sinks within the horn capsule as the connective tissue link becomes looser or lengthens. Weight is applied to the horn capsule as tension as the bone dangles within.

32.10 Increased Hoof Wear

White line disease and sole hemorrhage are substantially more common when animals stand for extended periods of time on hard floors. Numerous physiological changes occur in periparturient cows that result in an increase in standing, which in turn causes an increase in foot wear. The rate of wear subtracted from the rate of growth determines the thickness of the

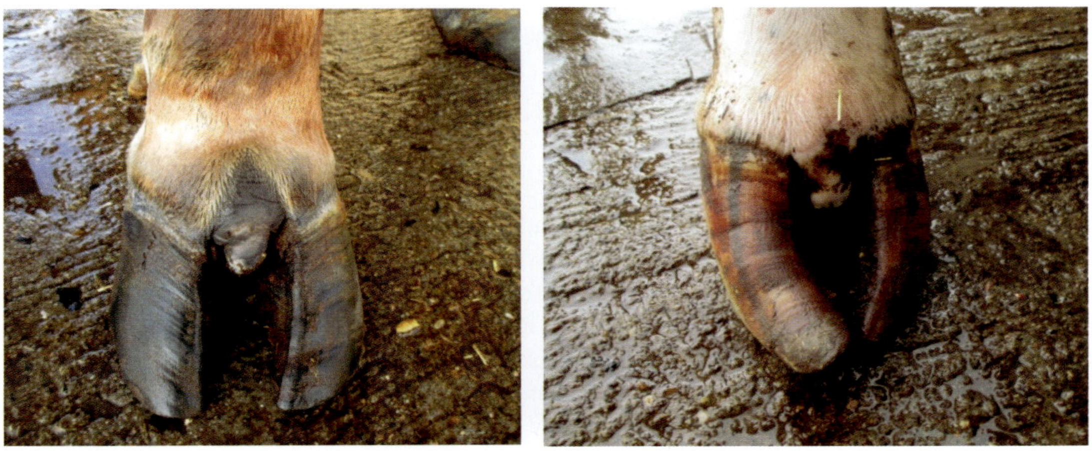

Figure 32.7 Interdigital hyperplasia.

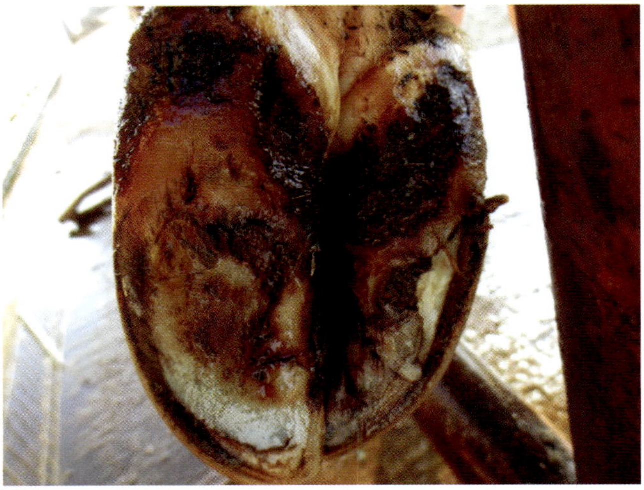

Figure 32.8 Heel horn erosion.

sole at any given time; therefore, higher wear combined with the typical decrease in growth at calving will result in a thinner sole. The likelihood that the corium will bruise and a poor quality hoof will subsequently form is further increased by thin soles (Bergesten and Frank 1996; Livesey et al. 1998) (Figure 32.8).

32.11 Excessive Standing

Heifers that are not used to cubicles and poor cubicle comfort (due to an inadequate size or a lack of bedding) will both cause more standing. A lack of areas for lounging and corridors with blind ends, which heifers find particularly difficult to access, make the issue worse. The postpartum heifer is especially vulnerable to these alterations since she is frequently introduced into the milking herd with little to no integration beforehand. She frequently has to wait to be fed and milked, and she also needs to establish her place in the herd's hierarchy of social dominance. All of these alterations take place right before calving, when sole horn growth is the smallest.

32.12 Calving

At the moment of calving, the corium is at its most vulnerable and bruise-prone state. The beef cows' horns, which have one ring on them for each calving, demonstrate that horn production is constantly disrupted at parturition. It also explains why the incidence of lameness peaks between 8 and 16 weeks after calving since it takes this long for the injured horn to develop from the sole's corium to the foot's bearing surface. At the time of calving, horn growth slows, but there is also increased wear, especially in heifers. This will happen if they spend too much time standing while they wait to be milked, feed, find a place to lay down, or engage in interactive movements with other herd members. Overall, there is a negative net growth because horn growth is slower than horn wear. The sole may become exceedingly soft due to this increase in wear compared to growth, which further damages the underlying corium and puts the foot at risk for sole ulcers and white line disease.

It is unknown whether the act of calving itself or the start of milk production causes the corium to become more fragile. Recent research has revealed that it might be the abrupt increase in milk production, which creates a huge need for amino acids that include sulfur, which could have a crucial role. The generation of milk and the synthesis of keratin, the primary component of horn, both depend on amino acids that include sulfur. Clearly, there is a quick distribution of resources toward milk production at the time of calving, and this may be what causes the development of low quality horn.

In addition to the corium being predisposed to harm upon calving, there is frequently a shift in nutrition, housing, and social grouping immediately following calving that can exacerbate the corium's vulnerability to damage and raise the prevalence of lameness.

32.13 Management

Strong evidence supports the association between lameness and moist and unclean surfaces, notably in the case of DD. Horn takes in moisture from its surroundings and is softer when damp than when dry. Therefore, it is important to manage and house cows in a way that keeps their feet as dry as possible. In free-stall systems, this can be very challenging. Hooves can be kept dry by regularly scraping the passages twice daily and adding a little lime to the free-stall bed to help control mastitis. It is best to treat cows gently. Rushing them down paths makes it impossible for them to avoid stepping on stones that can further bruise the corium, especially in young cows whose corium is already more delicate and whose sole is thin due to a negative net growth. It will help if there are designated "cow tracks" with a supple surface made of tree bark (Benz et al. 2002). To encourage increased sole thickness, cows and heifers should have access to hard surfaces throughout the dry time and their feet should not be over-trimmed when their feet are drying off.

It has been established that soft floors support the conditions necessary for the claw to work well and for cow behavior to be unhindered. Because it is likely that there is a close relationship between the biomechanics, microcirculation, and nutrition of the live cells that nourish the horn-producing tissues of the claw, the experiment also demonstrates that horn quality is heavily dependent on unhindered mobility. Installing rubber mats has the benefit of simultaneously addressing the issue of inadequate traction and the hardness of the floor in the walking area.

32.14 Diagnosis of Lameness

The fact that lameness is a clinical symptom and not an illness in and of itself must always be kept in mind. Therefore, the following steps should be used in order to determine the cause and grade (Table 32.1) of lameness. When interpreting the results of a broad clinical evaluation and a more thorough physical evaluation, the animal's history and environment should be taken into account (Cramer and Solano 2023).

a) **Evaluation of locomotion:** The goal of evaluating locomotion is to determine the anatomical site of discomfort and resultant lameness as well as to assess how well the patient has recovered from treatment. Assessing a cow's locomotion entails examining its posture (such as its back, shoulders, and pelvis) and movements (such as rising and reclining, when possible) as well as each limb and digit. Lameness in the front or rear limbs and occasionally in the upper limb can be identified through gait analysis. A thorough foot examination ought to always be carried out in most cases, particularly for dairy calves, before the upper limb is considered the cause of lameness (Desrochers 2017).
b) **Physical examination:** Animals should be carefully tied, and each limb and foot securely fastened after the afflicted limb has been identified in order to conduct a more thorough examination. The foot should be carefully examined for edema, lesions, and foreign objects, including the interdigital space and heel bulbs, unless there is an obvious visual lesion. Hoof testers should be used to measure the intensity of pain response in the hooves if no evident lesions are

Table 32.1 Lameness scoring system.

Anderson description (Anderson et al. 1976)	Greenough description (Greenough and Ferguson 1985)	Sprecher description (Wells et al. 1993)	Wells description (Sprecher et al. 1997)
0 – Normal gait	1 – Normal gait	1 – Normal: stands and walks normally, flat back topline	0 – Gait abnormality not visible at a walk; not reluctant to walk
1 – Mild: walks easily, readily; bears full weight on foot and mild limb but has an observable gait alteration; stands on all four limbs; line of back bone normal	2 – Slightly abnormal: stiff	2 – Mildly lame: stands with flat back topline; arches back during ambulation; slightly abnormal gait	1 – Mild variation from normal gait at walk; includes intermittent gait asymmetry of a mild bilateral or quadrilateral restriction in free movement
2 – Moderate: reluctant to walk and bear weight but does use the limb to ambulate; short weight bearing phase of stride; rests the affected limb when standing; increased periods of recumbency, may see arching of backbone	3 – Slight lameness: moderate and consistent lameness	3 – Moderately lame: stands and walks with arched back topline; shortened phase of stride	2 – Moderate and consistent gait asymmetry or symmetric gait abnormality but able to walk
3 – Severe: reluctant to stand; refuses to walk without stimulus, non-weight bearing on affected limb; "hoops" over limb rather than bear weight; does not use limb when standing and lies down most of the time; backbone arched with caudoventral tip to pelvis	4 – Obvious lameness: still weight bearing	4 – Lame: arched back topline when standing and walking; obvious diminished weight bearing in one or more limb(s)	3 – Marked gait asymmetry or severe symmetric abnormality
4 – Catastrophe: recumbent; unable to rise; humane euthanasia often indicated	5 – Severe lameness: non-weight bearing	5 – Severely lame: constantly arched back; difficulty moving	4 – Recumbent

visible during or following hoof trimming. A significant amount of pressure is applied using the hoof tester, and reactions such as kicking, withdrawing, tightening of the muscles, or flinching are observed. Functional hoof trimming can be followed by therapeutic trimming if the issue stems from the foot. If no foot lesion is found or no pain response to hoof testers is evoked, then an upper limb lameness will be suspected. To find the source of upper limb lameness, careful palpation of the joints, muscles, tendons, and bones as well as manipulation of the limb (flexion, extension, abduction, and adduction) will be necessary (Schlageter-Tello et al. 2014).

c) **Other diagnostic tools:** The use of ancillary diagnostics is indicated for lameness that is difficult to diagnose or when more information is needed to establish the prognosis or the best course of treatment. To aid distinguishing between foot lameness and upper leg lameness, digital nerve blocks or intravenous regional anesthesia (2% lidocaine, 20–30 ml) can be delivered distal to a tourniquet tied above the dewclaw. The tourniquet can be left on for up to 60 minutes, and the effects of anesthesia continue even after its removal. After the tourniquet is removed, lameness can be assessed. Advanced procedures like imaging, arthroscopy, arthrocentesis, and synovial fluid analyses are normally reserved for animals of higher value. If joint disease (such as septic arthritis, osteochondrosis, or trauma) is suspected, arthrocentesis can be employed together with synovial fluid studies. Diagnoses for fractures, luxations, septic arthritis, and osteochondrosis can be made with the aid of radiographic imaging. The musculoskeletal system's soft tissues can be examined by ultrasound to help with the diagnosis of conditions such septic arthritis, tendonitis, osteochondral fragments, and muscle injuries (Van Nuffel et al. 2015).

References

Anderson, J.F., Arnold, J.P., and Farnsworth, R.J. (1976). Amputation of bovine medial dew claws on hind-legs as an aid in controlling teat trauma. *Veterinary Medicine* 71: 73–76.

Benz, B., Wandel, H., and Jungbluth, T. (2002). Yielding walking areas in loose house systems. *Proceedings of the 12th International Symposium on Lameness in Ruminants*, Orlando, Florida, USA (9–13 January 2002), 280–282. Ithaca, New York, USA: International Veterinary Information Service.

Bergesten, C. and Frank, B. (1996). Sole haemorrhage in tied perimiparous cows as an indicator of peripaturient lameness: effect of diet, flooring and season. *Acta Veterinaria Scandinavica* 37: 383–394.

Blowey, R.W. (2002). Claw trimming–how it should be done? A comparison of two approaches. *Proceedings of the 12th International Symposium on Lameness in Ruminants*, Orlando, Florida, USA (9–13 January 2002), 122–126. Ithaca, New York, USA: International Veterinary Information Service.

Blowey, R.W. and Weaver, A.D. (1991). *A Color Atlas of Diseases and Disorders of Cattle*, 89–128. London: Wolf Publishing Ltd.

Campbell, J., Greenough, P.R., and Petrie, L. (1996). The effect of biotin on sandcracks in beef cattle, *Proceedings of the 9th International Symposium on Disorders of the Ruminant Digit and the International Conference on Lameness in Cattle*, Jerusalem, Israel (14–19 April 1996): 29–32. Israel: Conference Secretariat, Ortra Limited.

Cramer, G. and Solano, L. (2023). Detection and diagnosis of lameness in cattle. *Merck Veterinary Manual*. https://www.msdvetmanual.com/musculoskeletal-system/lameness-in-cattle/detection-and-diagnosis-of-lameness-in-cattle#v80036123 (accessed 22 January, 2024). New Jersey, USA: Merck and Co., Inc.

Dacosta Gomez, C., Al Masri, M., Steinberg, W. et al. (1998). Effect of varying hay/barley proportions on microbial biotin metabolism in the rumen stimulating fermentor. *Proceedings of the Nutrition Society* 7: 14–28.

Dehghani, S.N. (2008). Digital vascular variations in normal and laminitic foot in dairy cattle. *Lameness in Ruminants - International Lameness in Ruminants Symposium and Conference - Finland, 2008*, Kuopio, Finland (9–13 June 2008): 320–321. Ithaca, New York, USA: International Veterinary Information Services.

Dehghani, S.N., Sadeghi, A.M. (2006). Digital blood vessel alterations in normal and laminitic dairy cattle. *Proceedings of the 6th Iranian Symposium of Veterinary Surgery, Anesthesia and Radiology*, Mashhad, Iran (in Persian).

Desrochers, A. (2017). Diagnosis and prognosis of common disorders involving the proximal limb. *The Veterinary Clinics of North America. Food Animal Practice* 33: 251–270.

Greenough, P.R. and Ferguson, J.G. (1985). Alternatives to amputation. *The Veterinary Clinics of North America. Food Animal Practice* 1: 195–203.

Laven, R.A., Demirkan, I., Earter, S.D., et al. (2000). Relationship of antibodies to spirochaetes and the prevalence and severity of digital dermatitis. *Proceedings of the XI International Symposium on Disorders of the Ruminant Digit and III International*

Conference on Bovine Lameness (ed. C.M. Mortellaro and L. De Vecchis), Parma, Italy (3–7 September 2000):173–178. Italy: Parmalat.

Livesey, C.T., Harrington, T., Johnston, A.M. et al. (1998). The effect of diet and housing on the development of sole haemorrhages, white line haemorrhages and heel lesions in Holstein heifers. *Journal of Animal Science* 67: 9–16.

Mulling, C.K. and Lischer, C.J. (2002). New aspects on etiology and pathogenesis of laminitis in cattle. *Proceedings of the XXII World Buiatrics Congress* (ed. M. Kaske, H. Scholz, and M. Hölterschinken), Hannover, Germany: 237–247. Hannover, Germany: Klinik für Rinderkrankheiten, Veterinary University.

Nowrouzian, I. (1991). Digital dermatitis: An unrecognized epidemic in dairies in Iran. *Proceedings for 1990-91 British Cattle Veterinary Association*: 84–95.

Nowrouzian, I. (1992). Epidemiological patterns of lameness in dairies in Iran. *Proceedings of the 7th International Symposium on Disorders of the Ruminant Digit,* Rebild, Denmark (21–25 June 1992): 152–157.

Ossent, P. and Lischer, C. (2000). Bovine laminitis: The lesions and theories on their pathogenesis. *Proceedings of the XI International Symposium on Disorders of the Ruminant Digit and III International Conference on Bovine Lameness* (ed. C.M. Mortellaro and L. De Vecchis), Parma, Italy (3–7 September 2000): 31–36. Italy: Parmalat.

Rodriguez-lainz, A., Melendez-Retamal, P., Hird, D.W. et al. (1999). Farm and host-level risk factors for digital dermatitis in Chilean dairy cattle. *Preventive Veterinary Medicine* 42: 87–97.

Schlageter-Tello, A., Bokkers, E.A.M., Koerkamp, P.W.G.G. et al. (2014). Manual and automatic locomotion scoring systems in dairy cows: a review. *Preventive Veterinary Medicine* 116: 12–25.

Sprecher, D.J., Hostetler, D.E., and Kaneene, J.B. (1997). A lameness scoring system that uses posture and gait to predict dairy cattle reproductive performance. *Theriogenology* 47: 1179–1187.

Van Nuffel, A., Zwertvaegher, I., Pluym, L. et al. (2015). Lameness detection in dairy cows: part 1. How to distinguish between non-lame and lame cows based on differences in locomotion or behavior. *Animals* 5: 838–860.

Wells, S.J., Trent, A.M., Marsh, W.E. et al. (1993). Prevalence and severity of lameness in lactating dairy cows in a sample of Minnesota and Wisconsin herds. *Journal of the American Veterinary Medical Association* 202: 78–82.

Whay, H.R. and Shearer, J.K. (2017). The impact of lameness on welfare of the dairy cow. *The Veterinary Clinics of North America. Food Animal Practice* 33: 153–164.

33

Repeat Breeding

Reza Asadpour[1], Arash Kheradmand[2], and Morteza Taravat[1]

[1] *Department of Clinical Science, Faculty of Veterinary Medicine, University of Tabriz, Tabriz, East Azerbaijan, Iran*
[2] *Department of Clinical Sciences, School of Veterinary Medicine, Lorestan University, Khorram Abad, Lorestan, Iran*

33.1 Introduction

A repeat breeder (RB) cow, also known as a repeat breeder or repeat breeder syndrome, refers to a cow that fails to conceive and remains nonpregnant despite repeated breeding attempts (Smith et al. 2018). This condition can significantly impact the reproductive efficiency and profitability of a cattle operation (Martins et al. 2020). RB cows are a concern for farmers and veterinarians alike as they can lead to economic loss due to extended calving intervals and increased culling rates (Diskin and Sreenan 2016; DeJarnette 2020).

RB syndrome is a complex issue that can have multiple underlying causes (Figure 33.1) These causes can be attributed to various factors such as genetics, nutrition, management practices, and reproductive disorders. The condition can affect both dairy and beef cattle, although the prevalence may vary between different breeds and production systems.

Understanding and managing RB cows require a comprehensive approach that involves careful evaluation, diagnosis, and targeted interventions (Bisinotto et al. 2019). Identifying the underlying cause is crucial for effective treatment and prevention strategies. Common diagnostic techniques include thorough reproductive examinations, hormone analysis, and uterine health evaluations (Bisinotto et al. 2019; Pursley et al. 2021).

Effective management practices can help reduce the incidence of repeat breeders. These practices may include optimizing the cow's nutritional status, implementing appropriate breeding protocols, ensuring proper estrus detection, and addressing any underlying health issues (Carvalho et al. 2019; Santos et al. 2020). Additionally, advanced reproductive technologies such as artificial insemination (AI), embryo transfer (ET), and synchronization protocols can be employed to improve conception rates and increase the chances of successful pregnancy (Chebel et al. 2016; Sartori et al. 2020). Minimizing stress factors and providing a favorable environment for RB cows can contribute to improved fertility. This includes reducing heat stress, providing comfortable housing conditions, and implementing proper heat detection and estrus synchronization programs (Wathes et al. 2007).

While RB cows pose challenges to cattle producers, ongoing research and advancements in reproductive technologies offer promising solutions. By understanding the factors that contribute to RB syndrome and implementing appropriate management strategies, farmers can enhance reproductive performance and overall profitability in their herds.

33.2 Risk Factors and Management

33.2.1 Genetic or Congenital Defects in the Reproductive System

Defects in the reproductive system can contribute to RB cows via various abnormalities that affect the fallopian tubes, uterus, cervix, and vagina. These defects can hinder conception by impeding the sperm's ability to reach the egg. For instance, abnormalities in the fallopian tubes or the lack of a natural endometrium can prevent successful implantation of

Periparturient Diseases of Cattle, First Edition. Edited by Tanmoy Rana.

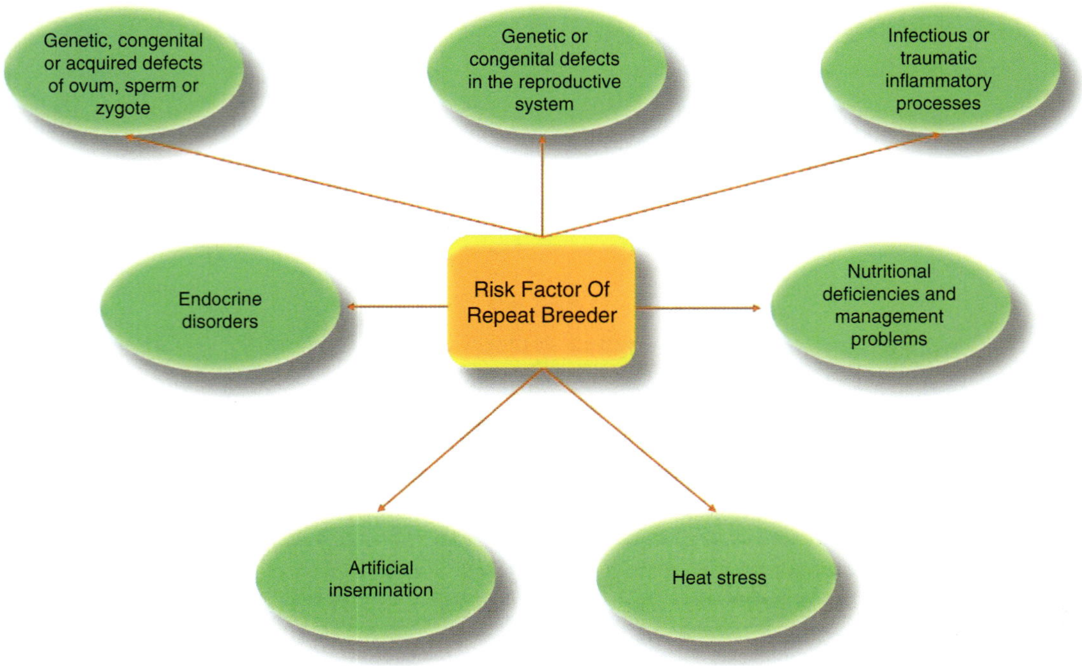

Figure 33.1 Etiology of repeat breeder syndrome in cattle.

the fertilized egg. Additionally, weakened uterine defense mechanisms, such as endometritis, can lead to embryo death (Smith et al. 2018).

While these defects are more commonly observed in heifers at puberty, they can also occur in adult cows. In some cases, adult cows may exhibit less severe symptoms, such as a unicorn uterus, where the frequency of estrus may be affected. However, natural pregnancies can still occur despite these defects, and the identification of such defects may only become apparent after subsequent mating (Diskin and Sreenan 2016).

Although genetic or congenital defects in the reproductive system are relatively rare causes of RB cows, they can be diagnosed through rectal or vaginal examinations. Ovarian abnormalities, including issues with the ovarian capsule, and fibrous adhesions in the reproductive tract have been observed more frequently in RB cows (Chebel et al. 2016).

33.2.2 Genetic, Congenital, or Acquired Defects of Ovum, Sperm, or Zygote

The incidence of ovum disorders in RB cows is approximately 5%, whereas it is around 2% in healthy heifers. Ovum defects may contribute to reduced fertility in older cows (Smith et al. 2018). In a study by Chebel et al. (2016), 37 blastocysts obtained from 23 RB heifers were examined, and only 30% of them were classified as normal. In contrast, 74% of the 31 blastocysts obtained from 18 healthy heifers were found to be normal. Another study also reported a higher prevalence of abnormal embryos in RB heifers during the early stages compared to healthy heifers (Chebel et al. 2016). The amount of apoptosis in the ovarian follicles of RB and healthy heifers was investigated in a study. The researchers found no differences in the granulosa and inner monolayer of preovulatory follicles between RB heifers and virgin heifers. However, there were significant differences in apoptotic cells in preovulatory follicles between RB heifers and healthy heifers. The density of apoptotic cells showed a strong and direct relationship with the degree of atresia. No differences were observed in the follicular wall and its morphology between RB and healthy heifers. These findings indicate that RB heifers during estrus have a follicular structure similar to that of healthy cows (Chebel et al. 2016).

The aging of the egg after ovulation in mammals primarily leads to defects in fertilization, polyspermy, and early embryonic death. This situation occurs when the animal is mated or inseminated long after the end of estrus. Consanguineous matings can cause infertility over time due to incompatibility between the zygote and the mother. However, inbreeding mating can dilute lethal genes. Morphological defects in sperm, sperm chromosomes, and abnormal nucleus can also hinder fertilization. Testicular hypoplasia and degeneration contribute to the production of infertile and abnormal sperm (Chebel et al. 2016). Moreover, when semen is stored at 5 °C for 5 days, its ability to fertilize the egg gradually declines, which results in an increase in early embryonic death. If frozen sperm is used within 30 days of collection, the fertility rate is approximately 66%. However, if it is used after 6 months, the fertility rate drops to around 55%. This decrease in fertility is likely due to chromosomal damage (Chebel et al. 2016).

33.2.3 Infectious or Traumatic Inflammatory Processes That Affect the Genital Tract

This process causes repeat breeding due to premature fetal death. In some cases, inflammatory processes can lead to partial or complete obstruction of the reproductive system, which hinders conception. Impaired conception can also occur in cows that suffer from acute salpingitis, metritis, and vaginitis, where inflammatory exudate and bacteria can be toxic to sperm, causing reduced motility and sperm death (Albihn 1991). Bacterial and viral agents such as *Campylobacter fetus*, *Tritrichomonas fetus, Brucella abortus*, and bovine viral diarrhea virus (BVDV), if introduced into the uterus during AI, can cause endometritis, which contributes to RB syndrome in cows. In some cases, viral infections can lead to salpingitis and sterility due to obstruction of the affected areas (Brooks 1998). Several nonspecific factors, including bacteria such as *Streptococcus*, *Staphylococcus*, *Haemophilus*, *Actinomyces pyogenes*, and *Pseudomonas aeruginosa*, can cause infertility by inducing endometritis. These bacteria can enter the uterus during AI, and their presence can contribute to RB syndrome (Albihn et al. 1991). In RB cows, the prevalence of bacterial factors in the uterus at 50 days post calving is similar to fertile cows, with over 50% of both groups being infected with at least one type of bacteria. The use of antibiotics in the uterus of RB cows is not recommended (Albihn et al. 1991). A study found that among 94 samples of cervical mucus, 59 samples were bacteria free, while 35 samples had isolated bacteria, including *Staphylococcus aureus*, *Streptococcus epidermidis*, and *Klebsiella*. Poor hygiene, overcrowding, severe weather changes (especially heat), and uterine infections can contribute to endometritis, metritis, RB, and infertility in cows. The presence of bacteria and the resulting inflammation compromise the health of the sperm, which leads to impaired fertility. The bacteria isolated in the study showed sensitivity to gentamicin and chloramphenicol, while being less sensitive to penicillin G and oxytetracycline (Ayalon 1978).

For successful growth and survival of the zygote, a suitable uterine environment is crucial. The uterus has local defense mechanisms, including antibody production, mucus flow, and uterine contractions, which can eliminate endometritis over one or more estrous cycles. However, in RB cows, there may be inflammatory and pathological changes in the uterus. The intrauterine injection of antibiotics and antiseptics has shown positive results in treating possible uterine infections and may be beneficial (Bage et al. 2001).

In a subset of RB cows, no pathogenic bacteria are isolated in uterine cultures. However, nonspecific bacteria may be present in the cervix or other posterior parts of the reproductive system and contaminate the uterus following mating. The pregnancy rate after ET is higher in healthy cows compared to RB cows, suggesting that the uterine environment in RB cows may affect the success of pregnancy (Sood et al. 2017). After parturition, endometritis is typically present in all cows but recovers spontaneously over time. Therefore, if the rectal examination shows a healthy genital tract in RB cows, there is no reason to avoid treatment. According to researchers from other studies, AI is considered inappropriate, and there are concerns about misdiagnosis and potential negative effects on fertility. Changes in timing include alterations in the luteal phase level, estrus occurring much earlier or later than expected, and irregular intervals. Cows induced before day 42 after calving have a lower pregnancy percentage compared to cows induced after day 60 (Meredith 1995). Biopsy samples from the uteruses of RB cows often reveal a high number of plasma cells and lymphocytes, which indicate concurrent endometritis. Mild reactions are typically observed in the endometrium, which suggests immunological adequacy due to a reaction with antigenic substances. Most of these antigens are bacteria that invade the uterus during parturition until the next estrus. One report recommended injecting 30–50 ml of Lugol's solution in 30–50 ml of distilled water into the uterus 24 hours after AI if the RB factor is not detected. If the animal becomes pregnant using this method, the procedure should be repeated. The timing of antiseptic inoculation into the uterus is crucial, and the most suitable time is after the sperm enters the oviduct. Allow a sufficient period to elapse before the embryo reaches the uterus to ensure the disappearance of any toxic effects of the antiseptic (Meredith 1995). Therefore, this should not be done more than 3 days after AI to avoid potential harm to the embryo and luteolysis of the corpus luteum (CL) on day 4 or 5. Antiseptics should not be used during times of stress for two reasons: (i) they can create unfavorable conditions in the uterus for the survival and transfer of sperm, and (ii) they may migrate from the uterus to the oviduct and ovarian bursa, causing inflammatory reactions such as blockage and adhesion of the ovarian bursa (Meredith 1995).

In another experiment, embryos were collected from healthy and RB heifers 7 days after insemination. The embryos were then transferred to the uterine horn of designated cows that did not have a CL on the other side of the ovary. Recipients were cultured on days 16–17 and 32–35 after insemination. The survival rate of embryos in RB heifers was lower compared to healthy heifers, which indicates that the uterine environment in RB heifers is less favorable for the support, maintenance, and development of the embryo (Gustafsson and Larsson 1985).

33.2.4 Endocrine Disorders

Endocrine disorders are not commonly observed in cows with retained fetal membranes (RB cows) due to the step-by-step pattern of their reproductive cycle (Figure 33.2). However, certain conditions such as the prolonged treatment of ovarian cysts with luteinizing hormone (LH), gonadotropin-releasing hormone (GnRH), or long term progesterone-based estrus synchronization can potentially lead to endocrine disorders and contribute to RB (Roberts 2004). During the examination of RB cows 24–36 hours after insemination, several possible observations may be made, including delayed ovulation, lack of ovulation, misdiagnosis of estrus, or the presence of ovarian cysts. Delayed or absent ovulation is rare, but if either of these conditions is detected, a prescription of 2000–5000 units of human chorionic gonadotropin (hCG) or 100 µg of GnRH is recommended, and the cow should be bred daily until ovulation occurs (Roberts 2004). Recent studies have shown that administering 100 µg of GnRH at the time of insemination in RB cows increases the pregnancy rate by 15% (Stevenson et al. 1984). Similarly, in heifers with RB, GnRH administration at insemination significantly enhances the pregnancy rate by 7% and the fertility rate by 18% (Stevenson et al. 1984). Another report suggests that administering GnRH during follicular development or shortly before it can increase the pregnancy rate by 6%. Administering GnRH 14 days after calving or during the first service after calving can also raise the pregnancy rate by 15–18% (Stevenson et al. 1990). The mechanism of action of GnRH has been explained as follows: when injected during the mid-luteal phase, it prevents the rise in estradiol concentration following the second follicular wave. GnRH also induces small pulses of prostaglandin from around day 12 onward, which sensitizes the CL to release larger amounts of prostaglandins in the subsequent days. This mechanism reduces follicular estradiol production, prevents an increase in oxytocin receptors in the CL, and inhibits the stimulation

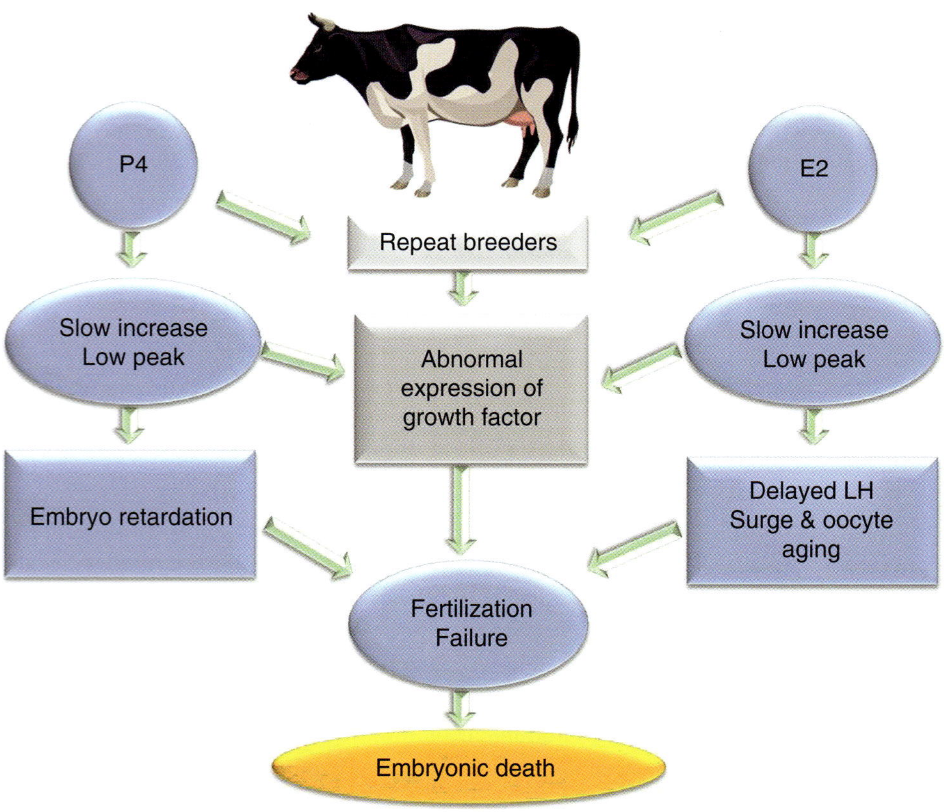

Figure 33.2 Endocrine disorders associated with repeat breeder syndrome in cattle.

of prostaglandin secretion by oxytocin. GnRH can stimulate ovulation of the dominant follicle during the luteal phase, usually occurring on days 4–7 and 14–16, which coincides with the maximum follicle diameter for 3 days. Additionally, administering GnRH on the sixth day of the cycle can induce ovulation in 75% of cows and lead to the formation of additional corpora lutea, which minimizes luteinization. The follicle becomes more responsive to progesterone, which reduces estradiol production and subsequently decreases oxytocin receptor levels. However, some reports suggest that buserelin, a form of GnRH, may not be effective at improving the pregnancy rate (Peters and Ball 1995). After fertilization, the balance of estrogen and progesterone is crucial for the uterus to be receptive to the embryo by day 4. Excessive levels of either estrogen or progesterone create unfavorable conditions for embryo survival. Inadequate progesterone secretion between days 8 and 17 can lead to fetal death. Administering exogenous progesterone at a pharmacologically appropriate dose has been found to increase the pregnancy rate in RB cows. However, excessive progesterone administration may inhibit LH release and potentially cause fetal death due to insufficient progesterone in the bloodstream. Administering progesterone to cows with low pregnancy rates significantly improves the rate of conception. For instance, using progesterone-releasing intravaginal devices (PRIDs) for 8 days or controlled intravaginal device release (CIDR) for 6–12 days results in higher pregnancy rates compared to other methods (Bilodeau-Goeseels, Kastelic 2003). Some researchers have reported that progesterone administration significantly, and sometimes insignificantly, increases the pregnancy rate in RB cows. Progesterone measurement is considered a practical and suitable method for assessing pregnancy status and ovarian activity in RB cows. Administering exogenous progesterone during the early stages of CL formation increases the plasma progesterone concentration and improves insemination success (Thuemmel et al. 1992). The plasma progesterone concentration varies during the estrous cycle in RB cows, which leads to changes in the synthesis and secretion of uterine proteins required for early-stage embryo development (Sood et al. 2017). In a study comparing healthy heifers to RB heifers, it was found that RB heifers have a longer duration of static estrus and a higher incidence of ovulation disorders compared to healthy heifers. However, the plasma progesterone levels were not significantly different between the two groups. Strict stress management and proper AI techniques are important factors in achieving higher pregnancy rates in RB heifers (Albihn 1991). Another study involving six heifers showed that RB heifers have a longer duration and interval between the initiation of estrus and ovulation compared to healthy heifers. RB heifers also exhibited higher plasma progesterone levels at the start of estrus, which normalized during pregnancy. Additionally, RB heifers displayed abnormal levels of prostaglandin (PG)F2α metabolites and progesterone at the time of CL disappearance, but these levels returned to normal during pregnancy (Albihn et al. 1991).

33.2.5 Nutritional Deficiencies and Management Problems

These factors have been identified as common causes of reduced fertility and frequent estrus in cows, particularly in larger herds and those utilizing AI. Insufficient daily observation of cows to detect estrus is one of the primary reasons for repeated breeding (Roberts 2004). Short estrus cycles can be attributed to the presence of ovarian or endometrial cysts. The average duration of cow estrus is 10–28 hours, and insemination typically occurs 10–15 hours after estrus ends. The optimal timing for insemination is 10 hours before and after the end of estrus, which necessitates strict herd management. The lifespan of sperm in the female reproductive tract is 48 hours, with peak fertility occurring 12–24 hours after mating. If estrus and ovulation are normal, performing two inseminations at the end of estrus and 12–20 hours later only marginally increases fertility rates by approximately 2% (Roberts 2004).

A report indicates that the pregnancy rates achieved through insemination at various stages of estrus are as follows: 44% at the onset of estrus, 82.5% in the middle of estrus, 75% at the end of estrus, 62.5% 6 hours after the end of estrus, 32% 12 hours after the end of estrus, 28% 18 hours after the end of estrus, 12% 24 hours after the end of estrus, and 8% 36 hours after the end of estrus. Fertilization does not occur beyond 48 hours after the end of estrus, which indicates the short lifespan of the ovulated egg. The accurate determination of cow estrus and appropriate timing of AI are crucial for optimizing fertility in the herd (Roberts 2004).

Nutritional deficiencies and management problems can play a significant role in the occurrence of RB cows. Several factors related to nutrition and management can contribute to reduced fertility and repeated breeding in cows. Here is an overview of the role of nutritional deficiencies and management problems in RB cows.

a) **Energy and nutrient imbalance:** Inadequate energy intake and imbalances in nutrients such as protein, minerals (like phosphorus, copper, manganese, and iodine), and vitamins (like vitamin A and β-carotene) can negatively affect reproductive performance in cows (Santos et al. 2004; Jaiswal et al. 2017)

b) **Total digestible nutrients (TDNs) and energy balance:** Insufficient TDNs and a negative energy balance can impair reproductive function and increase the likelihood of repeat breeding (Santos et al. 2004).
c) **Iodine deficiency:** In areas with iodine deficiency, supplementing the diet with organic iodine before mating has been shown to improve pregnancy rates in RB cows (Jaiswal et al. 2017).

Proper feeding, including adequate TDNs and maintenance of a positive energy balance, plays a significant role in fertility. In iodine-deficient regions, supplementing cow diets with organic iodine for 8–12 days prior to mating has shown to increase pregnancy rates compared to control groups (Roberts 2004). Hypoglycemia and deficiencies in phosphorus, copper, manganese, iodine, vitamin A, and β-carotene can contribute to infertility, although each factor alone may not cause estrous repetition frames (Meredith 1995).

33.2.6 Heat Stress

High ambient temperatures, particularly above 80 °F, and thermal stress can have detrimental effects on fertility in cows, including increasing the incidence of repeat breeding (Roth et al. 2001). Heat stress negatively impacts fertility by disrupting normal estrous cycles, reducing oocyte quality, and impairing embryo development. Implementing effective heat stress management strategies can help mitigate these adverse effects (Figure 33.3).

a) **Disruption of normal estrous cycles:** Heat stress can lead to irregular or shortened estrous cycles in cows, which results in reduced fertility and increased repeat breeding (West 2003).
b) **Reduced oocyte quality:** High temperatures during heat stress can impair oocyte quality, which leads to reduced fertilization rates and decreased embryo development (Roth et al. 2001; Hansen 2009).
c) **Impaired embryo development:** Heat stress can negatively affect various stages of embryo development, including reduced blastocyst formation and increased embryonic loss (Hansen 2019; Wolfenson et al. 2000).
d) **Suboptimal herd management:** Inadequate management practices, including a lack of proper shade, cooling facilities, and access to water during hot seasons, can contribute to heat stress and reproductive problems in cows (Roth et al. 2001).

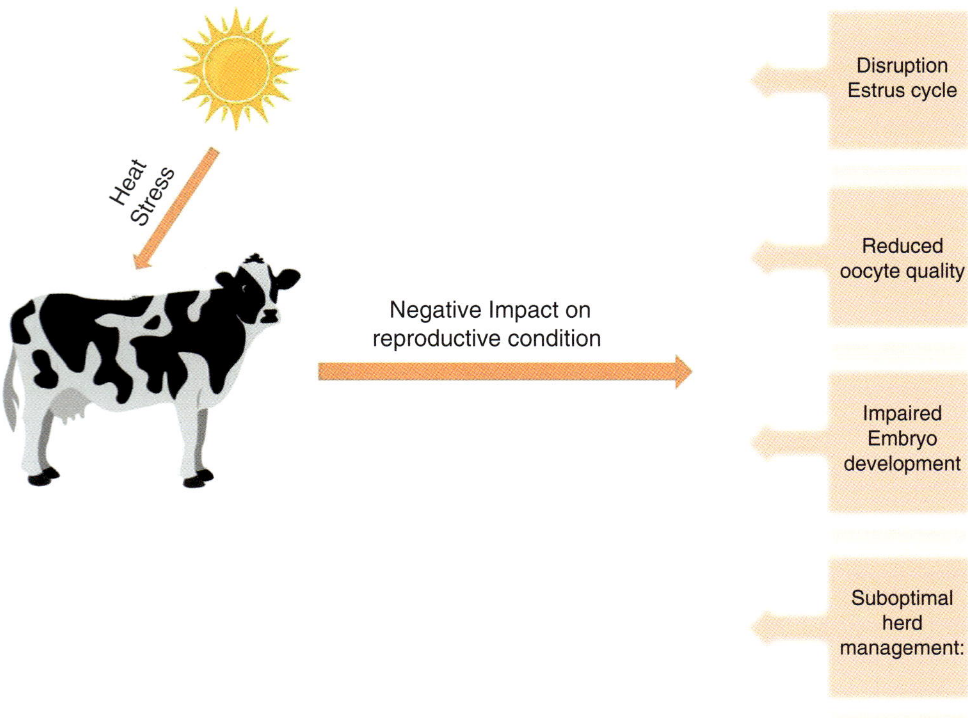

Figure 33.3 The effect of heat stress on the reproductive condition in cows.

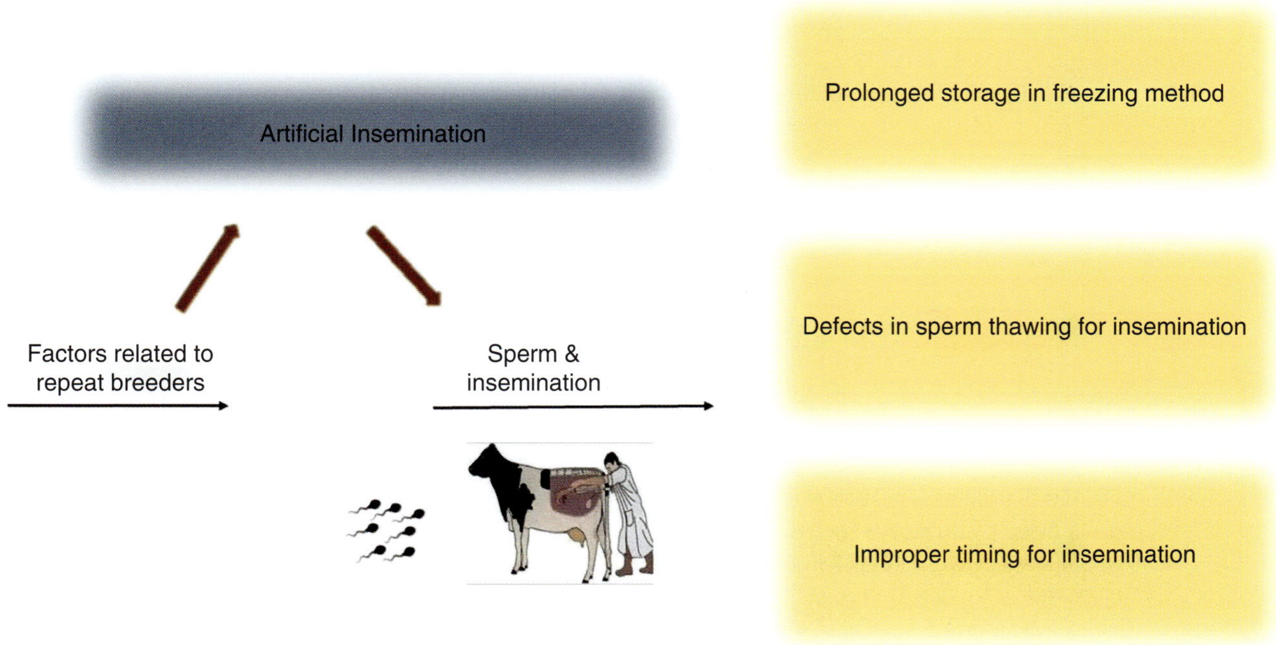

Figure 33.4 Role of artificial insemination in managing repeat breeder syndrome in cows.

33.2.7 Artificial Insemination

Several factors can contribute to the production of infertile sperm. These include prolonged storage and improper sperm freezing as sperm viability and fertility are severely affected when stored at temperatures higher than −79 °C. Improper thawing methods also harm sperm, which necessitate a quick and adequate thawing in warm or cold water. Timely insemination within a few minutes after sperm thawing is crucial as keeping them at a temperature of 5 °C for an hour or more negatively impacts sperm quality (Figure 33.4). To achieve optimal fertility rates, insemination should be performed at least 60 days or more after calving as pregnancy rates decrease before this period (Roberts 2004).

33.3 Conclusion

RB cows are those that have failed to conceive after repeated inseminations. Managing RB cows involves identifying the potential causes of infertility and implementing appropriate treatments. Common treatments for RB cows include:

- **Uterine therapy:** RB cows often experience uterine infections or inflammation, which can hinder conception. Uterine therapy involves the use of antibiotics or intrauterine infusions to treat infections and reduce inflammation, which improves the chances of a successful conception.
- **Hormonal treatments:**
  - Progesterone supplementation: Administering exogenous progesterone, such as through intravaginal progesterone devices or progesterone injections, can help synchronize estrus and enhance fertility in RB cows.
  - GnRH-based protocols: GnRH protocols that involve the administration of GnRH at specific intervals can help stimulate follicular development and increase the likelihood of ovulation in RB cows.
- **Nutritional management:** Ensuring proper nutrition is crucial for reproductive success in RB cows. Dietary adjustments, such as improving energy and nutrient balances, can enhance overall reproductive performance.
- **ET:** In cases where RB cows have persistent fertility issues, ETs can be considered. This technique involves transferring embryos from genetically superior cows or donors to RB cows to improve their reproductive success.

- **Heat stress management:** Heat stress negatively affects reproductive performance in RB cows. Implementing heat stress management strategies, such as providing shade, ventilation, and access to cool water, can help mitigate the adverse effects of heat stress on fertility.
  It is important to note that the specific treatment approach may vary depending on the underlying causes identified in individual RB cows. Consulting with a veterinarian or reproductive specialist is recommended to tailor the treatment plan to the cow's specific needs.

References

Albihn, A. (1991). Standing oestrus, ovarian function and early pregnancy in virgin and repeat breeder heifers. *Journal of Veterinary Medicine Series A* 38 (1–10): 212–221.

Albihn, A., Shamsuddin, M., Qunshan, H., and Kindahl, H. (1991). Plasma levels of prostaglandin F2α metabolite and progesterone in repeat breeder heifers. *Acta Veterinaria Scandinavica* 32 (3): 361.

Ayalon, N. (1978). A review of embryonic mortality in cattle. *Reproduction* 54 (2): 483–493.

Båge, R., Bosu, W.T., and Rodríguez-Martínez, H. (2001). Ovarian follicle apoptosis at the onset of standing estrus in virgin and repeat-breeder dairy heifers. *Theriogenology* 56 (5): 699–712.

Bilodeau-Goeseels, S. and Kastelic, J.P. (2003). Factors affecting embryo survival and strategies to reduce embryonic mortality in cattle. *Canadian Journal of Animal Science* 83 (4): 659–671.

Bisinotto, R.S., Ribeiro, E.S., Martins, C.M. et al. (2019). Update on the causes, consequences, and management of the repeat breeder cow syndrome. *Animal Reproduction* 16 (3): 353–364.

Brooks, G. (1998). Fertility of repeat breeder cows in subsequent lactations. *The Veterinary Record* 143 (22): 615–616.

Carvalho, P.D., Souza, A.H., Amundson, M.C. et al. (2019). Relationships between fertility and postpartum changes in body condition and body weight in lactating dairy cows. *Journal of Dairy Science* 102 (3): 2804–2815.

Chebel, R.C., Mendonça, L.G., Costa, P. et al. (2016). *Journal of Dairy Science* 99: 1–16.

DeJarnette, J.M. (2020). The reproductive impact of the repeat breeder cow. *Veterinary Clinics of North America: Food Animal Practice* 36 (2): 307–316.

Diskin, M.G. and Sreenan, J.M. (2016). Fertilization and embryonic mortality rates in beef heifers after artificial insemination. *Journal of Reproduction and Fertility* 81 (1): 23–32.

Gustafsson, H. and Larsson, K. (1985). Embryonic mortality in heifers after artificial insemination and embryo transfer: differences between virgin and repeat breeder heifers. *Research in Veterinary Science* 39 (3): 271–274.

Hansen, P.J. (2009). Effects of heat stress on mammalian reproduction. *Philosophical Transactions of the Royal Society of London. Series B, Biological Sciences* 364 (1534): 3341–3350. https://doi.org/10.1098/rstb.2009.0131.

Hansen, P.J. (2019). Reproductive physiology of the heat-stressed dairy cow: implications for fertility and assisted reproduction. *Animal Reproduction* 16 (3): 497–510. https://doi.org/10.21451/1984-3143-AR2019-0034.

Jaiswal, R., Selokar, N.L., Kumar, P. et al. (2017). Nutritional interventions for improving reproductive efficiency in repeat breeding cows. *Veterinary World* 10 (11): 1397–1402. https://doi.org/10.14202/vetworld.2017.1397-1402.

Martins, J.P.N., Cardoso, R.C., and Santos, J.E. (2020). Economic aspects of fertility in dairy cattle. *Journal of Dairy Science* 103 (7): 5966–5982.

Meredith, M.J. (1995). *Animal Breeding and Infertility*. Cambridge, MA, USA: Blackwell Science.

Peters, A.R. and Ball, P.J. (1995). *Reproduction in Cattle*, 2e. Oxford: Blackwell Science Ltd.

Pursley, J.R., Mee, M.O., and Wiltbank, M.C. (2021). Synchronization of ovulation in dairy cows using PGF2α and GnRH. *Theriogenology* 44 (7): 915–923.

Roberts, S.J. (2004). *Veterinary Obstetrics and Genital Diseases*, 2e. Location: New Delhi, India: CBS Publishers & Distributors Private Limited.

Roth, Z., Arav, A., Bor, A. et al. (2001). Improvement of quality of oocytes collected in the autumn by enhanced removal of impaired follicles from previously heat-stressed cows. *Reproduction* 122 (5): 737–744. https://doi.org/10.1530/rep.0.1220737.

Santos, J.E., Thatcher, W.W., Chebel, R.C. et al. (2004). The effect of embryonic death rates in cattle on the efficacy of estrus synchronization programs. *Animal Reproduction Science* 82-83: 513–535. https://doi.org/10.1016/j.anireprosci.2004.05.011.

Santos, J.E., Bisinotto, R.S., Ribeiro, E.S. et al. (2020). Applying nutrition and physiology to improve reproduction in dairy cattle. *Animal Reproduction* 17 (1): e20190091.

Sartori, R., Siqueira, L.G., Silva, T.E. et al. (2020). Individualized progesterone treatments improve fertility and timing of ovulation in cattle. *Journal of Dairy Science* 103 (1): 820–828.
Smith, M.F., Gonda, M.G., and Moss, G.E. (2018). The impact of repeat breeder cows on beef herd productivity. *Animal Reproduction Science* 189: 1–9.
Sood, P., Zachut, M., Dekel, I. et al. (2017). Preovulatory follicle characteristics and oocyte competence in repeat breeder dairy cows. *Journal of dairy science* 100 (11): 9372–9381.
Stevenson, J.S., Schmidt, M.K., and Call, E.P. (1984). Gonadotropin-releasing hormone and conception of Holsteins. *Journal of Dairy Science* 67 (1): 140–145.
Thuemmel, A.E., Gwazdauskas, F.C., Whittier, W.D., and McGilliard, M.L. (1992). Effect of progesterone supplementation in repeat-breeder cattle on conception and plasma progesterone. *Journal of Endocrinological Investigation* 15 (5): 393–396.
Wathes, D.C., Pollott, G.E., Johnson, K.F. et al. (2007). Heifer fertility and carry over consequences for life time production in dairy and beef cattle. *Animal* 1 (3): 347–356.
West, J.W. (2003). Effects of heat-stress on production in dairy cattle. *Journal of Dairy Science* 86 (6): 2131–2144. https://doi.org/10.3168/jds.s0022-0302(03)73803-x.
Wolfenson, D., Roth, Z., and Meidan, R. (2000). Impaired reproduction in heat-stressed cattle: basic and applied aspects. *Animal Reproduction Science* 60–61: 535–547. https://doi.org/10.1016/s0378-4320(00)00101-x.

34

Endometritis

Annadurai Thangamani[1], Ramasamy Rajkumar[2], Abdul Reshma[1], Sakthivel Manokaran[1], Sarath Thulasiraman[2], and Ayyasamy Elango[3]

[1] *Department of Veterinary Gynaecology and Obstetrics, Veterinary College and Research Institute, Tamil Nadu Veterinary and Animal Sciences University, Salem, Tamil Nadu, India*
[2] *Veterinary Clinical Complex, Veterinary College and Research Institute, Tamil Nadu Veterinary and Animal Sciences University, Salem, Tamil Nadu, India*
[3] *Dean, Veterinary College and Research Institute, Salem, Tamil Nadu Veterinary and Animal Sciences University, Tamil Nadu, India*

34.1 Introduction

Bovine species are considered to be the backbone of agriculture in India and some other low-income countries. Endometritis is defined as the presence of cloudy to milky muco-purulent vaginal discharge or a cervical diameter more than 7.5 cm after 26–30 days in milk. The occurrence of uterine infections in buffaloes is much more common than in cows, which might be due to improper closure of the vulval lips, poor hygienic management, vaginal stimulation for milk letdown, and wallowing habits that are considered predisposing factors (Azawi 2006). An infection of the uterus is one of the most important reproductive problems in buffaloes, moreover uterine infections cause high economic loss to the farming community due to medical therapy as well as extended (prolonged) days open and intercalving periods. Normal commensal organisms present in the reproductive tract become pathogenic if animals have weak defense mechanisms. Moreover, pathogenic bacteria frequently persist and become resistant to immune mechanisms, which makes uterine disease a key cause of bovine infertility (Sheldon and Dobson 2004). The most common inflammatory conditions of the uterus are endometritis and metritis, they share common causative agents, predispose the animal to one another, and largely share common treatment options (Noakes et al. 2009). In recent centuries, endometritis has arisen as a challenge to field veterinarians in terms of diagnosis and treatment criteria. Endometritis is a serious problem in bovines, especially in buffaloes, when it is associated with a cessation of cyclicity due to persistent corpus luteum (CL) and oxidative stress; however, early treatment with vitamin E and selenium has a good prognosis for buffaloes. The present review discusses recent advanced treatment protocols, including antibiotics and immunomodulators, used for endometritis in veterinary hospitals and teaching veterinary clinical complexes.

34.2 Diagnosis

Diagnostic methods include a clinical observation and history, a transrectal palpation (TRP), the whiteside test (WST), a transrectal ultrasonographic examination (TRUE), the vaginoscopy method, the vaginal speculum method, the endometrial biopsy and histopathological technique, the endometrial cytology method, and serum markers.

34.3 Treatment

Treatments for endometritis used to stimulate uterine muscle tone, blood supply, and flow of mucus of the uterus are varied. Assumptions and concepts regarding the optimal therapy for bovines with endometritis are controversial. The intrauterine douching of antiseptics or antibiotics and systemic injections of prostaglandins are the most frequently used treatments for endometritis.

Periparturient Diseases of Cattle, First Edition. Edited by Tanmoy Rana.

34.3.1 Intrauterine Douching

a) **1% or 2% Lugol's iodine solution:** Intrauterine douching with 2% Lugol's Iodine solution is considered the cheapest and best treatment protocol for estrual mucus with flakes. Intrauterine douching with Lugol's iodine solution will strongly stimulate uterine muscle contraction, tone, and greatly increase mucus secretions. Three consecutive days of treatment with Lugol's iodine solution and the intramuscular administration of a penicillin or fluroquinolone antibiotic was effective in endometritis cases.
b) **Antibiotics:** Several records indicate that the presence of either aerobic or anaerobic bacteria, or both, in the uterine epithelium contributes to a reduction in fertility of cows with uterine infections. The antibiotic selected should be active against both types of bacteria. Aminoglycosides are not recommended for the treatment of endometritis because the presence of an anaerobic environment is not suitable. Similarly, sulphonamide drugs are ineffective in the presence of tissue breakdown products, and moreover, they disturb the normal uterine defense mechanism. Oxytetracycline (OTC) therapeutic action is largely concentrated to the uterine lumen and endometrium because its absorption into the blood stream is relatively low. For that reason, the direct intrauterine douching of OTC produces a tremendous therapeutic concentration in the caruncles and endometrium of healthy and affected animals.

34.3.2 Prostaglandin (PG)F2α Therapy

Even though antimicrobials reduce the bacterial load, they also depress the activity of uterine neutrophils and interfere with the normal defense mechanisms of the uterus (Patra et al. 2014). For replacing antimicrobials, prostaglandin (PG) compounds like cloprostenol (500 μg) and dinoprost (25 mg) are utilized to treat endometritis; the mechanism of action is said to be the lysis of CL followed by a reduction of the progesterone concentration in the uterine progesterone (P4) receptor. A reduced concentration of P4 facilitates uterine contractions that lead to the expulsion of organic debris present in the uterus.

34.3.3 Stress Reduction Therapy

Endometritis is considered to be a serious issue when it corresponds with the cessation of cyclicity and involvement of oxidative stress. Vitamin E and selenium administration is indicated in severe chronic endometritis cases because the glutathione peroxidase level is reduced compared to healthy animals (Hanafi et al. 2010).

34.4 An Antibiotic Therapy Alternative

Immunomodulator therapy: Immunomodulator therapy is considered a novel method of treating immunocompromised animals with a suspicion of endometritis. Severe endometritis is a cause of stress in bovines that results in a reduction in appetite, followed by a decreased milk yield, and ultimately, a poor conception rate following insemination. To rectify that problem, immunomodulators were brought to the market. Bacterial colony counts were significantly reduced with the following immunomodulators: lipopolysaccharides (LPS), lysozymes, oyster glycogens (OGs), and PGF2α.

34.5 Characteristics of Ideal Immunomodulators

- **Nontoxic:** It should be nontoxic to the uterine tissues, even at higher concentration doses.
- **Side effects:** It should not have any side effects likes teratogenic or carcinogenic effects in animals.
- **Tissue residues:** It should leave no tissue residues and be followed by a short withdrawal period.
- **Transmission:** It should not be secreted in animal products like milk.
- **Immune response:** It should stimulate the cellular and humoral immunity defense mechanisms.
- **Environmental effects:** An immunomodulator and its metabolic products should be easily biodegradable without causing any pollution.

34.6 Immunomodulators and Their Mechanisms of Action

34.6.1 Hormones

- **Estrogen:** This hormone plays an important role in increasing natural uterine defense mechanisms through increasing blood flow to the genitalia, infiltration into the uterine epithelium of invader cells like leucocytes, uterine contraction, and mucus flow. It is currently not warranted in the treatment of clinical endometritis in either lactating cows or buffaloes as appreciable levels are secreted in milk that may make it unfit for human consumption. Furthermore, the use of estrogen in higher doses could lead to the development of cystic ovarian degeneration.
- **Prostaglandins:** Prostaglandin hormones play an important role in increasing natural uterine defense mechanisms through the induction of estrus through the lysis of CL followed by increased uterine contraction and secretions. There is a lot of research work that has demonstrated that prostaglandins can be used as an alternate therapy instead of the traditional use of antibiotics in clinical endometritis.

34.6.2 Cell Wall Extracts

- ***Escherichia coli* lipopolysaccharide (LPS):** The gram-negative bacterial cell wall contains an immunogenic material known as LPS. There is considerable research work confirming that *E. coli* LPS can be used as an alternate therapy to the traditional use of antibiotics in clinical endometritis and metritis.
  - Mechanism of action: It acts as a chemotaxis signal for polymorphonuclear cells and causes the influx of serum protein and immunoglobulin into the uterus to perform their immunogenic functions. *E. coli* LPS effectively improved the response of nonspecific cellular immunity at eliminating clinical endometritis and improving pregnancy rates following the intrauterine infusion of 100 μg *E. coli* LPS in cows and buffaloes with endometritis and repeat breeding syndrome.
- **Mycobacterial cell wall components:** Mycobacterial cell walls contain mycolic acid that induce the immune system.
  - Mechanism of action: Mycolic acid, which is a component of mycobacterial cell walls, has been shown to cause a rapid and widespread influx of polymorphonuclear (PMN) cells (which are chiefly responsible for the clearance of uterine infections) by stimulating immunological components like tissue necrosis factor (TNF)-α, interferon (INF)-γ, interleukins (IL-6, IL-2), and myeloperoxidase production as well as by suppressing IL-10 production (Korf et al. 2005).

34.6.3 Bodily Fluids

The addition of a small amount of autologous serum, plasma, or hyperimmune serum to uterine secretions can increase the opsonizing capacity and enhance the phagocytic ability of PMNs. In cattle and buffaloes, the use of autologous plasma has been tested to cure uterine infections like endometritis and metritis. There are no recent reports regarding the clinical use of serum, plasma, and hyperimmune serum for treating endometritis in bovines.

34.6.4 Polymorphonuclear Cell Extracts

Bovine neutrophil extract has bactericidal activity against both gram-positive and gram-negative bacteria. The extract of a PMN cell contains three small antibiotic peptides called defensins. These defensins kill many bacteria and viruses in vitro and could, therefore, be used as a possible immunotherapy for bovine clinical endometritis.

34.6.5 Monomeric Glycoproteins

- **Granulocyte macrophage colony stimulating factor (GM-CSF):** It is naturally secreted by macrophages during immune system stimulation by invading foreign antigens. Now GM-CSF is produced using genetic engineering techniques.
- **Mechanism of action:** Increases the PMNs in circulation by 12-fold and has a good scope for exploring its use to treat uterine infections in cows and buffaloes.

34.6.6 Arachidonic Acid Derivatives

Arachidonic acid metabolites like, leukotriene (LT)B4 are known to be physiologically produced by activated granulocytes, macrophages, and mast cells.

- **Mechanism of action:** Arachidonic acid metabolites stimulate the immune system and induce neutrophil accumulation during inflammation. They particularly stimulate the phagocytic capacity of PMNs in bovines and may also stimulate the activation, proliferation, and release of cytokines by B and T lymphocytes, monocytes, and natural killer cells. Moreover, the intrauterine administration of PGF2α increases the uterine production of LTB4, which seems to promote uterine immune defense mechanisms and improve uterine health, which is followed by improved conception rates.

34.6.7 Oyster Derivatives

Oyster glycogen has been used as an immunogenic agent to induce inflammation and to promote the activation of granulocytes and neutrophils. Moreover, it has been tried in designed animal models. The activation of granulocytes and neutrophils were observed after intraperitoneal and intrauterine administration. Glycogen also acts as a vascular permeability component.

34.6.8 Herbal Extracts

Herbal or plant extracts provide safe and cheap means of treating any uterine-related diseases in bovines. Commonly used herbal extracts are neem (*Azadirachta indica*), heart-leaved moonseed (*Tinospora cordifolia),* garlic extracts, rosemary (*Rosmarinus officinalis),* and German thyme *(Thymus vulgaris).*

Neem (*Aza. indica*) has been reported to possess different nonspecific immune stimulant properties; antimicrobial, antiviral, and antifungal activities; antioxidant; and immunomodulatory properties. It can be used efficiently. *Tin. cordifolia* was used extensively to treat clinical endometritis. Garlic extracts have been used as nonspecific immunomodulators, and a significant reduction in the bacterial load of the cervical discharge at the subsequent estrus was observed. Recently identified antifungal compounds from *Ros. officinalis* and *Thy. vulgaris* have a good curative effect with immunostimulant and free radical scavenger properties for treating clinical mycotic endometritis caused by *Candida albicans* (Hanafi et al. 2010).

34.6.9 Lysozyme and its Dimers

Therapeutic agents, like lysozyme applied as an intrauterine infusion, has led to an increased influx of neutrophils into the lumen (Kumar et al. 2013). The intrauterine administration of 2 mg lysozyme in 50 ml of phosphate-buffered saline or a 5% glucose solution increased the production of IFN-α and culminated in acute phagocytosis. Moreover, it had antiviral efficacy and could modulate TNF-α synthesis without any mutagenic or allergic reactions; hence, it could be used for prophylaxis and therapeutic purposes.

34.6.10 Antihelminthics

In recent years levamisole has also been utilized for the treatment of endometritis because it has immunomodulation characteristics when administered at 2.5 mg/kg, subcutaneously. The administration of levamisole significantly alters stress factors (malondialdehyde, catalase activity, superoxide dismutase).

34.6.11 α-Tocopherol

The bactericidal activity of levofloxacin combined with the immunostimulant activity of α-tocopherol is the basis behind its higher efficacy.

34.7 Conclusion

The incidence of clinical and subclinical endometritis remains at a significant level in commercial dairy farms as well as the farmers' fields. It has been challenging for field veterinarians with regards to the selection of antibiotics. However, advancements in diagnostic techniques and therapeutic strategies have emerged to deal with uterine disorders.

The diagnosis of subclinical endometritis in its early stages remains a challenge in the field and farm today. Therefore, the recent use of certain immunomodulators in the early stages of postpartum, when used following a standard set of diagnostic methods and the standard for managing herd hygiene, could minimize the problems of endometritis to nondetectable levels and reduce the resultant economic loss to dairy farms.

References

Azawi O I. (2006). Clinical, bacteriological and pathological studies of uterine infections in Iraqi buffaloes. Doctoral dissertation. University of Baghdad.

Hanafi, E.M., Abdel-khader, M.M., Kassem, S.S., and Danial, E.N. (2010). Aroma-therapy for endometritis induced by *Candida albicans*. *International Journal of Academic Research* 2: 112–119.

Korf, J., Stoltz, A., De Verschoor, J. et al. (2005). The mycobacterium tuberculosis cell wall component mycolic acid elicits pathogen-associated host innate immune response. *European Journal of Immunology* 35: 890–900.

Kumar, H., Singh, B., Goswami, T.K., and Rawat, M. (2013). Use of neem preparations for the treatment of endometritis cows. *Advances in Animal and Veterinary Sciences* 1: 194–196.

Noakes, D.E., Parkinson, T.Z., and England, G.C.W. (2009). *Arthur's Veterinary Reproduction and Obstetrics*, 403. Pennsylvania: W.B. Saunders Company.

Patra, M.K., Kumar, H., and Nandi, S. (2014). Differential cytokine expression profile in peripheral blood mononuclear cells of endometritic buffaloes. *The Indian Journal of Animal Sciences* 84: 1265–1269.

Sheldon, I.M. and Dobson, H. (2004). Postpartum uterine health in cattle. *Animal Reproduction Science* 82–83: 295–306.

35

Immunomodulation in Relation to Periparturient Diseases

Vivek K. Singh

Department of Veterinary Clinical Complex, Bihar Veterinary College, Bihar Animal Sciences University, Patna, Bihar, India

35.1 Introduction

A pivotal time in the life of a dairy cow occurs during a period that extends from the 2 to 3 weeks prior through the 2–3 weeks after calving; denoted as the transition period, this is when dairy cows face tremendous metabolic and physiologic changes that challenge the homeostatic mechanisms of the body (Morgante et al. 2012). The change from a gestational nonlactating to a nongestational lactating state (Leroy et al. 2008) dents both the metabolic and immune statuses of periparturient cows (Perryman et al. 1989). These alterations bestow transition cows with a high incidence of metabolic, infectious, and reproductive disorders that include parturient paresis, subclinical hypocalcemia, ketosis, mastitis, retained placentas, metritis, postpartum anestrus, displaced abomasa, and subacute ruminal acidosis (Duffield et al. 2009; Kegley et al. 2001; Spain 1993). Physiological changes during this period impose considerable challenges on homeostasis by altering normal metabolism and producing stressors that result in diverse disorders (Castillo et al. 2005; Sordillo et al. 1997). During the transition period, dairy cows undergo physiological stress preparing for and recovering from parturition, dramatically alter their metabolism to supply the mammary gland with nutrients necessary for milk synthesis (Sordillo et al. 1997), and deal with a reduced dry matter intake (DMI), negative energy balance (NEB) (Piccione et al. 2012), and immunosuppression (Shankar and Prasad 1998). Due to immunosuppression, the animal becomes susceptible to various diseases. Immunomodulation, the process of modifying immune responses, plays a crucial role in maintaining health and preventing diseases during this vulnerable period. This chapter explores the immunomodulatory mechanisms involved in periparturient diseases with a focus on dairy cows.

35.2 Immunological Changes During the Periparturient Period

Dairy cows enter a NEB that is further aggravated by nutrient prioritization toward the mammary gland (LeBlanc 2010). The NEB status is characterized by alterations in blood metabolite and hormone profiles (Perryman et al. 1989). During the periparturient period, shifts in the metabolic profile appear to reflect responses associated with inflammation (Bertoni et al. 2008). Inflammation is common in periparturient cows and is linked to health and performance in early lactation (Bradford 2011). One of the greatest challenges during the periparturient period is meeting the nutrient demands of the cow. In late gestation, the demands of the pregnant uterus are high, but the demands associated with early lactation are much greater. In addition to the metabolic changes seen in the transition cow, both neutrophil and lymphocyte functions are impaired (Esposito et al. 2014). Different cytokines play important roles in the immune functions of the animal. T helper-1 (Th1) lymphocytes mainly secrete interleukin (IL)-2 and interferon (IFN)-γ and promote the cell mediated immune response. T helper-2 cells mainly secrete IL-4, IL-10, IL-5, and promote humoral immunity (Roche et al. 2009). A balance between the Th1 and Th2 cell subpopulations and the production of cytokines coordinates the immune response to ensure pathogen elimination without causing disease (Carter and Dutton 1996).

Immunosuppression and the marked changes in endocrinological, nutritional, and metabolic status increase the concentrations of circulating cortisol around parturition (Vallee and Falchuk 1993). These dynamic changes seem to be central to

Periparturient Diseases of Cattle, First Edition. Edited by Tanmoy Rana.

the metabolic disturbances that favor the establishment of infections in the postpartum cow (Burton et al. 2005; Goff 2006). The severity of this immunosuppression is exacerbated by factors such as an NEB (Mutoni et al. 2012), hypocalcemia (Ducusin et al. 2003), and increased circulating levels of cortisol for prolonged periods around calving (Burton et al. 2005). One of the older and most promising technologies to boost the immunity of animals during peripartum periods of immunosuppression is the supplementation of various micronutrients. Vitamins and minerals play an important role in the growth of animals and their reproductive performance (El-Shahat and Abdel Monem 2011). Thus, supplementation with dietary immunomodulators is especially critical during the periparturient period (Weiss and Spears 2006). Further evidence has suggested that cows who suffer the greatest decline in feed intake just before calving are the most immunosuppressed and have a higher incidence of metritis and endometritis (Hammon et al. 2006; Tomlinson et al. 2008). Due to the diversity of proteins and enzymes that contain Zn, Cu, and Mn, these trace minerals are essential for a wide variety of physiological processes that regulate growth, production, reproduction, and health. Zinc is widely distributed throughout the body as a component of metalloenzymes and metalloproteins (Urton et al. 2005). Zinc finger proteins play an integral role in regulating gene expression that consequently impacts a wide variety of bodily functions including cell division, growth, hormone production, metabolism, appetite control, and immunity (Urton et al. 2005). Zinc has a catalytic, coactive, and/or structural role in a wide variety of enzymes that regulate many physiological processes including metabolism, growth, and immune function (Urton et al. 2005). Because Zn is required for the production of protective keratins in the hoof and teat, one area of recent attention has been evaluating the role Zn plays in maintaining structural integrity and health in the hoof and udder (Suthar et al. 2013). Zinc is an essential component of numerous enzymes, including enzymes involved in the synthesis of DNA and RNA. In the antioxidant system, Zn is a component of Cu–Zn superoxide dismutase (SOD). In addition to an antioxidant role, Zn may affect immunity via its important role in cell replication and proliferation (Waller 2000). Research in humans and laboratory animals has documented that a Zn deficiency impairs immune responses and reduces disease resistance (Seder 1994). Severe Zn deficiency in calves (Ohtsuka et al. 2006) and in lambs (Droke and Spears 1993) has also been shown to impair immunity. Plasma Zn concentrations decrease in dairy buffaloes at parturition and return to baseline values within 3 days (Goff and Stable 1990). Some research suggests that organic forms of Zn may affect mammary gland health status. The supplementation of dairy diets with zinc methionine has reduced somatic cell counts (SCCs) in some studies but not in others (Kellogg 1990). It was found that lactating buffaloes supplemented with zinc proteinate had a lower rate of new intramammary infections than those supplemented with inorganic zinc oxide (Sordillo and Raphael 2013). He suggested that zinc proteinate may enhance resistance to mammary infections by increasing keratin synthesis in the teat canal. It is well documented that Cu requirements of ruminants are greatly affected by dietary concentrations of Mo, S, and Fe. Studies examining the effect of dietary Cu on immune responses in cattle have been reviewed (Waller 2000). There is a remarkable increase in the phagocytic activities and lymphocyte proliferation response in the peripheral blood of transition Sahiwal cows provided prepartum supplementation of vitamin E, Cu, and Zn (Dang et al. 2013). Additionally, it has also been found that the prepartum supplementation of micronutrients boosts mammary health by reducing the SCC and percent neutrophils secreted in cow milk (Mulligan and Doherty 2008). Improvements in Ca homeostasis through dietary anionic salts are thought to be mediated by this compensated acidosis that makes the receptor site for parathyroid hormone more efficient. The parathyroid hormone is necessary for the mobilization of calcium from the bones. Improved calcium mobilization improves the availability of calcium stores at the time of parturition and minimizes the drop in blood calcium (Weiss et al. 1990).

35.3 Immunomodulatory Mechanism

35.3.1 Balance of Pro-inflammatory and Anti-inflammatory

During the periparturient period, the balance between pro-inflammatory and anti-inflammatory cytokines shifts. There is an upregulation of pro-inflammatory cytokines like IL-1, IL-6, and tumor necrosis factor (TNF)-α. These cytokines play essential roles in initiating and regulating the immune responses to infections. However, excessive pro-inflammatory responses can lead to tissue damage and exacerbate periparturient diseases. To counteract the potential harmful effects of excessive inflammation, anti-inflammatory cytokines like IL-10 and transforming growth factor (TGF)-β are up-regulated. These cytokines help dampen the immune response, prevent tissue damage, and promote tissue repair. Several trace elements and vitamins are potentially useful in maintaining an appropriately balanced immune status in dairy cows to cope with cytokine misregulation and NEB during the transition period. The list of potentially useful trace elements that function as or are key components of immune status includes copper, zinc, manganese, and selenium. There are substantial amounts of research data that indicate the valuable effects of these trace elements and vitamins on curtailing the pernicious effects of the transition period in European and crossbred dairy cows (Benzaquen et al. 2015; Chawla and Kaur 2004; Dermauw et al. 2015; Konviana et al. 2015).

35.3.2 Amelioration of Oxidative Stress

The periparturient period also leads to increased oxidative stress due to an imbalance between reactive oxygen species (ROS) production and antioxidant defense mechanisms. Oxidative stress can negatively impact immune function and increase the cow's susceptibility to infections. Zinc is an essential component of numerous enzymes, including enzymes involved in the synthesis of DNA and RNA. In the antioxidant system Zn is a component of Cu–Zn SOD. In addition to an antioxidant role, Zn may affect immunity via its important role in cell replication and proliferation (Waller 2000). Research in humans and laboratory animals has documented that Zn deficiency impairs immune responses and reduces disease resistance (Seder 1994). Copper is involved in the antioxidant system via its involvement in the enzymes Cu–Zn SOD and ceruloplasmin. Copper–zinc SOD is responsible for the dismutation of superoxide radicals to hydrogen peroxide in the cytosol (Halliwell and Gutteridge 1999). Ceruloplasmin is a Cu transport protein that also exhibits oxidase activity. It oxidizes ferric iron (Fe^{3+}) to ferrous iron (Fe^{2+}) without the production of free Fe^{3+} that can cause oxidation and peroxidation to tissues (Halliwell and Gutteridge 1999). Ceruloplasmin is an acute phase protein that increases during disease and may be important for scavenging superoxide radicals (Broadley and Hoover 1989).

35.3.3 Potentiation of Leukocyte Function

During the periparturient period, there are alterations in leukocyte function. It has been documented that a phosphorus deficiency and hypophosphatemia negatively affect cellular immune functions in various species (LeBlanc 2010). Calcium is also important for intracellular metabolism and signaling in most cell types, including the leukocytes of the immune system. Realizing the importance of calcium in leukocyte activation, low blood calcium around the time of calving could contribute to periparturient immunosuppression. Recently, it was reported that calcium stores in mononuclear leukocytes are depleted prior to the development of hypocalcemia in the blood and that this depletion of intracellular calcium potentially contributes to immunosuppression (Esposito et al. 2014). Neutrophil and macrophage activity may decrease, which reduces the cow's ability to combat pathogens effectively. Vitamin E, Cu, and Zn supplementation leads to a remarkable increase in the phagocytic activities and lymphocyte proliferation response in the peripheral blood of transition cows (Dang et al. 2013). Therefore, the supplementation of Ca, P, vitamin E, Cu, and Zn potentiate the leukocyte function and immune status of the transition cow.

35.4 Conclusion

A pivotal time in the life of a dairy cow occurs during a period that extends 2–3 weeks prior through 2–3 weeks after calving; denoted as the transition period, this is when they face tremendous metabolic and physiologic changes that challenge the homeostatic mechanisms of the body. The change from the gestational nonlactating state to the nongestational lactating state dents both the metabolic and immune statuses of transition cows. Production diseases of dairy cows are a manifestation of their inability to cope with the metabolic demands of high production and thus continue to be a cause of economic loss in the dairy industry as well as an animal welfare concern. Thus, the transition period of the dairy cow is by far the most important window of opportunity that the dairy farmer has to maximize the overall profitability of the dairy cow. Paying close attention to various management practices, including prepartum dietary supplementation, is paramount for minimizing the extent of metabolic alterations and immunosuppression that occurs during this critical time period. Many scientific studies have demonstrated remarkable oxidative and immunological alterations in parturient cows during transition period.

Cows supplemented prepartum with ammonium chloride and immunomodulators have exhibited the best amelioration of transition-induced metabolic alterations. Results of the present study clearly showed a remarkable amelioration of SCC and metabolic panels toward normalcy in cows supplemented prepartum with immunomodulators and anionic salt. This could be attributed to the positive effects of nutritional supplements on the health, metabolomics, and immune statuses of transition cows. Remarkable immunological changes, lipid mobilization, and alterations in serum metabolites occur in parturient cows that predispose them to immunosuppression and metabolic alterations for a few weeks postpartum. Prepartum immunomodulator and anionic salt supplementations could potentially ameliorate the metabolic and immunological alterations due to transition stress in parturient cows. Therefore, prepartum supplementation with immunomodulators and ammonium chloride could be one of the best strategies to curb transition-induced physiological aberrations and thus production diseases in cows.

References

Benzaquen, M., Galvão, K.N., Coleman, A.E. et al. (2015). Effect of oral mineral and energy supplementation on blood mineral concentrations, energetic and inflammatory profile, and milk yield in dairy cows affected with dystocia. *The Veterinary Journal* http://dx.doi.org/10.1016/j.tvjl.2015.03.001.

Bertoni, G., Trevisi, E., Han, X., and Bionaz, M. (2008). Effects of inflammatory conditions on liver activity in puerperium period and consequences for performance in dairy cows. *Journal of Dairy Science* 91 (9): 3300–3310.

Bradford, B.J. (2011). Inflammation and oxidative stress in transition cows. *Proceedings of the 73rd Cornell Nutrition Conference for Feed Manufacturers,* East Syracuse, New York, USA (18–20 October 2011): 8–17. Ithaca, New York, USA: Cornell University.

Broadley, C. and Hoover, R.L. (1989). Ceruloplasmin reduces the adhesion and scavenges superoxide during the interaction of activated polymorphonuclear leukocytes with endothelial cells. *The American Journal of Pathology* 135: 647–655.

Burton, J.L., Madsen, S.A., Chang, L.C. et al. (2005). Gene expression signatures in neutrophils exposed to glucocorticoids: a new paradigm to help explain 'neutrophil dysfunction' in parturient dairy cows. *Veterinary Immunology and Immunopathology* 105: 197–219.

Carter, L.L. and Dutton, R.W. (1996). Type 1 and type 2: a fundamental dichotomy for all T-cell subsets. *Current Opinion in Immunology* 8: 336–342.

Castillo, C., Hernandez, J., Bravo, A. et al. (2005). Oxidative status during late pregnancy and early lactation in dairy cows. *Veterinary Journal* 169: 286–292.

Chawla, R. and Kaur, H. (2004). Plasma antioxidant vitamin status of periparturient cows supplemented with α-tocopherol and β-carotene. *Animal Feed Science and Technology* 114: 279–285.

Dang, A.K., Jamwal, M., Kaur, M. et al. (2013). Effect of micronutrient supplementation around calving on the plasma cortisol levels of Murrah buffaloes and Sahiwal and Karan Fries cows. *Tropical Animal Health and Production* 45 (4): 1047–1050.

Dermauw, V., Dierenfeld, E., Du Laing, G. et al. (2015). Impact of a trace element supplementation programme on health and performance of cross-breed (Bos indicus x Bos taurus) dairy cattle under tropical farming conditions: a double-blinded randomized field trial. *Journal of Animal Physiology Animal Nutrition (Berl)* 99 (3): 531–541.

Droke, E.A. and Spears, J.W. (1993). In vitro and in vivo immunological measurements in growing lambs fed diets deficient, marginal or adequate in zinc. *Journal of Nutritional Immunology* 2: 71–90.

Ducusin, R.J., Uzuka, Y., Satoh, E. et al. (2003). Effects of extracellular Ca2+ on phagocytosis and intracellular Ca2+ concentrations in polymorphonuclear leukocytes of postpartum dairy cows. *Research in Veterinary Science* 75 (1): 27–32.

Duffield, T.F., Lissemore, K.D., McBride, B.W., and Leslie, K.E. (2009). Impact of hyperketonemia in early lactation dairy cows on health and production. *Journal of Dairy Science* 92 (2): 571–580.

El-Shahat, K.H. and Abdel Monem, U.M. (2011). Effects of dietary supplementation with vitamin E and/or selenium on metabolic and reproductive performance of Egyptian Baladi Ewes under subtropical conditions. *World Applied Sciences Journal* 12: 1492–1499.

Esposito, G., Irons, P.C., Webb, E.C., and Chapwanya, A. (2014). Interactions between negative energy balance, metabolic diseases, uterine health and immune response in transition dairy cows. *Animal Reproduction Science* 144 (3): 60–71.

Goff, J.P. (2006). Major advances in our understanding of nutritional influences on bovine health. *Journal of Dairy Science* 89 (4): 1292–1301.

Goff, J.P. and Stable, J.R. (1990). Decreased plasma retinol, a-tocopherol, and zinc concentration during the periparturient period: effect of milk fever. *Journal of Dairy Science* 73: 3195–3199.

Halliwell, B. and Gutteridge, J.M.C. (1999). *Free Radicals in Biology and Medicine*, 3e. New York, USA: Oxford University Press.

Hammon, D.S., Evjen, I.M., Dhiman, T.R. et al. (2006). Neutrophil function and energy status in Holstein cows with uterine health disorders. *Veterinary Immunology and Immunopathology* 113 (1–2): 21–29.

Kegley, E.B., Spears, J.W., and Auman, S.K. (2001). Dietary phosphorus and an inflammatory challenge affect performance and immune function of weanling pigs. *Journal of Animal Science* 79: 413–419.

Kellogg, D.W. (1990). Zinc methionine affects performance of lactating cows. *Feedstuffs* 62 (35): 15.

Konviana, J., Vargova, M., Paulíkova, V. et al. (2015). Oxidative stress and antioxidant status in dairy cows during prepartal and postpartal periods. *Acta Veterinaria Brno* 84: 133–140.

LeBlanc, S.J. (2010). Monitoring metabolic health of dairy cattle in the transition period. *The Journal of Reproduction and Development* 56 (S): 29–35.

Leroy, J.L.M.R., Vanholder, T., Van Knegsel, A.T.M., and Bols, P.E.J. (2008). Nutrient prioritization in dairy cows early postpartum: mismatch between metabolism and fertility? *Reproduction in Domestic Animals* 43 (S): 96–103.

Morgante, M., Gianesella, M., Casella, S. et al. (2012). Response to glucose infusion in pregnant and nonpregnant ewes: changes in plasma glucose and insulin concentrations. *Comparative Clinical Pathology* 21: 961–965.

Mulligan, F.J. and Doherty, M.L. (2008). Production diseases of the transition cow. *The Veterinary Journal* 176: 3–9.

Mutoni, G., Prasad, S., De, K. et al. (2012). Effect of supplementation of vitamin E, copper and zinc around peripartum on udder health, milk yield and composition of Sahiwal cows. *Livestock Research for Rural Development* 24: 220.

Ohtsuka, H., Watanabe, C., Kohiruimaki, M. et al. (2006). Comparison of two different nutritive conditions against the changes in peripheral blood mononuclear cells of periparturient dairy cows. *Journal of Veterinary Medical Science* 68: 1161–1166.

Perryman, L.E., Leach, D.R., Davis, W.C. et al. (1989). Lymphocyte alterations in zinc-deficient calves with lethal trait A46. *Veterinary Immunology and Immunopathology* 21: 239–248.

Piccione, G., Messina, V., Marafioti, S. et al. (2012). Changes of some haematochemical parameters in dairy cows during late gestation, post partum, lactation and dry periods. *Veterinary Medicine And Zootechnics* 58: 59–64.

Roche, J.R., Friggens, N.C., Kay, J.K. et al. (2009). Invited review: body condition score and its association with dairy cow productivity, health, and welfare. *Journal of Dairy Science* 92: 5769–5801.

Seder, R.A. (1994). Acquisition of lymphokine-producing phenotype by CD4+ T cells. *The Journal of Allergy and Clinical Immunology* 94: 1195–1202.

Shankar, A.H. and Prasad, A.S. (1998). Zinc and immune function: the biological basis of altered resistance to infection. *American Journal of Clinical Nutrition* 64: 447S–463S.

Sordillo, L.M. and Raphael, W. (2013). Significance of metabolic stress, lipid mobilization, and inflammation on transition cow disorders. *The Veterinary Clinics of North America Food Animal Practice* 29 (2): 267–278.

Sordillo, L.M., Shafer-Weaver, K., and DeRosa, D. (1997). Immunobiology of the mammary gland. *Journal of Dairy Science* 80 (8): 1851–1865.

Spain, J. (1993). Tissue integrity: a key defense against mastitis infection: the role of zinc proteinates and a theory for mode of action. In: Lyons, T.P. (Ed.), Biotechnology in the Feed Industry, Proceedings of the 9th Annual Symposium. Alltech Technical Publication, Nicholasville, KY, USA, pp. 53–58.

Suthar, V.S., Canelas-Raposo, J., Deniz, A., and Heuwieser, W. (2013). Prevalence of subclinical ketosis and relationships with postpartum diseases in European dairy cows. *Journal of Dairy Science* 96 (5): 2925–2938.

Tomlinson, D.J., Socha, M.T., and DeFrain, J.M. (2008). Role of trace minerals in the immune system. *Proceedings of the Pennsylvania State Dairy Cattle Nutrition Workshop*, Grantville, Pennsylvania, USA (12–13 November 2008): 39–52.

Urton, G., Keyserlingk, M.A., and Weary, D.M. (2005). Feeding behavior identifies dairy cows at risk for metritis. *Journal of Dairy Science* 88 (8): 2843–2849.

Vallee, B.L. and Falchuk, K.H. (1993). The biochemical basis of zinc physiology. *Physiology Review* 73: 79–118.

Waller, K.P. (2000). Mammary gland immunology around parturition. Influence of stress, nutrition and genetics. *Advances in Experimental Medicine and Biology* 480: 231–245.

Weiss, W.P. and Spears, J.W. (2006). Vitamins and trace mineral effects on immune function of ruminants. In: *Ruminant Physiology* (ed. K. Sejrsen, T. Hvelplund, and M.O. Nielsen), 473–496. Utrecht, The Netherlands: Wageningen Academic Publishers.

Weiss, W.P., Hogan, J.S., Smith, K.L., and Hoblet, K.H. (1990). Relationships among selenium, vitamin E, and mammary gland health in commercial dairy herds. *Journal of Dairy Science* 73: 381–390.

36

Application of Biosensors and Artificial Learning in Disease Diagnoses

Nasrul I. Shaikh[1], *R.S. Sethi*[2], *and Abhishek Bhardwaj*[3]

[1] *All Vet Diagnostic Solutions India, New Delhi, Delhi, India*
[2] *College of Dairy Science and Technology, Guru Angad Dev Veterinary and Animal Sciences University, Ludhiana, Punjab, India*
[3] *College of Veterinary Science, Guru Angad Dev Veterinary and Animal Sciences University, Ludhiana, India*

36.1 Introduction

Biosensors have emerged as powerful tools in veterinary science, revolutionizing the field of animal health monitoring and management (Bogdanov et al. 2018). These innovative devices combine the principles of biology and sensor technology to detect and quantify specific analytes, which provides real-time and accurate information about an animal's health status (Ahmadi et al. 2019). Biosensors have found widespread applications in veterinary medicine to enable the early detection of diseases, monitoring of physiological parameters, and personalized treatment approaches (Kamal et al. 2020).

The principle of biosensors is based on the recognition of a biological response and its conversion into a measurable signal (Pandey et al. 2017). They consist of a bioreceptor, which can be enzymes, antibodies, or microorganisms, and a transducer that converts the biological signal into an electrical, optical, or electrochemical output (Rodriguez-Mozaz et al. 2017). This integrated design allows biosensors to detect and measure various analytes of interest, such as metabolites, hormones, pathogens, and disease-specific biomarkers (Uddin et al. 2021).

In recent years, there have been significant advancements in biosensor technology that have made them more efficient, portable, and user-friendly. Miniaturization has played a crucial role in the development of biosensors and enabled their integration into small devices that can be easily used on-site or at the point of care. Additionally, the incorporation of wireless connectivity has revolutionized data transmission to allow for remote monitoring and real-time access to animal health information by veterinary professionals.

The applications of biosensors in veterinary science are diverse and wide-ranging. One notable application is disease detection and diagnosis (Lam et al. 2021). Biosensors can detect the presence of pathogenic microorganisms, antibodies, and disease-specific biomarkers in animal samples, which aids in the early identification of infectious diseases. This capability is particularly valuable in the diagnosis of conditions such as mastitis, parvovirus infection, and respiratory disorders as it allows for timely interventions and appropriate treatment strategies.

Biosensors also play a crucial role in monitoring metabolic parameters and overall animal well-being. By measuring blood glucose levels, lactate concentration, and other metabolites, biosensors provide valuable insights into metabolic disorders and nutritional imbalances. This information is vital in optimizing animal nutrition, preventing metabolic diseases, and ensuring the overall health and productivity of livestock.

Another significant benefit of biosensors in veterinary science is the continuous monitoring of physiological parameters. Biosensors can measure vital signs such as heart rate, body temperature, and respiratory rate, which provides valuable data for assessing animal health and detecting abnormalities or signs of distress. This real-time monitoring capability allows for the early detection of health issues and prompt intervention, which ultimately leads to improved animal welfare and better treatment outcomes.

Periparturient Diseases of Cattle, First Edition. Edited by Tanmoy Rana.

Despite the numerous benefits of biosensors in veterinary science, there are challenges that need to be addressed for their widespread adoption. Ensuring the accuracy and reliability of biosensor measurements, standardizing measurement protocols, and addressing regulatory considerations are critical aspects. Additionally, there are ethical concerns related to animal welfare, data privacy, and interdisciplinary collaborations between veterinarians.

36.1.1 Significance of Biosensors

Biosensors have emerged as invaluable tools in the scientific monitoring and management of periparturient diseases in cattle. The periparturient period, which encompasses the time surrounding parturition, poses significant challenges to the health and well-being of cows that make timely disease detection and effective management crucial (Bicalho et al. 2020a). Biosensors offer distinct advantages in this context by providing real-time and continuous monitoring of specific analytes relevant to periparturient diseases, thereby enabling early intervention and improved disease management strategies (Bicalho et al. 2020a; Sheldon et al. 2018).

One key benefit of biosensors is their ability to detect and quantify disease-specific biomarkers, metabolic markers, hormonal levels, and inflammatory markers (Sheldon et al. 2018). By accurately assessing these analytes, biosensors provide valuable insights into the health status of periparturient cows. The early detection of periparturient diseases, such as metritis, mastitis, reproductive disorders, and metabolic disturbances, is paramount for timely veterinary care and targeted management approaches that result in improved treatment outcomes (Bicalho et al. 2020a).

Furthermore, biosensors offer noninvasive or minimally invasive monitoring modalities, which minimizes stress to the animals (Ruegg 2017). Continuous data collection can be achieved without the need for manual intervention to ensure uninterrupted monitoring and the precise measurement of physiological parameters. This aspect is particularly advantageous during the periparturient period, as it allows for prolonged and accurate observation of cow health without causing additional discomfort or disturbances (Ruegg 2017).

Another notable advantage of biosensors is their capacity for remote monitoring through wireless connectivity (Oliveira et al. 2020). This capability enables veterinarians and farmers to access real-time data on cow health parameters from a central monitoring system. Remote monitoring enhances the ability to detect early warning signs, promptly intervene, and implement tailored management strategies, thereby improving overall health outcomes for periparturient cows (Oliveira et al. 2020).

By leveraging biosensors in the monitoring and management of periparturient diseases, researchers, veterinarians, and farmers gain valuable scientific insights into cow health and welfare. The ability to detect diseases at an early stage, continuously monitor vital parameters, and implement timely interventions contributes to reduced morbidity and mortality rates, improved treatment efficacy, and enhanced overall herd health.

In summary, biosensors provide a scientific approach to the monitoring and management of periparturient diseases in cattle. Their capacity to provide real-time and continuous monitoring of disease-specific analytes, along with noninvasive or minimally invasive measurement techniques and remote monitoring capabilities, facilitates early detection, intervention, and effective disease management. Incorporating biosensors in veterinary research and practice empowers stakeholders to enhance cow health, minimize economic loss, and optimize overall herd productivity.

36.1.2 Fundamentals of Biosensors

Biosensors are analytical devices that combine biological components with transducers to detect and measure specific analytes in a sample (Turner et al. 2013). They operate on the principle of converting a biological response, such as the binding of a biomolecule to a target analyte, into a measurable signal. The fundamental components of a biosensor typically include a biological recognition element (e.g. enzymes, antibodies, or nucleic acids) that selectively interacts with the target analyte, a transducer that converts the biological response into a detectable signal, and a signal processing unit for data analysis and interpretation (Turner et al. 2013; Singh et al. 2016).

The biological recognition element is the key component of a biosensor and imparts selectivity and specificity to the device. Different types of biological recognition elements can be used depending on the target analyte and application. For example, enzymes can be employed to catalyze specific reactions and generate a signal proportional to the analyte concentration, while antibodies or nucleic acids can bind to specific target molecules with high affinity and selectivity (Singh et al. 2016; Turner et al. 2013).

The transducer converts the biological response into a measurable signal that can be detected and quantified. Various transduction methods are employed in biosensors, including optical, electrochemical, piezoelectric, and thermal techniques. Optical biosensors utilize changes in light intensity, wavelength, or polarization upon analyte binding, while electrochemical biosensors measure changes in current or potential that result from the biochemical reaction (Turner et al. 2013; Singh et al. 2016).

Signal processing and data analysis are crucial in biosensor technology to ensure accurate and reliable measurements. The signal obtained from the transducer is typically amplified, filtered, and converted into a digital format for further analysis. Advanced algorithms and mathematical models are employed to interpret these data, compensate for interference or noise, and provide meaningful information about the analyte concentration or presence (Singh et al. 2016; Turner et al. 2013).

Biosensors operate based on the fundamental principles of recognition and transduction to detect and quantify specific analytes in a sample (Turner et al. 2013). The operation of a biosensor involves two main processes: recognition and signal transduction. The recognition process involves the specific interaction between the biological recognition element and the target analyte, while the signal transduction process converts this interaction into a measurable signal.

The recognition process relies on the specificity and selectivity of the biological recognition element, which can be enzymes, antibodies, nucleic acids, or whole cells. These elements bind to the target analyte through specific interactions such as antigen–antibody binding, enzyme–substrate reactions, or complementary base pairing in nucleic acids (Turner et al. 2013; Singh et al. 2016). The binding event occurs at the surface of the biosensor and is typically accompanied by a change in the physical or chemical properties of the recognition element.

The signal transduction process converts the recognition event into a measurable signal that can be detected and quantified. Various transduction mechanisms are employed in biosensors, including optical, electrochemical, piezoelectric, and thermal methods (Turner et al. 2013; Singh et al. 2016). For example, in an optical biosensor, the binding event may lead to a change in light absorption, emission, or scattering properties, which can be detected using photodiodes or spectrometers. In an electrochemical biosensor, the binding event may generate a current or potential change, which can be measured using electrodes.

The transduced signal is typically amplified, processed, and analyzed to obtain quantitative information about the target analyte concentration. Amplification techniques such as enzymatic reactions or signal amplifiers can be employed to enhance the detectability and sensitivity of the biosensor (Turner et al. 2013). Signal processing techniques, including filtering, data analysis, and calibration, are used to extract meaningful information from the raw signal and to compensate for interferences or background noise.

In summary, biosensors operate based on principles of recognition and signal transduction. The recognition process involves the specific interaction between the biological recognition element and the target analyte, while the signal transduction process converts this interaction into a measurable signal using various transduction mechanisms. Understanding the principles of biosensor operation and signal transduction is essential for the design and development of effective and reliable biosensing platforms for a wide range of applications.

36.2 Periparturient Diseases of Cattle

Periparturient diseases, also known as postpartum diseases or transition cow disorders, refer to a group of health issues that occur in dairy cattle during the period surrounding calving. This critical phase, which includes late pregnancy and early lactation, poses significant challenges to the cow's physiology and immune system. Periparturient diseases can have severe consequences on the cow's health and productivity as well as overall farm economics. It is crucial for farmers and veterinarians to understand these diseases, their causes, and effective preventive measures to minimize their impact on cattle health and farm profitability.

Periparturient diseases of cattle encompass a range of health conditions that occur during the periparturient period, which includes late pregnancy and early lactation. This critical phase is characterized by significant physiological changes as the cow prepares for calving and transitions into milk production. However, these changes can pose various challenges to the cow's overall health and well-being (Smith et al. 2019).

Hormonal fluctuations play a crucial role in the onset of periparturient diseases. As the cow approaches parturition, there is a decrease in calcium levels and an increase in stress hormones, which can disrupt the cow's metabolic balance.

This hormonal imbalance, particularly the drop in calcium levels, can lead to a condition called milk fever. Milk fever is characterized by hypocalcemia and can have severe consequences if left untreated.

Additionally, the increased stress hormones during the periparturient period can suppress the cow's immune system. This immunosuppression makes the cow more susceptible to infections, such as metritis and mastitis, which are common periparturient diseases. These infections can further exacerbate the cow's health issues and impact her milk production (Brown et al. 2017).

To mitigate the risks associated with periparturient diseases, it is crucial for farmers and veterinarians to implement proactive management strategies. Nutritional management during late pregnancy and early lactation is essential to meet the cow's increased energy and nutrient requirements. Providing a well-balanced diet, especially in terms of calcium and energy levels, can help minimize the occurrence of metabolic disorders like milk fever and ketosis.

Moreover, maintaining proper cow comfort and housing conditions is vital to reduce stress and promote the cow's overall well-being during the periparturient period (Haskell et al. 2018). Adequate ventilation, clean and comfortable resting areas, and appropriate space allowances are key considerations for creating an environment that supports the cow's health and immune function.

By implementing these management practices and closely monitoring cows during the periparturient period, farmers can detect early signs of diseases and promptly provide necessary treatments. Regular veterinary check-ups, along with vaccination programs and biosecurity measures, can further contribute to preventing and managing periparturient diseases effectively.

36.2.1 Significance of Periparturient Diseases

The significance of periparturient diseases in cattle cannot be overstated as they have considerable implications for both individual animals and the overall productivity and profitability of dairy farms. Understanding the significance of these diseases is crucial for implementing effective preventive measures and improving animal welfare.

First and foremost, periparturient diseases can have a direct impact on the health and well-being of individual cows. Affected cows may experience pain, discomfort, and a decreased quality of life. These diseases can lead to reduced milk production, compromised reproductive performance, and increased culling rates. Additionally, periparturient diseases can contribute to secondary complications, such as lameness, which further diminishes cow welfare (Smith et al. 2019).

The economic impact of periparturient diseases is substantial. Dairy farms rely on milk production for their revenue, and any decline in milk yield due to periparturient diseases can result in significant financial loss. Moreover, the cost of veterinary treatments, medications, and additional labor required to manage and treat these diseases can place a considerable burden on farm finances (Bicalho et al. 2020b).

Periparturient diseases also affect reproductive performance, which has long term consequences for dairy herd profitability. Fertility issues resulting from diseases like metritis and subclinical endometritis can delay or prevent cows from conceiving, which leads to longer calving intervals and reduced overall herd productivity (Sheldon et al. 2018).

Furthermore, the occurrence of periparturient diseases can affect the farm's reputation and consumer perception. Consumers are increasingly concerned about animal welfare and the use of medications in food production. Farms known to have high rates of periparturient diseases may face negative publicity, which can impact consumer trust and sales and market share as a consequence (Bennett et al. 2019).

Preventing and effectively managing periparturient diseases is therefore crucial for the sustainability and success of dairy farms. By implementing proactive management practices, such as optimized nutrition, adequate cow comfort, and timely veterinary care, farmers can reduce the incidence and severity of these diseases. This, in turn, leads to healthier cows, improved productivity, reduced veterinary expenses, and enhanced overall farm profitability (Smith et al. 2019).

In conclusion, periparturient diseases have significant significance in the dairy industry by impacting the health and welfare of individual cows, farm economics, and consumer perception. Recognizing the importance of these diseases and implementing preventive measures is essential for promoting animal well-being, sustaining farm profitability, and meeting consumer expectations.

36.2.2 Prevalence and Economic Impact

The prevalence and economic impact of periparturient diseases in cattle are significant concerns for the dairy industry. Understanding the extent of these diseases and their financial implications is essential for implementing appropriate management strategies and improving overall herd health.

The prevalence of periparturient diseases can vary depending on several factors, including farm management practices, nutrition, genetics, and overall herd health status. However, studies have consistently shown that a substantial proportion of dairy cows experience one or more periparturient diseases during the transition period. Estimates suggest that 40% or more of dairy cows are affected by periparturient diseases, which makes it a widespread issue (Bicalho et al. 2020b).

The economic impact of periparturient diseases can be significant and multifaceted. A primary consequence of these diseases is decreased milk production. Affected cows may experience reduced milk yields, both in the short term and in subsequent lactations. This decline in productivity directly translates to financial loss for dairy farms, as milk is the primary source of revenue. Moreover, cows that suffer from periparturient diseases may require additional veterinary treatments, medications, and extended recovery periods, which further increases expenses.

The economic impact extends beyond immediate milk loss and veterinary costs. Periparturient diseases can also have a detrimental effect on reproductive performance. Conditions such as metritis and endometritis can cause delays or failures in a cow's ability to conceive, which leads to extended calving intervals and reduced overall herd fertility. Longer calving intervals decrease the number of calves produced and increase the costs associated with maintaining nonproductive animals on the farm (Sheldon et al. 2018).

Furthermore, periparturient diseases can result in increased culling rates. Cows that suffer from severe or recurrent periparturient diseases may be more likely to be culled from the herd due to compromised health or reduced productivity. The replacement cost of these culled cows and the lost potential for genetic improvement can significantly impact farm economics (Bicalho et al. 2020a).

Beyond direct financial losses, periparturient diseases can also affect the farm's reputation and consumer perception. As consumers increasingly value animal welfare and sustainable agricultural practices, farms known for high rates of periparturient diseases may face reputational damage. Negative publicity or concerns regarding the use of medications and veterinary interventions in food production can impact consumer trust and influence purchasing decisions (Bennett et al. 2019).

In conclusion, periparturient diseases have a substantial prevalence and economic impact in the dairy industry. The decrease in milk production, additional veterinary costs, reduced reproductive performance, and increased culling rates collectively contribute to significant financial loss for dairy farms. Implementing effective preventive measures and management strategies are essential to reduce the prevalence of these diseases, improve herd health, and enhance farm profitability.

36.2.3 Role of Management Practices in Prevention

The role of management practices in preventing periparturient diseases is paramount in maintaining the health and well-being of dairy cattle during the critical transition period. Implementing effective management strategies can significantly reduce the incidence and severity of these diseases to ensure optimal cow health and productivity.

- **Nutrition:** Proper nutrition is crucial for preventing periparturient diseases. Providing a well-balanced diet that meets the cow's increased energy and nutrient requirements during late pregnancy and early lactation is essential. Adequate levels of energy, protein, minerals (including calcium), and vitamins support the cow's immune function, metabolic processes, and overall health. Working with a nutritionist to formulate appropriate rations based on the specific needs of a cow can help prevent metabolic disorders like milk fever and ketosis.
- **Cow comfort and housing:** Ensuring optimal cow comfort and housing conditions plays a vital role in preventing periparturient diseases. Comfortable and clean resting areas promote resting and reduce stress, which can positively impact the cow's immune system and overall health. Proper ventilation and temperature control help mitigate heat stress and respiratory issues. Sufficient space allowance, access to clean water, and appropriate flooring surfaces contribute to cow comfort and reduce the risk of injuries, such as lameness.
- **Transition cow management:** Implementing a comprehensive transition cow management program is crucial for minimizing the risk of periparturient diseases. This includes closely monitoring cows during the periparturient period, observing them for early signs of disease, and promptly providing necessary interventions or treatments. Regular health checks, including monitoring the body condition score (BCS), rumen fill, and assessing udder health, help identify potential issues and enable timely intervention.
- **Biosecurity measures:** Implementing biosecurity measures can reduce the introduction and spread of infectious agents that can cause periparturient diseases. These include quarantine and testing protocols for new additions to the herd, strict hygiene practices, and effective biosecurity protocols for visitors and equipment. Minimizing exposure to pathogens can help prevent diseases such as metritis and mastitis.

- **Vaccination programs:** Vaccinations can play a crucial role in preventing certain periparturient diseases. Consultation with a veterinarian and implementing a targeted vaccination program based on the specific disease risks of the herd can help protect cows from infectious diseases. Vaccines for diseases such as bovine viral diarrhea (BVD), leptospirosis, and infectious bovine rhinotracheitis (IBR) can help reduce the incidence and severity of these diseases.
- **Record keeping and data analysis:** Maintaining detailed records and analyzing data related to periparturient diseases can provide valuable insights into herd health and enable the early identification of trends or potential issues. Keeping track of calving dates, reproductive performance, disease incidence, and treatment outcomes allows for targeted interventions and adjustments to management practices as needed.

By implementing these management practices, dairy farmers can significantly reduce the occurrence of periparturient diseases, which leads to healthier cows, improved productivity, reduced veterinary expenses, and enhanced overall farm profitability.

36.2.4 Hormonal Changes and Immunological Challenges

The periparturient period in cattle is characterized by significant hormonal changes and immunological challenges that can have profound effects on the cow's health and well-being. Understanding these dynamics is crucial for effective management and prevention of periparturient diseases.

I) **Hormonal changes:** As cows approach parturition, there are distinct hormonal fluctuations that occur in preparation for calving and the initiation of lactation. One of the most notable changes is the decrease in blood calcium levels, known as hypocalcemia or "milk fever." This drop in calcium is attributed to the cow's high demand for calcium to support milk production. Hypocalcemia can lead to muscle weakness, impaired immune function, and increased susceptibility to other periparturient diseases.

   Additionally, there is an increase in stress hormones, such as cortisol, during the periparturient period. These stress hormones play a vital role in preparing the cow for the upcoming challenges associated with calving and lactation. However, the excessive or prolonged elevation of stress hormones can have negative consequences. Prolonged stress hormone exposure can lead to immunosuppression, which hinders the cow's ability to mount an effective immune response against pathogens.

II) **Immunological challenges:** The periparturient period poses significant immunological challenges for cows. Immune function is naturally suppressed during this time, which makes cows more susceptible to infections and diseases. This immunosuppression is thought to be mediated by the high levels of stress hormones as well as the influence of certain metabolic factors and nutritional changes (Jones et al. 2020).

   The decreased immune function during the periparturient period can increase the risk of uterine infections, such as metritis and endometritis. These infections occur due to the invasion of bacteria into the uterus during calving or postpartum. The compromised immune response makes it more difficult for the cow to clear these infections, which leads to prolonged inflammation and potential reproductive issues.

   Furthermore, immunosuppression can also impact the cow's susceptibility to mastitis, a common and economically significant periparturient disease. Mastitis is primarily caused by bacterial infections of the udder, and the weakened immune system during the periparturient period can compromise the cow's ability to defend against these pathogens. This can result in increased somatic cell counts (SCCs), reduced milk quality, and potential damage to mammary tissue.

   Managing these immunological challenges during the periparturient period involves implementing strategies to support and enhance the cow's immune function. This includes providing the appropriate nutrition to ensure the cow's immune system has the necessary nutrients to function optimally. Vaccination programs, administered prior to the periparturient period, can also help stimulate an immune response and provide protection against specific pathogens.

In conclusion, the periparturient period in cattle is marked by significant hormonal changes and immunological challenges. The hormonal fluctuations, including decreased calcium levels and increased stress hormone levels, can impact the cow's health and make her more susceptible to periparturient diseases. The immunosuppression during this time further increases the risk of infections and compromises the cow's ability to mount an effective immune response. By understanding and addressing these hormonal and immunological dynamics, appropriate management strategies can be implemented to reduce the incidence and severity of periparturient diseases and promote cow health and productivity.

36.2.4.1 Overview of Hormonal Changes

During late pregnancy and parturition in cattle, there are significant hormonal changes that occur in preparation for calving and the initiation of lactation. These hormonal fluctuations play a crucial role in facilitating a successful transition from pregnancy to lactation and ensuring the well-being of the cow and her offspring.

- **Relaxin:** One of the key hormones involved in the periparturient period is relaxin. Relaxin is produced by the corpus luteum and placenta and acts to relax the pelvic ligaments and soft tissues in the birth canal. This hormone allows for easier passage of the calf during parturition, which facilitates a smooth and less stressful calving process (Bartol et al. 2015).
- **Progesterone:** Progesterone, produced by the corpus luteum, maintains pregnancy and inhibits uterine contractions. However, as parturition approaches, progesterone levels decrease, which allows for the initiation of the calving process. The decline in progesterone is thought to be triggered by the release of fetal cortisol, which stimulates the production of enzymes that break down progesterone.

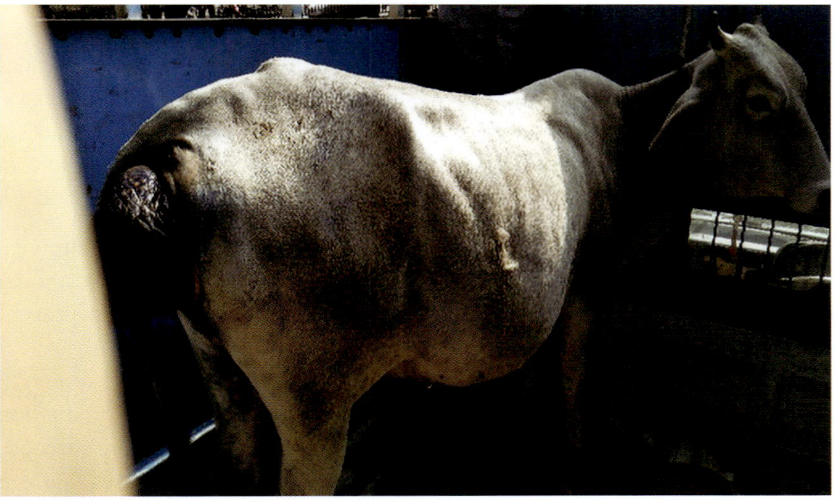

Ante-partum prolapse.

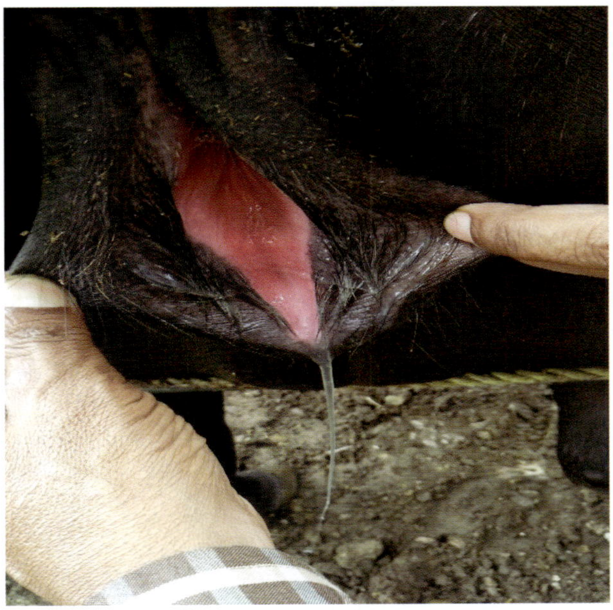

Normal effect of estrogen on the vaginal mucous membrane, note the pinkish color and clear discharge.

- **Estrogens:** Estrogens play a vital role in preparing the reproductive tract for calving and lactation. As parturition nears, estrogen levels increase, which leads to changes in the cervix and increased blood flow to the udder. These changes help facilitate cervical dilation and prepare the udder for milk production.
- **Oxytocin:** Oxytocin is a key hormone involved in milk letdown and uterine contractions during parturition. It is released in response to the suckling or stimulation of the teats to cause the contraction of smooth muscles in the udder and uterus. This facilitates milk flow and expulsion of the placenta, which contribute to the successful establishment of lactation.
- **Prolactin:** Prolactin is a hormone responsible for milk production and lactation. During late pregnancy and parturition, prolactin levels increase in preparation for the onset of milk synthesis. Prolactin promotes the development of mammary tissue, stimulates the initiation of lactogenesis, and plays a crucial role in maintaining milk production throughout the lactation period (Capuco et al. 2019).

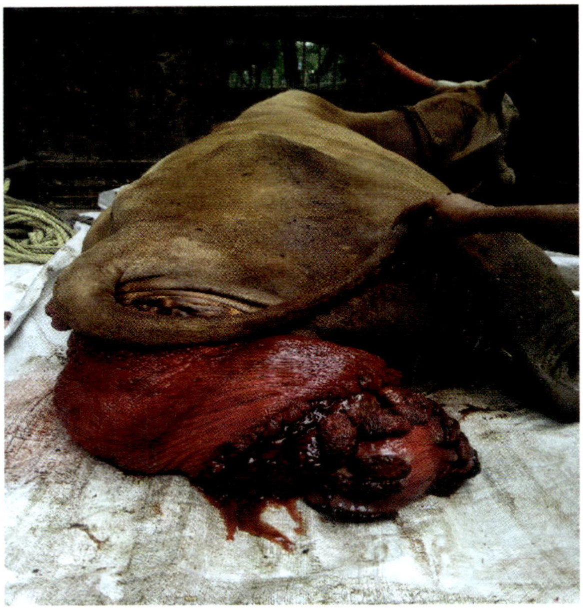

Postpartum prolapse due to hypocalcemia.

These hormonal changes work together to ensure a smooth transition from late pregnancy to parturition and the subsequent establishment of lactation. The precise timing and coordination of these hormonal fluctuations are critical for the cow's reproductive success, calf survival, and milk production.

It is important to note that disruptions or imbalances in these hormonal changes can lead to complications during parturition or impact the cow's subsequent lactation performance. Proper management, including regular monitoring, nutritional support, and veterinary assistance when necessary, can help optimize the hormonal balance and ensure a successful transition for both the cow and her calf.

36.2.4.2 Impact of Hormonal Changes on the Immune System

The hormonal changes that occur during the periparturient period in cattle have a significant impact on the immune system. These hormonal fluctuations can affect immune function and responsiveness, which makes cows more susceptible to infections and diseases during this critical transition period.

- **Immune suppression:** One of the notable effects of hormonal changes during the periparturient period is the suppression of the immune system. The increase in stress hormones, such as cortisol, as well as the influence of other hormonal factors can contribute to immune suppression. This suppression is thought to be an adaptive response to prevent immune-mediated reactions against the developing fetus and ensure successful pregnancy (Burton et al. 2017).
- **Impaired immune response:** The periparturient period is characterized by a reduced ability of the immune system to mount an effective response against pathogens. This impaired immune response can result in the decreased production of immune cells, reduced phagocytic activity, and diminished cytokine production. As a result, cows are more susceptible to infections, including uterine infections like metritis and mastitis, and other periparturient diseases (Burton et al. 2017; Gilbert et al. 2019).
- **Alteration of inflammatory responses:** Hormonal changes during the periparturient period can also affect the inflammatory response. Inflammation is a crucial defense mechanism against infections, but the hormonal fluctuations can disrupt the balance of pro-inflammatory and anti-inflammatory cytokines. This can lead to excessive inflammation or an inadequate inflammatory response, both of which can impact the cow's ability to effectively combat pathogens (Sordillo and Raphael 2013).
- **Metabolic stress and immune function:** Hormonal changes during the periparturient period are closely linked to metabolic changes, and these metabolic stressors can further impact immune function. The high energy demands for lactation coupled with hormonal imbalances can lead to a negative energy balance and metabolic disorders such as ketosis. Metabolic stress negatively affects immune cell function and compromises the cow's ability to mount an effective immune response (Sordillo and Raphael 2013).

It is important to note that the immunosuppression and altered immune responses during the periparturient period are transient and generally resolve as cows transition into lactation. However, during this vulnerable period, management strategies that support and boost immune function are crucial for preventing and minimizing the incidence and severity of periparturient diseases.

Strategies such as providing proper nutrition, ensuring an adequate energy intake, optimizing cow comfort, and implementing biosecurity measures can help mitigate the impact of hormonal changes on the immune system. Additionally, timely vaccinations and preventive measures against specific diseases can help strengthen the cow's immune defenses during this critical period.

36.2.4.3 Immunological Challenges

During the periparturient period, cows face significant immunological challenges that can impact their health and increase their susceptibility to infections and diseases. These challenges arise from changes in the hormonal milieu, metabolic stress, and alterations in the cow's immune response.

- **Immunosuppression:** One of the primary immunological challenges during the periparturient period is the temporary suppression of the immune system. This suppression is believed to be an adaptive response to prevent immune-mediated reactions against the developing fetus and to allow for a successful pregnancy. However, this immunosuppression also makes cows more vulnerable to infections and compromises their ability to mount an effective immune response (LeBlanc 2014).
- **Impaired neutrophil function:** Neutrophils are crucial immune cells responsible for the recognition and elimination of pathogens. However, during the periparturient period, there is a decline in neutrophil function and activity that leads to an impaired ability to combat bacterial infections. Reduced neutrophil migration, phagocytosis, and oxidative burst contribute to the increased susceptibility of cows to diseases such as mastitis and metritis (Sheldon et al. 2018).
- **Dysregulated inflammatory responses:** The periparturient period is marked by altered inflammatory responses in cows. There is a shift toward a more anti-inflammatory state that is characterized by elevated levels of anti-inflammatory cytokines and reduced levels of pro-inflammatory cytokines. This dysregulation can impair the cow's ability to effectively respond to infections and resolve inflammation, which leads to prolonged and chronic inflammation.
- **Disrupted gut microbiota:** The gut microbiota plays a vital role in maintaining immune homeostasis and defending against pathogens. However, hormonal changes and metabolic stress during the periparturient period can disrupt the balance of the gut microbiota. This disruption can lead to an imbalance in microbial populations, the increased translocation of harmful bacteria across the gut barrier, and heightened systemic inflammation (Mach et al. 2017).
- **Metabolic stress and immune function:** Metabolic stress, characterized by a negative energy balance and elevated concentrations of non-esterified fatty acids and ketone bodies, further challenges the cow's immune system. Metabolic stressors can directly affect immune cell function and compromise the cow's ability to mount an effective immune response. This can result in reduced antibody production, impaired phagocytosis, and diminished immune cell proliferation.

These immunological challenges during the periparturient period increase the susceptibility of cows to various diseases, including mastitis, metritis, and retained placentas. Effective management strategies are essential to support the cow's immune system and minimize the negative impacts of these challenges. Providing proper nutrition, optimizing cow comfort, implementing preventive measures, and ensuring a clean and hygienic environment are important steps to reduce the incidence and severity of periparturient diseases and promote the health and productivity of cows.

36.2.5 Metabolic Disorders

The periparturient period in dairy cows is a critical phase characterized by significant metabolic changes to support the transition from late pregnancy to lactation. However, these metabolic adaptations can sometimes lead to metabolic disorders that can negatively impact cow health, fertility, and milk production. Some common metabolic disorders observed during this period include ketosis, fatty liver syndrome, and displaced abomasa.

- **Ketosis:** Ketosis, also known as acetonemia or pregnancy toxemia, is a metabolic disorder characterized by elevated levels of ketone bodies (acetone, acetoacetate, and β-hydroxybutyrate) in the blood. During the periparturient period, cows experience a negative energy balance as the demands for milk production exceed their energy intake. This triggers the mobilization of stored body fat, which results in the excessive production of ketone bodies. Ketosis can lead to reduced feed intake, weight loss, decreased milk production, and increased susceptibility to other health issues.
- **Fatty liver syndrome:** Fatty liver syndrome, also known as hepatic lipidosis, occurs when the liver accumulates excessive amounts of fat during the transition period. The negative energy balance and increased mobilization of body fat contribute to the accumulation of fat in the liver. Fatty liver syndrome can impair liver function and lead to a reduced appetite, decreased milk production, and compromised immune response. If left untreated, it can progress to liver failure and have severe consequences for cow health (Drackley 1999).
- **Displaced abomasum:** Displaced abomasum (DA) is a condition in which the abomasum (the fourth compartment of the cow's stomach) shifts from its normal position. DA is often associated with metabolic changes during the periparturient period, particularly a negative energy balance. The reduced feed intake and rumen function can cause the abomasum to become distended and displaced. DA can result in reduced appetite, weight loss, reduced milk production, and predispose cows to other complications such as ketosis and metritis.

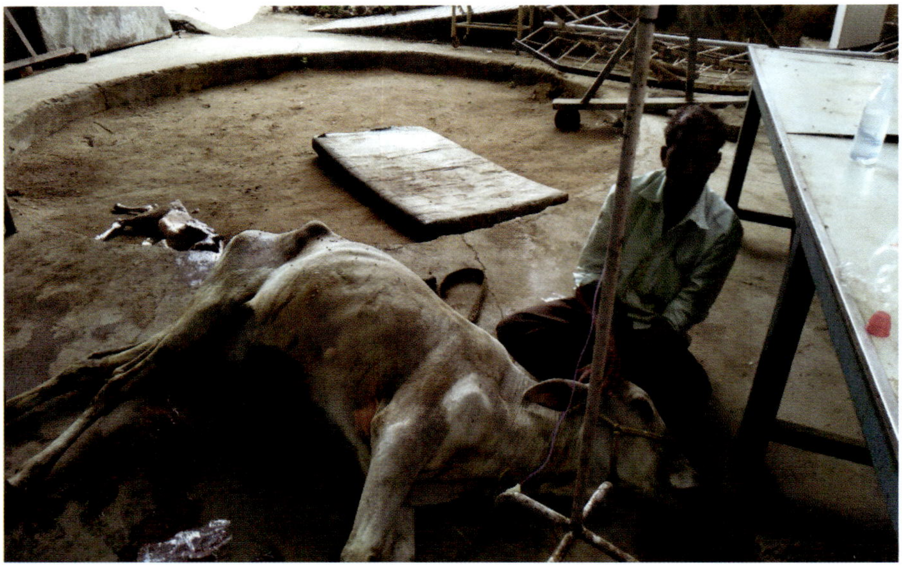

Treating a cow with ketosis.

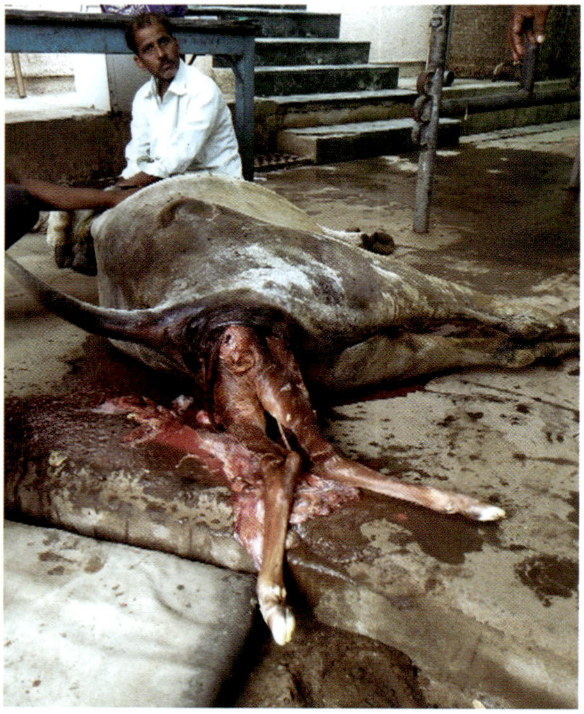

Veterinarian assisting a cow with dystocia due to breech presentation of the calf.

These metabolic disorders can have a significant impact on cow health, reproductive performance, and overall productivity. Proper management and preventive measures are essential to minimize the occurrence and severity of these conditions. Key strategies include:

- **Balanced nutrition:** Providing a well-balanced diet that meets the cow's energy requirements during the periparturient period is crucial. Ensuring a smooth transition from a dry cow ration to a lactation diet and maintaining a consistent feeding regimen can help prevent a negative energy balance and reduce the risk of metabolic disorders.
- **Body condition scoring:** Regular monitoring of the BCS can help identify cows at risk of metabolic disorders. Maintaining an appropriate BCS through proper nutrition and managing body condition changes can help mitigate the occurrence of these conditions.
- **Transition management:** Implementing effective transition management practices, such as gradual diet changes, minimizing stress, and providing a comfortable environment, can support the cow's adaptation to the demands of lactation and reduce the risk of metabolic disorders.
- **Veterinary support:** Working closely with a veterinarian is crucial for identifying and managing metabolic disorders. Routine health checks, blood testing, and the early detection of metabolic issues can help prompt intervention and the appropriate treatment.

By implementing comprehensive management strategies and maintaining optimal cow health during the periparturient period, the incidence and severity of metabolic disorders can be minimized, which results in improved cow welfare, reproductive success, and milk production.

36.2.6 Reproductive Disorders

The periparturient period, which includes the time immediately before and after calving, is a critical phase for reproductive health in dairy cows. During this period, cows are susceptible to various reproductive disorders that can negatively impact their fertility and reproductive performance. Some common reproductive disorders observed during the periparturient period include metritis, retained placentas, and subclinical endometritis.

- **Metritis:** Metritis is an inflammatory condition of the uterus that commonly occurs within the first 21 days after calving. It is characterized by an infection and inflammation of the uterine lining. Metritis is often associated with the entry of bacteria into the uterus during calving, compromised immune function, and hormonal changes. Cows with metritis typically exhibit clinical signs such as a foul-smelling vaginal discharge, fever, decreased appetite, and reduced milk production. A timely diagnosis and treatment are crucial to minimize its negative impact on fertility and reproductive success (Sheldon et al. 2009).
- **Retained placenta:** Retained placenta refers to the failure of the placenta to be expelled within 12–24 hours of calving. It is often associated with insufficient uterine contractions during the calving process. Retained placentas can lead to uterine infections, delayed uterine involution, and increased risk of metritis. It can also result in reduced fertility, as the presence of retained placental membranes can hinder the cow's ability to conceive and maintain pregnancy (Kasimanickam et al. 2004).
- **Subclinical endometritis:** Subclinical endometritis is a condition characterized by inflammation of the uterine lining without visible signs of infection. It is a common reproductive disorder that often goes unnoticed without proper diagnostic tools. Subclinical endometritis is associated with impaired uterine defense mechanisms, altered immune responses, and hormonal changes during the periparturient period. It can negatively affect fertility, as the inflamed uterine environment can hinder sperm transport, fertilization, and embryo development (Gilbert et al. 2005).

These reproductive disorders can have detrimental effects on cow fertility, subsequent reproductive performance, and overall herd productivity. Effective management strategies to minimize the occurrence and impact of these disorders include:

- **Hygiene and sanitation:** Maintaining a clean calving environment, including proper bedding and hygiene practices, can reduce the risk of uterine infections and the incidence of reproductive disorders.
- **Timely intervention and treatment:** Prompt detection and intervention are crucial for reproductive disorders. The timely administration of appropriate treatments, such as antibiotics for metritis or the manual removal of retained placentas, can help prevent complications and optimize cow fertility.
- **Postpartum monitoring:** Regular postpartum monitoring, including uterine health assessments, can aid in the early detection of reproductive disorders. Techniques such as uterine cytology or bacterial culture can be used to identify subclinical endometritis or uterine infections.
- **Nutrition and body condition:** Proper nutrition, maintaining an optimal body condition, and managing the energy balance during the periparturient period are important for reproductive health. Nutritional imbalances and excessive body condition loss can increase the risk of reproductive disorders.
- **Breeding management:** Optimizing breeding management practices, including accurate heat detection, timely insemination, and appropriate synchronization protocols, can improve conception rates and minimize the impact of reproductive disorders on herd fertility.

Effective reproductive management, in collaboration with veterinary support, is crucial during the periparturient period to minimize the occurrence of reproductive disorders and ensure optimal reproductive performance in dairy cows.

36.2.7 Periparturient Mastitis

Periparturient mastitis is a common and significant health issue that affects dairy cows during the periparturient period, which encompasses the time just before and after calving. It refers to the inflammation and infection of the mammary gland that leads to clinical or subclinical mastitis. This condition poses considerable challenges for dairy producers as it can have detrimental effects on milk quality, cow welfare, and farm profitability (Schukken et al. 2003).

1) **Clinical mastitis:** Clinical mastitis is characterized by visible signs of inflammation in the udder, such as swelling, heat, redness, and abnormal milk. It is often accompanied by systemic signs of illness in the cow, such as fever and reduced appetite. Clinical mastitis during the periparturient period can be caused by a variety of bacteria, including

environmental pathogens that contaminate the cow's environment as well as contagious pathogens that spread from other infected cows. Prompt detection and treatment are crucial to prevent the progression of clinical mastitis and minimize its impact on milk production and cow health (Sordillo and Streicher 2002).

2) **Subclinical mastitis:** Subclinical mastitis is a hidden form of mastitis that lacks visible signs but is characterized by inflammation and infection within the udder. It can be challenging to detect without specific tests, such as an SCC analysis. Subclinical mastitis is prevalent during the periparturient period due to various factors that include hormonal changes, compromised immune function, and the stress associated with calving. Subclinical mastitis can lead to an increased SCC in milk, reduced milk production, and an increased risk of clinical mastitis if left untreated (Rajala-Schultz et al. 1999).

36.2.7.1 Risk Factors

- **Cow hygiene:** Maintaining proper cow hygiene and providing a clean and dry environment are crucial to reduce the exposure of the udder to environmental pathogens that can cause mastitis.
- **Teat preparation:** Proper teat preparation before milking, including premilking teat disinfection and post-milking teat dipping, helps reduce the risk of mastitis by minimizing the entry of bacteria into the teat canal.
- **Immune function:** The periparturient period is associated with immunological changes that can affect the cow's ability to resist mastitis-causing pathogens. Strategies to support immune function, such as proper nutrition and minimizing stress, can help enhance the cow's resistance to mastitis.
- **Milking management:** Effective milking management practices, including proper milking machine function, regular maintenance, and proper milking procedures, are crucial to minimize the risk of mastitis. Ensuring consistent and gentle milking routines can reduce the potential for teat-end damage and bacterial entry.
- **Dry cow management:** Implementing appropriate dry cow management protocols, such as dry cow therapy with intramammary antibiotics and teat sealants, can help prevent new intramammary infections and reduce the risk of periparturient mastitis.

The timely identification of mastitis cases, proper treatment with antibiotics based on culture and sensitivity testing, and adherence to withdrawal periods are essential to effectively manage mastitis during the periparturient period. Regular monitoring of the SCC in milk can help detect subclinical mastitis and guide management decisions.

Periparturient mastitis poses significant economic and animal welfare implications for dairy farms. Effective mastitis control programs, including proper management practices, regular monitoring, and appropriate treatment protocols, are necessary to reduce the incidence and impact of mastitis during the periparturient period and ensure the production of high quality milk while safeguarding cow health and welfare.

36.2.8 Management and Prevention of Periparturient Diseases

Effective management and prevention strategies play a crucial role in reducing the incidence and impact of periparturient diseases in cattle. By implementing appropriate management practices, dairy farmers can enhance the overall health and well-being of their cows during this critical period. Here are some key management and prevention strategies:

- **Nutritional management:** Providing proper nutrition is essential during the periparturient period to support the cow's immune system and overall health. It involves formulating well-balanced diets that meet the cow's energy, protein, mineral, and vitamin requirements. Care should be taken to prevent excessive body condition loss as it can increase the risk of metabolic disorders. Close attention should also be given to transition cow diets by ensuring a smooth transition from the dry period to lactation (Overton et al. 2004).
- **Housing and environment:** Maintaining a clean, comfortable, and well-ventilated housing environment is critical in preventing periparturient diseases. Proper ventilation helps reduce humidity and the concentration of pathogens, which minimizes the risk of respiratory and udder infections. Bedding material should be clean and dry to prevent the buildup of bacteria and reduce the likelihood of mastitis (Wells et al. 2018).
- **Vaccination programs:** Implementing appropriate vaccination protocols can help prevent infectious diseases that are prevalent during the periparturient period. Consultation with a veterinarian can aid in determining the necessary vaccines based on the farm's specific disease risks and geographic location. Vaccinations against diseases such as IBR, BVD, leptospirosis, and clostridial infections can be beneficial (Raboisson et al. 2016).

- **Biosecurity measures:** Implementing biosecurity measures helps minimize the introduction and spread of infectious diseases within the herd. This includes controlling visitor access to the farm, quarantining new animals before introducing them to the herd, and maintaining strict hygiene practices. Regular testing and monitoring for common pathogens can help identify and address any emerging issues (Martin et al. 2015).

36.3 Role of Biosensors in Periparturient Disease Management

Biosensors play a crucial role in the management of periparturient diseases in cattle by facilitating metabolic monitoring and early detection of metabolic disorders. Metabolic monitoring is essential for assessing the metabolic status of cows during the periparturient period and allows for timely interventions in metabolic disorders. Biosensors enable the measurement of blood glucose levels and ketone bodies, which are critical indicators of metabolic health (Bicalho et al. 2020a). Continuous monitoring of these parameters using biosensors provides real-time data and enables the early detection of metabolic disorders such as ketosis and hypocalcemia. This early detection allows for prompt intervention, targeted management strategies, and improved treatment outcomes (Bicalho et al. 2020a).

The measurement of blood glucose levels and ketone bodies using biosensors provides valuable insights into the metabolic state of periparturient cows. Elevated blood glucose levels can indicate metabolic stress, while increased ketone body levels may suggest a state of ketosis. Biosensors offer the advantage of real-time and continuous monitoring, which allows for accurate and frequent assessments of these metabolic parameters (Bicalho et al. 2020b). The timely measurement of blood glucose and ketone bodies using biosensors helps identify cows at risk of metabolic disorders, which enables early interventions and tailored management approaches.

Continuous monitoring for the early detection of metabolic disorders is a key role of biosensors in periparturient disease management. Biosensors provide a noninvasive and real-time monitoring method that allows for the continuous assessment of metabolic parameters over an extended period (Bicalho et al. 2020b). By continuously monitoring blood glucose levels and ketone bodies, biosensors enable the early detection of metabolic imbalances, which is crucial for preventing severe metabolic disorders. This continuous monitoring approach enhances the ability to intervene promptly, implement targeted management strategies, and improve overall cow health during the periparturient period.

36.3.1 Detection of Somatic Cell Counts, Electrical Conductivity, and pH Levels in Milk

Biosensors play a vital role in the management of periparturient diseases in cattle by facilitating udder health monitoring through the detection of SCCs, electrical conductivity, and pH levels in milk. Udder health is of utmost importance during the periparturient period, and biosensors offer valuable insights into the health status of the mammary gland (Bicalho et al. 2020a). By measuring SCCs, biosensors can identify elevated levels, which are indicative of udder inflammation and commonly associated with mastitis. The early detection of mastitis through biosensors allows for its prompt treatment and minimizes the negative impact on udder health.

In addition to SCCs, biosensors enable the measurement of electrical conductivity and pH levels in milk, which further contribute to udder health monitoring. Electrical conductivity is a parameter that reflects the ionic concentration of milk, and changes in conductivity can indicate subclinical mastitis or udder health abnormalities (Bicalho et al. 2020b). By continuously monitoring electrical conductivity, biosensors provide a real-time assessment of udder health and enable early interventions to prevent the progression of udder disorders.

The measurement of pH levels in milk using biosensors is another valuable tool for udder health monitoring. An increase in milk pH can indicate the presence of mastitis-causing bacteria as they can alter the milk's acidity (Bicalho et al. 2020a). Biosensors allow for accurate and frequent pH measurements to provide a reliable indicator of udder health status. The early identification of pH level changes using biosensors allows for timely interventions, thereby minimizing the severity of mastitis and its impact on milk quality and cow well-being.

In summary, biosensors play a significant role in monitoring udder health during the periparturient period. Through the detection of SCCs, electrical conductivity, and pH levels in milk, biosensors provide valuable information for the early identification of udder inflammation and mastitis. This early detection enables prompt treatment, which ensures the preservation of udder health, milk quality, and overall cow welfare.

36.3.2 Early Disease Identification for Prompt Treatment and Monitoring

The early identification of mastitis is vital for prompt treatment and the prevention of further complications. Biosensors offer a valuable tool for this purpose by enabling the early detection of mastitis through various parameters, including SCCs, electrical conductivity, and pH levels in milk (Bicalho et al. 2020b). By continuously monitoring these parameters, biosensors can detect subtle changes indicative of udder inflammation and the onset of mastitis. Early identification allows for timely intervention, such as antibiotic treatment, and helps minimize the impact of mastitis on cow health and milk production.

Biosensors also play a significant role in monitoring reproductive health in periparturient cows. They enable the measurement of hormonal changes, such as progesterone levels, which are critical for assessing reproductive health (Bicalho et al. 2020b). Monitoring progesterone levels using biosensors provides insights into the estrous cycle and helps identify potential reproductive disorders or irregularities. By tracking progesterone levels, biosensors help determine the optimal timing for insemination or breeding, which improves the chances of successful reproduction and maximizes herd productivity.

Furthermore, biosensors assist in the detection of irregularities in the estrous cycle and ovulation. Through the continuous monitoring of hormonal fluctuations, biosensors can identify deviations from normal reproductive patterns in periparturient cows (Bicalho et al. 2020b). The early detection of irregularities allows for timely veterinary interventions and the implementation of appropriate management strategies. Biosensors enable real-time monitoring and an accurate assessment of hormonal changes, which provides valuable information to optimize reproductive health and maximize breeding success rates.

36.3.3 Remote Monitoring and Data Analytics

Remote monitoring and data analytics are essential components of biosensor technology that enable the efficient and effective utilization of biosensors in various applications. Remote monitoring allows for real-time data collection and analysis from biosensors placed on animals, which eliminates the need for manual intervention and provides continuous insights into animal health and behavior (Oliveira et al. 2020). Biosensors equipped with wireless connectivity can transmit data to a central monitoring system, which can be accessed remotely by veterinarians and farmers. This capability revolutionizes the way periparturient diseases are managed by providing timely access to critical health information and facilitating proactive decision making.

The remote monitoring of biosensors offers several advantages in periparturient disease management. It allows for the early detection of disease markers or abnormalities, which enables prompt interventions and improves treatment outcomes. By continuously monitoring analytes and parameters relevant to periparturient diseases, biosensors provide a wealth of data that can be analyzed to detect patterns, trends, and anomalies. These data can be processed and analyzed using advanced data analytics techniques, such as machine learning algorithms and predictive modeling, to derive valuable insights into cow health and disease management strategies.

Data analytics plays a pivotal role in leveraging the wealth of information collected from biosensors during remote monitoring. It involves the processing, interpretation, and extraction of meaningful information from the raw data generated by biosensors (Oliveira et al. 2020). By applying sophisticated analytics algorithms, patterns and trends can be identified to allow for the early detection of diseases, prediction of health outcomes, and optimization of management practices. Data analytics also enables the integration of biosensor data with other relevant information, such as environmental data or animal records, to provide a more comprehensive understanding of the factors that influence periparturient diseases.

The combination of remote monitoring and data analytics in biosensor technology provides a powerful toolset for periparturient disease management. It allows for the real-time monitoring of cow health, facilitates the early detection of diseases, and enables evidence-based decision making. Moreover, the continuous stream of data collected from biosensors can contribute to the development of data-driven models and algorithms that improve disease prediction and support personalized management approaches.

Wireless biosensors have emerged as a valuable technology for the remote monitoring of periparturient cows. These biosensors are designed to be attached to the animals and can wirelessly transmit real-time data to a central monitoring system, which allows for the continuous monitoring of cow health parameters (Ruegg 2017). By utilizing wireless connectivity, veterinarians and farmers can remotely access these data and monitor the health status of periparturient cows without the need for their physical presence.

The use of wireless biosensors enables real-time data collection and provides immediate access to vital information about the health and well-being of periparturient cows. These real-time data can include various parameters such as temperature, heart rate, activity level, and rumination behavior. By continuously monitoring these parameters, wireless biosensors provide valuable insights into the cow's health status and allow for the early detection of potential health issues (Ruegg 2017).

The real-time data obtained from wireless biosensors plays a crucial role in informed decision making regarding periparturient disease management. By accessing and analyzing the collected data, veterinarians and farmers can make timely and evidence-based decisions regarding disease prevention, treatment, and management strategies. For example, if a wireless biosensor detects abnormal temperature or heart rate patterns in a periparturient cow, it can alert the stakeholders to potential health problems and prompt them to take immediate action (Ruegg 2017).

Furthermore, real-time data from wireless biosensors can be used to identify trends and patterns in cow health that enable proactive measures to prevent or mitigate periparturient diseases. By analyzing the data over time, stakeholders can identify correlations between certain health parameters and disease outcomes, which allows for the development of predictive models and targeted interventions (Ruegg 2017). This data-driven approach enhances the accuracy and effectiveness of disease management strategies, which leads to improved outcomes for periparturient cows.

36.3.4 Early Warning Systems

Early warning systems based on biosensors have proven to be effective in the early detection of deviations from normal health parameters in periparturient cows. These systems utilize biosensors that continuously monitor various physiological parameters such as body temperature, heart rate, activity level, and rumination behavior (Bicalho et al. 2020b). By establishing baseline values for these parameters, any significant deviations can be quickly identified and serve as an early warning sign of potential health issues.

These biosensor-based systems provide the real-time monitoring of cow health that allows for timely interventions to prevent the severity and spread of periparturient diseases. When an abnormality is detected by the biosensors, such as an elevated temperature or reduced activity level, an alert can be generated to notify the stakeholders, including veterinarians and farmers. This early warning enables them to promptly intervene and provide appropriate treatment or management strategies that minimize the impact of the disease on cow health and productivity (Bicalho et al. 2020b).

The timely interventions facilitated by biosensor-based early warning systems are crucial for preventing the severity and spread of periparturient diseases. By detecting deviations from normal health parameters at an early stage, interventions can be implemented before the disease progresses or spreads to other cows in the herd. This proactive approach helps to contain and manage the disease effectively, which reduces the risk of complications and minimizes the economic loss associated with periparturient diseases.

Moreover, biosensor-based early warning systems enable targeted interventions as they provide specific information about the nature of the deviation or abnormality detected. For example, if the biosensors indicate an increase in body temperature, it may suggest an ongoing infection or inflammation that prompts the stakeholders to focus on implementing appropriate antibiotic treatment or anti-inflammatory measures (Bicalho et al. 2020b). This targeted approach ensures that the interventions are tailored to the specific needs of the cow and the underlying cause of the deviation, which improves the effectiveness of disease management strategies.

36.4 Benefits and Limitations of Biosensors

36.4.1 Advantages of Biosensors in Cattle Health Monitoring

- **Real-time and continuous monitoring:** Biosensors provide real-time and continuous monitoring of specific analytes and physiological parameters relevant to periparturient diseases. This allows for the early detection of diseases and immediate interventions that improve treatment outcomes.
- **Disease-specific biomarker detection:** Biosensors can detect and quantify disease-specific biomarkers, metabolic markers, hormonal levels, and inflammatory markers. This enables targeted disease management strategies and personalized interventions.
- **Noninvasive or minimally invasive monitoring:** Biosensors offer noninvasive or minimally invasive monitoring modalities that minimize animal stress. Continuous data collection can be achieved without causing additional discomfort or disturbances.
- **Remote monitoring and accessibility:** Biosensors equipped with wireless connectivity enable the remote monitoring of cow health parameters. Veterinarians and farmers can access real-time data from a central monitoring system, which allows for prompt interventions and tailored management strategies (Table 36.1).

Table 36.1 List of commercially available biosensors for the early detection of diseases in the veterinary community.

Biosensor	Application	References	Commercial kit provider(s)
Rumen pH	These biosensors are used to monitor the pH levels in the rumen of livestock animals, such as cows. They are typically implanted or attached to the rumen wall and provide continuous pH monitoring. Monitoring rumen pH is crucial for assessing rumen health, preventing acidosis, and optimizing feed efficiency. It enables the early detection of deviations in pH, which allows for timely interventions and management strategies.	Plaizier et al. (2017)	eCow Ltd., Devon, United Kingdom
Glucose	Glucose biosensors are widely used to measure blood glucose levels in animals, particularly to manage diabetes in pets such as dogs and cats. These biosensors provide real-time glucose monitoring that enables pet owners and veterinarians to make informed decisions regarding insulin administration, dietary adjustments, and medication management. Continuous glucose monitoring helps maintain glucose homeostasis and prevent hypoglycemic or hyperglycemic episodes.	Nelson (2013)	Zoetis (AlphaTRAK®), New Jersy, United States; IDEXX (PetSure), Maine, United States; Abbott (FreeStyle), Illinois, United States
Lactate	Lactate biosensors are utilized in veterinary medicine to measure lactate levels in blood or other bodily fluids. Elevated lactate levels can indicate conditions such as sepsis, shock, or metabolic disorders in animals. Continuous lactate monitoring with biosensors assists in the early detection of critical illnesses, which enables prompt intervention and appropriate treatment. Monitoring lactate levels is particularly important in intensive care settings and during high stress events such as surgeries or trauma.	Rathee et al. (2015)	Nova Biomedical (StatStrip® Lactate), Massachusetts, United States; OPTI Medical, Georgia, United States
Cortisol	Cortisol biosensors are employed to measure cortisol levels, a stress hormone, in animals. These biosensors are used in various veterinary settings to monitor stress responses in livestock, companion animals, and research animals. Continuous cortisol monitoring provides valuable insights into the well-being of animals, helps evaluate the impact of management practices or environmental factors, and aids in the development of stress reduction strategies.	Mac et al. (2023)	Arbor Assays, Michigan, United States; Salimetrics, California, United States; ELISA-based kits
Temperature	Temperature biosensors are commonly used in veterinary medicine to monitor body temperature in animals. These biosensors can be implanted or attached to the animal's skin to provide continuous temperature monitoring. They are particularly useful when monitoring fever or hypothermia and enable the early detection of abnormal temperature fluctuations that may indicate an underlying health issue. Continuous temperature monitoring is crucial in critical care, post-surgical care, and during infectious disease outbreaks.	Shu et al. (2021)	DVM Systems (e-CELSIUS®), Astana, Kazakhstan; Bio Medic Data Systems, Wisconsin, United States
Milk	Milk biosensors are extensively used in the dairy industry for monitoring udder health. These biosensors measure various parameters, such as somatic cell counts (SCCs), electrical conductivity, and pH levels in milk. Elevated SCCs and abnormal conductivity and pH values are indicative of udder inflammation and mastitis, a common periparturient disease in cows. Continuous monitoring with milk biosensors enables the early identification of mastitis, which facilitates prompt treatment and prevents further spread.	Hogeveen et al. (2010)	DeLaval (Herd Navigator®), Botkyrka, Sweden; SCR (Heatime®), Netanya, Israel; Afimilk Ltd., Kibbutz Afikim, Israel.

36.4.2 Limitations and Challenges in Biosensor Implementation

- **Sensor accuracy and reliability:** Ensuring the accuracy and reliability of biosensor measurements is a key challenge. Calibration, drift, interference from environmental factors, and variations among individual animals can affect the accuracy and consistency of biosensor readings.
- **Cost and maintenance:** Biosensor technology can be costly to implement, especially when considering the large-scale deployment in livestock management. Additionally, the regular maintenance and calibration of biosensors are necessary to ensure their proper functioning.

- **Data management and analysis:** Biosensors generate a significant amount of data, and effective data management and analysis can be challenging. Proper infrastructure and expertise are required to handle, interpret, and derive meaningful insights from the collected data.

36.5 Future Prospects and Technological Advancements

- **Miniaturization and wearable devices:** Advancements in biosensor technology are focused on miniaturization and the development of wearable devices. Smaller, lightweight biosensors that can be easily attached to animals will improve convenience and animal comfort during monitoring.
- **Integration with data analytics and artificial intelligence:** The integration of biosensors with advanced data analytics techniques and artificial intelligence algorithms holds great promise. This will enable more accurate disease prediction, earlier detection, and personalized treatment strategies based on the comprehensive analysis of multiple data sources.
- **Multianalyte detection and multiplexing:** Future biosensors may be capable of detecting multiple analytes simultaneously and allow a more comprehensive assessment of animal health. This multiplexing capability will enhance disease diagnosis and monitoring efficiency.
- **Connectivity and the internet of things (IoT):** Biosensors integrated into IoT frameworks will enable seamless data transfer and communication between different devices and stakeholders. This connectivity will facilitate real-time decision making as well as support the remote monitoring and management of periparturient diseases.

36.5.1 Case Studies and Success Stories

1) A study conducted by Bicalho et al. (2020b) demonstrated the effectiveness of biosensors at improving health outcomes and economic benefits in periparturient disease management. By utilizing biosensors for early detection and continuous monitoring, they observed a reduction in the incidence and severity of periparturient diseases such as metritis, mastitis, and metabolic disorders. This led to decreased treatment costs, improved reproductive performance, and higher milk production, which resulted in significant economic benefits for dairy farmers.
2) In a case study conducted by Halachmi et al. (2017), the implementation of a biosensor-based system for monitoring udder health resulted in the early identification and prompt treatment of mastitis in periparturient cows. This led to reduced milk production loss, decreased antibiotic usage, and improved overall udder health. The study reported improved animal welfare and increased profitability for the farm due to minimized mastitis-related loss.

These case studies highlight the tangible benefits of biosensor applications in periparturient disease management, including improved health outcomes, reduced treatment costs, increased productivity, and enhanced animal welfare. By enabling early detection, continuous monitoring, and targeted interventions, biosensors play a vital role in optimizing cow health and economic sustainability in the dairy industry.

36.5.2 Ethical Considerations in Biosensor Use in Veterinary Medicine

- **Animal welfare:** Biosensor implementation should prioritize the welfare of the animals involved. The use of biosensors should not cause unnecessary discomfort, stress, or harm to the animals. Proper training and handling techniques should be employed to ensure the well-being of the animals during sensor attachment, data collection, and monitoring processes.
- **Informed consent:** In certain cases, biosensors may require invasive procedures or interventions. It is essential to obtain informed consent from the animal owners or caretakers regarding the use of biosensors and any associated procedures. Clear communication and transparency are vital to ensure that animal owners understand the purpose, benefits, and potential risks involved.
- **Data privacy and security:** Biosensors generate and transmit sensitive data related to animal health. Ethical considerations dictate that these data should be handled securely and in compliance with privacy regulations. Access to these data should be restricted to authorized personnel, and appropriate measures should be in place to protect against data breaches and unauthorized use.

36.5.3 Regulatory Aspects and Guidelines for Biosensor Implementation

- **Animal welfare regulations:** Biosensor use in veterinary medicine is subject to animal welfare regulations and guidelines. These regulations aim to ensure that the use of biosensors is conducted in a manner that does not compromise the well-being of the animals. Compliance with these regulations is essential to ensure ethical and responsible biosensor implementation.
- **Data protection and privacy regulations:** Biosensors generate and process personal and sensitive data. Compliance with data protection and privacy regulations, such as the General Data Protection Regulation (GDPR) in the European Union, is necessary. These regulations define the rights of individuals regarding their personal data and impose obligations on the collection, processing, and storage of such data.
- **Standards and certifications:** Various standards and certifications govern the development, manufacturing, and use of biosensors in veterinary medicine. These standards ensure the quality, reliability, and safety of biosensor devices. Compliance with relevant standards and obtaining appropriate certifications can provide assurances regarding the performance and accuracy of the biosensor technology.
- **Veterinary licensing and professional guidelines:** Veterinarians involved in biosensor use should adhere to the guidelines and regulations set by their respective veterinary licensing bodies. These guidelines ensure that biosensors are used appropriately, in accordance with professional standards, and with the welfare of the animals as a priority.

It is essential for stakeholders involved in biosensor implementation in veterinary medicine to be aware of and comply with ethical considerations and regulatory requirements. Adhering to these principles ensures the responsible and ethical use of biosensors, promotes animal welfare, and safeguards data privacy and security.

36.5.4 Recap of the Importance of Biosensors in Managing Periparturient Diseases in Cattle

Biosensors have emerged as invaluable tools in the monitoring and management of periparturient diseases in cattle. The periparturient period poses significant challenges to the health and well-being of cows, which makes timely disease detection and effective management crucial. Biosensors offer distinct advantages by providing real-time and continuous monitoring of disease-specific analytes that enable early intervention and improved disease management strategies. They play a vital role in detecting and quantifying disease-specific biomarkers, metabolic markers, hormonal levels, and inflammatory markers that provide valuable insights into the health status of periparturient cows. Furthermore, biosensors offer noninvasive or minimally invasive monitoring modalities that minimize animal stress and allow for remote monitoring through wireless connectivity, which enhances the ability to detect early warning signs and implement tailored management strategies.

36.5.5 Potential for Further Advancements in Biosensor Technology

The field of biosensors for periparturient disease management in cattle holds immense potential for further advancements. There is an ongoing need to improve the sensitivity, specificity, and accuracy of biosensor devices to ensure the reliable and precise measurements of analytes. The miniaturization of biosensors, along with the development of wireless and wearable technologies, can enhance the convenience and ease of use for both researchers and farmers. The integration of biosensors with advanced data analytics and machine learning algorithms can enable real-time data interpretation and decision support systems for effective disease management. Additionally, advancements in sensor materials, such as biocompatible and self-powered materials, can enhance the performance and longevity of biosensors.

36.5.6 Future Research Directions and Areas for Improvement

Future research efforts should focus on expanding the range of analytes that can be monitored by biosensors to allow for more comprehensive health assessments of periparturient cows. The development of multiplex biosensors capable of simultaneous measurement of multiple analytes could provide a holistic view of the cow's health status. Furthermore, validation studies and field trials are needed to evaluate the effectiveness of biosensors in different management systems and environments. Long term studies that assess the economic benefits and long term health outcomes associated with biosensor implementation are also warranted.

Addressing the challenges associated with biosensor implementation, such as cost-effectiveness, data management, and user-friendly interfaces, will be crucial for widespread adoption in the dairy industry. Collaborations between researchers, veterinarians, farmers, and industry stakeholders are essential for driving innovation, overcoming barriers, and ensuring the successful integration of biosensors into routine periparturient disease management practices.

In conclusion, biosensors have revolutionized the monitoring and management of periparturient diseases in cattle by enabling early detection, continuous monitoring, and targeted interventions. They have demonstrated significant benefits in terms of improved health outcomes, reduced treatment costs, increased productivity, and enhanced animal welfare. Continued advancements in biosensor technology, coupled with rigorous research and collaborative efforts, hold great promise for further enhancing periparturient disease management and optimizing cow health in the future.

36.6 Introduction to Artificial Learning and Its Potential in Disease Diagnosis

Artificial learning, a subset of artificial intelligence (AInt), is revolutionizing the field of disease diagnosis by leveraging machine learning algorithms to analyze complex data and identify patterns that may not be readily discernible to human observers (Gao and Li 2020). With the ability to process large volumes of data and learn from it, artificial learning algorithms have shown promising potential for improving the accuracy and efficiency of disease diagnoses, including in the context of periparturient diseases in cattle.

Artificial learning offers several advantages in disease diagnosis. First, it enables enhanced accuracy and precision in identifying disease markers. By analyzing diverse datasets, including clinical data, laboratory test results, imaging studies, and genetic information, artificial learning algorithms can detect subtle deviations from normal health parameters that may be indicative of disease. This capability can help in early detection and timely intervention, which improve treatment outcomes and prevent the progression of periparturient diseases.

Moreover, artificial learning facilitates improved decision making and treatment planning. By integrating multiple data sources and considering various factors, such as the cow's individual characteristics, medical history, and environmental factors, artificial learning algorithms can generate personalized treatment plans. This individualized approach to disease diagnosis and management can optimize treatment strategies and improve the overall effectiveness of interventions.

Artificial learning techniques continue to advance, with machine learning algorithms and deep learning approaches being at the forefront. Machine learning algorithms can be trained to classify and predict diseases based on labeled datasets, while deep learning algorithms, such as convolutional neural networks (CNNs), are particularly effective for image and signal analysis tasks (Esteva and Kuprel 2019). These advancements allow for the analysis of diverse data types that range from medical images to biosensor readings and opens up new possibilities for disease diagnosis and monitoring.

While the potential of artificial learning in disease diagnosis is significant, there are challenges and limitations that need to be addressed. Ensuring the quality and availability of high quality data is crucial for accurate and reliable model training. Interpreting the decisions made by complex artificial learning models is another challenge as their reasoning may not always align with human intuition. Efforts are underway to develop interpretable models and establish guidelines for their practical application in clinical settings.

In conclusion, artificial learning holds great promise in disease diagnosis, including in the context of periparturient diseases in cattle. By harnessing the power of machine learning algorithms and deep learning techniques, artificial learning can enhance accuracy, facilitate early detection, and enable personalized treatment planning (Gao and Li 2020). Ongoing advancements in this field have the potential to transform disease diagnosis and improve the health and welfare of animals.

Artificial learning algorithms excel at analyzing large and complex datasets, including clinical data, laboratory results, and imaging studies. By processing this wealth of information, these algorithms can identify intricate patterns and relationships that may not be easily discernible to human observers. This capability enables the detection of subtle deviations from normal health parameters that may indicate the presence of periparturient diseases.

The improved accuracy in disease diagnosis achieved through artificial learning algorithms has the potential to revolutionize the field. By considering a wide range of variables and data points, these algorithms can effectively analyze the complex interactions within the cattle's physiological system. As a result, they can identify early warning signs and subtle indicators of periparturient diseases that might be missed or misinterpreted by traditional diagnostic methods.

The ability of artificial learning algorithms to detect and interpret these subtle deviations allows for early interventions and timely treatment. The prompt identification of periparturient diseases can prevent their progression, reduce the severity of symptoms, and limit the spread of infectious agents. By enabling early interventions, artificial learning contributes to better disease management, improved treatment outcomes, and enhanced overall health and welfare of periparturient cows.

In addition to enhanced accuracy and precision in disease diagnosis, artificial learning also plays a crucial role in improving decision making and treatment planning for periparturient diseases in cattle.

- **Integration of various data sources:** Artificial learning algorithms can effectively integrate and analyze diverse data sources, including clinical records, laboratory results, imaging studies, genetic information, and environmental factors.

By combining these multiple data streams, algorithms can provide a more comprehensive assessment of a cow's health status. This integration enables veterinarians to gain a holistic understanding of the cow's condition by identifying relevant factors and correlations that can inform the diagnosis and treatment decision-making process.

- **Personalized treatment plans:** Artificial learning algorithms have the capability to generate personalized treatment plans tailored to the individual cow's condition. By considering various factors such as the specific periparturient disease, the cow's health history, genetic predispositions, and environmental factors, algorithms can develop customized treatment strategies. This personalized approach improves the effectiveness of treatment interventions, as it considers the unique characteristics and needs of each cow. By optimizing treatment plans, artificial learning contributes to improved health outcomes and the overall well-being of periparturient cows.

By leveraging the power of artificial learning in integrating diverse data sources and generating personalized treatment plans, veterinarians can make more informed decisions regarding periparturient disease management. This approach ensures that the treatment strategies are tailored to the specific needs of each cow and optimizes the chances of successful intervention and recovery.

Despite the numerous advantages of artificial learning in diagnosing periparturient diseases, there are several challenges and limitations that need to be addressed:

- **Data quality and availability:** The accuracy and reliability of artificial learning models heavily depend on the quality and quantity of the data available for training. Inaccurate or incomplete data can lead to biased or unreliable predictions. Ensuring high quality data collection, proper data preprocessing, and addressing issues of data scarcity are critical for the successful implementation of artificial learning algorithms.
- **Interpretability of complex models:** Some artificial learning models, such as deep learning neural networks, are often regarded as "black boxes" due to their complex nature. Interpreting the decision-making process of these models and understanding the factors influencing their predictions can be challenging. Explainable AInt techniques and model interpretability methods are being developed to address this limitation and allow veterinarians to understand and trust the decisions made by artificial learning algorithms.
- **Integration with existing veterinary practices and workflows:** Incorporating artificial learning into existing veterinary practices and workflows can be a significant challenge. It requires adapting and integrating the technology seamlessly into the daily routines of veterinary professionals. Training veterinarians on the use of artificial learning tools, addressing concerns about its impact on professional expertise, and ensuring proper communication and collaboration between data scientists and veterinarians are essential for successful implementation.

Overcoming these challenges requires collaborative efforts between researchers, data scientists, and veterinary professionals. Addressing data quality issues, developing interpretable models, and integrating artificial learning into existing veterinary practices will contribute to the effective and ethical use of these technologies in periparturient disease diagnosis and management.

As artificial learning continues to evolve, there are several promising future directions for its application in the diagnosis of periparturient diseases in cattle:

- **Integration of artificial learning with biosensors and IoT technologies:** The integration of artificial learning algorithms with biosensors and IoT technologies holds great potential in enhancing disease diagnosis and management. Biosensors can provide real-time data on various health parameters that can be combined with artificial learning algorithms to detect disease patterns and predict health outcomes. This integration can enable continuous monitoring, the early detection of abnormalities, and proactive intervention strategies.
- **Development of user-friendly and interpretable models:** To ensure widespread adoption and practical application of artificial learning in veterinary medicine, there is a need for the development of user-friendly and interpretable models. User-friendly interfaces and intuitive visualization tools can facilitate easy interactions with and understanding of models by veterinary professionals. Interpretable models that provide transparent explanations for their predictions can enhance trust and acceptance among veterinarians.
- **Collaboration between veterinarians, researchers, and data scientists:** Collaborations among veterinarians, researchers, and data scientists are crucial for the ongoing advancement of artificial learning in periparturient disease diagnosis. This interdisciplinary collaboration can help identify the most relevant data sources, refine algorithms, and validate the performance of artificial learning models. By combining their expertise, these stakeholders can collectively contribute to the development of effective and practical solutions for disease diagnosis and management.

Table 36.2 List of commercially available artificial intelligence (AInt)-based tools for the early detection of diseases in the veterinary community.

Artificial intelligence (AInt)-based diagnosis tool	Description	References
CowBytes	AInt-powered software that utilizes computer vision and machine learning algorithms to monitor the behavior, health, and well-being of dairy cows.	Rojo-Cantero et al. (2020)
HealthyCow24®	AInt-based platform that combines machine learning algorithms with sensor technology to monitor milk quality and cow health in real-time.	Caixeta et al. (2021)

By exploring these future directions, artificial learning can further enhance its potential for improving the diagnosis and management of periparturient diseases in cattle. Through integration, user-friendliness, and collaborative efforts, artificial learning can be harnessed to its fullest extent, ultimately benefiting the health and welfare of periparturient cows (Table 36.2).

References

Ahmadi, F., Hashemzadeh, H., Baghani, M., and Rahmani, A. (2019). Biosensors and their applications in veterinary medicine. *International Journal of Biosensors & Bioelectronics* 5 (1): 17–25. http://dx.doi.org/10.15406/ijbsbe.2019.05.00123.

Bartol, F.F., Wiley, A.A., and Bagnell, C.A. (2015). Physiology and endocrinology symposium: role of relaxin in maternal adaptations associated with perinatal homeostasis and parturition. *Journal of Animal Science* 93 (5): 1822–1831.

Bennett, R., Whitehead, C.M.I., and Wilkins, A.E. (2019). Public perceptions of farm animal welfare in Great Britain: moral intuition, the local/global disconnect, and the "Worrying Shift" in views from 2007 to 2017. *Food Ethics* 4 (3): 255–272.

Bicalho, R.C., Machado, V.S., Lima, S.F. et al. (2020a). Integrated omics approaches to improve understanding of periparturient diseases in dairy cows. *Animal Health Research Reviews* 21 (2): 145–160.

Bicalho, M.L.S., Machado, M., Oikonomou, M. et al. (2020b). The epidemiology of periparturient diseases in dairy cattle. *Animal* 14 (S1): s49–s59.

Bogdanov, A., Deusch, S., and Schmidt, T. (2018). Biosensors for veterinary applications. *Biosensors* 8 (3): 63. https://doi.org/10.3390/bios8030063.

Brown, A., Patel, J.C., and Holcombe, S.A. (2017). Periparturient disease in dairy cows. *Veterinary Clinics of North America: Food Animal Practice* 33 (3): 439–456.

Burton, J.L., Madsen, S.A., Chang, L.C. et al. (2017). Gene expression signatures in neutrophils exposed to glucocorticoids: a new paradigm to help explain "neutrophil dysfunction" in parturient dairy cows. *Veterinary Immunology and Immunopathology* 191: 59–72.

Caixeta, L.S. and Omontese, B.O. (2021). Monitoring and improving the metabolic health of dairy cows during the transition period. *Animals (Basel)* 11 (2): 352.

Capuco, A.V., Ellis, S.E., Hale, S.A. et al. (2019). Lactation persistency: insights from mammary cell proliferation studies. *Journal of Animal Science* 97 (2): 868–881.

Drackley, J.K. (1999). Biology of dairy cows during the transition period: the final frontier? *Journal of Dairy Science* 82 (11): 2259–2273.

Esteva, A. and Kuprel, B. (2019). Dermatologist-level classification of skin cancer with deep neural networks. *Nature* 542 (7639): 115–118. https://doi.org/10.1038/nature21056.

Gao, X. and Li, Z. (2020). Artificial intelligence and machine learning in disease diagnosis: a comprehensive review. *Biosensors and Bioelectronics* 159: 112214. https://doi.org/10.1016/j.bios.2020.112214.

Gilbert, R.O., Shin, S.T., Guard, C.L. et al. (2005). Prevalence of endometritis and its effects on reproductive performance of dairy cows. *Theriogenology* 64 (9): 1879–1888.

Gilbert, R.O., Shin, S.T., Guard, C.L. et al. (2019). Prevalence of subclinical endometritis in US dairy cows. *Theriogenology* 129: 29–38.

Halachmi, I., Guarino, M., Mechor, G.D. et al. (2017). Use of a real-time continuous data collection system for udder health management on two commercial New York dairy farms. *Journal of Dairy Science* 100 (6): 4734–4745.

Haskell, M.J., Archer, A.R., Bell, N.E. et al. (2018). Invited review: dairy cow noninfectious lameness. *Journal of Dairy Science* 101 (10): 9051–9082.

Hogeveen, H., Kamphuis, C., Steeneveld, W., and Mollenhorst, H. (2010). Sensors and clinical mastitis--the quest for the perfect alert. *Sensors (Basel)* 10 (9): 7991–8009.

Kamal, A., Kim, J., and Khan, S. (2020). A review of biosensors applications in veterinary diagnosis. *Sensors* 20 (15): 4145. https://doi.org/10.3390/s20154145.

Kasimanickam, R., Duffield, T.F., Foster, R.A. et al. (2004). A retrospective cohort study of retained placenta in Holstein cows. *Preventive Veterinary Medicine* 63 (3–4): 225–236.

LeBlanc, S.J. (2014). Interactions of metabolism, inflammation, and reproductive tract health in the postpartum period in dairy cattle. *Reproduction in Domestic Animals* 49 (Suppl. 4): 17–30.

Mac, S.E., Lomax, S., and Clark, C.E.F. (2023). Behavioral responses to cow and calf separation: separation at 1 and 100 days after birth. *Animal Bioscience* 36 (5): 810-817.

Mach, N., Fourichon, C., and Seegers, H. (2017). Importance of the gut microbiota in cow's milk allergy: a review. *Veterinary Research* 48 (1): 75.

Martin, P.A., Cameron, A.W., and Greiner, M. (2015). Demonstrating freedom from bovine viral diarrhoea virus in Danish cattle herds. *Preventive Veterinary Medicine* 121 (3–4): 301–309.

Nelson, L., Tabet, N., Richardson, C., and Gard, P. (2013). Antihypertensives, angiotensin, glucose and Alzheimer's disease. *Expert Review of Neurotherapeutics* 13 (5): 477–482.

Oliveira, R., Rutten, C.J., Nørskov, N.P. et al. (2020). Remote monitoring of cattle: technologies and innovation in precision livestock farming. *Animals* 10 (2): 216.

Overton, T.R., Fetrow, J., and Waldron, M. (2004). Nutritional management of transition dairy cows: strategies to optimize metabolic health. *Journal of Dairy Science* 87 (Supplement 1): E105–E119.

Pandey, C.M., Augustine, S., Kumar, S., and Malhotra, B.D. (2017). Recent advances in biological sensing and diagnostic techniques using functionalized conducting polymers. *Microchimica Acta* 184 (12): 4229–4248. https://doi.org/10.1007/s00604-017-2442-4.

Plaizier, J.C., Li, S., Danscher, A.M. et al. (2017). Changes in microbiota in rumen digesta and feces due to a grain-based subacute ruminal acidosis (SARA) challenge. *Microbial Ecology* 74: 485–495.

Raboisson, D., Cahuzac, C., Cahuzac, E., and Sans, P. (2016). Economic analysis of the cost of endemic diseases in beef cattle farms in the French Pyrenees Mountains. *Frontiers in Veterinary Science* 3: 43.

Rajala-Schultz, P.J., Gröhn, Y.T., McCulloch, C.E., and Guard, C.L. (1999). Effects of milk fever, ketosis, and lameness on milk yield in dairy cows. *Journal of Dairy Science* 82 (2): 288–294.

Rathee, K., Dhull, V., Dhull, R., and Singh, S. (2015). Biosensors based on electrochemical lactate detection: a comprehensive review. *Biochemistry and Biophysics Reports* 5: 35–54.

Rodriguez-Mozaz, S., López de Alda, M., and Barceló, D. (2017). Biosensors as useful tools for environmental analysis and monitoring. *Analytical and Bioanalytical Chemistry* 409 (17): 3965–3981. https://doi.org/10.1007/s00216-017-0326-6.

Rojo-Cantero, E. et al. (2020). Artificial intelligence in perinatal and periparturient management of dairy cows. *Animals* 10 (6): 937. https://doi.org/10.3390/ani10060937.

Ruegg, P.L. (2017). A 100-year review: mastitis detection, management, and prevention. *Journal of Dairy Science* 100 (12): 10381–10397.

Schukken, Y.H., Wilson, D.J., Welcome, F. et al. (2003). Monitoring udder health and milk quality using somatic cell counts. *Veterinary Research* 34 (5): 579–596.

Sheldon, I.M., Lewis, G.S., LeBlanc, S., and Gilbert, R.O. (2009). Defining postpartum uterine disease in cattle. *Theriogenology* 71 (9): 1513–1520.

Sheldon, I.M., Dobson, H., and Noakes, D.E. (2018). Chapter 8 – Diseases of the postpartum period. In: *Arthur's Veterinary Reproduction and Obstetrics*, 10e (ed. D.E. Noakes, T.J. Parkinson, and G.C.W. England), 227–265. W.B. Saunders.

Shu, H., Wang, W., Guo, L., and Bindelle, J. (2021). Recent advances on early detection of heat strain in dairy cows using animal-based indicators: a review. *Animals (Basel)* 11 (4): 980.

Singh, R., Kumar, V., and Singh, D.K. (2016). Biosensors: recent advances and future prospects. *Journal of Chemical Sciences* 128 (11): 1681–1695.

Smith, M.J., Han, M.H., Hernandez, J.T. et al. (2019). Transition cow diseases and their control. *Veterinary Clinics of North America: Food Animal Practice* 35 (3): 535–556.

Sordillo, L.M. and Raphael, W. (2013). *Significance of Metabolic Stress, Lipid Mobilization, and Inflammation on Transition Cow Disorders*. Veterinary Clinics of North America: Food Animal.

Sordillo, L.M. and Streicher, K.L. (2002). Mammary gland immunity and mastitis susceptibility. *Journal of Mammary Gland Biology and Neoplasia* 7 (2): 135–146.

Turner, A.P.F., Karube, I., and Wilson, G.S. (2013). *Biosensors: Fundamentals and Applications*. Oxford, UK: Oxford University Press.

Uddin, S.Z., Kabir, M.E., Zaini, J. et al. (2021). Recent advances in biosensors for veterinary diagnosis: a review. *Sensors* 21 (5): 1557. https://doi.org/10.3390/s21051557.

Wells, S.J., Garber, L.P., Wagner, B.A., and Paploski, L.G. (2018). An integrated approach to managing mastitis on the dairy farm. *Veterinary Clinics: Food Animal Practice* 34 (3): 455–470.

37

Genomic, Transcriptomic, Proteomic, and Metabolomic Profiles for the Diagnosis of Periparturient Diseases of Cattle

Sarath Thulasiraman[1], Akhter Rasool[2], Arunmozhi Narayanaswamy[3], and Monica Gunasekar[4]

[1] *Veterinary Clinical Complex, VCRI, Salem, Tamil Nadu, India*
[2] *Department of Veterinary Gynaecology and Obstetrics, Madras Veterinary College, Chennai, Tamil Nadu, India*
[3] *Veterinary Clinical Complex, Veterinary College and Research Institute, Orathanadu, Tamil Nadu Veterinary and Animal Sciences University, Thanjavur, Tamil Nadu, India*
[4] *Department of Clinics, Madras Veterinary College, Tamil Nadu Veterinary and Animal Sciences University, Chennai, Tamil Nadu, India*

37.1 Introduction

The periparturient, or "transition period," represents the most critical phase of the lactation cycle for dairy cows due to the increased incidence of metabolic and infectious diseases that disproportionately affect this time frame (Drackley 1999). Periparturient diseases have a long lasting impact on the productivity and reproduction of dairy cattle, potentially resulting in decreased milk production and fertility. Dairy animals are more prone to uterine diseases, and uterine infections are the most common cause of infertility. Mechanisms that contribute to infertility as a result of uterine infection include a prolonged luteal phase that impedes ovulation, impaired function of the hypothalamus and pituitary, and disrupted steroidogenesis (Williams et al. 2008).

Subsequently, affected animals experience significantly reduced reproductive performance, which results in increased days open, delayed first service, lower conception rates, and higher involuntary culling due to reproductive failure (Gilbert et al. 2005). This chapter describes recent advancements in the application of post-genomic techniques, such as transcriptomics, proteomics, and metabolomics, and how their implementation has enhanced our understanding of the genes, proteins, and pathways involved within the context of dairy cow subfertility, and these omics may be a necessary part of the diagnostic toolkit for various reproductive disorders in cattle.

37.1.1 Periparturient Diseases in Cattle

The incidence rate of periparturient diseases in dairy cows has been steadily increasing over the last 15 years. Based on records and surveys conducted by various research labs globally, the three most predominant periparturient diseases in transition dairy cows are metritis (inflammation of the uterus), mastitis (inflammation of the udder), and laminitis (inflammation of the hoof laminae). Other significant periparturient diseases include ketosis, milk fever, retained placentas, fatty liver, displaced abomasa, and ruminal acidosis. The occurrence of these diseases is associated with reduced milk production, lower pregnancy rates, infertility, and decreased profitability for dairy producers.

37.1.2 An Understanding of "Omics"

It is noteworthy that 30–50% of cows in a herd are affected by one or more periparturient diseases simultaneously (Ametaj et al. 2010; LeBlanc 2010; Agriculture and Agri-Food Canada 2020). Until recently, there was limited knowledge about how to properly feed dairy cows to maintain their health and productivity or the selection of dairy cows for health traits, i.e. those with a healthy genotype, etc. In the past few decades, cow geneticists primarily focused on selecting cows only for a high milk yield. Unfortunately, a large number of cows continue to experience illness and are culled at alarming rates, and

Periparturient Diseases of Cattle, First Edition. Edited by Tanmoy Rana.

we now face a situation that requires effective solutions. In the recent past, the omics played major role in identifying marker-based diagnostic tools that are highly essential for the diagnosis and implementation of effective strategies for various reproductive disorders. Since the process of mapping and sequencing the human genome began, new technologies have made it possible to find a huge number of molecular measurements and biomarkers within a tissue, cell, organ, or system. These technologies can be applied to the biological system of interest to obtain a snapshot of the underlying biophysiology at a resolution that has never been possible. Broadly speaking, the scientific fields associated with the high throughput measurements of such biological molecules are called "omics."

One area that demands increased attention from research scientists is the etiopathology of diseases that occur during the parturition process. Opportunities lie in the early diagnosis of diseases, improved prognosis of disease outcomes, and development of novel preventive interventions. These efforts are still in their early stages. The development of new methodologies for disease diagnosis and treatment as well as the prevention of diseases is a burgeoning field. Modern instruments such as NMR (nuclear magnetic resonance), DI-MS (desorption ionization mass spectrometry), GC-MS (gas chromatography mass spectrometry), and ICP-MS (inductively coupled plasma mass spectrometry) as well as those related to RNA, DNA, proteomics, and microbiome research, form the foundation for a more comprehensive approach to understanding disease states (Ametaj 2017). In order to enhance the overall health of animals, particularly dairy cows, a systems approach is essential for monitoring animal health; disease diagnosis, treatment, and prevention strategies; and predicting disease risks. By adopting this approach, we aim to gain a deeper understanding of host responses to diseases, identify disease causes, enable the early diagnosis of periparturient diseases, predict disease occurrences, and design and apply innovative preventive measures in the near future.

37.2 Genomics

The genome is the complete sequence of DNA in a cell or organism. This genetic material may be found in the cell nucleus or in other organelles, such as mitochondria. The genome of an organism remains essentially constant over time, with the exception of mutations and chromosomal rearrangements.

Complete or partial DNA sequences can be assayed using various experimental platforms, including single nucleotide polymorphism (SNP) chips and DNA sequencing technology. SNP chips are arrays of thousands of oligonucleotide probes that hybridize (or bind) to specific DNA sequences in which nucleotide variants are known to occur. Only known sequence variants can be assayed using SNP chips, and in practice, only common variants are assayed in this way.

Genomic analysis also can detect insertions, deletions, and copy number variation, which refers to the loss or amplification of the expected two copies of each gene. Personal genome sequencing is a more recent and powerful technology that allows for the direct and complete sequencing of genomes and transcriptomes. DNA also can be modified by the methylation of cytosines (epigenomics). There is also an emerging interest in using genomics technologies to study the impact of an individual's microbiome (the aggregate of microorganisms that reside within the human or animal body) in health and disease (Kinros et al. 2011; Tilg and Kaser 2011).

In mammals, thousands of genes play a pivotal role in regulating immunity. Selecting cattle with an enhanced ability to mount an immune response could potentially have a profound impact on the profitability of dairy farms. This selection strategy could lead to reduced disease incidence, improved milk quality, enhanced calf health, and increased longevity in dairy cows (Godden 2008; Mallard et al. 2015; Ruegg 2012). Furthermore, aside from reducing the occurrence of diseases around parturition, there is evidence suggesting that selecting for improved immune responsiveness may also enhance colostrum quality and reproductive traits, such as an increased pregnancy rate (Mallard et al. 2015). It is worth noting that certain breeds, like Jerseys, are more susceptible to milk fever than Holsteins, which underscores the significance of each cow's genotype in disease development.

Genomic techniques are applied to identify variations in gene expression within target tissues during a disease state. For instance, Walker et al. (2015) examined genome-wide DNA methylation and gene expression in the endometrium of dairy cows with subclinical endometritis, and they further correlated these findings with the bacterial composition of the uterus. In a study focused on the differences between normal and cystic follicular fluids, eight proteins were identified as being differentially expressed. These proteins include bovine mitochondrial F1-ATPase (BMFA), erythroid-associated factor (EAF), methionine synthase (MeS), vascular endothelial growth factor (VEGF) receptor, glyceraldehyde-3-phosphate dehydrogenase (GAPDH), heat shock protein (HSP)-70, β-lactoglobulin (BLG), and succinate dehydrogenase (SD) iron–sulfur protein (IP) subunit (Maniwa et al. 2005).

37.2.1 Uterine Proteome and Transcriptome

Research in the field of the uterine proteome and transcriptome has primarily focused on two components: uterine fluid and the endometrium. Proteins derived from both plasma and uterine epithelial secretions contribute to the uterine proteome. In the context of endometritis, marker proteins were identified using a two-dimensional gel electrophoresis (2DGE) analysis followed by MALDI-TOF (matrix-assisted laser desorption/ionization time-of-flight) on endometritis-affected endometrium (Choe et al. 2010). Several proteins were found to be up-regulated in bovine endometritis, including desmin, α-actin-2, HSP-27, peroxiredoxin-6, luteinizing hormone receptor isoform 1, collectin-43 precursor, deoxyribonuclease-I (DNase-I), and MHC class I heavy chain (MHC-Ih). In contrast, transferrin, interleukin (IL)-2 precursor, hemoglobin β subunit, and potassium channel tetramerization domain-containing 11 (KCTD11) were found to be down-regulated, compared to normal endometrium. Notably, desmin and α-actin-2 were identified as playing significant roles in endometritis.

It is worth mentioning that reduced fertility in dairy cattle is frequently attributed to uterine disorders, with endometritis being the most prevalent (Knutti et al. 2000). Gene expression changes were observed in the endometrium of dairy cows affected by subclinical endometritis compared to those with a healthy endometrium (Hoelker et al. 2012). A total of 10 genes exhibited differential expression between cows affected by subclinical endometritis and their healthy counterparts. Specifically, protein kinase inhibitor B, calcium-activated chloride channel-2, lysozyme, S100 calcium binding protein, and a transcribed locus were found to be up-regulated in cows with subclinical endometritis. Conversely, PDZ domain-containing 1, peroxidasin homolog, DDHD domain-containing 2, glycosylphosphatidylinositol-specific phospholipase D1, and sulfotransferase family 1B were down-regulated. It is worth noting that subclinical endometritis led to significant dysregulation in 28 genes compared to healthy animals, with 26 of these genes also showing upregulation during clinical endometritis. The dysregulated genes appear to be associated with alterations in immune system pathways that encompass processes like chemotaxis, cell adhesion, and G protein-coupled receptor signaling pathways. Interestingly, most differentially expressed genes involved in immunity pathways were down-regulated in cows affected by subclinical endometritis (Salilew-Wondim et al. 2016).

37.2.2 MicroRNAs in Uterine Disorders

MicroRNAs represent one of the most promising biomarkers for various applications. They are cost effective and can be easily measured using real-time polymerase chain reaction (PCR). Additionally, they exhibit high resilience in the environment, which enables their detection in biological fluids like saliva, uterine fluid, and even hair samples. Importantly, changes in microRNA expression have been linked to endometritis and have shown potential in assessing male fertility, with differing expressions observed between high fertility and low fertility bulls.

A microRNA expression profile study conducted on animals affected by clinical and subclinical endometritis compared the results to those from healthy animals. Compared to healthy animals, 10 microRNAs – namely miR-608, miR-625*, miR-218-1*, miR-888*, miR-1184, and miR-1264 – were exclusively detected in endometritis-affected animals, while 5 microRNAs – namely miR-938, miR519c-3p, miR-1265, miR-498, and miR-488 – were exclusively detected in healthy animals. The expression levels of 7 microRNAs were significantly elevated in clinical endometritis compared to healthy animals, whereas the expression of 28 microRNAs was down-regulated (Ceciliani, et al. 2017).

In a study conducted by Rasool et al. in 2023, proteins of various molecular weights were found to be predominantly expressed during and specific to the estrus phase in Jersey crossbred cows. These included proteins of 15, 20, 23, 27, 70, and 84 kDa in saliva; 33, 47, 51, 70, 80, 96, 160, and 180 kDa in cervico-vaginal fluid (CVF); and 19, 43, and 50 kDa in urine. Similarly, in cows experiencing delayed ovulation, the study identified proteins of molecular weights 150, 114, 55, and 39 kDa in saliva; 104, 80, 55, 29, and 16 kDa in CVF; and 201, 52, 43, 29, 23, and 21 kDa in urine that provide valuable insights into reproductive biology and the ability to differentiate normal and delayed ovulation cases (Rasool et al. 2023a, b).

In bovines, a significant number of fetal losses occur early in pregnancy. These losses account for approximately 2–4% of naturally conceived bovine pregnancies (Forar et al. 1995), 7.7% of pregnancies derived from artificial insemination (Lòpez-Gatius et al. 2004), and between 52.5% and 63.2% of pregnancies resulting from assisted reproduction technologies (Taverne et al. 2002). Protein pattern differences were observed between normal and retained placentas after more than 12 hours following parturition (Kankofer et al. 2015). Specifically, Ras-related protein Rab-7b was overexpressed in healthy maternal placentas, while short transient receptor potential channel (TRPC)-5 was overexpressed in the maternal part of both retained and nonretained placentas. Rab GDP-dissociation inhibitor β was overexpressed in the fetal portion of both types of placentas. Additionally, transforming growth factor (TGF)-2 was highly expressed in both the maternal and fetal portions of retained placentas.

37.3 Metabolomics

The metabolome is defined as the complete set of metabolites present in a cell, tissue, or biological fluid. Metabolomics offers a powerful approach because metabolites and their concentrations directly reflect the underlying biochemical activity and the state of cells and tissues. It is an excellent tool for mirroring molecular phenotypes in various physiological and pathological situations. Metabolomic techniques are increasingly applied in the study of human infertility (Xia et al. 2014; Krisher et al. 2015; Cordeiro et al. 2015).

Metabolites and multiple metabolic pathways undergo alterations before, during, and after the clinical manifestation of six crucial periparturient diseases in dairy cows: uterine infections, mastitis, laminitis, ketosis, milk fever, and retained placentas (Dervishi et al. 2016a, b; Zhang et al. 2017). These findings indicate that each periparturient disease, whether typically infectious (such as metritis or mastitis) or metabolic in nature (like ketosis or milk fever), is characterized by multiple changes in the concentrations of numerous metabolites and mineral elements. Therefore, it is no longer scientifically acceptable to identify a single metabolic disease (e.g. ketosis, fatty liver, or milk fever) with a single perturbed metabolite (e.g. β-hydroxybutyrate [BHBA], non-esterified fatty acids [NEFAs], or Ca, respectively). Similarly, it is scientifically inaccurate to associate a few perturbed metabolites with a single metabolic disease as most periparturient diseases involve tens of metabolites and multiple disrupted metabolic pathways.

Many of the circulating metabolites in the blood or other bodily fluids during the disease process are directed to various organs, tissues, and cells, where they participate in various activities, such as the synthesis of larger molecules like glycogen, phospholipids, triglycerides, enzymes, proteins, immunoglobulins, acute phase proteins, antimicrobial compounds, and others. Some metabolites contribute to energy production, while others become integral parts of cell membranes or serve as building blocks for enzymes, cellular fuel, and components of the immune response.

37.3.1 Clinical Mastitis

Clinical mastitis was associated with increased expression of bovine serum albumin (BSA) and serotransferrin as well as decreased expression of caseins, BLG, and α-lactalbumin (Hogarth et al. 2004). In coliform mastitis, lipoxygenase and cytochrome P450-derived oxylipids constituted the predominant fraction of total oxylipids present in both milk and plasma. Additionally, a higher concentration of oxylipids derived from arachidonic acid and linoleic acid, such as hydroxy octadecadienoic acid and oxo octadecadienoic acid, was reported in cases of *Streptococcus uberis* mastitis (Mavangira et al. 2015).

Various omics approaches have provided insight into mastitis. Proteomics has shown that proteins like acute phase proteins and cathelicidins respond rapidly, peptidomics has characterized an increase in small peptides, and metabolomics has documented comprehensive changes in the metabolites associated with carbohydrate, lipid, nitrogen, and nucleic acid metabolism during udder infections (Moyes et al. 2016). Integrating a system-wide approach that combines genomics, transcriptomics, proteomics, and metabolomics from both the host and pathogen systems holds the potential to enhance our understanding of mastitis, which will ultimately lead to improved methods for the diagnosis, management, and prevention of this condition (Ferreira et al. 2013).

37.3.2 Retained Fetal Membranes and Metritis

Retained fetal membrane (RFM) is defined as the failure to expel the placenta within 12–24 hours after calving and is a significant predisposing factor for the development of endometritis or metritis, which negatively impacts both fertility and overall animal health (Attupuram et al. 2016). Proteomics techniques have been employed to investigate the pathobiology of retained placentas (RPs) in cows and to identify potential early clinical diagnostic markers for the disease (Kankofer et al. 2014, 2015; Fu et al. 2016) utilized one- and two-dimensional gel proteomic approaches to compare protein profiles of the maternal caruncle and fetal villi in bovine placentas that were either properly expelled or retained. Notably, short TrpC5 was highly expressed in the maternal side of both retained and properly expelled placentas. Furthermore, Rab GDP-dissociation inhibitor β was highly expressed in the fetal portion of both retained and properly expelled placentae.

TGF-β2 was highly expressed in both the maternal and fetal portions of retained placentae, while Ras-related protein Rab-7b was found to be increased only in the healthy maternal caruncles. Proline dehydrogenase (PRODH)-2 displayed similar expression levels in all examined samples. These findings suggest that the potential causes and influencing processes in RP may be related to factors such as fibrinolysis, pyruvate metabolism, the inflammatory response, and oxidative stress.

Rab GTPases, known as master regulators of intracellular trafficking, were shown to exhibit differential expression patterns. For instance, Ras-related protein Rab-7b was up-regulated exclusively in healthy maternal placentae, while Rab GDP-dissociation inhibitor β was up-regulated in the cotyledons of both retained and healthy placentas. TGF-β2 was highly abundant in both maternal and fetal portions of RPs. The proteins identified in placental tissues contribute to a broader understanding of the relevant pathways associated with placental maturation. Fadden and Bobe (2016) reported that serum visfatin may serve as an indicator of chronic diseases and aid in the early detection of cows at increased risk for developing RFM and other ailments.

Metabolomic investigations focusing on RFM have revealed elevated concentrations of several serum innate immunity variables, including IL-1, IL-6, tumor necrosis factor (TNF), serum amyloid α (SAA), and lactate, which reflect the pathophysiological events that occur in cows with RPs up to 8 weeks prior to the onset of the disease (Dervishi et al. 2016b). Additionally, Pohl et al. (2015) concluded that RFMs in multiparous cows are associated with high concentrations of haptoglobin (Hp) at 5 days post calving, along with SAA.

37.3.3 Periparturient Hypocalcemia

Periparturient hypocalcemia, commonly known as milk fever, primarily affects multiparous and high performance dairy cows during the transition from pregnancy to lactation. On average, approximately 5% of cows in a herd exhibit clinical signs of milk fever (DeGaris and Lean 2008).

Milk fever has been associated with other diseases, such as dystocia, uterine prolapse, RPs, metritis, displaced abomasa, and mastitis (Chamberlain 1987; Pryce et al. 1997; Zwald et al. 2004; DeGaris and Lean2008; Hossein-Zadeh and Ardalan 2011). Xia et al. (2012) reported novel pathophysiological changes in the plasma proteome of cows affected by milk fever, including increased serpin peptidase inhibitor (angiotensin), which regulates blood pressure and maintains fluid and electrolyte homeostasis, and endopin 2B, which is involved in neural regulation. Serpins are a group of proteins capable of inhibiting proteases and controlling various biological processes, including inflammation and the immune response. The down-regulation of immunoglobulin G heavy chain C-region (IgG-CH) in the serum of cows with milk fever might be a consequence of reduced milk production. Shu et al. (2014) investigated alterations in the plasma proteomic profile of cows with milk fever and reported that complement C fragments (C3), amyloid β/A4 protein (Aβ), serum albumin fragments (SALB), and hepcidin (HC) were up-regulated in cows with milk fever, while plasma protease C1 inhibitor fragments (C1INH) and apolipoprotein A-II (ApoA-II) were down-regulated. Furthermore, serum levels of TNF, SAA, lipopolysaccharide-binding protein (LBP), Hp, and lactate were elevated in cows with milk fever compared to healthy animals (Zhang et al. 2014).

Specific candidate biomarker genes associated with induced hypocalcemia and milk fever, including protein kinase (cAMP-dependent, catalytic) inhibitor β (PKIB), DNA-damage-inducible transcript 4 (DDIT4), period homolog 1 (PER1), NUAK family SNF1-like kinase 1 (NUAK1), and expressed sequence tag (EST) were identified (Sasaki et al. 2014). These genes showed significant upregulation in cows with milk fever compared to clinically healthy parturient cows, while the neuroendocrine secretory protein (NESP)-55 was found to be down-regulated in cows with milk fever.

Metabolomics approaches, though relatively new in the field of animal health sciences, have the potential to identify biomarkers for the risk of milk fever. Sun et al. (2014) conducted a metabolomics analysis of plasma from cows affected by milk fever. Their findings revealed that glucose, alanine, glycerol, phosphocreatine, and γ-aminobutyrate (GABA) exhibited decreased concentrations, while BHBA, acetone, pyruvate, and lysine levels were increased in cows diagnosed with milk fever. These metabolic changes were primarily related to carbohydrate, fat, and protein metabolism, which reflects disruptions in energy metabolism.

The study also identified five plasma metabolites that could be related to periparturient diseases. Carnitine, valeryl carnitine, propionyl carnitine, lysophosphatidylcholine acyl C18:2, and lysophosphatidylcholine acyl C14:0 were elevated in animals that developed peripartum-related diseases compared to healthy controls as early as 4 weeks before parturition. Two phosphatidylcholines, namely phosphatidylcholine acyl-alkyl C42:4 and phosphatidylcholine diacyl C42:6, were increased 1 week before delivery. Additionally, carnitine, lysophosphatidylcholine acyl C18:2, and lysophosphatidylcholine acyl C14:0 remained elevated for 1 week postpartum, while carnitine levels decreased after 4 weeks. These results are significant as they suggest the potential use of three metabolites, namely carnitine, propionyl carnitine, and lysophosphatidylcholine acyl C14:0, as potential predictors of peripartum-related diseases up to 4 weeks before delivery (Hailemariam et al. 2014; Huber et al. 2016; Li et al. 2014). Consequently, carnitines have emerged as potential biomarkers for metabolic diseases associated with the transition period.

References

Agriculture and Agri-Food Canada (2020). Statistics of the Canadian Dairy Industry. https://publications.gc.ca/collections/collection_2020/aac-aafc/A71-18-2020-eng.pdf (accessed 23 January 2023).

Ametaj, B.N. (2017). Demystifying the myths: switching paradigms from reductionism to systems veterinary in approaching transition dairy cow diseases. In: *Periparturient Diseases of Dairy Cows: A Systems Biology Approach* (ed. B.N. Ametaj), 9–29. Springer Cham.

Ametaj, B.N., Zebeli, Q., and Iqbal, S. (2010). Nutrition, microbiota, and endotoxin-related diseases in dairy cows. *Revista Brasileira de Zootecnia* 39: 433–444.

Attupuram, N.M., Kumaresan, A., Narayanan, K., and Kumar, H. (2016). Cellular and molecular mechanisms involved in placental separation in the bovine: a review. *Molecular Reproduction and Development* 83: 287–297.

Ceciliani, F., Vecchio, D., De Carlo, E. et al. (2017). A systems biology approach to dairy cattle subfertility and infertility. In: *Periparturient Diseases of Dairy Cows: A Systems Biology Approach* (ed. B.N. Ametaj), 93–119. Springer Cham.

Chamberlain, A.T. (1987). The management and prevention of the downer cow syndrome. *Proceedings of the British Cattle Veterinarians Association*, Nottingham, England: 20–30.

Choe, C., Park, J.W., Kim, E.S. et al. (2010). Proteomic analysis of differentially expressed proteins in bovine endometrium with endometritis. *Korean Journal of Physiology and Pharmacology* 14 (4): 205–212.

Cordeiro, F.B., Cataldi, T.R., Perkel, K.J. et al. (2015). Lipidomics analysis of follicular fluid by ESI-MS reveals potential biomarkers for ovarian endometriosis. *Journal of Assisted Reproduction and Genetics* 32 (12): 1817–1825.

DeGaris, P.J. and Lean, I.J. (2008). Milk fever in dairy cows: a review of pathophysiology and control principles. *Veterinary Journal* 176: 58–69.

Dervishi, E., Zhang, G., Hailemariam, D. et al. (2016a). Occurrence of retained placenta is preceded by an inflammatory state and alterations of energy metabolism in transition dairy cows. *Journal of Animal Science and Biotechnology* 7: 26–39.

Dervishi, E., Zhang, G., Hailemariam, D. et al. (2016b). Alterations in innate immunity reactants and carbohydrate and lipid metabolism precede occurrence of metritis in transition dairy cows. *Research in Veterinary Science* 104: 30–39.

Drackley, J.K. (1999). Biology of dairy cows during the transition period: the final frontier? *Journal of Dairy Science* 82: 2259–2273.

Fadden, A.N. and Bobe, G. (2016). Serum visfatin is a predictive indicator of retained placenta and other diseases in dairy cows. *Journal of Veterinary Science and Medical Diagnosis* 5: 1.

Ferreira, A.M., Bislev, S.L., Bendixen, E., and Almeida, A.M. (2013). The mammary gland in domestic ruminants: a systems biology perspective. *Journal of Proteomics* 94: 110–123.

Forar, A.L., Gay, J.M., and Hancock, D.D. (1995). The frequency of endemic fetal loss in dairy cattle: a review. *Theriogenology* 43 (6): 989–1000.

Fu, S., Liu, Y., Nie, T. et al. (2016). Comparative proteomic analysis of cow placentas with retained foetal membranes. *The Thai Journal of Veterinary Medicine* 46: 261–270.

Gilbert, R.O., Shin, S.T., Guard, C.L. et al. (2005). Prevalence of endometritis and its effects on reproductive performance of dairy cows. *Theriogenology* 64 (9): 1879–1888.

Godden, S.M. (2008). Colostrum management for dairy calves. *Veterinary Clinics of North America. Food Animal Practice* 24 (1): 19–39.

Hailemariam, D., Mandal, R., Saleem, F. et al. (2014). Identification of predictive biomarkers of disease state in transition dairy cows. *Journal of Dairy Science* 97: 2680–2693.

Hoelker, M., Salilew-Wondim, D., Drillich, M. et al. (2012). Transcriptional response of the bovine endometrium and embryo to endometrial polymorphonuclear neutrophil infiltration as an indicator of subclinical inflammation of the uterine environment. *Reproduction, Fertility, and Development* 24 (6): 778–793.

Hogarth, C.J., Fitzpatrick, J.L., Nolan, A.M. et al. (2004). Differential protein composition of bovine whey: a comparison of whey from healthy animals and from those with clinical mastitis. *Proteomics* 4 (7): 2094–2100. https://doi.org/10.1002/pmic.200300723.

Hossein-Zadeh, N.G. and Ardalan, M. (2011). Bayesian estimates of genetic parameters for metritis, retained placenta, milk fever, and clinical mastitis in Holstein dairy cows via Gibbs sampling. *Research in Veterinary Science* 90: 146–149.

Huber, K., Dänicke, S., Rehage, J. et al. (2016). Metabotypes with properly functioning mitochondria and antiinflammation predict extended productive life span in dairy cows. *Scientific Reports* 6: 24642.

Kankofer, M., Wawrzykowski, J., and Hoedemake, M. (2014). Profile of bovine proteins in retained and normally expelled placenta in dairy cows. *Reproduction in Domestic Animals* 49: 270–274.

Kankofer, M., Wawrzykowski, J., Miller, I. et al. (2015). Usefulness of DIGE for the detection of protein profile in retained and released bovine placental tissues. *Placenta* 36: 246.

Kinros, J.M., Darzi, A.W., and Nicholson, J.K. (2011). Gut microbiome-host interactions in health and disease. *Genomic Medicine* 3 (3): 14.

Knutti, B., Küpfer, U., and Busato, A. (2000). Reproductive efficiency of cows with endometritis after treatment with intrauterine infusions or prostaglandin injections, or no treatment. *Journal of Veterinary Medicine A, Physiology, Pathology, Clinical Medicine* 47 (10): 609–615.

Krisher, R.L., Schoolcraft, W.B., and Katz-Jaffe, M.G. (2015). Omics as a window to view embryo viability. *Fertility and Sterility* 103 (2): 333–341.

LeBlanc, S.J. (2010). Health in the transition period. *Advances in Dairy Technology* 22: 97–110.

Li, C., Xu, C., Xia, H. et al. (2014). Plasma metabolic profiling of dairy cows affected with clinical ketosis using LC/MS technology. *The Veterinary Quarterly* 34: 152–158.

Lòpez-Gatius, F., Murugavel, K., Santolaria, P. et al. (2004). Pregnancy rate after timed artificial insemination in early post-partum dairy cows after Ovsynch or specific synchronization protocols. *Journal of Veterinary Medicine A, Physiology, Pathology, Clinical Medicine* 51 (1): 33–38.

Mallard, B.A., Emam, M., Paibomesai, M. et al. (2015). Genetic selection of cattle for improved immunity and health. *The Japanese Journal of Veterinary Research* 63 (1): S37–S44.

Maniwa, J., Izumi, S., Isobe, N., and Terada, T. (2005). Studies on substantially increased proteins in follicular fluid of bovine ovarian follicular cysts using 2-D PAGE and MALDI-TOF MS. *Reproductive Biology and Endocrinology* 3: 23.

Mavangira, V., Gandy, J.C., Zhang, C. et al. (2015). Polyunsaturated fatty acids influence differential biosynthesis of oxylipids and other lipid mediators during bovine coliform mastitis. *Journal of Dairy Science* 98 (9): 6202–6215. https://doi.org/10.3168/jds.2015-9570.

Moyes, K.M., Sorensen, P., and Bionaz, M. (2016). The impact of intramammary Escherichia coli challenge on liver and mammary transcriptome and cross-talk in dairy cows during early lactation using RNAseq. *PLoS One* 11 (6): e0157480.

Pohl, A., Burfeind, O., and Heuwieser, W. (2015). The associations between postpartum serum haptoglobin concentration and metabolic status, calving difficulties, retained fetal membranes, and metritis. *Journal of Dairy Science* 98 (7): 4544–4551.

Pryce, J.E., Veerkamp, R.F., Thopson, R. et al. (1997). Genetic aspects of common health disorders and measures of fertility in Holstein Friesian dairy cattle. *Animal Science* 65: 353–360.

Rasool, A., Sarath, T., Krishnakumar, K., and Porteen, K. (2023a). Protein profiling of saliva, cervicovaginal fluid and urine in delayed ovulatory condition of jersey crossbred cows. Master thesis. Tamil Nadu Veterinary and Animal Sciences University.

Rasool, A., Sarath, T., Krishnakumar, K., and Porteen, K. (2023b). Novel approaches to diagnose reproductive disorders in Bovine. In: *Advanced Molecular Techniques in Animal Disease Diagnosis* (ed. A. Pathak, M. Bharadwaj, D. Sharma, and S.P. Singh), 167–177. Delhi: Narendra Publishing House.

Ruegg, P.L. (2012). New perspectives in udder health management. *The Veterinary Clinics of North America. Food Animal Practice* 28 (2): 149–163.

Salilew-Wondim, D., Ibrahim, S., Gebremedhn, S. et al. (2016). Clinical and subclinical endometritis induced alterations in bovine endometrial transcriptome and miRNome profile. *BMC Genomics* 17 (1): 218.

Sasaki, K., Yamagishi, N., Kizaki, K. et al. (2014). Microarray-based gene expression profiling of peripheral blood mononuclear cells in dairy cows with experimental hypocalcemia and milk fever. *Journal of Dairy Science* 97: 247–258.

Shu, S., Xia, C., Zhang, H. et al. (2014). Plasma proteomics analysis of dairy cows with milk fever using SELDI-TOF-MS. *Asian Journal of Animal and Veterinary* 9: 1–12.

Sun, Y., Xu, C., Li, C. et al. (2014). Characterization of the serum metabolic profile of dairy cows with milk fever using 1H-NMR spectroscopy. *The Veterinary Quarterly* 34: 159–163.

Taverne, M.A., Breukelman, S.P., Perényi, Z. et al. (2002). The monitoring of bovine pregnancies derived from transfer of in vitro produced embryos. *Reproduction, Nutrition, Development* 42 (6): 613–624.

Tilg, H. and Kaser, A. (2011). Gut microbiome, obesity, and metabolic dysfunction. *Journal of Clinical Investigations* 121 (6): 2126–2132.

Walker, C.G., Meier, S., Hussein, H. et al. (2015). Modulation of the immune system during postpartum uterine inflammation. *Physiological Genomics* 47 (4): 89–101.

Williams, E.J., Sibley, K., Miller, A.N. et al. (2008). The effect of Escherichia coli lipopolysaccharide and tumour necrosis factor alpha on ovarian function. *American Journal of Reproductive Immunology* 60 (5): 462–473.

Xia, C., Zhang, H.Y., Wu, L. et al. (2012). Proteomic analysis of plasma from cows affected with milk fever using two-dimensional differential in-gel electrophoresis and mass spectrometry. *Research in Veterinary Science* 93: 857–861.

Xia, L., Zhao, X., Sun, Y. et al. (2014). Metabolomic profiling of human follicular fluid from patients with repeated failure of in vitro fertilization using gas chromatography/mass spectrometry. *International Journal of Clinical and Experimental Pathology* 7 (10): 7220–7229.

Zhang G, Hailemariam DW, Dervishi E et al (2014) Activation of innate immunity in transition dairy cows before clinical appearance of milk fever. In: *2014 Joint Annual Meeting Abstract Book*, Kansas City, Missouri, USA (20–24 July 2014)/ *Journal of Animal Science* 92(e-supplement 2)/*Journal of Dairy Science* 97(e-supplement 1): 434.

Zhang, G., Dervishi, E., Dunn, S.M. et al. (2017). Metabotyping reveals distinct metabolic alterations in ketotic cows and identifies early predictive serum biomarkers for the risk of disease. *Metabolomics* 13: 43–58.

Zwald, N.R., Weigel, K.A., Chang, Y.M. et al. (2004). Genetic selection for health traits using producer recorded data. II. Genetic correlations, disease probabilities, and relationships with existing traits. *Journal of Dairy Science* 87: 4295–4302.

38

Management of Periparturient Disorders

Haritha Gurram S.

Department of Veterinary Clinical Complex, College of Veterinary Science (SVVU), Garividi, Vizianagaram, Andhra Pradesh, India

38.1 Peripartureint Period

The term "periparturient" arises from the word "parturition" and the prefix "peri," which literally but vaguely means "around" (Mather Edward and Melancon 1981). It is also termed the transition period and is defined as the period from 3 weeks prepartum to 3 weeks postpartum. This period is marked by several changes in the immune and endocrine systems in preparation for colostrogenesis, parturition, and lactogenesis (Sordillo et al. 2009). During this period, the dam undergoes nutritional, metabolic, physiological, immunological, and hormonal changes that have an impact on the incidence of infections and metabolic diseases. Mostly, during the periparturient period, cows are in a state of negative energy balance because the demand for nutrients is either not met or demand exceeds the availability of nutrients provided in the feed. This negative energy balance results in lower blood glucose levels and the mobilization of body reserves to provide energy, which leads to elevated blood concentrations of non-esterified fatty acids (NEFA) and β-hydroxybutyric acid (BHBA) (Busato et al. 2002). After calving, the cow is prone to severe stress and immunosuppression, which increases its susceptibility to uterine and mammary infections. The cow demands increased nutrients for maintenance and milk production. Calcium and phosphorus are also mobilized for milk synthesis, which leads to a decrease in their blood concentrations (Drackley et al. 2005). All these changes can lead to metabolic disorders, viz. hypocalcemia, hypomagnesemia, ketosis, hypophosphatemia, and hepatic lipidosis (Figure 38.1). These may coincide with the resumption of ovarian activity, the development of follicles that supply oocytes for fertilization, and uterine involution and remodeling. Thus, these processes and metabolic states can together affect pre- and post-ovulatory reproductive function (Braganca and Zangirolamo 2018) (Figure 38.2). Thus, significant occurrences during the periparturient period are often determined by events initiated earlier and may alter events far into the future.

Periparturient diseases are costly in terms of their effect on milk production, reproduction, and the cow's susceptibility to other concurrent diseases. Proper management during the transition period affects the well-being of the animal by decreasing the incidence of metabolic and infectious diseases, increasing production, and improving reproductive performance during the subsequent lactation. Intensive management of the nutrition, feeding system, and environment of the periparturient cow reduces the odds of disease and increases the odds of success.

38.1.1 General Feeding Management During Periparturient Period

a) The cows should be fed a minimum of four times a day with 6-hour intervals.
b) From the seventh month of gestation, cows should be fed 1–2 kg concentrate feed in addition to their nutritional requirements. The cows may gain 20–25 kg of body weight during this period.
c) A 10-kg milk producer must gain 500 g/day in the last 2 months of the dry period.
d) For challenges during feeding: 2 weeks before the expected date of calving, start feeding 0.5 kg of concentrate mixture and increases this amount by 300–400 g daily until the cow is consuming 0.5–1 kg concentrate for every 100 kg body weight.

Periparturient Diseases of Cattle, First Edition. Edited by Tanmoy Rana.

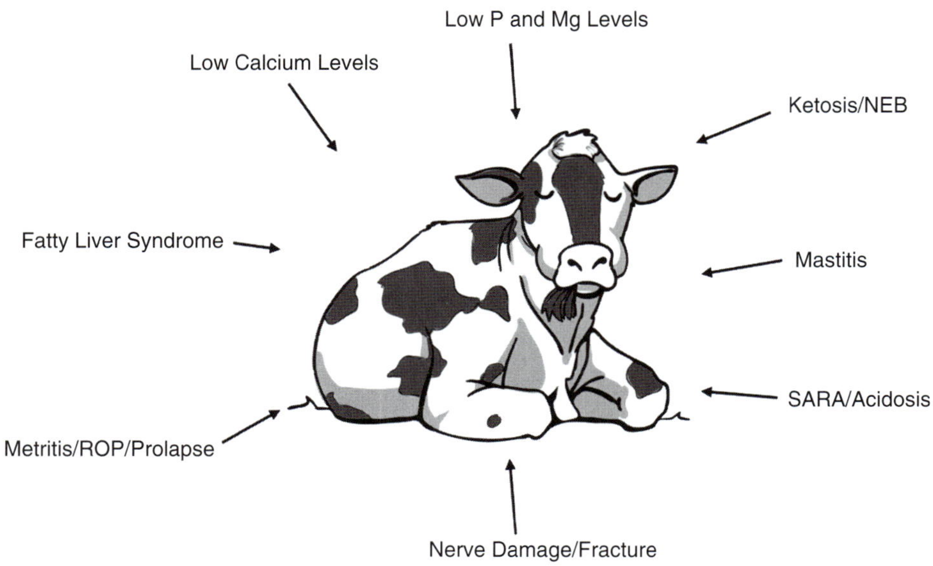

Figure 38.1 Multifactorial causes of downer-cow syndrome.

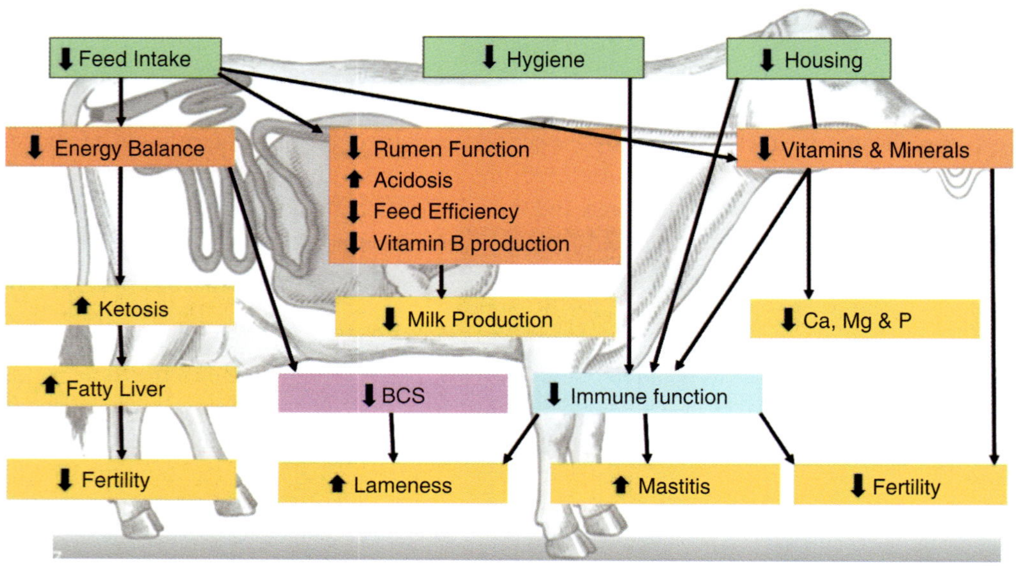

Figure 38.2 Pictorial representation of the predisposing factors for periparturient disorders.

e) Feed dairy animals on a leguminous or a mixture of leguminous and nonleguminous diet supplemented with concentrate, ensuring that they derive 30–40% of the feed units from grains and 60–70% from forages.
f) To maximize income, dairy animals must be fed individually, according to their individual milk production and nutritional requirements.
g) Liberal feeding and an abundant supply of clean drinking water is necessary for continued high production and its persistence throughout lactation (Manzoor et al. 2017, 2021).

38.2 Hypocalcemia (Milk Fever)

This is a metabolic disease of adult female cattle that occurs most commonly about the time of parturition and/or after parturition and is characterized by hypocalcemia, severe muscular weakness, sternal and lateral recumbency (Figure 38.3), circulatory collapse, and depression. Older animals are more susceptible to milk fever because of decreased calcium

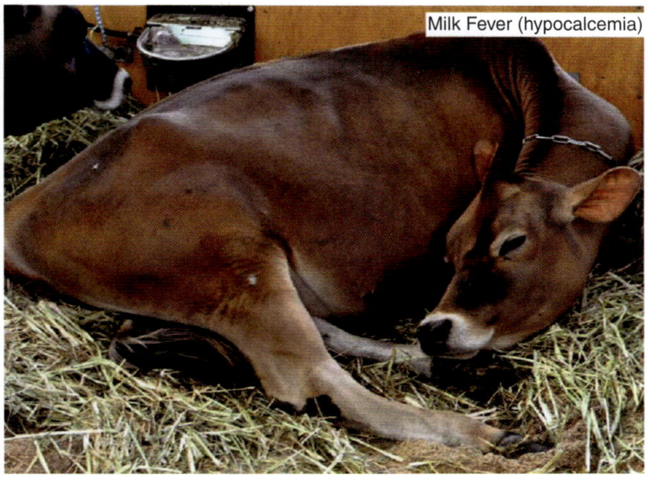

Figure 38.3 Lateral kink of the head in a hypocalcemic cow.

mobilization, a decrease in the number of osteoblasts that could delay the ability of bone to contribute Ca to the plasma Ca pool, decreased absorption efficiency (i.e. a decline in intestinal 1,25-dihydroxy vitamin D [1,25$(OH)_2$D] receptors with age is coupled with a lowered ability of older cows to respond to the vitamin D hormone to cause a longer adaptation to intestinal Ca absorption), increased milk yield, and decreased exchangeable Ca in the skeleton. Conversely, first calf heifers rarely develop milk fever because they are able to adapt rapidly to the high demands of Ca for lactation. Jersey cows, Jafarabadi buffaloes, and crossbred cattle are found to be more susceptible. High yield animals are mostly affected because of the excess drain of Ca through milk (1.2 g/kg) or colostrum (2.3 g/kg). About 6% of cases occur just a few hours before or at the time of parturition, and about 91% of cases occur in the post-parturient stage. Milk fever can also be concurrent with retained placentas, metritis, uterine prolapse, ketosis, etc.

38.2.1 Dietary Risk Factors

a) **Dietary Ca:** Excessive Ca intake during the dry period, feeding more than 100 g/day of Ca, is associated with an increased incidence of milk fever.
b) **Dietary P:** High levels of P (780 g/day) also increases the incidence of milk fever because it inhibits renal enzymes that catalyze the production of 1,25$(OH)_2$D.
c) **Dietary anion–cation balance:** Recent studies indicate that the anion–cation balance in the prepartum diet is more important than dietary Ca as a risk factor for milk fever. A prepartum diet high in cations such as sodium and potassium is associated with an increase in the incidence of milk fever, while a diet high in anions, viz. chlorides and sulfur, is associated with a decrease in the incidence of milk fever. A high anion diet increases the plasma levels of 1,25$(OH)_2$D prior to parturition. Most forages, viz. legumes and grasses, are high in potassium and are alkaline.

38.2.2 Management of Milk Fever

Treatment with a parenteral injection of calcium is standard practice and very effective. Calcium borogluconate is the preparation of choice as it causes less tissue irritation. The addition of boric acid increases the solubility of calcium gluconate.

Dose and route: Calcium borogluconate 25% at 400–800 ml or 1 ml/kg body weight, intravenously (IV), or 1 g/45 kg body weight, IV.

38.2.2.1 Reasons for a Failure to Response to Ca Therapy

i) Incomplete or incorrect diagnosis.
ii) Delay in treatment (if treated during stages I and II – a good response; and if treated during stage III – a poor [50%] response).
iii) Underdosing.
iv) Concurrent hypophosphatemia/hypomagnesemia.
v) Other complications (displaced abomasum, ketosis, metritis, mastitis, hypokalemia, etc.).

Table 38.1 Calcium requirements during the periparturient period.

	Calcium requirements		
Weight of cow	**Maintenance (g)**	**Pregnancy (g)**	**Milk production (g)**
400	17	23	For both, 2–3 per kg of milk
500	20	29	

38.2.2.2 Control Measures

Hypocalcemia can be controlled to some extent with better managemental practices. For controlling milk fever incidence, a low Ca diet should be given during early pregnancy, whereas a diet rich in Ca at the time of parturition would minimize milk fever cases. The parenteral administration of vitamin D_3 at 10 million IU, i.e. 1 million IU/45 kg body weight, intramuscularly (IM), 1 week before calving and prophylactic injections of calcium soon after calving is effective. Oral calcium gel dosing should be done after calving in cows that are predisposed due to hypocalcemia in previous calvings.

Provide 25 g ammonium chloride to pregnant animals with their grain during the last few weeks of gestation and increase it to 100 g/day at calving. Provide good shelter to protect pregnant/lactating animals from cold stress. Exercise the animals to maintain normal rumen function and stimulate bone metabolism. Avoid long distance transportation during pregnancy and early lactation. Keep animals under observation for 48 hours before and 48 hours after calving. Feed roughages to animals that are about to deliver to stimulate rumen contractions as concentrate causes stasis. In lactating/pregnant animals, regular dietary Ca supplementation is essential (Table 38.1). Give mineral mixtures regularly as required by each animal.

38.3 Post-parturient Hemoglobinuria (PPH)

This is a metabolic disease that occurs in phosphorous-deficient, high producing dairy cows and buffaloes, and it is characterized by intravascular hemolysis, hemoglobinuria, and profound anemia. Buffaloes are more susceptible than cows. It is more common during the third to eighth lactation. In cows, the disease occurs in the post-parturient period, while in buffaloes it mostly occurs during advanced pregnancy and early lactation. The higher incidence of disease was recorded in buffaloes fed exclusively dry roughages or with a negligible quantity of concentrate compared to those receiving either a good amount of concentrates or ad lib greens. Fodder deficient in phosphorus, impaired phosphorus absorption from the gut, the increased requirement of phosphorus (as there is a heavy drain of P through milk [0.93–1 g/kg] in recently calved animals), the increased phosphorous requirements for fetal development during advanced pregnancy, and the feeding of cruciferous plants like rape, kale, turnip, etc. make an animal susceptible to deficiency. Recently calved or advanced pregnancy buffaloes maintained on dry roughages and exposed to cold climates are usually affected.

38.3.1 Management of PPH

Sodium acid phosphate at 80 g, IV as a 20% solution in dextrose or distilled water, for 2–4 days is highly effective. Tonoricin®(Vetoquinol, Maharashtra, India)/Tonophosphan® (Intervet India, Maharashtra, India) at 30 ml, IV, daily for 2–4 days is also effective. Ascorbic acid at 15–20 mg/kg, IV, daily for 2–4 days is also used as it is an antioxidant that relieves the oxidative stress on red blood cells (RBCs). Supportive treatment includes 20% dextrose at 500–1000 ml, IV, daily for 2–3 days as it provides energy and helps the utilization of P by RBCs. Hematinics like iron-dextran (Imferon®, Shreya Life Sciences, Maharashtra, India) or a hematinic mixture ($FeSO_4 + CuSO_4 + CoSO_4$) is supplemented to correct anemia. Blood transfusions are warranted in severe cases.

The regular provision of a mineral mixture that contains phosphorus, as required for maintenance and production, is advisable. Protect recently calved or advanced pregnancy animals from cold stress. The provision of an adequate quantity of concentrates and greens ad lib are recommended as control measures (Table 38.2).

Table 38.2 Phosphorus requirements during the periparturient period.

	Phosphorus requirements		
Weight of animal (kg)	Maintenance (g)	Pregnancy (g)	Milk production (g)
400	13	18	1.7–2.4 per kg of milk
500	15	22	

38.4 Hypomagnesemia

Hypomagnesemic tetany is a highly fatal metabolic disease of ruminants characterized by hypomagnesemia, tetany, and hyperesthesia. Both pregnant and lactating females are affected. It usually occurs in high yielding cows during the first 2 months of lactation. Hypomagnesemia is common during the winter due to depressed appetites and a negative energy balance during bad weather. Although an effective treatment is available, the case-fatality rate is high because of the short course of the disease. The worst combination of causative factors is a low dietary intake (lush pasture) in recently calved cows during a spell of cold windy weather.

The treatment is administering the Ca and Mg-containing solution that gives a satisfactory result. The safest general recommendation is to use a Ca–Mg combination preparation, IV, followed by subcutaneous (SC) injections of magnesium sulfate. E.g Mifex® (Elanco, Indiana, United States) or Miphocal® (Indian Immunologicals Ltd., Telangana, India) at 300–450 ml, IV, followed by magnesium sulfate 10% at 100–150 ml, SC; or magnesium sulfate (20%) at 200–300 ml, IV; or as 10% at 400–600 ml, IV (1 ml/kg body weight), are all found to be effective.

Magnesium gluconate and magnesium lactate maintain serum levels of magnesium for a longer duration. The symptomatic usage of a sedative to control convulsions (chlorpromazine hydrochloride or diazepam) is helpful. A deficiency in magnesium can be managed by feeding magnesium salts (magnesium oxide, 60 g daily in cattle) during dangerous periods. Top dressing of the pasture with magnesium-rich fertilizers like calcined magnesite at 1125 kg/hectare is satisfactory. The magnesium content of the pasture can be increased by spraying a 2% magnesium sulfate salt at fortnightly intervals. The provision of magnesium sulfate at 500 g/100 l through the water during risk periods is effective. Animals should be provided with comfortable shelter during the winter. The provision of hay along with greens is advisable.

38.5 Ketosis

Ketosis is a metabolic disease of high yielding animals characterized by hypoglycemia, ketonemia, and ketonuria. It is the accumulation of an abnormal amount of ketone bodies in the tissues and fluids that is a multifactorial disorder of energy metabolism. The disease in cattle responds to treatment and is often self-limiting with feed intake.

Primary ketosis is caused due to starvation, underfeeding, or the feeding of an unbalanced diet and is often uncomplicated, whereas secondary ketosis is caused by various associated systemic or infectious diseases, viz. mastitis, metritis, etc. In secondary ketosis, animals consume inadequate feed due to a loss of appetite even though sufficient feed is offered. It commonly occurs within 10 days and 2 months of calving. High yielding crossbred cows are more susceptible. Milk production is reduced from 25% to 100%, and about 30–40% of cases are complicated by concurrent diseases like metritis, traumatic reticuloperitonitis (TRP), abomasal diseases, etc.

Ketosis is associated with underfed cattle that experience a metabolic shortage of gluconeogenic precursors followed by excessive fat mobilization. Secondary ketosis in very early lactation (1–2 weeks postpartum) is usually associated with fatty liver. Cows in early lactation have low insulin–glucagon ratios and are in a lipolytic and catabolic state. A low insulin–glucagon ratio stimulates lipolysis in adipose tissue with consequent increases in the serum concentrations of NEFAs and subsequently, BHBA, acetoacetic acid, and the decarboxylation products of acetone and isopropanol (Manzoor et al. 2021). Normal cows have plasma BHBA concentrations less than 1000 μmol/l, cows with subclinical ketosis have concentrations greater than 1400 μmol/l, and cows with clinical ketosis have concentrations often in excess of 2500 μmol/l

(Risco and Retamal 2011). Both fatty liver and ketosis are probably part of a spectrum of conditions associated with intense fat mobilization in cattle. The clinical signs of ketosis are considered digestive form/wasting, nervous form, and subclinical/spontaneous, and it is sometimes associated with hypocalcemia.

38.5.1 Management of Ketosis

The rationale for managing ketosis is to relieve the need for glucose formation in tissues and to allow normal ketone body utilization, which can be achieved by glucose replacement therapy.

Replacement therapy includes 20% glucose, IV, for 2–3 days (repeated treatments are required). Glucose precursors, viz. sodium propionate at 80 g, by mouth (PO), for 3–6 days and propylene glycol or glycerine at 225 g, PO, twice daily (BID) for 2 days, followed by 110 g, PO, daily for 2 days are also beneficial. Glucose at 500 g, orally as a drench, following premedication with a 30 g sodium bicarbonate solution, orally, helps immediately. Fructose/xylitol or a mixture of glucose and fructose are also useful but should be administered with caution. Glucocorticoids help in the successful management of ketosis. Glucose (20%) along with corticosteroid therapy is more effective than therapy with glucose or corticosteroids alone. Glucose with insulin (0.5 U/kg, IV or SC) therapy is highly useful in cases of recurrent ketosis or in cases that are unresponsive to glucose or corticoid therapy. Insulin with corticosteroid therapy can also be used to treat ketosis. A single dose of anabolic steroids like nandrolone decanoate (Deca-Durabolin®, Organon and Co., New Jersy, United States) or trenbolone acetate at 60–120 mg is also suggested. Miscellaneous therapy with niacin (antilipolytic), vitamin B12 (converts propionate to glucose), and chloral hydrate (breaks down starch in the rumen and stimulates the production of propionate) aids in management.

Following the standard management practices in rearing cattle and feeding them as required helps control metabolic diseases. To control ketosis, precautionary measures should be taken, such as conducting blood glucose estimations at least twice during the second to sixth weeks of lactation to identify the subclinical form of disease. Perform the Rothera's test on urine/milk samples at weekly intervals until 6–8 weeks after calving. However, in problematic herds, daily PO administration of glucose precursors, like sodium propionate at 110 g for 6 weeks and propylene glycol 200–400 ml from 5 days before to 10 days after calving, is advisable.

38.6 Fatty Liver

Fatty liver results from a state of negative energy balance and is one of the important metabolic diseases of postparturient dairy cows. Although often considered a postpartum disorder, it usually develops before and during parturition. Fatty liver syndrome is characterized by a high hepatic triacylglycerol infiltration in early lactation that commonly occurs in high milk yielders. The periparturient depression of feed intake and endocrine changes associated with parturition and lactogenesis contribute to the development of fatty liver. Cows that are over conditioned at calving are at highest risk. Fatty liver can develop within 24 hours of an animal going off feed (Bobe et al. 2001). Fatty liver at calving is commonly associated with ketosis (Mulligan and Doherty 2008). Although lipid accumulation in the liver is a reversible process, the slow rate of triglyceride export as lipoproteins causes the disorder to persist for an extended period. The depletion of the liver lipid content usually begins when the cow reaches a positive energy balance and may take several weeks to fully subside.

The metabolic consequences of triglyceride accumulation in the liver include reduced gluconeogenesis, ureagenesis, hormone clearance, and hormone responsiveness. Consequently, hypoglycemia, hyperammonemia, and altered endocrine profiles may accompany fatty liver. Fatty liver is likely to develop concurrently with other diseases like metritis, mastitis, abomasal displacement, or hypocalcemia.

38.6.1 Management of Fatty Liver

Reducing the severity and duration of a negative energy balance is crucial to prevent fatty liver. This can be achieved by avoiding the over conditioning of cattle, rapid diet changes, unpalatable feeds, periparturient diseases, and environmental stress. The critical time for prevention of fatty liver is from 1 week before through 1 week after parturition, which is when cows are most susceptible. Glucose or glucose precursors are effective because they may cause an insulin response.

Propylene glycol, 300–600 ml/day, given as an oral drench during the final week prepartum, has effectively reduced plasma NEFAs and the severity of fatty liver at calving. Glucagon (10 mg/day, IV, for 14 days) is effective at reducing liver triglycerides. Minimizing stress is important for the prevention of fatty liver. Sudden changes in the environment should be avoided. For example, changes in ration, housing, temperature, herd mates, etc. may cause a reduction in feed intake and trigger the catecholamine-mediated increase in fat mobilization. The repeated IV bolus administration of 500 ml of a 50% dextrose solution is commonly used in dairy practice and can be combined with the administration of propylene glycol 250 ml, PO, BID.

38.7 Ruminal Acidosis

This is an acute ruminal dysfunction caused by the ingestion of a large amount of carbohydrate-rich feeds and is clinically characterized by severe toxemia, dehydration, ruminal stasis, weakness, recumbency, and high mortality. During the transition period, the farmers feed livestock ad libitum or with excess carbohydrates, i.e. the ingestion of excess grains or highly fermentable carbohydrates causes a marked change in the microbial population that results in increased fermentation with excess lactic acid production. The speed of onset of signs is faster with ground feed than whole grains. Ruminal acidosis, when it occurs in an acute form, is acute ruminal acidosis, whereas in its chronic form it is called subacute ruminal acidosis (SARA). SARA is considered a major threat to the welfare of lactating dairy cows and may affect up to 20% of cattle in early to mid-lactation. SARA is defined as a condition where the rumen fluid pH is below 6, while acute rumen acidosis is when the rumen pH is below 5.5 and associated with rumen motility that is weak or ceased. Acute rumen acidosis is common in feedlots, whereas SARA is more common on dairy farms. Often, ruminal acidosis and SARA are confused with each other, but they vary in their occurrence as ruminal acidosis classically occurs when an animal consumes an excess of grain or due to lactate accumulation, while SARA is due to excessive volatile fatty acid (VFA) production that exceeds the absorption ability of rumen papillae. This reduced ability of VFA absorbance is commonly seen at calving when a dry cow is switched to a grain ration (in the dry period, rumen papilla are adapted to high fiber feeds and are smaller and less distinct in size) because neither rumen papilla nor ruminal microbes are adapted to high grain rations (Haq et al. 2016).

The most common diagnostic techniques are based on rumen pH determination. The most widespread methods used are the indwelling pH data logger method, rumenocentesis, the oral-stomach tube technique, and the rumen cannula method. Dairy cows experiencing an episode of SARA will reduce their feed intake in order to reduce the acid load in their rumen. Cows will start eating again when the ruminal pH is above 5.6 (Stone 2004). This results in erratic feed intake that often goes unnoticed in individual cows experiencing SARA. Reduced ruminal efficiency, liver and lung abscesses, and laminitis all can be related to SARA. One method for the field diagnosis of SARA is to examine the hair around the skin of the rectum, i.e. the perianal region; due to chronic acid damage to the skin, hairless shiny skin indicates SARA. A low rumen pH can cause rumenitis, metabolic acidosis, lameness, hepatic abscesses formation, pneumonia, and even death (Bramley et al. 2008). It can be prevented by balancing the diet. Also, sudden changes in feed and the feeding of grain and/or molasses should be avoided. Feed buffers such as sodium bicarbonate or ionophores also counteract acidosis.

38.7.1 Management of SARA

There is no specific treatment for SARA. However, Humer et al. (2018) has suggested certain practical management indications that include:

a) Check the particle size distribution of the diet. An appropriate distribution of small and large feed particles will result in a less selective feeding behavior and in a more stable rumen pH.
b) Provide sufficient space at the feeding lane (at least 60 cm/cow), which avoids feed competition and the consumption of large meals.
c) Do not overmix the total mixed rations (TMR; a maximum of 3–5 minutes after the last ingredient is added). Over mixing decreases the structure of the ration.
d) Add water to a dry TMR until a dry matter content of 55% is reached, to minimize sorting.
e) Deliver feed more often and increase the number of feed pushups to encourage small and frequent meals.

38.8 Laminitis

Laminitis is a pathophysiologic disturbance of the microstructure of the dermis or corium of the claw. Due to its prevalence, lameness is probably the primary animal welfare issue that affects the species (Hoblet and Weiss 2001). The highest incidence of lameness is seen in high production, intensively managed dairy cattle. It is probably equal in importance to reproductive inefficiency, which it is now known to be closely related to, and it causes huge economic loss. Inflammation is primarily associated with a dysfunction in the digital vasculature system that results in hypoxia and malnutrition of the sensitive laminar structure in the hoof wall (Mendes et al. 2013). The etiology of the circulatory disturbance is not fully understood, and there are some possible explanations related to nutrition. Laminitis has been associated with nutrition and specifically with ruminal acidosis either in its acute or subacute (SARA) form. The exact relationship between laminitis and SARA is not known. One theory states that acidosis-induced damage to the ruminal epithelium allows the absorption of histamine and endotoxins into the blood that come from the lysis of gram-negative bacteria in the rumen due to the low pH. Histamine and endotoxins cause vasoconstriction and inflammation in the lamella of the hoof, which causes laminitis (Stone 2004). Cows fed a higher level of crude protein may have an increased incidence and duration of lameness. It is possible that the products of excess protein degradation in the rumen may be the causative agents for lameness. It has also been shown that nutritional supplements such as biotin and zinc can help reduce lameness through improving claw horn quality (Baird and Muelling 2009). Other trace minerals that impact claw conditions include iodine (I), selenium (Se), copper (Cu), manganese (Mn), and cobalt (Co).

38.9 Displaced Abomasa

The abomasum is a movable organ and because of this, the organ is easily displaced from its original position. The displacement may be on the left or right side. Left-displacement of the abomasum (LDA) is more common (80%) than a right-displaced abomasum (RDA; 15%). It usually occurs in large sized, high producing dairy cows immediately after parturition and is more common in exotic and crossbred cattle. Hypomotility of the abomasum in cattle fed higher concentrate and lower fiber diets, during parturition, and due to hypocalcemia are important contributing factors. Nutrition is a major risk factor in the etiology of displaced abomasa, but the precise cause is still unclear. A low feed intake and increased negative energy balance prepartum have been found to be common causes of the increased risk for displaced abomasa in cows. VFAs in the abomasum have also been reported to reduce abomasal motility. The effects of VFA on motility may be exacerbated by the low ruminal absorption of VFAs during the transition period, and hypocalcemia may also play a role. Due to reduced feed consumption, slow contractions, and inadequate filling of the rumen, which, therefore, does not reach the ventral abdominal wall, empty space appears that allows for movement of the abomasum. Then, usually, more fatty acids escape absorption in the rumen and reach the abomasum. Those VFAs, along with hypocalcemia and accumulated gases, contribute to reducing abomasum contractility and the development of atony. Thus, inadequate feed consumption and insufficient rumen fill along with reduced motility and the strength of abomasal contractions contribute to the onset of a displaced abomasum.

Conservative treatment is not effective. Roll the animal on its back and massage the anterior part of the abdomen from left to right. Symptomatically treat with dextrose and antibiotics. A surgical correction (abomasoplexy, i.e. fixing the abomasum to the wall) will prevent recurrence of the condition. Displaced abomasa can be prevented by maintaining the forage–concentrate ratio of the diet fed in late gestation and early lactation.

38.10 Mastitis

Bovine mastitis is a persistent, inflammatory reaction of the udder tissue due to physical trauma or microbial infections and is frequently associated with poor udder hygiene. Mastitis is considered the most common disease that leads to economic loss in dairy industries due to reduced yield and poor milk quality. Mastitis may appear as a mild to potentially fatal mammary gland infection in dairy cattle. Bovine mastitis can be grouped into three classes based on the degree of inflammation, namely clinical, subclinical, and chronic mastitis. Clinical bovine mastitis is evident and easily detected by visible abnormalities, such as a red and swollen udder and fever, in dairy cows (Manzoor et al. 2021). The milk of the cow appears watery with the presence of flakes and clots. Clinical mastitis can be further subdivided into peracute, acute, and subacute, depending on the degree of inflammation. Severe cases of clinical mastitis can also be fatal. Contrary to clinical mastitis, subclinical mastitis (SCM) has no visible abnormality in the udder or milk, but milk production decreases along with an increase in the somatic cell count (SCC). There is a large cohort of microbial species that are known to cause mastitis. These range from viruses to mycoplasmas, fungi, and bacteria. Bacteria known to cause mastitis include *Pasteurella multocida, Staphylococcus aureus, Streptococcus zooepidemicus, Str. agalactiae, Str. pyogenes, Str. faecalis, Mycobacterium bovis, Klebsiella* spp., *Brucella abortus, Pseudomonas aruginosa, Escherichia coli, Leptospira pomona*, etc. Fungal entities responsible for mastitis are *Aspergillus fumigatus, Candida* spp., *Trichosporon* spp., etc. Physical injury to the mammary region, poor hygiene, and/or trauma also cause this condition. Predisposing factors include the environment, personnel hygiene, hygiene of the udder (animal), and any trauma or stress to the animal. A clear sign of mastitis is inflammation of the udder, swelling, change in color of the udder, pain upon palpation, and hardness of the udder in clinical cases, comparted to a normal udder with only changes to the milk in SCM. In SCM, the udder and the milk appear physically normal but the SCC is higher, which eventually results in a drop in milk yield.

38.10.1 Management of Mastitis

The earlier the diagnosis and treatment, the lower the treatment cost and loss of milk yield. Keeping this in mind, fortnightly test milk samples with the following tests, i.e. Californian mastitis test (CMT; equal quantities of milk and CMT reagent are mixed by rotating, SCM milk will form a gel), strip cup test (small flakes are present in SCM milk when viewed against a black surface, flake size increases with the degree of SCM), pH paper test (a green color is indicative of SCM), and surf field mastitis test (like CMT but using concentrated detergent solution instead of CMT reagent) to help detect SCM. Mild clinical mastitis cases may not require treatment, but all clinical mastitis cases require antimicrobial agents (intramammary infusion or parentally). It is always better to do a bacterial culture and antibiotic sensitivity test (ABST) of the milk before selecting the antibiotic to prevent antimicrobial resistance. Acute and peracute mastitis cases also require supportive therapy (fluid and electrolytes) and nonsteroidal anti-inflammatory drugs (NSAIDs) (Radostits et al. 2007). Antimicrobial treatment is not usually effective for chronic cases, it is better to dispose of or cull the animal. It is better to prevent mastitis before it becomes a problem. Treatment regimens are not discussed here as there are many vagaries based on location, sensitivity of organism, type of mastitis, etc., and recommendations are based on ABST results. These measures can go a long way in prevention:

a) Provide clean, dry and adequate bedding for cows to lie on.
b) Cows should be clean while entering the milking area.
c) Use a different cloth or towel to clean the teats on each cow.
d) Teats should be completely dry and clean before milking.
e) Completely remove the milk and use germicidal teat dips after milking.
f) Feed the cows after milking so that they do not immediately lie down. This prevents the entry of microbes into teat canals that are still open from milking.
g) Intramammary antimicrobial therapy is advised for a localized single teat infection or during the dry period.

38.11 Reproductive Abnormalities

Reproductive disorders like anoestrum, pyometra, metritis, prolapses (uterine and vaginal), abortion, dystocia, retained fetal membranes (RFMs), and repeat breeding have been reported to be major problems that cause serious economic loss. Cows with puerperal metritis, dystocia, and RFMs have delayed uterine involution, which increases the incidence of uterine infection, increases the postpartum interval to conception, and reduces milk production. Cows with RFMs were at twice the risk of metritis, and the conception rate is 20% lower in cows with endometritis. About 35% of animals were culled as they failed to conceive due to postpartum disorders (LeBlanc et al. 2002). A negative energy balance increases the incidence of metabolic disorders like hypocalcemia, acidosis, ketosis, fatty liver, and displaced abomasa. Milk fever and ketosis affect uterine contractions, delay calving, and increase the risk of RFMs and endometritis (Lean and De Garis 2010). Due to a slower uterine involution, reduced reproductive rate, prolonged interconception and calving interval, negative effect on fertility, increased cost of medication, drop in milk production, reduced calf crop, and early depreciation of potentially useful cows, the farmers face economic loss in the dairy sector. It is very difficult to diagnose these problems by one particular disorder or symptom because the predisposing factors are interrelated, such as the management of calving, hygiene, parity, stage of gestation, nutrition, etc. (Seid 2020).

38.11.1 Management of Uterine Infections

The management of uterine infections includes intrauterine or systemic antibiotic administration, supportive therapy, and hormone therapy. Penicillin is most commonly recommended (20 000–30 000 IU/kg, BID). The systemic administration of ceftiofur hydrochloride (2.2 mg/kg body weight, IM) improves clinical signs of metritis; an intrauterine treatment with 5 g chlortetracycline, twice weekly for 2 weeks prevented the negative effects of metritis on fertility and milk yields in multiparous cows. An intrauterine ozone flush is an efficacious and cost-effective treatment for metritis and endometritis that has an overall positive effect on fertility and the host tissues (Duricic et al. 2014).

A sexual health control program, which is a mandatory part of any reproductive management program, should always accompany an artificial insemination program. A few important aspects that should be considered in maintaining good sexual health are as follows:

a) Proper feeding and management.
b) Elimination of reproductive diseases like brucellosis, vibriosis, and trichomoniasis, etc. from the herd.
c) Prompt action should be taken when cows show an abnormal discharge, continual or continuous heat, anoestrum, failure to settle with more than two inseminations, etc.
d) Regular pregnancy examinations.
e) Isolate animals with communicable diseases.
f) Cull cows that have proven to be sterile.
g) Well-maintained records.
h) Sanitary practices.
i) Getting the cows to calve at intervals of 12–14 months.

The recognition of subclinical stages in periparturient diseases is difficult as the clinical signs are not typical and most of the time they may occur as concurrent infections. The periparturient condition may be confirmed by analyzing blood, milk, or sometimes urine. Blood and milk analyses of the nutritional and disease statuses of animals in herd help when making decisions to improve nutritional strategies and production management. Metabolic profile testing (MPT) refers to the use of a battery of tests to diagnose of subclinical nutritional and metabolic disease in dairy cows on a herd basis. MPT is most useful in the diagnosis and management of periparturient disease (Tables 38.3 and 38.4).

Table 38.3 Nutrient imbalances (deficiency or excess) and their associated metabolic and reproductive disorders.

Potential disease process	Nutrient deficiency	Associated diseases
Milk fever	Calcium (Ca)	P, K, Mg, ketosis
Hypomagnesemia	Magnesium (Mg)	P, Ca, K
Hypophosphatemia	Phosphorus (P)	Mg, Ca, anemia
Ketosis	Energy, protein	Ca, fatty liver, left-displaced abomasa, mastitis, reproductive disorders
Displaced abomasa	Fiber, energy	Ketosis, reproductive disorders, Ca, mastitis
Downer-cow syndrome	Ca, P, potassium (K)	Ketosis, mastitis, reproductive disorders, dystocia
Reproductive disorders	Ca, energy, cobalt (Co), copper (Cu), iron (Fe), selenium (Se), vitamins A and E, protein	Fatty liver, Ca, ketosis

Source: Haq et al. (2016).

Table 38.4 Reference values for biochemical parameters related to periparturient diseases.

Parameter	Reference range
Calcium (mg/dl)	9.7–12.4
Phosphorus (mg/dl)	5.6–6.5
Magnesium (mg/dl)	1.8–2.3
Glucose (mg/dl)	45–75
Triglycerides (mg/dl)	0–14
Potassium (mmol/l)	3.9–5.8
Total protein (g/dl)	6.7–7.4
Albumin (g/dl)	3–3.6
Creatinine kinase (U/l)	4.8–12.1
Alkaline phosphatase (ALP; U/l)	0–488
Alanine transaminase (ALT; U/l)	11–40
Aspartate aminotransferase (AST; U/l)	78–132

References

Baird, L.G. and Muelling, C.K.W. (2009). Risk factors, pathogenesis and prevention of subclinical laminitis in dairy cows. *Proceedings of the CanWest Veterinary Conference*, Alberta, Canada (17–20 October 2009): 1–10.

Bobe, G., Young, J.W., and Beitz, D.C. (2001). Invited review: pathology, etiology, prevention, and treatment of fatty liver in dairy cows. *Journal of Dairy Science* 87 (10): 3105–3124.

Braganca, L.G. and Zangirolamo, A.F. (2018). Strategies for increasing fertility in high productivity dairy herds. *Animal Reproduction* 15: 256–260.

Bramley, E., Lean, I.J., Fulkerson, W.J. et al. (2008). The definition of acidosis in dairy herds predominantly fed on pasture and concentrates. *Journal of Dairy Science* 91 (1): 308–321.

Busato, A., Faissler, D., Kupfer, U., and Blum, J.W. (2002). Body condition scores in dairy cows: associations with metabolic and endocrine changes in healthy dairy cows. *Journal of Veterinary Medicine. A, Physiology, Pathology, Clinical Medicine* 49: 455–460.

Drackley, J.K., Dann, H.M., Douglas, G.N. et al. (2005). Physiological and pathological adaptations in dairy cows that may increase susceptibility to periparturient diseases and disorders. *Italian Journal of Animal Science* 4: 323–344.

Duricic, D., Lipar, M., and Samardzija, M. (2014). Ozone treatment of metritis and endometritis in Holstein cows. *Veterinarski Arhiv* 84: 103–110.

Haq, Z., Khan, N., Rastogi, A. et al. (2016). Nutrition and metabolic diseases in dairy cattle – a review. *International Journal of Agriculture Sciences* 8 (12): 1154–1159.

Hoblet, K.H. and Weiss, W. (2001). Metabolic hoof horn disease, claw horn disruption. *The Veterinary Clinics of North America. Food Animal Practice* 17: 111–127.

Humer, E., Petri, R.M., Aschenbach, J.R. et al. (2018). Invited review: practical feeding management recommendations to mitigate the risk of subacute ruminal acidosis in dairy cattle. *Journal of Dairy Science* 101 (2): 872–888.

Lean, I. and De Garis, P. (2010). *Transition Cow Management: A Review for Nutritional Professionals, Veterinarians and Farm Advisers*, 1–56. Dairy Australia.

LeBlanc, S.J., Duffield, T.F., Leslie, K.E. et al. (2002). Defining and diagnosing postpartum clinical endometritis and its impact on reproductive performance in dairy cows. *Journal of Dairy Science* 85: 2223–2236.

Manzoor, A., Nazir, T., Dar, Z.A. et al. (2017). Transition mismanagement compromises production potential of dairy animals. Vet Helpline India, Ltd. https://www.vethelplineindia.co.in/transition-mismanagement-compromises-production-potential-of-dairy-animals/ (accessed 23 January 2024).

Manzoor, A., Ahuja, R., Kalkal, H. et al. (2021). Chapter 5: Production diseases and its management in dairy animals. In: *Advanced Research in Veterinary Sciences*, 1e (ed. N. Patra), 91–102. New Delhi: Scripown Publications.

Mather Edward, C. and Melancon, J.J. (1981). The periparturient cow – a pivotal entity in dairy production. *Journal of Dairy Science* 64 (6): 1422–1430.
Mendes, H.M.F., Casagrande, F.P., Lima, I.R. et al. (2013). Histopathology of dairy cows' hooves with signs of naturally acquired laminitis. *Pesquisa Veterinaria Brasileira* 33 (5): 613–619.
Mulligan, F.J. and Doherty, M.L. (2008). Production diseases of the transition cow. *The Veterinary Journal* 176: 3–9.
Radostits, O.M., Gay, C.C., Hinchcliff, K.W., and Constable, P.D. (2007). Diseases of the mammary gland. In: *Veterinary Medicine:A Textbook of the Diseases of Cattle, Horses, Sheep, Pigs, and Goats*, 10e, vol. 15 (ed. O.M. Radostits, C.C. Gay, K.W. Hinchcliff, and P.D. Constable), 673–749. Endinburg: Saunders, Ltd & 1670–1672.
Risco, C.A. and Retamal, P.M. (2011). *Diseases that Affect the Reproductive Performance of Dairy Cattle*, 1e, 123–131. Dairy Production Medicine.
Seid, H.A. (2020). Review on major reproductive health problems of dairy cattle in Ethiopia. *International Journal of Advanced Research in Biological Sciences* 7 (6): 81–90.
Sordillo, L.M., Contreras, G.A., and Aitken, S.L. (2009). Metabolic factors affecting the inflammatory response of periparturient dairy cows. *Animal Health Research Reviews* 10: 53–63.
Stone, W.C. (2004). Nutritional approaches to minimize subacute ruminal acidosis and laminitis in dairy cattle. *Journal of Dairy Science* 87: 13–26.

Index

Page numbers followed by *f* and *t* indicate figures and tables.

c

d

g

h

i

t

w

x

y

z